Medical Transcription Fundamentals

SECOND EDITION

Medical Transcription Fundamentals

Where Success Takes Root

SECOND EDITION

Diane Gilmore, CMT, AHDI-F

From the Publisher of Stedman's

 Wolters Kluwer | Lippincott Williams & Wilkins
Health

Philadelphia · Baltimore · New York · London
Buenos Aires · Hong Kong · Sydney · Tokyo

Senior Publisher: Julie Stegman
Acquisitions Editor: Peter Sabatini
Product Director: Eric Branger
Senior Product Manager: Amy Millholen
Marketing Manager: Shauna Kelley
Copyeditor: Kristin Wall
Compositor: Aptara, Inc.
Printer: C&C Offset – China

Library of Congress Cataloging-in-Publication Data

Gilmore, Diane M. (Diane Marie), 1957- author.
  Medical transcription fundamentals : where success takes root / Diane Gilmore,
CMT, AHDI-F. – Second Edition.
    p. ; cm.
  Includes bibliographical references and index.
  Summary: "Unlike other textbooks that discuss medical concepts in complex and
abstract terms, this book outlines the fundamentals of medical specialties in a
format that is easy to understand"–Provided by publisher.

  ISBN 978-1-60913-866-0 (pbk. : alk. paper)
1. Medical transcription–Programmed instruction. I. Title.
  [DNLM: 1. Forms and Records Control–methods–Programmed Instruction.
2. Medical Secretaries–Programmed Instruction. 3. Vocational Guidance–
Programmed Instruction. W 18.2]
  R728.8.G55 2012
  653′.18–dc22

                                                    2010052802

12
1 2 3 4 5 6 7 8 9 10

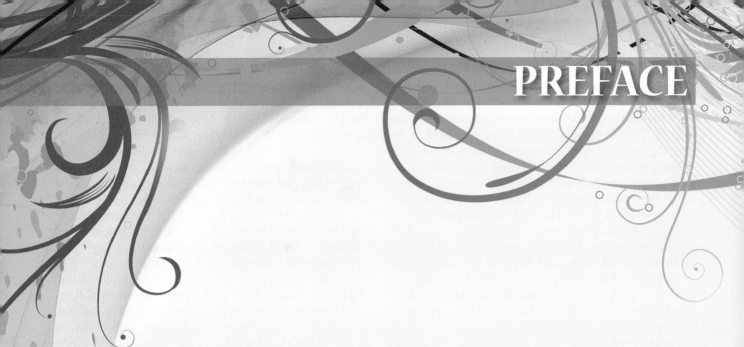

PREFACE

A medical transcriptionist, whether working in an office or in a home-based environment, is an integral part of a healthcare team. Far more than a typist in the medical field, a medical transcriptionist must be familiar with the terminology used in every medical specialty and must be able to produce the documents and reports required by each specialty in a professional and competent manner. These reports are the foundation of patient care and not only comprise a patient's complete record, but also track a patient's medical history and determine any future treatment.

Medical Transcription Fundamentals, Second Edition, a holistic approach to the study of medical transcription, is a comprehensive, yet concise, manual *written by a practicing medical transcriptionist for student medical transcriptionists*. This conversational approach, filled with practical, "from-the-trenches" tips and advice, makes this book particularly valuable to the new transcriptionist entering the field. Compatible with the Association for Healthcare Documentation Integrity (AHDI) Model Curriculum and designed with the adult-vocational and postsecondary school student in mind, this product meets the needs of both students and instructors. It can serve as the primary textbook in a short-term medical transcription course. Alternatively, it can be incorporated into a more comprehensive medical skills program in which a course in medical transcription may be one component of the curriculum. This text can also be used for independent, on-line study. After completing the exercises and activities in this book, students will be able to prepare standard medical reports accurately and efficiently. They will also be well versed in the fundamentals of anatomy and medical terminology as used in various medical specialty practices.

The majority of medical transcription textbooks currently on the market focus on general simulation and transcription activities. Most are not written by medical transcription practitioners and do not cover the issues relevant to students entering this field. Those textbooks that do, typically do more flexing of vocabulary prowess rather than simply explaining the topic in a manner that students can easily comprehend. Furthermore, these texts fail to follow up with adequate skill-building exercises to reinforce an understanding of the concepts and terms associated with each specialty.

Medical Transcription Fundamentals identifies the specific knowledge, skills, and education required for medical transcriptionists and outlines the responsibilities associated with the occupation. With a light, conversational writing style that is easy to read and understand, this product lays a solid foundation for a medical transcription career by providing a conceptual understanding of general medical terms and various medical specialties in a way that is easily remembered. It further encourages independent thinking and provides practice in working with the concepts covered in each chapter through a variety of challenging exercises and activities.

NEW TO THIS EDITION

The second edition of *Medical Transcription Fundamentals* builds on the original edition of learning tools with the addition of two new chapters not covered very thoroughly in other products: *Surgery* and *Pharmacology*. The surgical chapter serves as a foundation on which to build a student's knowledge of preparing surgery reports in the acute care setting. This chapter covers the general concepts of surgery, along with terms typically encountered by a medical transcriptionist in transcribing operative reports, including patient positioning, anesthesia, fluids, tools and instruments, wound closures and coverings, formatting issues, and common surgical phrases, all of which will enable students to produce accurate, grammatically correct documentation of surgical procedures. The pharmacology chapter contains a comprehensive review of the purpose and history of drugs, medication descriptions, regulation, development, and the terminology used to indicate drug forms, types, and routes of administration that are transcribed regularly by medical transcriptionists in nearly every medical report.

In addition, as the transition to general use of the electronic health record (EHR) is being mandated by the federal government as an effective means of lowering the nation's healthcare costs, it is vital that medical transcriptionists become proficient in the use of speech recognition technology, and this is a highly desirable skill for medical transcriptionists. To that end, this edition provides hands-on practice with speech recognition editing exercises for each of the specialty chapters using authentic speech-recognized drafts so that the student can develop these skills. The experience provided by exposure to this new technology can help students develop the confidence that these new skills will serve them well when they begin working.

In addition, the specialty sections now offer special ancillary activities called cloze exercises to help students test listening and reading comphrension. Simply put, a cloze exercise is a "fill-in-the-blank" document that consists of sentences of a report with several words missing. Instead of transcribing the report, students listen to the report as it is being dictated and supply the missing word or words by listening and comprehending the context of what is being said from the sentences dictated. These exercises enable students to use critical thinking skills to supply words that are missing from text by understanding the story being told. One of the skills of a competent medical transcriptionist who encounters terms they are not familiar with is to try to determine the missing word from the context of the report, or to be able to streamline researching for the word by understanding the topic being discussed. These exercises give students practicing in hearing and researching challenging medical terms.

Finally, this edition incorporates the latest styles, forms, and grammar and usage specific to the profession from *The Book of Style, Third Edition* by AHDI.

ORGANIZATION OF TEXT AND TASKS

The text is divided into three main sections. Part I, "Medical Transcription Fundamentals," describes the skills required in the medical transcription field, profiling a typical medical transcriptionist career. This profile details the responsibilities of the medical transcription professional and describes the various environments in which a medical transcriptionist might choose to work. This section also delineates the techniques and tools that are an integral part of the medical transcriptionist's daily work. Basic medical terminology is presented in this section, introducing students to terms that will appear in medical reports across the spectrum of specialties. Chapter exercises and activities develop and enhance students' understanding of general medical terminology and word-building skills. The basic structure of medical reports used in every field of medicine is analyzed and broken down into component parts, with an explanation of the type of information that belongs in each section. One entire chapter is devoted to editing and proofreading techniques, providing standard guidelines and helpful tips that students will use throughout the course and can continue using throughout their careers.

Part II, "Medical Specialties," is a comprehensive study of the specialized fields of medicine that students are most likely to encounter in the workplace, beginning with the most common specialties and progressing to more complex and esoteric areas of medical practice. Each chapter begins with an in-depth exploration of a particular anatomic/physiologic system, followed by a discussion of the diseases common to that part of the body; the standard diagnostic studies used to detect these diseases; and the relevant procedures, protocols, and pharmacology typically used to treat them. Beautifully rendered illustrations, most in full color, accompany the text to promote understanding of the subject matter. A variety of self-study exercises and activities interspersed throughout the chapters, including "real life" transcription of medical reports, provides opportunities for students to apply the concepts learned while simultaneously improving their computer skills. Each chapter contains a comprehensive listing of commonly used combining forms along with abbreviations and terminology relevant to the topic, *each fully defined and discussed in the chapter.*

Finally, Part III, "Your New Career," is a primer both for finding employment in the field and for starting a home-based medical transcription business. This section outlines approaches and techniques that can help to maximize the efficiency of searching for a position as a medical transcriptionist. In addition to explaining the fundamentals of a winning resume and an eye-catching cover letter, this portion of the textbook also explores various strategies for successfully passing online recruitment tests and impressing potential employers in the interview process, followed by a discussion of appropriate behaviors and attitudes for new medical transcriptionists in the workplace, with tips on becoming a valuable employee. In addition, considerations for operating a home-based medical transcription business are discussed in detail.

FEATURES OF THE BOOK

Unlike other textbooks that discuss medical concepts in complex and abstract terms, this book outlines the fundamentals of medical specialties in a format that is easy to understand. Comprehensive, yet concise, *Medical Transcription Fundamentals* explores each specialty from the perspective of a medical transcriptionist, with an emphasis on the information and knowledge base required by a new medical transcriptionist entering the field for transcribing the reports and documents used in a particular field.

Reference Tables and Review Questions

Each chapter includes a comprehensive collection of combining word forms as well as a list of fully defined abbreviations and medical terms associated with a particular specialty. These end-of-chapter resources provide a wealth of information that can be used by students in the classroom and on the job. In addition, each chapter concludes with a set of insightful questions designed to encourage class discussion and to test and reinforce the student's understanding of the chapter topics.

Transcription Tips and "On-the-Fly" Concept Reinforcement

Helpful "Transcription Tips," which alert students to common transcription mistakes, appear throughout each chapter. Short questions and quizzes are also interspersed throughout the text to test a student's immediate comprehension of the material presented.

Insight

Each chapter contains an informative "Insight" that presents up-to-date medical views and reviews, which present actual situations and events and help to broaden students' knowledge of the topics and promote insightful class discussion.

Computer Activities Using CD-ROM

The most significant feature of this text is the seamless integration of the information provided about various medical specialities with the opportunity for hands-on experience in transcribing dictation and preparing documents commonly used in the given fields of specialty from audio files. This package introduces the fundamental concepts associated with each field of medicine, and then reinforces these concepts with creative chapter activities found on the CD-ROM included with each student textbook.

The CD-ROM features a variety of supplemental activities designed to review the terms and concepts introduced in the chapter. The material is structured to strengthen an overall understanding of concepts; and learning is fun as students tackle different activities to reinforce the topics presented.

Additional questions, including fill-in-the-blanks, matching, true/false, and multiple choice (with answers for self-check), test students' retention and understanding of the material presented. Sample reports containing common errors provide proofreading practice. Games, quizzes, and puzzles help making learning fun and interesting.

Additional dictation contained in computer .mp3 files for supplemental transcription practice provides an opportunity for the student to practice "real life" transcription of authentic medical reports dictated by physicians practicing a variety of medical specialities. The .mp3 file format allows students to listen to and transcribe dictation using keyboard controls. In addition, the dictation files reflect the voices of not only real doctors in many places, but a variety of dialects and accents, allowing students to experience and practice transcribing material dictated by English-as-a-second-language (ESL) clinicians and to be well prepared when encountering these types of reports on the job.

In addition to these chapter activities, the CD-ROM contains a comprehensive reference section, which includes an alphabetical compilation of the medical terminology and abbreviations referenced and defined throughout the text and a complete list of all the transcription tips presented.

INSTRUCTOR'S RESOURCES

The instructor's resources available for use with *Medical Transcription Fundamentals*, include a variety of helpful teaching tools that encourage active learning:

- Complete lesson plans, in *.doc* format for easy viewing and printing, which provide an outline of the lesson presented, textbook page references, figure and table references, PowerPoint slide numbers, and a list of creative class activities and teaching suggestions for the instructor to help reinforce the topics discussed, *all in one convenient view.*
- Answers to exercises and transcription activities.
- PowerPoint slide presentations to assist in reinforcing concepts.
- An image bank containing the art from the textbook that may be used in the classroom.
- A test generator program that can create chapter or cumulative tests from hundreds of test questions in a snap.
- Supplemental games and quizzes.

In summary, students who complete the exercises and activities in *Medical Transcription Fundamentals* will be well prepared for careers in the medical transcription field, whether they choose to work in private physicians' offices, clinics or hospital settings, or as self-employed medical transcription entrepreneurs. Students receive a comprehensive understanding of the basic concepts as taught by a working medical transcription and instructor in the field. This valuable and timely information, associated with various medical specialties and reinforced with "real life" activities involving actual medical reports and documents, will provide students with the confidence and competence necessary to secure a position as a medical transcriptionist in this rewarding profession.

This User's Guide introduces you to the many features of *Medical Transcription Fundamentals*. Taking full advantage of these features, you not only read about medical transcription, you become engaged in exercises and activities that boost your ability to learn and put your knowledge and skills into practice.

TEXT FEATURES

Each chapter is loaded with features that enable you to concentrate on key points, quickly build transcription skills, and assess your knowledge as you progress through the text.

Objectives

Objectives focus your studies as you progress through the chapter by setting forth what you will know upon successful completion of the chapter.

Introduction

The Introduction summarizes the chapter contents and explains why the material is essential for successful medical transcription practice.

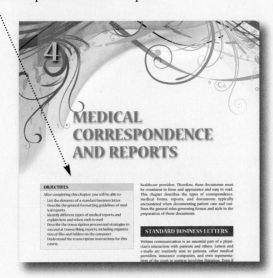

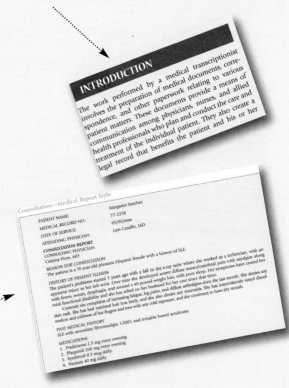

Sample Medical Documents

Sample Medical Documents serve as models that you can use for the text's transcription exercises and later on in your own professional practice.

Quick Check

Quick Checks are interspersed throughout the text to let you quickly test and reinforce your comprehension.

Chapter Summary

The Chapter Summary reinforces the key points of the chapter and their relevance to medical transcription practice.

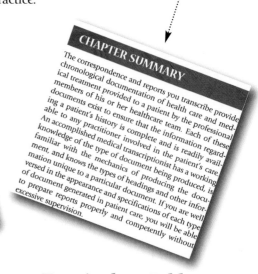

Insight

Insight at the end of each chapter offers additional perspectives and deepens your understanding of the chapter.

Terminology Tables

Combining forms, abbreviations, and terminology are listed and defined at the end of each chapter.

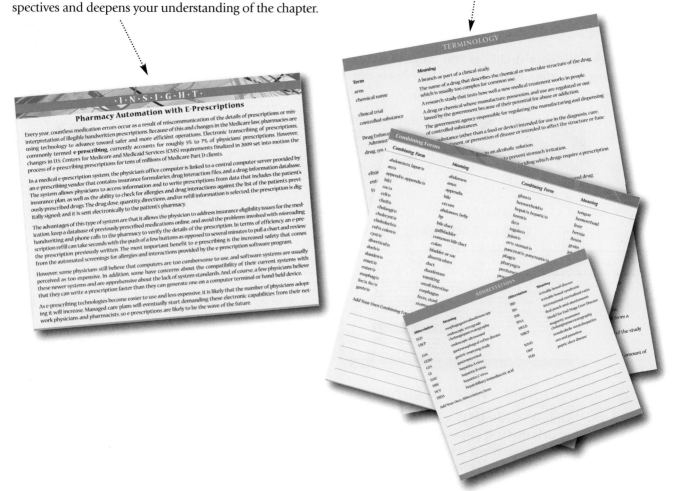

Color Illustrations

Detailed illustrations enable you to better understand and visualize the medical terminology that transcriptionists need to know.

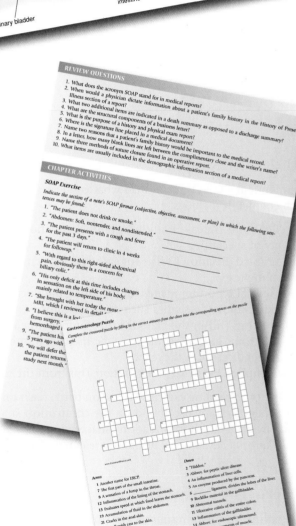

Transcription Tips

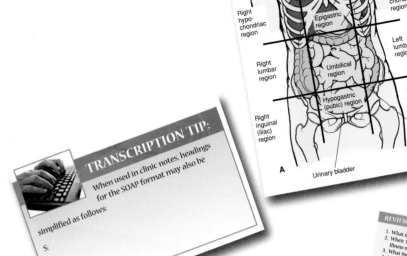

TRANSCRIPTION TIP:
When used in clinic notes, headings for the SOAP format may also be simplified as follows:

S:

O:

A:

P:

Transcription Tips throughout the text help you avoid common errors and offer helpful hints based on the author's first-hand experience.

Review Questions and Chapter Activities

Review questions, exercises, and activities provide a variety of opportunities for you to apply concepts learned in each chapter and improve your skills.

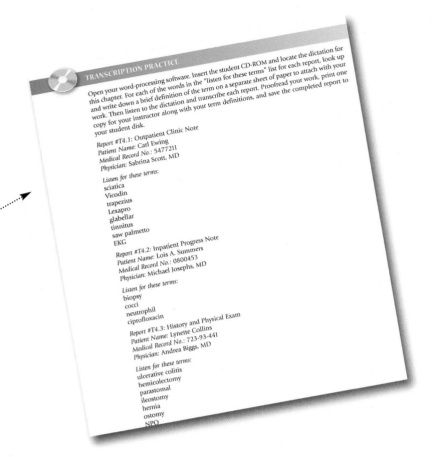

TRANSCRIPTION PRACTICE

Open your word-processing software. Insert the student CD-ROM and locate the dictation for this chapter. For each of the words in the "listen for these terms" list for each report, look up and write down a brief definition of the term on a separate sheet of paper to attach with your work. Then listen to the dictation and transcribe each report. Proofread your work, print one copy for your instructor along with your term definitions, and save the completed report to your student disk.

Report #T4.1: Outpatient Clinic Note
Patient Name: Carl Ewing
Medical Record No.: 5477211
Physician: Sabrina Scott, MD

Listen for these terms:
sciatica
Vicodin
trapezius
Lexapro
glabellar
tinnitus
saw palmetto
EKG

Report #T4.2: Inpatient Progress Note
Patient Name: Lois A. Summers
Medical Record No.: 0800453
Physician: Michael Josephs, MD

Listen for these terms:
biopsy
cocci
neutrophil
ciprofloxacin

Report #T4.3: History and Physical Exam
Patient Name: Lynette Collins
Medical Record No.: 723-93-441
Physician: Andrea Biggs, MD

Listen for these terms:
ulcerative colitis
hemicolectomy
parastomal
ileostomy
hernia
ostomy
NPO

Transcription Practice

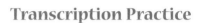

Transcription Practice at the end of most chapters lets you put your knowledge into practice by creating medical documents using dictation you'll find on the Student CD-ROM.

Student Resources

Your Student CD-ROM reinforces what you learn in the text with a variety of creative exercises corresponding to each chapter. It includes:

- Ten hours of real dictation by physicians who have distinct accents and dialects and who practice in a variety of specialties
- Scripted dictation (3 files for each specialty chapter) as a companion to the Transcription Practice exercises in the text
- Medical report templates for preparing the documents discussed in the text
- Skill-building activities such as proofreading exercises, question bank, speech recognition exercises, cloze exercises (fill-in-the-blank with accompanying audio reports), and flash cards
- Electronic glossary containing the medical terminology used in the text
- Appendices from the text
- Compiled list of all Transcription Tips from the text

The proofreading exercises, question bank, flash cards, glossary, medical report templates, transcription tips, and appendices are also found on the companion student site at http://thepoint.lww.com/gilmore2e. See the inside front cover for information on accessing the student resources on thePoint.

Taking full advantage of the student resources allows you to make a successful transition from student to professional!

Instructor Resources

The online instructor resources available for use with *Medical Transcription Fundamentals, Second Edition*, include lesson plans and activities; test generator; PowerPoints; image bank; extra exercises; and answers to chapter exercises, Transcription Practice, real dictation, and proofreading exercises.

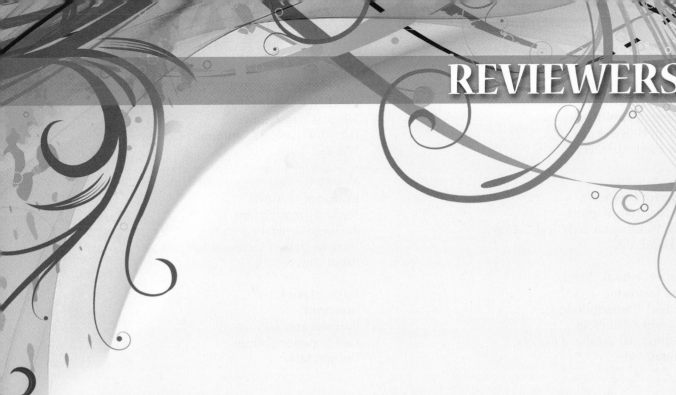

REVIEWERS

Peter Austin-Zacharias, PhD
Director
Medical Transcription
Sumner College
Portland, OR

Lenora Binegar
Medical Coordinator
Washington County Career Center
Marietta, OH

Cindi Brassington, MS CMA
Professor
Allied Health
Quinebaug Valley Community College
Danielson, CT

Mary Elizabeth W. Browder, MEd
Associate Professor
Office Information Technology
Medical Assisting Services
Raymond Walters College|UC Blue Ash
Cincinnati, OH

Jean Bucher, BA, MSEd
Adjunct Faculty
Clark College
Vancouver, WA

Cindy Conley
Instructor
Health Information Technology
Ozarka College
Melbourne, AR

Debbie Gilbert
Health Unit Coordinator
Department of Technology
Dalton College
Danton, GA

Janice Hess
Program Director
Health Information Management
Metropolitan Community College
Omaha, NE

Lisa D. Ijames, BA
Instructor
Health Information Management
Fountainhead College of Technology
Knoxville, TN

Lynn Jennings
Program Director, Medical Assisting
Allied Health
College of the Albemarle
Elizabeth City, NC

Loreen MacNichol
Professor
Office Administration
Kaplan University
South Portland, ME

Barbara Marchelletta,
AS, BS, CMA (AAMA), CPC, CPT
Program Director
Allied Health
Beal College
Bangor, ME

Rebecca C. Martinez, PharmD, MS, RPh
Associate Dean
School of Health Sciences
Kaplan University
Fort Lauderdale, FL

Ann Minks
Program Director
Medical Transcription
Lake Washington Technical College
Kirkland, WA

Elaine Nowak, MEd
Lead Instructor
Medical Transcription
Business Technology
Northcentral Technical College
Wausau, WI

Elizabeth M. Sprinkle, CMA (AAMA), BA
Program Coordinator
Medical Transcription
Forsyth Technical Community College
Winston-Salem, NC

Nancy L. Stephenson, MEd Admin
Instructor (Retired)
Medical Transcription
Business/General Education
Western Dakota Technical Institute
Rapid City, SD

Barb Struck
Instructor
Business and Technology
Lake Superior College
Duluth, MN

CONTENTS

Preface   v
User's Guide   ix
Reviewers   xiii

PART I
Medical Transcription Fundamentals   1

CHAPTER 1   A Career Profile   3
Introduction   3
What is a Medical Transcriptionist?   3
Required Knowledge and Skills   4
History and Principles of Medical
    Record Keeping   7
Electronic Medical Record and
    Electronic Health Record   8
Patient Confidentiality, HIPAA, and
    HITECH   9
Work Environments   11
Professional Affiliation   13
Chapter Summary   14

**CHAPTER 2   Technology, Tools, and
                Techniques   20**
Introduction   20
Understanding Information
    Technology   21
Computer Systems   23
Computer Applications   24
The Internet   26
Transcription Methods   27
Transcription References and Tools   30
Special Word-Processing Features   32
File Management   34
Chapter Summary   35

**CHAPTER 3   The Basics of Medical
                Terminology   42**
Introduction   42
Medical Word Building   42
Word-Confusion Problems   48
Slang and Medical Jargon   49
Medical Abbreviations   51
Anatomic Terms   53
Clock Body Positions   57
Chapter Summary   57

**CHAPTER 4   Medical Correspondence
                and Reports   66**
Introduction   66
Standard Business Letters   66
Medical Reports   68
The Transcription Process   82
Strategies for Success   82
Transcription Instructions   84
Chapter Summary   85

CHAPTER 5   Mechanics of Editing   93
Introduction   93
Grammar Review   93
Punctuation Review   96
Capitalization   102
Numbers   104
Symbols   105
Eponyms   105
Acronyms   106
Proofreading Techniques   106
Chapter Summary   109

PART II
Medical Specialties   117

CHAPTER 6   **Surgery   119**
  Introduction   119
  General Surgery Concepts   119
  The Surgical Process   120
  Common Surgical Terminology   122
  Surgical Prefixes, Suffixes, and
      Combining Forms   127
  Chapter Summary   128

CHAPTER 7   **Pharmacology   134**
  Introduction   134
  Overview of Pharmacology   134
  History of Pharmacology   135
  Drug Regulation and
      Development   136
  Drug Administration   137
  Types of Drugs   139
  Controlled Substances   139
  Transcribing Drug Nomenclature   141
  Chapter Summary   141

CHAPTER 8   **Laboratory Studies and
  Medical Imaging   148**
  Introduction   148
  Understanding Pathology   148
  Laboratory Studies   151
  Radiologic Imaging   158
  Chapter Summary   164

CHAPTER 9   **Dermatology   177**
  Introduction   177
  Anatomy of the Integumentary
      System   177
  Common Dermatologic Diseases and
      Treatments   180
  Diagnostic Studies and
      Procedures   190
  Chapter Summary   190

CHAPTER 10   **Ophthalmology   202**
  Introduction   202
  Anatomy of the Eye   202
  Visual Process   205
  Chapter Summary   216

CHAPTER 11   **Otorhinolaryngology   229**
  Introduction   229
  What is Otorhinolaryngology?   229
  Anatomy of the Ears, Nose,
      and Throat   230
  The Process of Hearing   234
  Common Otolaryngologic Diseases
      and Treatments   235

  Diagnostic Studies and
      Procedures   239
  Chapter Summary   244

CHAPTER 12   **Pulmonology   258**
  Introduction   258
  Anatomy of the Respiratory
      System   259
  Respiratory Process   260
  Mechanical Ventilation   263
  Common Pulmonary Diseases and
      Treatments   263
  Diagnostic Studies and
      Procedures   270
  Chapter Summary   273

CHAPTER 13   **Cardiology and the
  Cardiovascular System   288**
  Introduction   288
  The Cardiovascular System   289
  Anatomy of the Heart   289
  Cardiovascular Circulation   291
  Cardiac Cycle   292
  Heart Sounds   293
  Heart Rate and Rhythm   294
  Blood Pressure   295
  Common Cardiac Diseases and
      Treatments   295
  Diagnostic Studies and
      Procedures   301
  Chapter Summary   304

CHAPTER 14   **Gastroenterology   319**
  Introduction   319
  Anatomy of the Gastrointestinal
      System   319
  The Digestive Process   323
  Common Gastrointestinal Diseases and
      Treatments   324
  Diagnostic Studies and
      Procedures   333
  Chapter Summary   336

CHAPTER 15   **Urology   352**
  Introduction   352
  Anatomy of the Genitourinary
      System   352
  Process of Urination   355
  Common Genitourinary Diseases and
      Treatments   356
  Diagnostic Studies and
      Procedures   368
  Chapter Summary   371

CHAPTER 16 **Obstetrics and Gynecology 386**
Introduction 386
Anatomy of the Female Reproductive
    System 386
Fundamentals of Human
    Reproduction 390
Common Gynecologic Diseases and
    Treatments 395
Diagnostic Studies and
    Procedures 400
Chapter Summary 403

CHAPTER 17 **Orthopaedics 420**
Introduction 420
Anatomy of the Musculoskeletal
    System 421
Anatomic Regions of the Body 428
Anatomic Terms of Motion 429
Common Musculoskeletal Diseases and
    Treatments 429
Diagnostic Studies and
    Procedures 437
Chapter Summary 441

CHAPTER 18 **Neurology 457**
Introduction 457
Anatomy of the Nervous System 458
Common Neurologic Diseases and
    Treatments 463
Diagnostic Studies and
    Procedures 472
Chapter Summary 478

CHAPTER 19 **Immunology 495**
Introduction 495
Overview of the Immune System 496
Self and Nonself 496
Anatomy of the Immune System 497
Common Immunologic Diseases and
    Treatments 500
Diagnostic Studies and
    Procedures 510
Chapter Summary 513

CHAPTER 20 **Oncology 527**
Introduction 527
Cell Structure 528

How Cancer Develops 529
Cancer Risk Factors 532
Cancer Classification Systems 534
Diagnostic Studies and
    Procedures 536
Cancer Treatments 541
Chapter Summary 545

CHAPTER 21 **Endocrinology 558**
Introduction 558
Anatomy of the Endocrine
    System 558
Common Endocrine Diseases and
    Treatments 562
Diagnostic Studies and
    Procedures 569
Chapter Summary 570

PART III
Your New Career 585

CHAPTER 22 **Career Management 587**
Introduction 587
Job Search Strategies 587
Industry Terminology 590
Effective Resumés and Application
    Letters 593
Online Testing 599
Interview Success 601
Personal and Professional
    Development 603
Owning Your Own Business 608
Chapter Summary 612

APPENDICES
Appendix 1: ISMP'S List of Error-Prone
    Abbreviations, Symbols, and
    Dose Designations 619
Appendix 2: Selected Normal Laboratory
    Values 623
Appendix 3: Common Medical Abbreviations 634
Appendix 4: Suggested Web Sites 642
Appendix 5: Suggested List of References 643

Index 645

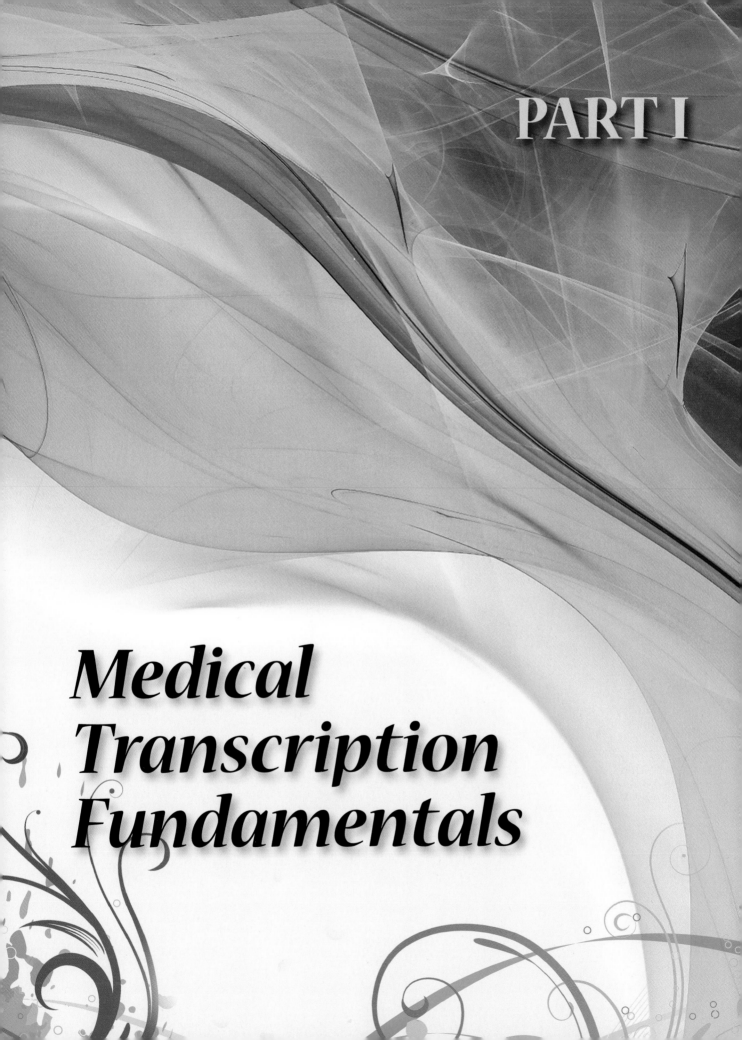

PART I

Medical Transcription Fundamentals

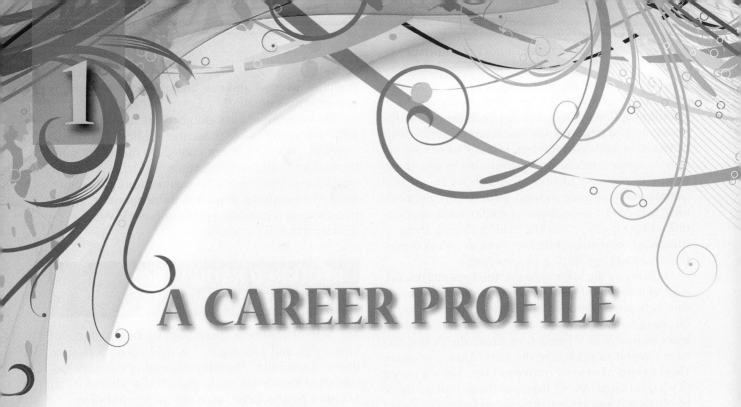

A CAREER PROFILE

INTRODUCTION

The health information management staff is an integral part of any successful medical office, from a small suburban office of a single physician to a large city hospital system. A medical transcriptionist, whether working at a medical facility or in a home-based environment, is a vital part of the medical records staff. Far more than a typist in the medical field, a medical transcriptionist must be familiar with the terminology used in every medical specialty and must be able to produce the documents and reports required by each specialty in a professional and competent manner. These reports comprise a **medical record**, a series of documents that track a patient's medical history. This chapter profiles the profession and details the required skills, responsibilities, and work environments in the field of medical transcription.

WHAT IS A MEDICAL TRANSCRIPTIONIST?

By definition, a **medical transcriptionist** (MT) is a person who converts medical information spoken by a healthcare provider into a written text document that can be printed or retained as a permanent record of a patient's medical care. A medical transcriptionist is *not* a typist, word processor, or medical secretary. Although the profession still uses the term "medical transcriptionist," MTs today are actually skilled medical language specialists, whose work documents patient care and helps facilitate the delivery of healthcare services.

According to the *Occupational Outlook Handbook* published by the U.S. Bureau of Labor Statistics, employment opportunities for MTs are expected to increase well into the next decade as the profession grows to accommodate a larger aging population. Medical transcription services will also be in demand as the need grows for electronic documentation that can easily be shared by multiple providers. MTs will be needed not only to create medical records but also to edit documents, review and identify discrepancies in medical records, and transmit medical information electronically. MTs have a wide choice of employment opportunities in a rapidly expanding field, including those in supervisory or management positions, as well as opportunities in writing, editing, and teaching.

Success as an MT requires a fundamental knowledge of a variety of skills that encompass the relationship between a physician and a transcriptionist in the dictation-transcription process. Whenever a patient seeks treatment at a hospital or clinic, the doctor dictates a report to document the facts of the encounter. These reports need to be converted into a written record of what occurred. An MT listens to the recordings made by physicians and other healthcare professionals, called **medical providers** (or, simply, **providers**). The MT transcribes the recordings into detailed patient reports, notes, correspondence, and other administrative materials. After the reports are reviewed and approved by the healthcare provider who dictated them, each transcribed report or record, along with its date of service, becomes part of the patient's permanent health record, either in print form or electronically in a computer database. This documentation is used by physicians and other healthcare providers to determine the care a patient will receive. Therefore, the MT must understand what is dictated and compose a healthcare record that is grammatically correct and accurate. In addition, while transcriptionists are required to record exactly what they hear, they are also expected to think about what is really being said and correctly interpret a physician's meaning.

Dictation is a collective word that encompasses the speech that is **transcribed**, or put into written form. Dictation in the medical field may include reports covering diagnostic studies, operative reports, letters, history and physical examinations, discharge summaries, inpatient progress reports, and outpatient clinic notes. A transcriptionist may transcribe this information directly from voice recordings heard through headphones or may edit reports created by the computer from a voice recognition program. Professionals who dictate reports into a patient's medical record can include doctors, nurse practitioners, nurses, residents, and other medical professionals who may all individually report about a specific encounter with a patient on a specific date of service. Because of this, one patient's visit can generate several reports from several providers, such that even a small medical practice or hospital can generate hundreds of reports in a day. An MT performs the duties of typing and formatting dictated accounts of these encounters into a written, easily readable form that

complies with all policies and procedures regarding patient confidentiality.

However, more than just good listening and typing skills are required to transcribe medical documents accurately. It simply is not enough to memorize some medical terms heard on television and to be a fast typist. Although there are no "formal" educational requirements for becoming a medical transcriptionist, an MT must possess certain skills and attributes in order to be successful in this profession.

REQUIRED KNOWLEDGE AND SKILLS

The field of medicine encompasses a huge volume of knowledge, and working in this field entails a tremendous responsibility. The following outlines the very specific set of knowledge, skills, and self-discipline skills an MT must possess to be successful in the profession:

- Skill in the use of personal computers, word-processing software, and various electronic means of transmitting finished reports to the medical provider. Software programs such as MS Word have dramatically transformed the way MTs work and are a dominant presence in the production of medical documents. Physicians and other healthcare providers employ state-of-the-art electronic technology to dictate and transmit highly complex and confidential information about their patients. These medical professionals rely on skilled MTs to use the corresponding technology to create accurate medical records. This technology is always changing. Advances in speech technology and the electronic transfer of data continue to shape the changing role of an MT. Therefore, it is essential to keep abreast of advances in computer technology.
- Expert knowledge of the English language, including rules governing punctuation and capitalization. You must be able to construct a proper sentence, using words, capitalization, and punctuation according to the standard rules of English-language grammar. You must also be able to proofread work for typographical and grammatical errors to make sure that the final report is accurate, complete, and grammatically correct.
- Knowledge of medical terminology as it applies to anatomy and physiology, diagnostic procedures, and treatments. A practical knowledge of the complex language of medicine enables you to transcribe a healthcare provider's dictation accurately and in a clear and comprehensible report format. Our collection of medical knowledge increases and changes every day, and you must always be ready to learn the latest words and

phrases of medical terminology. Achieving familiarity and fluency with medical terminology across a range of specialties is a formidable task, but this knowledge will set you apart from the rest as a quality MT.

- Have you ever listened to a song you love, read the lyrics, and then discovered just how far off you really were when you compared your notes to the writer's actual words? In medicine, words can sound deceptively alike, and inaccuracies can have dire consequences. An MT must have a thorough understanding of words to distinguish between terms that sound alike but are spelled differently and which have completely different meanings. He or she must be familiar with the terms used to describe anatomy, disease processes, medical procedures, and diagnostic studies. An MT must enjoy working with words and must have excellent reference skills to locate unusual and obscure terms. An MT not only transcribes words to create reports that are factually accurate but also is responsible for the correct format, punctuation, capitalization, and spelling of the text of these reports.
- Excellent listening skills to understand and correctly transcribe patient assessments and treatments which reduces the chance of patients receiving ineffective or even harmful treatments and ensures a high quality of patient care. In addition, you must be able to discern different accents and dictation styles, especially when English is not a dictator's first language. Dictators who speak English as a second language (ESL) may pronounce words differently or put emphasis on words or syllables in the wrong place. They may pronounce English letters differently, especially when their native language does not have similar letters and sounds. Some ESL dictators forget to say articles such as *a, an,* or *the,* which do not exist in their native languages.
- Critical thinking skills to understand the context of what is being dictated. Medical transcription is not simply typing words. You must pay strict attention to the minute details of the story unfolding in dictation and catch inconsistencies that may occur during dictation. For example, a diagnosis inconsistent with the patient's history and symptoms may be mistakenly dictated. The medical transcriptionist questions, seeks clarification, verifies the information, and enters the correct information into the report. Physicians frequently give inaccurate patient statistical information, mispronounce medications, and dictate without the patient's chart readily available (such as at home or from a cell phone), thereby furnishing data that is sometimes incorrect or simply unintelligible. An MT interprets the data as it is being dictated, listens for inaccuracies in information, and creates a document that is technically accurate in the context of the medical situation.
- A high level of concentration. Dictation is not always smooth and clear. Physicians often whisper, mutter, and sometimes talk to themselves or other people, forgetting a transcriptionist is listening and attempting to transcribe every word. They talk over screeching ambulance sirens, wailing babies, phones, and beepers. They chew gum, eat, interchange item numbers in a list, and often repeat key portions of dictation because they forget they have already dictated this information. Through all these distractions, an MT must be able to concentrate on the words being dictated.
- An interest in the field and the language of medicine. An MT must have a genuine interest in understanding the physiology of the human body and learning how body systems work. You need to be familiar with the drug names, dosages, and uses for hundreds of commonly prescribed medications in order to detect inconsistencies. For example, you should know or be able to look up the correct drug dosage when it is unclear whether "50 mg" or "15 mg" is being dictated. You also must have a desire to learn about the latest advances in pharmaceutical treatments for illnesses. You must desire to learn more about the laboratory and diagnostic studies used in the evaluation of diseases and remember normal laboratory values so as not to transcribe an inaccurate figure when an erroneous value is dictated. Learning all you can about the medical field, the latest advances in diagnostic and treatment protocols, and the terminology used to describe them will enable you to be the best MT you can be.
- Professional keyboarding skills. As a medical transcriptionist, you must be able to type materials that regularly include medical or legal terminology as well as words that derive from foreign languages. In addition, although keyboarding accuracy is emphasized over speed in creating medical reports, you should be aware of your typing speed. You should strive to maintain a typing speed of 60 words per minute or better in order to type documents and reports and transmit them to the medical provider in a timely manner. This is important because most MTs are paid by the total number of lines produced, as opposed to "dollars per hour." A line count is a measurement of lines typed, and the number of lines typed determines how much you are paid. Your value as an MT has a lot to do with your line count; a higher line count indicates that you can produce more typed lines, and hence, more reports, which is discussed in more detail in Chapter 22.

QUICK CHECK 1.1 ✓

Indicate whether the following statements are true (T) or false (F).

1. A medical transcriptionist does not have to know English very well in order to prepare medical reports.   T   F

2. A medical transcriptionist must be able to think critically.   T   F

3. A medical transcriptionist must have excellent listening skills.   T   F

4. The Hippocratic Oath outlines ethics for physicians' pastimes.   T   F

5. Medical television shows are a good source of education in medical transcription.   T   F

- Skill in creating a variety of reports, each of which may have its own formatting requirements. Reports outlining the details of patient care take many forms, including histories and physical examinations, progress reports, emergency room notes, consultations, operative reports, discharge summaries, clinic notes, referral letters, radiology reports, pathology reports, and other documents. These reports cover a variety of medical specialties. Therefore, it is essential that you be familiar with the formatting requirements of different types of reports and the information they must contain.

- Self-discipline. Contrary to the television and print ads glamorizing medical transcription as a profession in which you can work "whenever you feel like it," to be a successful MT you must have the discipline to work the hours required and to turn in your work on time. In fact, dependability is the number one factor that medical transcription service owners look for—even more than top grades and perfect attendance in school—when hiring a new employee. "Dependability" means transcribing work accurately and efficiently while blocking out the distractions of children, televisions, pets, ringing telephones, or neighbors who want to stop by simply because "you are home." No one can effectively transcribe complex medical reports in a state of distraction. You will need to block out periods of time that can be devoted solely to transcription and put off tasks such as cooking dinner, playing with the kids, or folding laundry until after your work is finished. Some at-home MTs hire a babysitter to come in and watch the kids while they work and make it clear to everyone in the house that "when mom (or dad) is working, do not disturb unless there is an emergency."

- Knowledge of medical ethics and the self-discipline to abide by the rules of ethical conduct. When most people think of ethics, or moral conduct, they think of rules for distinguishing between right and wrong, such as the Golden Rule ("Do unto others as you would have them do unto you"). **Ethics** are the norm for conduct that distinguish between acceptable and unacceptable behavior. The **Hippocratic Oath**, one of the most famous pieces of writing in the history of medicine, outlines the tenets of ethical conduct of physicians. The oath was written by the Greek physician Hippocrates, called the Father of Medicine because of his discoveries and contribution to modern medicine. Originally translated from Greek, the oath included rules of conduct for doctors that physicians still honor today in caring for their patients. The oath should also guide you as an MT in your conduct as a representative of the medical profession. This means being a vigilant advocate for quality patient documentation and adhering to the highest level of privacy and security provisions. You should strive to uphold moral and legal rights of patients, safeguard patient privacy, and approach your work with a focus on ensuring patient safety and quality of care. This means exercising integrity in work practices as well as abiding by all laws and standards governing the practice of patient documentation. Ethical conduct for an MT means fostering an environment that facilitates integrity, professionalism, and safeguarding of patient information at all times.

In short, the primary characteristics and skills an MT must possess are extensive knowledge of medical terminology and a high level of understanding of how it is used across a variety of medical specialties; deductive reasoning; self-discipline; and the ability to pay attention to details—in order to transform spoken words into a comprehensive record that accurately details a person's medical history. In addition, an MT always must be mindful of patient confidentiality and security of medical information.

Read the list of questions in Table 1.1 and consider your answers. Whether you can answer yes to these

TABLE 1.1   Do I Have What It Takes?

Ask yourself the following questions that pertain to the characteristics of a successful medical transcriptionist. Can you answer "yes" to them all?

Do I have good spelling, verbal communication, and memory skills?

Do I have a good memory?

Do I have good listening skills?

Do I have good critical thinking skills?

Do I have the ability to sort, check, count, and verify numbers accurately?

Can I use computer equipment and software well? Do I know computer-related terminology?

Can I navigate the Internet quickly and efficiently?

Do I love typing different types of documents?

Am I able to follow written and oral instructions?

Do I have excellent English grammar, punctuation, and capitalization skills?

Do I have good or above-average typing skills (at least 60 wpm)?

Am I willing to learn basic-to-advanced medical terminology?

Am I interested in learning about human anatomy and physiology as well as the latest developments in medical treatments for diseases?

Am I proficient at listening to and understanding people for whom English is their second language?

Am I not afraid to ask questions of information I do not know?

Am I particular about the documents I create in terms of quality and accuracy?

Am I interested in professional development and mastering the knowledge and skills of my profession so I may grow and learn in my day-to-day work life?

Am I a detail-oriented individual?

Do I follow through with tasks, even if they sometimes take longer than usual to accomplish?

Can I maintain a high level of concentration for long periods of time?

Do I enjoy learning new things and challenging concepts?

Am I dedicated to professional development and being the best I can be at whatever I choose to do in my career?

Am I discrete and careful about not disclosing information that is confidential?

HISTORY AND PRINCIPLES OF MEDICAL RECORD KEEPING

As evidenced by ancient cave drawings, people have attempted to keep records of some sort since the beginning of human existence. Although the medium changed from cave walls to stone tablets, from papyrus to parchment, and now from paper to electronic files, the reason for maintaining records remains the same: to document an individual's history and achievements. In the days when few people could read or write, those who could, called **scribes**, were hired to copy and interpret the spoken words of others. They transcribed sacred orations into the written rules and procedures by which a society governs its citizens.

Medical transcription originated in the early 1900s when medical stenographers helped physicians document all of the interactions between a physician and a patient. A **stenographer**, a person skilled in the transcription of speech, accompanied the physician during visits with patients, listening and taking down the physician's dictation in shorthand to document the medical record on a manual typewriter, as illustrated in Figure 1.1.

During World War I, when dictation recording equipment first became available, physicians began to use this equipment to dictate their findings and treatment plans so that a transcriptionist might produce a

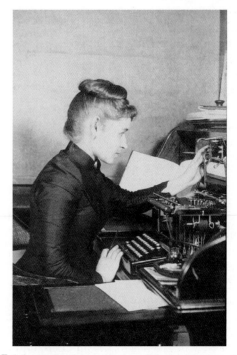

FIGURE 1.1. Medical Transcription of the Past. In the early 1900s, a stenographer took down the physician's dictation in shorthand and used a typewriter to document the medical record. Photo Credit: US National Oceanic and Atmospheric Administration.

questions now or are working toward this objective as you complete your coursework, an awareness of the skills and characteristics of a competent medical transcriptionist will help you focus on your goal.

written record at a later time. As physicians came to rely on the judgment and reasoning of experienced MTs to safeguard the accuracy and integrity of medical dictation, the MT evolved into a medical language specialist. As technology improves, the role of the MT will evolve into that of a medical language editor who reviews and corrects reports generated by voice recognition software to ensure the accurate processing of patient health information.

ELECTRONIC MEDICAL RECORD AND ELECTRONIC HEALTH RECORD

In the last decade, the US healthcare industry has embraced the use of technology for the entry and storage of patient information. An electronic storage system of patient data provides a secure, real-time electronic record of a patient's medical and health information generated by one or more medical providers during encounters in a care-delivery setting, such as a hospital, doctor's office, or clinic. Two terms, the **electronic medical record** (EMR) and the **electronic health record** (EHR), have come to be used interchangeably. However, these terms describe different concepts and procedures, both of which are crucial to improving the quality and efficiency of documenting patient information.

By definition, the electronic medical record is an individual application repository of a patient's medical encounters with a single provider. It consists of the provider's documentation of those encounters, including letters, chart notes, pharmacy record, allergies, billing information, and so on, as shown in the example screen shot from a patient's hospital EMR provider in Figure 1.2. The electronic health record (EHR), on the other hand, is a compilation of all the EMRs contained in the repository for a particular patient. This is a secure and private lifetime record of key health history and care

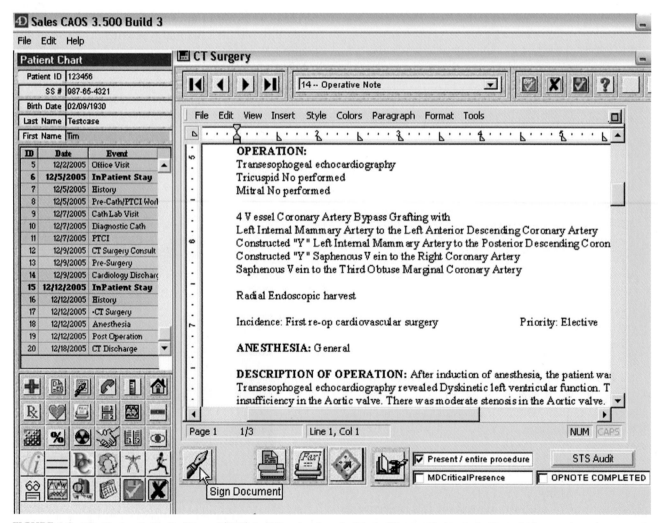

FIGURE 1.2. **The Electronic Medical Record (EMR).** An EMR system in a physician's office uses electronic charting, which promotes a clear, accurate record of patient care as opposed to a paper chart. Reprinted with permission from MediNotes Corporation, West Des Moines, IA.

for each person contained in one repository. This inter-operable, multi-provider, multi-speciality, and multi-disciplined electronic record is the organized collection of *all* records about an individual stored in the computer systems and databases of *all* the providers who have cared for that patient, including data documented during hospital stays, such as operative notes, laboratory data, and imaging studies. An individual's electronic health record is assembled using data supplied by the patient's doctors and other providers, making every form of clinical information available in a standardized electronic format. The EHR environment relies on functional EMRs that allow medical providers and organizations to exchange information with other providers within the community, the region, or even the nation.

The concept of an electronic patient record originated in the early 1990s with the growing popularity of the desktop computer, but high cost and the lack of uniform technological standards prevented the widespread use of this system. The advent of high-tech digital and specially-coded technology, high-speed Internet access, and more cost-effective options in the field of electronics have combined to make the use of an EMR/EHR system a viable option for the majority of healthcare providers.

The mandate to create a national patient record electronic database was signed into law in 2005 by the Bush administration. The purpose of the EHR is to automate and streamline the flow of a patient's medical information from all healthcare providers into one repository accessible by all the patient's providers. Patients would have access to, and ultimate control over, the contents of their medical records. Under this system, when a patient who has authorized the use of an EHR sees a new physician or other healthcare provider, the patient's entire medical history, including all current and past conditions, treatments, and medications, would be available to the new physician through the EHR database.

The EHR enables continuity of care among all of a patient's medical providers. Typically, patient information moves between providers by mail, phone, or fax, or it may even be hand-carried by the patient. Each provider a patient sees creates a separate set of records in a chart that includes scribbled phone messages, handwritten physician notes, and laboratory reports. The older or more ill the patient, the thicker the folder is likely to be, and the more jumbled and confusing the information becomes. Frequently this results in incomplete and contradictory reports in the records of the different medical providers.

The proposed system reduces the need for physicians to buy new hardware or software and makes maintaining the EHR much simpler. A portal, or single sign-on point of access via the Internet, enables the provider to locate a patient's information on a web-based company's site and allows the information to be displayed within a set of pages that the user can view in a browser. The patient's privacy and security of information is maintained and protected through the use of special coding and other technical tools that specify the names of the patient's physicians who have been granted access to the record.

Using the EHR's search and analysis tools, all of the patient's healthcare providers have access to the patient's complete medical record 24 hours a day. This eliminates the delays that can result when a patient's record has to be pulled and sent by fax. A physician can review and edit information online, have electronic signature capability, and distribute the requested information via secure e-mail. The record is not stored on any individual computer, but is assembled from the information in the database when accessed in a provider's computer memory for viewing purposes; it does not remain accessible on a provider's computer after the provider has logged off the main database.

In addition, when properly configured, the EHR can provide tailored alerts and notices to help healthcare professionals provide the most appropriate treatments. The EHR program has the ability to search all information in a patient's record and, based on the latest medical practices, can alert the healthcare provider to additional factors he or she may consider when making treatment decisions. For example, an EHR might alert a physician to an allergy to a particular medication being prescribed or identify the need for additional tests prior to making a diagnosis or treatment recommendation based on the patient's history or family history.

Evidence consistently shows that paper-based medical record systems do not provide the sufficiently safe, high-quality, and cost-effective exchange of patient information required in today's healthcare environment. Computer-based records are quickly replacing their paper-based counterparts as the consumer and political demand for change becomes stronger.

PATIENT CONFIDENTIALITY, HIPAA, AND HITECH

Confidentiality always has been, and always should be, central to the relationship between the patient and his or her healthcare provider. The **Health Insurance Portability and Accountability Act of 1996** (HIPAA, pronounced *HIP-aa*) is perhaps the single most significant piece of federal legislation affecting the healthcare industry since the inception of Medicare. The primary purpose of HIPAA was to ensure the portability and continuity of health insurance coverage if a person changed jobs, but it also gives patients greater access to their own medical records and more control over how their personally identifiable health information is used.

HIPAA also addresses the obligations of healthcare providers and health plans to provide privacy of health information transactions and for the confidentiality and security of patient data.

Part of HIPAA's provisions require the US Department of Health and Human Services (DHHS) to provide safeguards to protect individuals from having their private health information made available to whomever requests it. The DHHS wrote the **Security Rule** and the **Privacy Rule** as part of HIPAA to publicize standards for the privacy of all health information. The goal of the Security Rule is to protect personal information while still allowing for the efficient flow of health information needed to treat patients effectively. The Privacy Rule requires covered entities to protect individuals' health records and other identifiable health information by requiring appropriate safeguards to protect privacy and by setting limits and conditions on the uses and disclosures that may be made of such information. It also gives individuals certain rights with respect to their health information. These rules apply to health plans, healthcare clearinghouses, and those healthcare providers who conduct electronically certain financial and administrative transactions that are subject to the transactions standards adopted by the DHHS.

The Privacy Rule has reformed the industry's management of healthcare insurance, mandating that all insurance claims follow the same format, thereby simplifying administrative paperwork. More important, due to the enormous increase in the electronic transmission of health information, these federal privacy and security regulations enhance the privacy protections and security measures for health information. These provisions require healthcare plans and providers to establish procedural, administrative, and record-keeping policies that protect against misuse of an individual's health information, including protection against the improper use or disclosure of such information in any format—oral, written, or electronic. MTs are subject to the requirements set forth under HIPAA's Privacy Rule because they perform a function on behalf of healthcare providers that includes the use and disclosure of a patient's medical information. As a medical transcriptionist, you are required by the Privacy Rule to give every sincere, willful effort to preserve, protect, and defend the privacy and confidentiality of the records (audio files, transcribed reports, patient and/or job log sheets, etc.) that you handle during the transcription process, and to prevent theft or loss of this information while that information is in your possession or being transmitted to or from you.

In February 2009, as part of the American Recovery and Reinvestment Act of 2009 (ARRA), President Obama signed the Health Information Technology for Economic and Clinical Health (HITECH) Act, providing government funding to encourage the widespread adoption of the EHR in US healthcare systems. The Act has spurred the adoption of EHR systems across the country, which in turn improves coordination of patient care by increasing patient safety and reducing errors. The HITECH Act, devised by Congress primarily to address the adoption of electronic medical records nationwide, has added a tough data-breach notification requirement to the long list of HIPAA privacy rules. Together, both laws provide for punishments and fines by the US Department of Health and Human Services and the Federal Trade Commission (FTC) against organizations and other providers (as defined under HIPAA) who violate the rules regarding the breach of such information.

Medical transcriptionists and medical transcription services are regarded under the Act as **business associates**. The Act defines a business associate to include persons who, on behalf of a covered entity (but other than as members of the covered entity's workforce), perform or assist in performing a function or activity that involves the use or disclosure of individually identifiable health information. This includes transcription services, billing services, attorneys, accountants, technology vendors, and many other types of businesses that are directly regulated by the Act and by HIPAA. While not subjecting business associates to all of the obligations of covered entities (such as providing privacy notices), the Act requires them to comply with the HIPAA provisions mandating administrative, physical, and technical safeguards of patient information.

Whether working at home or in an on-site office, a competent MT recognizes the importance of patient confidentiality even without the provisions required by HIPAA and the HITECH Act. Most transcription services or companies have administrative and technical safeguards in place to protect patient confidentiality, but it is vital that an MT, especially one working at home, take the security of the patient record seriously. The following guidelines will help you to protect the privacy and electronic security of the health information at an individual workstation and to adhere to regulations set forth by HIPAA and the HITECH Act. Some points seem silly or over-compensating, but you would not want to be involved in any breach that is interpreted as willful neglect or noncompliance on your part under the federal guidelines.

1. If you transcribe from home, separate your workspace or office space from the rest of the home and restrict access by visitors and family members. If other family members do have access to your work area, discourage them from physically accessing your computer, which should be used for transcription alone.
2. Create strong passwords for all computers, including laptops, that are used for work purposes to discourage unauthorized access to your machine. Use passwords containing upper and lowercase letters,

numbers, and symbols with a length of more than 14 characters to ensure the highest security. Commit the password to memory and do not share it with anyone. Change the password periodically.

3. Do not have family members or friends help you with your work. Requests such as, "Honey, can you listen to this dictation and tell me what the doctor said?" or "Son, can you drop this completed work off at my employer's office on your way to football practice?" can jeopardize the confidentiality of a patient's information.

4. Log off the computer when leaving your workstation, or protect your files by using a screen saver that comes on after five minutes of inactivity, protected by a screen saver password.

5. Ensure that the computer display with access to patient information is not visible to unauthorized individuals.

6. Never leave sensitive or confidential information in a trash can. Do not write down patient details on papers or sticky notes at your desk. If you must write down the information, destroy the papers that contain patient information by using a document shredder.

7. Keep confidential patient information out of sight. Place this information in a locked file drawer or cabinet when not in use.

8. Avoid copying patient data to a personal laptop computer, any removable devices like a flash drive, external hard drive, CDs, DVDs, etc., as there is a chance that these devices could get lost or stolen.

9. Know how to protect your computer system. Firewalls, spyware protection, and virus protection programs should be a part of your vocabulary and areas of expertise. Nothing can be worse than having confidential patient information stolen by a computer hacker or an entire system brought down by the latest deadly computer virus.

When using communication resources such as e-mail, the fax machine, or the telephone, observe the following guidelines:

1. Assume that e-mail systems are not secure unless the messages will be transmitted in a special code that cannot be intercepted by others when they are sent. In any case, take precautions and use common sense when sending e-mail. Do not send confidential information unless the patient's identity has been blocked or removed. Do not send attachments with e-mails that are not specially coded to prevent being intercepted or read by others during transit.

2. Create a confidential message footer for e-mail messages, such as:
   NOTICE: This electronic mail communication contains confidential information intended only for the person(s) designated above. Any use, distribution, reproduction, or disclosure, or any other use of this transmission by any party is strictly prohibited. If you are not the intended recipient of this e-mail, promptly and securely delete it and all attachments.

3. Do not reveal any patient details or send voice or transcribed files, patient logs, or any other such individually identifiable patient health information through an instant-messenger window or cell phone text-message feature.

4. Limit access to voice mail or answering machines so that other family members do not access patient health information that may be left there. Take care in wording messages you leave on answering machines or voice mail.

5. Exercise care if using a speaker phone; be aware of the sensitive nature of conversations and of messages that may be overheard.

6. When using a fax machine, never fax information to an unsecured fax machine. Call ahead to ensure that the intended recipient will be on-hand to pick up the fax. Double-check the destination fax number before sending the fax. Use a fax cover sheet containing the previously noted confidentiality statement that is used for electronic transmissions.

Finally, respecting patient privacy and confidentiality includes the awareness that conversations might be overheard by others. Do not share information about patient reports with others, not even family or friends. The same precaution should be applied to online forums, message boards, Facebook, Twitter, and other places where confidential information could be seen or heard by others. Most issues of broken confidentiality result from MTs talking to friends about an unusual medical problem encountered in a patient's record. There is a remote, although real, possibility that a friend or relative of the patient could overhear the discussion, or that the person to whom the story is told could spread the news further.

The civil penalties for violations of HIPAA and HITECH include high monetary fines. There are also federal criminal penalties that include jail time for health-plan employees and providers and other employees who knowingly and improperly disclose patient information under false pretenses; and these penalties are even higher if such disclosure is used for monetary gain. Therefore, all MTs, even those who work at home, must make every effort to comply with all security regulations.

WORK ENVIRONMENTS

MTs may choose among a wide variety of work environments and opportunities for advancement. Many MTs are employed in settings such as hospitals, physicians' offices, clinics, laboratories, medical libraries, and government medical facilities. Full-time transcriptionists work a 40-hour week, although some work irregular schedules, such as swing or graveyard shifts, part-time, or on-call. Self-employed and home-based MTs have more flexible hours. Some transcriptionists work only on an on-call basis, depending on the amount of work needed to be done. Fringe benefits may include paid vacation, holidays, sick leave, medical insurance, and pension plans; however, transcriptionists who work only on-call and self-employed transcriptionists usually do not get these benefits.

Hospitals and Clinics

There are solid advantages associated with a position in a hospital or other healthcare institution. A new transcriptionist may find it more comfortable to work in a setting that offers the security of a supervisor on-hand to provide assistance if needed. In addition, it might be easier for a new MT to find work in a local hospital or large clinic. Because many qualified MTs work at home, hospitals and other institutions encounter difficulties in hiring capable employees and so are often willing to train new MT graduates in-house. Institutional employees may also enjoy better quality benefits, including health insurance, sick leave, and overtime. Finally, many people enjoy working in an office where they can interact daily with other people, create new friendships, and be involved in various employee functions and social events. MTs who work at home sometimes feel isolated from their peers.

Working at Home

Most MTs work at home, and this type of work is a dream for many people. There are also advantages to this form of work. Vast improvements in both computing and communications technology make it fast, efficient, and relatively inexpensive for medical institutions to contract work outside of their facilities. Therefore, an increasing number of MTs now work from home as employees or subcontractors for hospitals and transcription services, or as self-employed independent contractors. Those MTs with children find they can work their schedules around school, activities, meals, or naps. Working from home allows for greater flexibility in a work schedule as sometimes it is not necessary to conform to a brick-and-mortar facility's workday or preset hours. The savings in not having to commute to an office, maintain a business wardrobe, purchase meals outside the home, or pay for parking can add up quickly. In fact, many people are attracted to the medical transcription industry because it offers this unique opportunity to manage time and money to their advantage by working from their homes.

However, working at home has its own inherent issues to overcome in order to successfully work in this environment. In many cases, the MT is responsible for having his or her own equipment, which might include a computer, Internet access, keyboard, desk, chair, foot pedal, headset, mouse, reference materials, and lighting. In addition, the issue of establishing boundaries is

QUICK CHECK 1.2

Circle the letter corresponding to the best answer to the following questions.

1. An individual's health record maintained electronically is referred to as an
    A. EGD.
    B. EHR.
    C. ERR.
    D. EER.

2. When leaving your workstation, you should take the following action with respect to your computer
    A. log off.
    B. set the password.
    C. log in.
    D. turn off the computer.

3. The civil penalties for violations of HIPAA include
    A. an IRS audit.
    B. a reprimand from the boss.
    C. getting fired.
    D. monetary fines.

4. A fax sheet transmitting patient information should contain
    A. the patient's medical record number.
    B. your workstation number.
    C. a photo of the patient.
    D. a confidentiality statement.

5. A patient's EHR record is stored
    A. at the physician's office.
    B. in the physician's car.
    C. in a remote database.
    D. in the hospital file room.

probably the biggest hurdle for an at-home MT to learn. There may be distractions abound with family members who do not always understand that a home employee has a work schedule like an on-site employee. Telephone calls from friends, the needs and priorities of children, or even the lure of the television can interfere with productivity. The same smart work habits that spell success for any job, such as being focused, self-disciplined, self-motivated, and self-starting, apply to the at-home MT as they do the on-site one.

In whatever work environment, either at an office or at home, MTs usually work alone at individual workstations. A great degree of concentration and care are essential because of the potentially serious consequences transcription errors might have for a patient's care. Speed is also required for prompt placement of information in hospital reports or in patients' charts. Production standards are often set by employers for performance evaluation, and some employers base pay on production if the transcriptionist is not paid an hourly wage or straight salary.

PROFESSIONAL AFFILIATION

One of the important things you can do to enhance your career, either while a student or after completing training, is to join a professional association of MT peers. Since its inception in 1978, the **Association for Healthcare Documentation Integrity** (AHDI) is the organization that represents the interests of MTs and other healthcare documentation providers. AHDI sets standards of practice and offers medical transcription program approval, which encourages compliance with *AHDI's Model Curriculum* for Medical Transcription. In addition to establishing a code of ethics for MTs, the association administers credentialing programs and advocates on behalf of the profession with governmental and regulatory agencies.

Belonging to the national organization, as well as to regional and local chapters, will help you meet other MTs and make new friends while keeping up to date on the latest trends in the industry. AHDI, as well as its state and local components, provides magazines and newsletters for members that focus on continuing medical education as well as industry news, events, and articles of interest to MTs. AHDI emphasizes continuing education for its members and holds an annual conference for MTs, educators, supervisors and managers, and business owners. The association's local and state component associations also hold regular educational meetings and symposia. MTs receive quality medical education from local speakers at area and state meetings and have opportunities to learn about the newest trends in medicine and technology from guest speakers.

Mentoring programs are in place to help guide new transcriptionists in their career aspirations. Meetings and seminars provide opportunities for MTs to socialize and network with each other, making connections that help further individual careers. At many of these meetings, vendors exhibit products and services of interest to MTs or provide an opportunity for MTs to speak with company representatives about potential employment.

In the past, an MT's credential was simply a personal bonus or a "trophy" awarded for hard work and a willingness to pursue continuing education as the industry grew. However, the ongoing evolution of new technology in healthcare documentation as well as the global outsourcing of work has made education and credentialing a critical factor in achieving professional excellence. AHDI endorses credentialing to protect the public interest by promoting high professional and ethical standards and to recognize those MTs who demonstrate competency in medical transcription through the fulfillment of stated requirements. AHDI offers two credentials: **Registered Medical Transcriptionist** (RMT) and **Certified Medical Transcriptionist** (CMT), as well as one designation: **Fellow of the Association for Healthcare Documentation Integrity** (AHDI-F).

Registered Medical Transcriptionist

The RMT examination, first offered in 2006, is designed to assess competency in core knowledge and skills needed to practice medical transcription. Unlike the CMT exam, described later in this chapter, this exam will allow recent graduates of a transcription program to measure their level of competency in the field. The test is designed to cover basic core knowledge of anatomy and physiology, medical terminology, proper use of English language and grammar, disease processes, and medicolegal issues pertaining to the healthcare record. This exam was developed for new medical transcription program graduates and for MTs who do not have the years or variety of experience to be eligible for the CMT exam.

The first section of the exam is a set of multiple-choice questions covering topics such as medical language (prefixes, suffixes, root woods, terminology, and spelling), anatomy and physiology, disease processes, English language and usage, and confidentiality issues. The second half of the exam covers transcription performance. The audio portions to be transcribed are very short, usually no longer than a sentence. Other questions in this section refer to the audio and require editing or proofreading against it. If an MT fails the test, he or she is eligible to retake it after six months. Earning this credential illustrates that a person is a trained MT and has the base of knowledge required to perform well in a new job.

Certified Medical Transcriptionist

The CMT exam tests an MT in areas covering both medical transcription knowledge and transcription performance.

QUICK CHECK 1.3 ✓

Fill in the blanks of the following sentences.

1. The year AHDI first began was _____.

2. To become a Fellow, a medical transcriptionist must be an AHDI member in _____.

3. CMT is an abbreviation for _____.

4. The only organization that represents the interests of medical transcriptionists is the _____.

5. A CMT must recertify every _____ years.

At least two years of transcription experience in the acute care (or equivalent) setting is strongly recommended to take the CMT examination in order to allow for sufficient time to acquire a wide range of knowledge pertaining to specialty fields. For exam purposes, "acute care" is defined as incorporating medical center dictation to include many dictators, including a variety of English-as-a-second-language (ESL) dictators, many formats and report types. It encompasses all the major specialties as well as surgery dictation of all types, and some minor specialties.

Like the RMT exam, the CMT exam consists of both medical transcription-related knowledge items and transcription performance items. The transcription performance items include transcribing dictation, editing, and proofreading. If one does not pass the exam, a report will be given, indicating the objective areas where improvement is needed. Once a medical transcriptionist has achieved the CMT credential, he or she is required to maintain certification. In order to maintain certification, a certified medical transcriptionist must earn a minimum of 30 continuing education credits in each three-year cycle and pay a recredentialing fee. AHDI's recredentialing policies can be found at www.ahdionline.org.

AHDI's purpose in offering the CMT credential is to promote high professional and ethical standards, to improve the practice of medical transcription, and to recognize those professionals who demonstrate their competency in medical transcription through the fulfillment of stated requirements. Although credentialing is not mandatory to obtain employment, it conveys an elevated level of value to prospective employers. Because the exam is challenging and extensively tests the skills of an MT, the CMT credential tells an employer that the individual is knowledgeable about the profession and motivated to increase his or her knowledge of medicine and improve transcription skills.

AHDI Fellowship

AHDI also provides the opportunity for experienced MTs to earn the AHDI-F (Fellow of the Association for Healthcare Documentation Integrity) designation, which recognizes an MT's involvement in both work-related and community activities. This designation requires an MT to broaden his or her experience and to get involved in mentoring, community activities, and association events.

To become a Fellow, an MT must be member in good standing with AHDI and must earn a specific number of "points" for activities performed in different service categories in the five years preceding the application. These categories include membership in AHDI, attendance at professional meetings, obtaining CMT certification, writing articles for AHDI or other publications, and making presentations, acting as a mentor, demonstrating leadership skills, and being involved in civic activities.

CHAPTER SUMMARY

Medical transcription, like medicine itself, is both a science and an art. It is one of the most sophisticated of the allied health professions, creating an important partnership between healthcare providers and those who document patient care. There is no question that the work of a qualified MT has a significant impact on the quality of the documentation of care provided by a healthcare facility. Medical records are the foundation of health care and serve as a main medical reference for all healthcare decisions made by a patient and his or her physicians. MTs take great pride in producing these documents with timeliness, accuracy, and, of course, confidentiality.

·I·N·S·I·G·H·T·

Lessons from Katrina

Major weather events such as Hurricane Katrina, which struck New Orleans in 2005, were the wake-up call for anyone who questioned the need for electronic health records (EHRs). Floods from Katrina destroyed the medical records of hundreds of patients along the Central Gulf Coast of the United States because they were written on paper and stored in boxes in hospitals and physicians' offices. In addition, there were no records available to help identify the bodies of the victims. The government has now enacted legislation requiring EHRs to be a part of our national healthcare system.

ABBREVIATIONS

Abbreviation	Meaning	Abbreviation	Meaning
AHDI	Association for Healthcare Documentation Integrity	EMR	electronic medical record
		FDA	Food and Drug Administration
AHDI-F	Fellow of the Association for Healthcare Documentation Integrity	FTC	Federal Trade Commission
		HIPAA	Health Insurance Portability and Accountability Act of 1996
ARRA	American Recovery and Reinvestment Act of 2009		
CMT	Certified Medical Transcriptionist	HITECH	Health Information Technology for Economic and Clinical Health (Act)
DHHS	Department of Health and Human Services	RMT	Registered Medical Transcriptionist
EHR	electronic health record		

Add Your Own Abbreviations Here:

_____

_____

_____

_____

_____

TERMINOLOGY

Term	Meaning
Association for Healthcare Documentation Integrity (AHDI, formerly American Association for Medical Transcription, AAMT)	The organization that represents the interests of medical transcriptionists and other healthcare documentation providers.
business associate	Persons who, on behalf of a covered entity (but other than as members of the covered entity's workforce), perform or assist in performing a function or activity that involves the use or disclosure of individually identifiable health information, such as transcription services, billing services, attorneys, accountants, technology vendors, and many other types of businesses that are directly regulated by the HITECH Act and by HIPAA.
Certified Medical Transcriptionist (CMT)	A designation awarded by AHDI to those with greater than two years of experience in the field, who earn a passing score on a credentialing examination.
dictation	Speech that is put into written form.
electronic health record (EHR)	A secure, real-time electronic record of a patient's medical and health information generated by one or more encounters in any care-delivery setting, such as a hospital, doctor's office, or clinic.
electronic medical record (EMR)	An individual application repository of a patient's medical encounters with one provider consisting of the provider's documentation of encounters with that patient.
ethics	The norms for conduct that distinguish between acceptable and unacceptable behavior.
Fellow of the Association for Healthcare Documentation Integrity (AHDI-F)	A designation awarded by AHDI that signifies a balance of successful activities in the medical transcription profession in a variety of core areas involving practice duties, professional experience, leadership, and community involvement.
Health Insurance Portability and Accountability Act of 1996 (HIPAA)	A federal law that ensures the continuity of health insurance coverage if a person changes jobs, but also provides a national standard for the privacy of health information transactions and the confidentiality and security of patient data.
Health Information Technology for Economic and Clinical Health (HITECH) Act	An Act of Congress that has spurred the adoption of EHR systems across the country, which in turn, improve coordination of patient care by increasing patient safety and reducing errors.
Hippocratic Oath	A writing that outlines certain guidelines of ethical conduct to be taken by physicians.
medical provider	A term referring to a physician or other healthcare professional.
medical record	A series of documents that track a patient's medical history.
medical transcriptionist	A person who transcribes medical reports.
Privacy Rule	A provision of the Health Insurance Portability and Accountability Act of 1996 (HIPAA) that mandates nationwide standards to protect private health information.
provider	A shortened term for *medical provider*.
Registered Medical Transcriptionist (RMT)	A designation awarded by the AHDI to those with less than two years of experience in the field who earn a passing score on a credentialing examination.
scribe	A person employed to copy and interpret the spoken word of others.

Term	Meaning
stenographer	A person skilled in the transcription of speech.
transcribed	Information that is taken down in writing which has been dictated or recorded.

Add Your Own Terms and Definitions Here:

_____

_____

_____

_____

_____

_____

_____

_____

REVIEW QUESTIONS

1. How do the provisions of HIPAA affect medical transcriptionists?
2. What is the Hippocratic Oath?
3. What issues caused Congress to pass the HIPAA in 1996?
4. Why is it important for a medical transcriptionist to have strong listening skills?
5. What are the advantages of implementing an EHR system? Can you think of any disadvantages to such a system?
6. What are three skills needed to be a successful medical transcriptionist?
7. What is the recommended amount of time for a medical transcriptionist to work in the field before taking the CMT exam? The RMT exam?
8. How is the AHDI-F designation different from the CMT credential?
9. How will voice recognition technology affect the medical transcriptionist in the future?
10. Compare the advantages of working in a hospital or clinic-based setting to the advantages of working at home.

CHAPTER ACTIVITIES

Fill In The Blanks

Fill in the blanks with the correct answers.

1. _____ is an Act passed by Congress that provides a national standard for the privacy of health information transactions and confidentiality and security of patient data.

2. A _____ is a person who listens to the dictated recordings made by physicians and other healthcare professionals and transcribes them into patient reports.

3. Physicians and other healthcare professionals are commonly called _____.

4. The _____ is a secure, real-time electronic record of a patient's medical and health information generated by one or more encounters in any care-delivery setting,

5. The _____ provision of HIPAA requires healthcare plans and providers to establish procedural, administrative, and record-keeping policies that protect against misuse of an individual's health information.

6. The collective word for speech that is converted to written text by a medical transcriptionist is known as _____ .

7. A medical transcriptionist with acute care experience can take the _____ exam.

8. In ancient times, a person who could read and write was referred to as a _____.

9. _____ is the professional association that represents the interests of medical transcriptionists.

10. "Involvement in civic activities" is one of the categories of the _____ designation.

Multiple Choice

Circle the letter corresponding to the best answer for the questions below.

1. A breach of patient confidentiality can take place
    A. when an MT listens to the dictation through a headset.
    B. when the MT's computer is turned off.
    C. when a physician dictates a patient's report into the MT's answering machine.
    D. when the door to the MT's office is locked.

2. HIPAA stands for
    A. Health Insurance Portability and Accountability Act.
    B. Health Information Portability and Accident Act.
    C. Health Insurance Portability and Affordability Act.
    D. Health Installment Payment and Affordability Act.

3. An MT's home-based computer is not secure if
    A. the computer is used by the entire family.
    B. the computer is password protected.
    C. the computer is kept in a locked cabinet.
    D. none of the above.

4. What is NOT an advantage of an EHR system?
    A. the ability to provide tailored alerts and notices to providers
    B. convenient access to the patient's records at any time
    C. continuity of care
    D. the ability to share a patient's medical information with anyone over the Internet

5. A medical transcriptionist
    A. is a kind of medical provider.
    B. converts dictated medical information into readable text.
    C. is permitted to show her family a patient's medical reports if working at home.
    D. does not need to know how to punctuate a sentence; the computer does that automatically.

6. A medical transcriptionist should strive to maintain a typing speed of
    A. 50 wpm or less.
    B. 60 wpm or greater.
    C. exactly 45 wpm.
    D. up to 60 wpm.

7. What qualification must a medical transcriptionist possess?
    A. excellent listening skills
    B. the ability to talk fast
    C. a two-year college degree
    D. the ability to dictate according to company requirements

8. When did medical transcription originate as a profession?
    A. in the Egyptian era
    B. during the Middle Ages
    C. in the 1900s
    D. in the year 2000

9. One advantage of working in a hospital or clinic is
    A. the ability to work around the kids' ball games.
    B. more flexibility in work schedules.
    C. the savings in gas and wear-and-tear on the car.
    D. more social contact with co-workers.

10. The original Hippocratic Oath was translated from
    A. English.
    B. Latin.
    C. German.
    D. Greek.

2

TECHNOLOGY, TOOLS, AND TECHNIQUES

OBJECTIVES

After completing this chapter, you will be able to:

- Identify the basic components of a computer and explain how the computer processes and stores information.
- Describe different computer systems and the software applications used with each.
- Describe different methods of dictating, transcribing, and submitting work via the Internet.
- Identify reference tools most often accessed by medical transcriptionists and explain how each is used in the preparation of reports.
- Compare special word-processing features used by medical transcriptionists to aid in producing work more efficiently.

INTRODUCTION

Can you imagine a world without computers? Computers have changed everyday life in infinite ways that we would have never imagined 50 years ago. Not long ago, computers were primarily used to compute statistics and communication parameters for the military or those in higher education. The introduction of the first desktop computer by IBM in the 1980s changed the world's information-processing capabilities forever. Predictably, the computer has become one of the most valuable assets in both home and business communications. Software programs, also called **applications**, are sets of instructions that enable the computer to perform a variety of tasks, such as word processing, accounting, or creating spreadsheets and graphic designs.

The growth of information technology has had significant ramifications for the role of the medical transcriptionist, as the computer and printer quickly replaced the typewriter and carbon paper. A medical transcriptionist's work now revolves around the computer and the speed in which it can create, store, and transmit medical documents.

A medical transcriptionist produces a tremendous number of medical reports and other documents on a daily basis; therefore, powerful computers are essential tools of the trade. It is vital for medical transcriptionists to have a thorough understanding of the basic physical makeup of a personal computer and to understand some of the basic concepts of information technology to use this powerful tool effectively. Familiarity with the process of data storage and memory, the context for computer-based software applications in medical transcription, and the use of information networks in facilitating the production, storage, and retrieval of medical documents will help you attain maximum efficiency in producing a larger number of documents in a shorter period of time.

UNDERSTANDING INFORMATION TECHNOLOGY

Information technology (IT) is the general term that refers to the processing, storage, and/or transfer of information via the computer. A computer is really not one machine or device, but actually a system of many parts working together to store and process information. Computers work by analyzing and processing data according to a set of instructions (a program). **Data** is a collective term that encompasses facts and information. Data are entered, stored, and manipulated by the computer to provide information to the user.

Hardware

Computer hardware (or simply **hardware**) is the term used to describe the equipment that makes up the computer system. These are the physical parts of the system that you can see and touch and that allow information to be entered and retrieved from the computer. Many parts of the computer are housed in a case, sometimes referred to as the **tower**. The case usually stands on a desk or the floor and contains the circuitry needed for the computer to operate. Inside the computer, the **motherboard** is a large circuit board with connections for other components of the computer. The motherboard allows these components to exchange data. The **central processing unit** (CPU) is a small but very advanced microprocessor chip that sits on the motherboard. It processes data that is entered into the computer.

Almost every part of the computer provides data or receives data from the CPU and is connected to the computer case using cables. These cables plug into specific openings, called **ports**, typically located on the back of the case. The standard connector that plugs into these ports is called a **universal serial bus** (USB) connection. USB connectors allow you to attach every type of device quickly and easily, including headsets and foot pedals used by medical transcriptionists. The development of USB ports eliminated more cumbersome ways of connecting devices to the computer (such as special circuit boards or cards that had to be installed in the computer case itself). The USB provides a single, standardized, easy-to-use way to connect over 100 devices to a single computer.

The **mouse** is a small device used to point to and select items on your computer screen. It is connected to the computer by a long wire with a USB connection, but many newer models are wireless. A mouse typically has two buttons: a primary button (usually the left-sided button, which you "click" to select items) and a secondary button (usually on the right side of the mouse, which you "right-click" to select items). Many mice also have a wheel between the two buttons, which allows you to scroll smoothly through computer screens of information when you roll your finger across it. When you want to select an item, you point to the item and then "click" (press and release) the primary button. Pointing and clicking with your mouse is the main way to interact with your computer. You can also click on the item two times in succession, called "double-clicking," to activate the item, as when you open (or "execute") a program.

The **keyboard** is a device used mainly for typing text into your computer. Like the keyboard on a typewriter, it has keys for letters and numbers, but it also has extra keys that have special uses:

- **Function keys**, found on the top row and numbered F1 through F12, perform different functions depending on how they are used (or programmed) in different software programs.
- The **numeric keypad**, located on the right of the keyboard, which allows you to enter numbers quickly.
- The **navigation keys**, such as the arrow keys, the "home" key and "end" key, reposition your cursor quickly within a document.

The **monitor** is the device that displays viewable images generated by the computer. There are two basic types of monitors: **cathode-ray tube** (CRT) monitors and **liquid crystal display** (LCD) monitors. Both monitors produce sharp images, but the CRT monitor is large and cumbersome, whereas the LCD monitor has the advantage of being much thinner and lighter and is sometimes called a *flat screen* display monitor.

Software

Computer software (or simply **software**) refers to one or more computer programs that provide instructions to the computer to perform a particular task. Software is often divided into two categories. **Systems software** is the software that runs the computer itself. Also known as the *operating system*, this program coordinates all the data received by the computer and instructs the computer on how to process that data. It directs the flow of traffic inside the computer, telling it what to do and when to do it. In short, the operating system is the software that the rest of the software programs depend on to make the computer functional. A computer cannot function without an operating system. The operating system is activated as soon as the computer is turned on. Each time the computer is started, the operating system is also started. Although there are a number of operating systems in use, such as the Apple operating system for MacIntosh computers, Microsoft Windows is the operating system on most computers today.

Windows gets its name from the "windows," or informational boxes, it places on the computer's monitor. Each window shows information, such as an icon, a program, or a file you might be working on. You can have several windows open, or displayed, on the computer monitor at the same time, and jump from window to window; this enables you to complete tasks faster. In addition, you can size the windows to fit your needs, from very small to full-screen. Windows controls every window and each part of the computer. When you turn on your computer, Windows also starts and supervises any running programs or tasks.

Windows, or any operating system, has three basic functions:

- It coordinates the activities of the components attached to the computer, such as the keyboard, printer, monitor, and other hardware components.
- It manages all of the information entered into the computer, storing the data and commands to ensure that it will be able to find whatever information it needs to perform optimally.
- It executes the instructions given to perform specific tasks.

Applications software, also called computer programs, consists of instructions that enable the computer to perform a specific work task such as word processing, accounting, or use of spreadsheets and databases. These instructions are written by computer programmers in a language the computer can understand, placed on a storage medium, and then sold to users to install into their computers.

How a Computer Processes Information

Processing is the "thinking" that the computer does—the calculations, comparisons, and decisions it makes based on the information entered by the user. The CPU is where this "thinking" takes place. The CPU receives instructions from the computer's software via an input device such as a keyboard, mouse, or scanner and can process many millions of instructions per second. After processing the information, the results are displayed on a monitor, or display screen. The monitor displays the current process or application of the CPU.

Storing and Transferring Data

After data is entered into a computer and processed, it must be saved to preserve its contents after the computer is shut off. **Storage** is the term used to describe the device that stores and transfers data. The computer has one or more **disk drives**, which are devices that store information on a metal or plastic disk. The disk preserves the information that can be retrieved later, even when the computer is turned off. A **hard disk drive** is a storage device that is fixed inside the computer and stores large volumes of data, which can be accessed and retrieved quickly. The drive consists of a stack of small but rigid magnetic platters (disks) in a protective casing. Data is recorded magnetically onto circular tracks on these disks and stored for later retrieval. Because the hard disk can hold massive amounts of information, it is usually the computer's primary means of storage, holding almost all of the computer's programs and files.

Files can also be saved to a **Compact Disk-Read Only Memory** (CD-ROM) drive. This disk drive reads and/or saves data to and from a **compact disk** (CD), which is a metallic disk coated with a special dye that allows data to be recorded onto it by a laser. A **Compact Disk-Recordable** (CD-R) disk allows data to be recorded, or written, onto it for backup and duplication purposes. Once the CD-R disk is placed within the computer, the laser records, or "burns," the data onto the CD. Because of this method of creating a CD, CD-R drives are capable of recording to each CD only once. Unfortunately, this means that new data cannot be added to the CD once the initial set of information is saved onto it; however, data can be read and copied from the disk if needed. A **Compact Disk-Rewritable** (CD-RW) disk, on the other hand, has the capability of both reading data and saving it to the same disk multiple times. Data can be deleted and overwritten so that the same CD can be reused to store data. CDs are advantageous in that they can be used as a removable storage medium for transporting files or transferring files from one computer to another. Although the disk drive for this medium is called a CD-ROM drive, the drives in computers today are used to both read data and record data to CDs placed in them.

A **flash drive** is a small, stick-shaped memory drive about the size of a highlighter pen, which can hold the same amount of data as dozens or more CDs. As illustrated in Figure 2.1, a flash drive, also called a *jump drive* or a *memory stick*, is very lightweight, very portable (some models are the size of your thumb and also called "thumb drives") and compatible with any computer using a Windows operating system. A flash drive has a faster transfer rate than other drives because, unlike zip drives or hard drives, it has no moving parts; it uses solid-state circuitry that can be electrically erased and reprogrammed. In addition, it does not require a separate power source or batteries. The drive is plugged into a USB port on the computer's case and Windows will automatically recognize it as an additional drive. Files can then be immediately copied onto this tiny

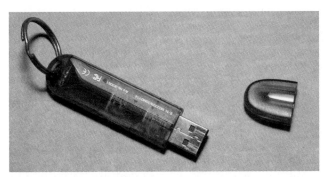

FIGURE 2.1. **Flash Drive.** Flash drives are so small that many people use them as key chains. Reprinted from Derek Lilly, Somerset, UK, Morgue-file.com.

drive. When the transfer is completed, the drive is simply unplugged from the computer and can be carried in a pocket or on a key chain to another location.

A flash drive is useful for quickly backing up files (i.e., accounts, spreadsheets, word documents, music, and slideshows) and safely storing data away from a desktop or laptop computer. Large files can be transported to another office or computer without worrying about compatibility. And unlike a CD-R disk, the data stored on a flash drive can be edited and stored an unlimited number of times. A flash drive also includes tools to recover data, and provides system updates and diagnostic utilities. Because a flash drive has no moving parts, it is more durable than other forms of removable media (such as CD-Rs) in environments that produce a lot of dust or humidity.

COMPUTER SYSTEMS

A computer can be connected to other computers via a network or set up as a stand-alone system.

Local Area Networks

Computers in and of themselves provide tremendous benefits in terms of efficiency, but computer capability and document accessibility increase greatly when individual computers are connected to one another using a **local area network** (LAN), or *network*. A network is a large computer capable of serving a vast number of users at the same time. Users do not sit down in front of the mainframe itself; rather, they connect to it using smaller individual computers called **workstations**. A network can connect computers in one building or in separate buildings miles apart. Networks can even be found in homes, connecting the computers of different family members. Many networks today are wireless and can connect computers all over the world to transmit and receive data.

The mainframe computer that contains the hardware and technology that connects the individual com-

puters to the system is the **file server**. The file server stores centrally shared data and programs that are used by all the individuals whose computers are attached to it. In a medical transcription setting, your computer may be connected to the file server of the medical transcription company for which you work, enabling you to send and receive reports from your employer.

Most business computers are connected to a network-based system. This enables documents, as well as hardware and software components, to be shared. For example, a document prepared by one medical transcriptionist at a hospital in California can be accessed and edited by another medical transcriptionist at a workstation in New York. Several users on the network can share the same printer or hard drive, and all can communicate with each other via electronic mail, or e-mail. Wireless LAN systems, such as those that drive the Internet, have even enabled hospitals and other healthcare providers to outsource some of their transcription needs overseas.

Smaller facilities and clinics can also use a network system to keep track of patient information. In a smaller office, a network can be used to make patient charting easier. As shown in Figure 2.2, the physician can then take an electronic tablet-type device into the exam room and enter patient information during the course of an examination. The information can then be uploaded to the patient's file on the computer, creating clear, accurate entries without the need for paper charting.

Stand-Alone Systems

In smaller physicians' offices and clinics, a **stand-alone system**, or a computer that is not connected to any other computer in the office, is the common choice. A stand-alone system includes the CPU, which contains all of the processing circuitry necessary to run the computer. Peripheral components—such as a keyboard, display screen, printer, mouse, or scanner—are attached to the CPU. The stand-alone system may be used by one employee or several, each using the system individually at different times. This type of system is usually more limited in its storage and processing facility than a network system but is often adequate to run a small clinic's document processing and payroll or calendar programs.

One advantage of a stand-alone system is the added security it can provide for private patient information. All information contained in the computer stays in one place and is not accessible from other computer workstations. In addition, a password can be applied to patient documents or to an entire software program. This controls access to the data contained in the computer, preventing other employees or even people who are not a part of the physician's medical staff, such as housekeeping personnel or outside delivery people, from accessing it.

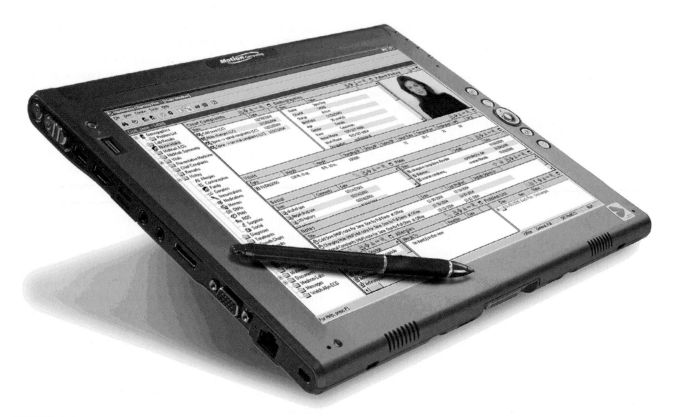

FIGURE 2.2. **Electronic Charting.** A computer network can enable a physician to take an electronic tablet-type device into the exam room and enter patient information during the course of the patient's visit. Reprinted with permission from MediNotes Corporation, West Des Moines, IA.

COMPUTER APPLICATIONS

The computer and its software components provide an efficient system of organizing files and documents for effective management of patients' records. Over the course of a patient's medical care, which can span from birth to death, the computer is essential in preparing documents and reports, recording dates in the office calendar, maintaining patient billing records, and keeping track of telephone numbers and other important information relevant to the patient's care. Various software programs, including word-processing programs used almost exclusively by medical transcriptionists, accomplish these tasks quickly and efficiently.

Windows

Microsoft Windows is integral to the operating system of virtually all computers. Although a software program itself, **Windows** is also the platform that makes it easier to execute commands to the computer. Windows can make learning and using software programs

QUICK CHECK 2.1 ✓

Indicate whether the following sentences are true (T) or false (F).

1. The CPU is the "brains" of the computer.   T   F

2. Microsoft Windows is a kind of systems software.   T   F

3. The motherboard is responsible for processing data.   T   F

4. Applications software is also known as "computer programs."   T   F

5. The operating system has to be started separately after the computer is turned on.   T   F

easier because it displays graphic images, called **icons**, and pull-down menus to execute commands. Windows enables the user to run several programs simultaneously to display multiple files and to execute commands from an on-screen list of menus or graphic icons by using a mouse. Windows also provides visual features so that documents can appear on the computer screen exactly as they will when printed, eliminating the guesswork needed to format more complex documents.

Windows publishes several versions of its software, each with a unique name such as Windows 2000, Windows Millennium, Windows NP and Windows XP, Vista, and most recently, Windows 7, each with unique features to enhance computer performance and web browsing for home or business use.

When you start your computer, Windows will load automatically. The view on your screen is called the **desktop**. You can think of this area on the screen as a regular desk with a work surface. The icons on the desktop are also called **shortcuts**. The shortcut "points" to a real file on the hard drive. The name comes from the fact that by creating a shortcut to a program or file directly on the desktop, you can save time and effort searching for the file on the computer. You can double-click the shortcut to open the program, and you can also click on the icon and, holding down the left-click button on the mouse, drag it to a new position on the desktop.

The **Start button** (and the **Start menu** that pops up after pressing it) serve as the central launching point for applications and tasks. The Start menu provides a customizable nested list of programs to launch as well as a list of most recently opened documents, a way to find files and get help, and access to the system settings. There is a bar that runs across the bottom of the screen called the **Task bar**. The Task bar displays software programs that are open and running simultaneously. Every time you start a new program, the computer puts a button on the Task bar to let you know that program is running. You can use the Task bar to switch back and forth between different open programs with a simple one click of the mouse. Finally, the small bar area at the far right of the Task bar is called the **System tray**. The System tray contains miniature icons for easy access to system functions such as fax, printer, modem, sound volume, etc. You can double-click or right-click on the icon to view the details and controls of each of the system functions in the System tray.

Word-Processing Applications

Many young people today probably do not remember the days when a typewriter was used to prepare documents. Word-processing software enables people not only to mass-produce documents, but also to edit work quickly and save it for future retrieval, if needed.

Word-processing programs are designed so that the appearance of documents may be easily enhanced with type styles and formatting features; formatting details that used to be difficult to manage efficiently on a typewriter, such as headers and footers, can be easily applied to any document using a word-processing program.

Microsoft (MS) Word quickly became the most popular word-processing software application because of its availability in all computer-system packages sold by retailers. Although other software manufactures have followed suit to "bundle" their programs into new computers, MS Word is by far the most commonly used program of this type. Like Windows, made by the same manufacturer, MS Word is the first software program to feature pull-down menus and text-enhancement icons that can be selected with a click of the mouse.

Microsoft published several versions of its popular word-processing software, Word, which is used almost exclusively by medical transcription companies today. Each version performs the same way, with menus, toolbars, task panes, and other menus and boxes.

In 2007, Microsoft released Word 2007. The striking difference with this version of Word compared to previous versions is its appearance, in that it displays no menus or toolbars. Replacing the menus and tool bars is a tabbed system called the Ribbon. The Ribbon contains a panel of commands that are organized into a set of tabs called the Tab Bar. Each task-oriented tab on the Tab Bar opens into a display of buttons representing groupings of tasks and their associated subtasks.

The Microsoft *Office* button replaces the traditional *File* pull-down menu of most Word programs. Clicking the *Office* button displays the *Office* button menu, a list of commands that deal with files and documents. In addition, Live Preview, a new feature of Word 2007, temporarily applies formatting on the selected text or object when you move your mouse over any of the formatting buttons. This temporary formatting is removed once the mouse pointer is moved away from the button, allowing you to preview how the text would appear without having to actually apply the formatting command. Mini toolbars appear whenever text is selected that contains the most commonly used formatting commands and other shortcuts in Word.

Medical Billing Applications

The computer is used extensively to keep track of patient billing. Medical billing software ensures that reimbursement claims are processed in a secure and efficient manner. It also tracks a patient's medical and insurance billing and accounting, showing at-a-glance information on the computer screen about a patient's charges, payments, and account adjustments.

Claims are transmitted electronically to insurance carriers using standard health insurance claim forms and billing codes already contained in the software program. Fewer errors are committed in the billing process and computerized billing simplifies and accelerates the claims process. In addition, most medical billing software programs are compliant with the sections of HIPAA that specify increased security standards and billing formats. Upon receiving the insurance claim, the carriers process the claim and can send payment directly to the medical provider or patient, as instructed.

THE INTERNET

The Internet is a global computer network system that consists of millions of LANs and computers connected to them. No one knows exactly how many computers are connected to the Internet, but it is certain that they number in the hundreds of millions, and this number is growing.

No one is "in charge" of the Internet. There are organizations that develop technical aspects of this network and set standards for creating applications on it, but no governing body is in control. The Internet backbone, through which Internet traffic flows, is owned by private companies.

Three vital functions of the Internet are the following:

- The **World Wide Web** (WWW). Also referred to simply as the *Web*, this refers to all the web pages and web sites on the Internet that contain some form of information. The Web was created to make it easier to find information on the Internet by linking information pages together. A web site's address on the Internet is called its **Uniform Resource Locator** (URL).
- **E-mail**. This refers to the way in which messages can be sent over the Internet.
- **File Transfer Protocol** (FTP). This is the method by which files are transferred from one computer to another over the Internet.

Sometimes the terms *Internet* and *World Wide Web* are used interchangeably. However, to be strictly correct, the Internet refers to all the computers that make up the network called the Internet, and the World Wide Web refers to the pages of information that are stored on those computers.

Computers on the Internet use a **client/server architecture**. This means that the remote file server computer system provides files and services to the client user's local computer. Software can be installed on a client's computer to access and take advantage of the newest technology. In medical transcription, for example, one hospital server system can serve several of its branch hospitals located around the country. Medical transcription companies can be connected to the system

in order to provide access for all of their employee transcriptionists to prepare and return reports pertaining to that hospital system.

An Internet user has access to a wide variety of services: e-mail, file transfer, vast information resources, interest-group membership, interactive collaboration, multimedia displays, real-time broadcasting, breaking news, shopping opportunities, and much more. In the medical field, the Internet enables doctors and other providers to conduct medical research without leaving the office—or, indeed, even the desk—by providing access to countless clinical trials, reports of studies in peer-reviewed medical journals, and new trends in medicine. On-line research services index a wider scope of up-to-date material and current clinical trials than that which could be found in any medical library, enabling a physician to have access to the very latest findings, protocols, and information even before they can be published and distributed in hard-copy form. Many Internet sites are devoted exclusively to specialized areas of medicine. For example, some medical research web sites help healthcare professionals and patients by providing the results of early cancer treatment trials in order to evaluate the risks and benefits of the newest therapies available.

With the advent of remote access and wireless technology, doctors have been able to use the Internet to view diagnostic images and charts or communicate with hospital staff from home or other off-site locations. However, the increased convenience was offset by the problem of protecting confidential patient information while permitting off-site healthcare providers to access the information.

The need for a solution that maintains the confidentiality and security of that information while complying with the strict privacy requirements of HIPAA led to the digital encryption of information when transmitted via the Internet. **Encryption** is a process whereby transmitted information is converted into a special coded computer language designed to protect the electronic transfer of data over the Internet. Companies that specialize in this technology create secure, encrypted connections, known as **tunnels**, between two locations, bypassing the open and often insecure public networks found on the Internet. This technology can also be used to control access within a single location to prevent unauthorized access to sensitive information on a large network. Data encryption enables healthcare providers and medical transcriptionists to use the Internet to view sensitive patient information and to receive and transmit patient reports securely.

As an MT, you may hear a term describing a company's computer system setup as VPN. A **virtual private network** (VPN) is a computer network that uses a public telecommunication infrastructure, such as the Internet, to provide remote offices or individual users with secure access to their organization's network. The goal of a VPN is to enable distant colleagues to access the company's secure network by using the Internet to carry the traffic, at much lower cost than a company having to expend the cost of creating leased lines and connections for each user on its network.

A VPN works by providing information security features such as authentication and confidentiality and are often used to secure traffic traveling over the Internet. This type of network enables users (such as the company's employees) to network together securely using the Internet to send and receive information by encrypting data at the sending end and decrypting it at the receiving end through special VPN tunnels. An additional level of security involves encrypting not only the data, but also the originating and receiving network addresses.

TRANSCRIPTION METHODS

Dictation has long been the standard means by which physicians document their encounters with patients. Medical transcriptionists use a variety of methods and technologies to transcribe this dictation.

Transcribing Machines

A **transcriber** is a machine that makes it possible to listen to dictated tape recordings in order to transcribe them into written documents. Although technology has progressed to allow a medical transcriptionist to transcribe dictation directly from the Internet, and some physicians prefer the information to be recorded digitally, or using no tapes, many physicians still dictate their reports onto cassette tapes. A medical transcriptionist listens to these tapes on a transcribing machine.

Transcribers have many convenient features to help make transcription fast and easy. The "Rewind" and "Fast Forward" functions move the tape recording backward and forward, respectively, pausing at each cue tone that starts a new dictated item. At the beginning of the tape, total dictation length is displayed. Alert tones play when the dictation ends, the tape recorder is broken, no tape is loaded, or some other error is detected.

Earphones, also called *headsets*, plug into a transcriber, allowing dictation to be heard. Medical transcriptionists use earphones both to hear dictation more easily and to maintain patient confidentiality. Earphones are available in a wide variety of styles and connect directly to the computer via a USB port. The earpieces themselves vary from those that fit snugly over the ear to those that look like small microphones and rest inside the external ear canal. When using earphones to transcribe, be sure to keep them clean and sterilized between uses, as they tend to collect debris and wax.

The **foot pedal** is a device that allows the transcriptionist to keep both hands on the keyboard to type while controlling the flow of dictation played back. Like USB earphones, USB foot pedals connect directly to the computer case with the use of a USB connection. Pressing the center of the foot pedal starts the playback of dictation; removing pressure from the center of the foot pedal stops the playback. Pressing the right side of the foot pedal rewinds the dictation; pressing the left side of the foot pedal fast forwards the dictation. Most transcriber machines can be adjusted to rewind automatically every time the foot pedal is released so that a few words are repeated when the playback begins again. This feature can help to ensure that no words are omitted in the final document.

Digital Dictation Platforms

Digital dictation is the recording and storing of dictation in a digital format on a chip, disk, or computer's hard drive instead of a tape or similar media. A **transcription platform** is a software information-processing program that enables providers to dictate reports using a digital format and medical transcriptionists to retrieve, transcribe, and return those reports directly from a central computer networking system using the Internet, as illustrated in Figure 2.3. This process involves a physician dictating a report into a hand-held recorder or call-in system. When the recorded dictation is ready to be retrieved by a transcriptionist or editor, the audio file is streamed securely from the platform directly to the MT who is logged onto the server. The voice and associated text files are transmitted via secure Internet connection that also complies with HIPAA standards. The dictated work is queued to the transcriptionists presently working on the system based on priority, return times, and other parameters defined by the company. Patient information and other demographics from the provider's information

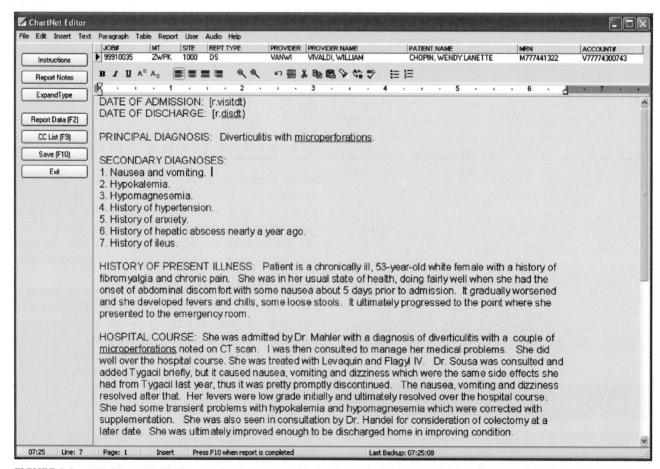

FIGURE 2.3. Digital Dictation Platforms. A digital dictation and transcription platform, such as ChartNet® (above), enables medical transcriptionists to retrieve, transcribe, and return medical reports directly from a central system using proprietary software. Reprinted with permission from Hudson Medical Systems, Inc., Hudson, Ohio.

system are inserted into report-specific document templates automatically, saving the MT time in locating and verifying the information. The report templates may also contain headings and some routine phraseology used by the physician whose dictation is being transcribed, eliminating the need to format each and every document before transcribing the report.

With the audio file automatically queued into the platform, the dictation is ready to be transcribed. A transcribing machine is not necessary for the transcription of digital dictation, saving time in fast-forwarding and rewinding tapes to find dictation starting points. The foot pedal is attached to the computer through a USB port, and the headset plugs into the computer's speakers. Because digital dictation is easier, faster, and less expensive than older, traditional tape transcriber systems, most companies use some type of digital dictation system.

Speech-Recognition Technology

Speech-recognition technology (SRT), also called *voice recognition* (VR), allows computers with a source of sound input, such as a microphone or hand-held dictation device, to interpret human speech, word for word, for transcription of medical documents.

SRT technology combines sophisticated software and powerful computing hardware to electronically convert speech to text. There are two methods of using SRT: The first, called **front-end speech** recognition, is a process whereby speech-recognized text is generated on-screen from dictation in real-time, allowing physicians to edit and correct the final document themselves. This method generally requires the physician or dictator to continually correct the mistakes the software makes. This is because, unlike grammar-constrained and natural-language recognition, voice recognition does not possess semantic understanding. The computer, through the use of SRT, only identifies individual words; it does not "understand" what is being said and cannot evaluate the logic of the flow of words it strings together. Many words, both "regular" English and medical terms, sound alike. If the dictation system does not understand the context for one of these words, it will not be able to identify the correct spelling. SRT also tends to pick up background voices, pausative sounds like "um" and "uh," and other unnecessary verbiage that must be edited out of the report, which makes this method of SRT too cumbersome and time-consuming for physicians to use efficiently.

The second method, called **back-end SRT**, is a method in which the audio file is retrieved at some point after the actual dictating has taken place (thus, on the *back end*). The medical transcriptionist accesses the draft report created by SRT along with the corresponding audio file through the Windows platform he or she is working on, and listens to the dictation. Following along with the dictation, the medical transcriptionist makes corrections to formatting, punctuation, or grammar, and might even correct errors in medical terminology. After making these corrections in the document, the medical transcriptionist returns the edited document to the facility. The document is then re-fed into the SRT program after corrections are made so that the system can "learn" how to address such items as abbreviations or slang terms often dictated by physicians. Back-end SRT is the method used most often by the medical transcription profession.

SRT has made vast inroads into the realm of healthcare documentation, thus affecting the way medical transcriptionists perform their work. However, this technology will not eliminate the need for qualified MTs in the foreseeable future. For example, much work still needs to be done to achieve a high rate of accuracy in converting what the SRT system hears to words on paper. Because dictators all pronounce words differently, the SRT sometimes does not convert speech to text accurately, as indicated in Table 2.1. Another concern being addressed with speech recognition is the confusion that may result as SRT systems evolve and "learn" as they progress in back-end SRT. Problems can result when an abbreviation is "remembered" by the SRT program and inserted incorrectly into a future document. For example, if a physician dictates the abbreviation, *DC*, and the medical transcriptionist edited the abbreviation in context of the report to the word "discontinue," the SRT program will learn that when it hears *DC*, it means the word "discontinue," even if the context of the sentence calls for another word or phrase, such as "discharge," "dilation and curettage," "discomfort," or "dressing change." Thus, the role of the transcriptionist as proofreader and editor of the documents generated by SRT remains vital.

SRT greatly improves productivity, enabling a medical transcriptionist to produce more reports in a shorter period of time. SRT-generated documents can be edited faster than they could have been transcribed, thus producing more lines in a given period of time for the MT and the company. SRT has become so popular that speech-recognition software is included with the Windows operating system software. As this technology may relieve some of the repetitive typing for the MT in the future, the role of the transcriptionist will become more knowledge-oriented and less task-oriented.

Even with its shortcomings, SRT is destined to become part of an increasingly complex dynamic that will make up the healthcare documentation process in the future. Therefore, strive to sharpen your skills by keeping up to date on advances in SRT, learn how it is being used in the industry, and understand how it is likely to affect the work you will be doing as an MT. While you do not have to become a computer specialist, keeping abreast of technological developments will increase the potential to play an even bigger and more productive role in medical documentation delivery in the future.

TABLE 2.1	Actual Automated Speech Errors
	"What Did You Say??"

Dictated	SRT
"She was given Dilaudid."	"She was given a lot of dirt."
"Famvir 500 mg daily."	"Some beer 500 mg daily."
"The patient has a prostate the size of an orange."	"The patient has a prostate the size of an RN."
"Geriatric Clinic"	"genital ache clinic"
"The patient was given 250 mg of Keflex."	"The patient was given 250 grand Catholics."
"I am going to hold her Decadron until the patient . . ."	"I am going to hold her Decadron and kill the patient . . ."
"The contents of the e-mail are self-explanatory."	"The contents of this e-mail are selfish lavatory."
"I would like to refer the patient to a board-certified sleep specialist."	"I would like to refer the patient to a board-certified sleaze specialist."
"He was introverted . . ."	"He was intervertebral . . ."
". . . their relationship . . ."	". . . will he she and she . . ."

TRANSCRIPTION REFERENCES AND TOOLS

For help in the identification and appropriate use of medical terms, a medical transcriptionist refers to standard medical reference materials, both in print and electronic forms. A comprehensive reference library is essential. Although the list of available resource materials from a variety of companies is immense, most transcriptionists agree on a basic set of "must haves" for a beginner to the field.

Style Book

The ability to structure and punctuate sentences correctly is vital to the production of quality medical reports. A **style book** is a manual that provides information on medical transcription styles, forms, and grammar and usage specific to medical terms. In addition, the style book also functions as a reference for the proper use of punctuation, hyphenation, capitalization, subject-verb agreement, and basic document formatting. *The Book of Style for Medical Transcription, 3rd ed.*, is known as the "gold standard" of style manuals among medical transcriptionists and is available for purchase at the AHDI web site. It has a comprehensive index prepared by a professional indexer. Practical hints about the topics discussed are placed in the margins and examples are provided for added clarity.

Medical Dictionary

A medical dictionary is an invaluable resource for understanding the language of contemporary medicine. It provides complex definitions of terms listed in alphabetical order and includes not just words but also abbreviations, eponyms, and acronyms. Many dictionaries include illustrations and charts, and electronic medical dictionaries that are loaded onto the computer with a CD-ROM also may contain audio clips of the word to provide correction pronunciation. There are many medical dictionaries available to transcriptionists. Most contain popular features including an extensive A-to-Z list of multiple-word entries to help readers find definitions quickly, color-coded synonyms, three-dimensional art images, and examples of common diagnostic imaging methods used today.

Spell-Checker Software

A medical spell checker is invaluable to a medical transcriptionist, and there are many products on the market from which to choose. A specialized medical spell-checker program integrates thousands of medical, pharmaceutical, and other life-science words into the standard spell checker of MS Word or other word-processing programs. The spell checker verifies correctly spelled words and provides suggested spellings for incorrectly spelled words. Some spell checkers also allow users to verify the spelling of a medical or pharmaceutical term by phonetic or typographical search while typing. Wild card keys of "?," indicating a one-letter wildcard character, or "*" for multiple characters, can be inserted into the spell checker to look up words that match the possible spelling of a word. Most spell checkers will also flag words that should be capitalized, such as days of the week or brand names as opposed to generic names of drugs.

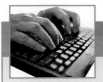

Text-Expanding Software

Text-expanding software programs can assist in the preparation of the large volume of dictation medical transcriptionists typically produce, while helping the transcriptionist avoid repetitive stress injury to wrists and/or hands from high-volume typing. These programs can reduce the number of actual keystrokes by up to 70%, enabling a medical transcriptionist to prepare more documents in a shorter period of time.

These programs go one step further than the Auto-Correct and AutoText features available in MS Word, but they work on the same principle. They automatically expand certain keystroke combinations into whatever word, phrase, sentence, or paragraph is assigned to that keystroke combination. However, unlike MS Word, in which the number of keystrokes allowed for AutoCorrect or AutoText is limited by the program's memory capabilities, there is virtually no limit to the numbers of entries that can be entered into the software. For example, the typed letters "cwc" might expand into the words "chest was clear." A typical sentence, "text expanded," could read as follows:

Original sentence: "SUBJECTIVE: This 67-year-old male with a history of cirrhosis, which is complicated by ascites and encephalopathy, presents for followup." Using text expander: "subj. Ths 67 yom w a ho cir, wi cb asc and ence, prss for fp."

Any number/letter combination can be used. For example, *2u* could expand to read, "2 units of packed red blood cells." A text-expanding program can even be used to produce entire paragraphs, such as a patient's entire physical examination if a physician repetitively dictates the same sentences and phrases. One entry in an expander dictionary can even yield a nearly-complete report. Many text-expanding programs have a built-in library of expansions whereby the program will display a window that allows the medical transcriptionist to select from a list of pertinent words or phrases.

These programs also enable you to create more than one set of abbreviations or dictionary of entries, so you can create one for each of your different accounts and/or medical specialities. This will enable you to use the same keystroke abbreviations in several dictionaries, but the keystrokes can have a different meaning in each. For example, the entry *ster* can mean "sternocleidomastoid" for an orthopedic clinic account you might be working on but can also be used to mean "stereotactic" for a neurosurgery account you may be assigned to as well.

Strive to create as many expander entries as possible to increase your document production as much as possible. As a rule of thumb, if you hear the same word or phrase three times or more in one day, create an expander entry for it, because you will probably hear it again. Take the time to stop transcribing and create the entry while you remember it. If there is no time at that moment, jot down the word or phrase to add later. It will take time at first to create a library of entries, but if you get into the habit of creating entries each and every time you hear a repetitive word or phrase (medical or otherwise), the time saved later will be invaluable.

Although you can never have too many expander entries, be very careful to proofread your work for expansion errors. A simple typographical error could activate a text expansion entry in the wrong place that the spell checker may overlook. For example, you may have a text expansion entry for the word "carcinoma" as "ca," but miss the entry being inadvertently expanded in the sentence, "The patient was from Modesto, CARCINOMA," when you meant "CA" for California. First names are often overlooked for text expansion errors. The entry "ben" for "benign" can wind up in the patient's name, Ben Smith, or "idarubicin" for the first name Ida.

Pharmaceutical Word Books

A pharmaceutical word book, commonly called a "drug book" by medical transcriptionists, provides a comprehensive cross-referenced list of individual brand name and generic drugs, along with the usual dosages for each. Many drug books also include over-the-counter remedies, natural and homeopathic medications, investigational drugs awaiting US Food and Drug Administration (FDA) approval, chemotherapy protocols, trademarked dosage forms (such as "Diskus" or "Dosepak"), discontinued drugs, and the drug categories and classes by which each drug is classified. Some drug books also contain additional information on proper uses of the drug, side effects, and other names by which the drug is known. Some word books contain an alphabetized list of medical problems or conditions, along with a list of the drugs used for treatment. This feature is especially useful when a transcriptionist needs to verify a drug name that was dictated for a particular illness or indication but which is not readily verifiable by spelling.

Book of Abbreviations

There are countless abbreviations used in medicine. A book of abbreviations lists both common and obscure medical abbreviations, acronyms, and symbols covering all medical specialties, along with their meanings.

QUICK CHECK 2.3 ✓

Indicate which transcription reference tool would be used to locate the following.

1. What ABG stands for:
   _____.

2. The spelling of an antidepressant medication:
   _____.

3. The meaning of the word "epiphysis":
   _____.

4. The word "tetralogy" in order to verify spelling or validity of context usage:
   _____.

5. Where to place a comma after an introductory phrase: _____.

An index for reverse search is often included to help the medical transcriptionist find the correct expansion for a medical abbreviation.

Medical Word Books

Medical word books are references that list alphabetically (but do not define) specific words—including diseases, syndromes, tests, abbreviations, and eponyms—commonly used in a variety of medical specialties and laboratory procedures. There are specialty word books for specific specialities such as gastroenterology, cardiology, surgery, orthopedics, neurology, and so on. There are also specialty word books on such topics as medical equipment and laboratory tests. A word book is used to look up a word dictated in order to verify spelling and verify validity in the context being stated, not to ascertain the word's meaning.

The advantage of using a medical word book over researching a word over the Internet is, first and foremost, the trustworthiness of the source. Words in these references have been researched and verified and can be looked up quickly. An Internet search engine may produce thousands of hits for the word, as well as a variety of sources, that will require time to investigate and verify. A medical transcriptionist should have a collection of word books published by a well-known medical publishing house and specific to as many medical specialties as he or she can afford.

Internet Resources

The Internet provides hundreds of web sites that can prove useful to a medical transcriptionist who is searching for information that is not readily available in reference books. Many medical transcriptionists have a "favorites" list in their Internet browser that has links to lists of physicians' names by state, names of hospitals, geographic locations that are not spelled by the dictator, particular brands of surgical equipment or healthcare products, or the correct spelling of recently approved drugs.

A caveat: Understand how to ascertain the legitimacy of your Internet source before using the information found on a particular web site. Many MTs use the Internet almost exclusively as a medical resource when researching information about which they are unsure. However, anyone can create a web site without having its contents verified as factual, and even a "reliable" medical site may contain information about a particular item or field of study that turns out to be false or in conflict with another. This is why many medical transcription service providers prohibit the use of the Internet as a transcriptionist's sole source of reference, even banning certain sites outright. Always verify your findings with a second reference (such as a medical word book or dictionary). For example, entering a search for the word "permacath," the way many dictators pronounce this term in dictation, will produce thousands of hits, even those considered to be reliable medical sites, with the spelling "permacath," when the correct spelling is PermCath.

SPECIAL WORD-PROCESSING FEATURES

MS Word offers some handy built-in tools to help make medical transcription easier.

Document Templates

The purpose of a template is to create readable, uniform documents. A **template** is a document with preset formatting and settings that acts as a basic structure for a document such as a fax, invoice, or business letter. It contains standard text that is common to all documents of a particular type as well as predefined document settings, such as margins and fonts. The template keeps these preferences "memorized," and each document of a particular type looks the same. It becomes a custom document after you fill in the blanks with your data and save the resulting document with a new name. You can edit the "new" document and make changes, but the template file remains intact.

Every word-processing program, including MS Word, contains document templates. Most programs feature a variety of built-in preset templates that can be used immediately or altered to meet the needs of the user. For example, blank MS Word documents are based on the *Normal* template, which uses the following preset options:

- font type and size (usually *Times New Roman* at *12 points*).
- language (usually *US English*).
- alignment (usually *flush left*).
- line spacing (usually *single*).
- **widow/orphan control**, a feature that prevents a paragraph from being broken in such a way that a single line appears at the top or bottom of a page (usually set to *on*).

New templates can also be created to function as a custom design for frequently used documents. Most healthcare providers use templates for reports so that they are all uniform in features such as appearance of headings, font size, and page settings.

Macros

A **macro** is a series of commands that is recorded in a single command so it can be played back, or executed, later. Macros are useful for automating complex or repetitive tasks or actions. Macros are recorded as a sequence of actions and then played back later, similar to a tape recorder.

Some typical uses for macros include:

- Speeding up editing and formatting of routine documents.
- Combining multiple commands; for example, performing a spell check on a document, then saving and printing the document, and then closing the document window.
- Automating complex tasks, such as opening a document template and positioning the cursor at each insertion point to add text automatically, and then saving the document.

Once a macro is created, you can activate it by using the *Macro* dialog box from the Word pull-down menu. You can also assign a keyboard shortcut to the macro and activate it by pressing the appropriate keyboard combination.

AutoCorrect

AutoCorrect is a feature of MS Word that automatically corrects common spelling mistakes as they are typed.

The AutoCorrect feature can save you time during editing. Some features of AutoCorrect include:

- Capitalizing the next word after a period and a space.
- Correcting two initial capital letters.
- Capitalizing names of days of the week.
- Correcting common typing errors, for example, "recieve" to "receive."
- Capitalizing first letters of words in table cells.
- Creating "smart quotes" (which turn toward the text) for regular quotation marks in text.

Because this feature was intended to correct errors as they occur, it is always active, meaning that whenever an "error" is typed, it will be corrected without the user having to think about it. However, Word does allow you to record exceptions or to turn off certain features of AutoCorrect, so you can take advantage of the feature without worrying about words or phrases particular to your work that may conflict with the rules of AutoCorrect. If you use a hospital name that has two initial capital letters, you would not want that text to be corrected.

AutoText

The AutoText feature is useful for saving keystrokes while typing in your document. An AutoText entry is composed of an abbreviation and an associated phrase. Similar to a text-expander program, AutoText stores and quickly inserts text, graphics, fields, tables, or other items used frequently in a document. This is useful for inserting standard or often-used text in a document so that you do not need to type it repeatedly. AutoText retains the formatting of the entry (such as font, size, or justification) used when you created the entry or matches the entry to the current document's formatting. Once an entry is created, it can be used throughout the current document and other documents associated with the same template. To make entering text easier, Word offers the AutoText toolbar. In addition to the entries you create, Word's AutoText entries include some standard entries to be used as they are or reformatted to your specifications.

Although AutoText performs like a text expander, it should not be used as a substitute for standard text-expanding software for medical transcriptionists. An

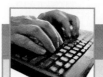

TRANSCRIPTION TIP:

If possible, add only lowercase words with AutoCorrect. When you add a word with an initial capital letter, such as *Apin* for *pain*, AutoCorrect replaces only words with an initial capital letter. When you use AutoCorrect on a word that is all lowercase, AutoCorrect will fix the word every time.

QUICK CHECK 2.4 ✓

Indicate which special word processing feature would be used for the following tasks.

1. Saving keystrokes while typing in a document: _____.

2. Using one command to spell check a report, print, and save: _____.

3. Correcting typographical errors as they happen: _____.

4. Using preset formatting and document settings to act as a basic structure for all fax cover sheets: _____.

5. Automatically capitalizing days of the week: _____.

---

excessively large AutoText list can affect the performance of the computer as well as the response time, causing the computer to "freeze up" or to delete the entire library of entries. Text-expanding software programs specially designed for document production like medical transcription allow for an unlimited amount of entries to be added to their databases without any threats of glitches.

Headers and Footers

A **header** is text printed at the top of each page of a document. A **footer** is text printed at the bottom of every page of a document. In MS Word, headers print in the top margin one-half inch from the top of every page, and footers print in the bottom margin one-half inch from the bottom of each page. Headers and footers can include text and graphics as well as the page number, total number of pages, current date, and current time.

In medical documents, headers can appear on every page of a medical report, or may be used from the second page onward, to indicate reference items pertaining to a patient's statistical information, such as the patient's name, medical record number, name of the report, date, page number, and physician's name. Footers may also be used to indicate page numbers in a multiple-page report.

FILE MANAGEMENT

Knowing how to organize, locate, and save the documents you create and use will make you more productive in class and on the job. In class, you will create a document on a blank screen, print the document, and save it using a new file name either on a CD or another location as indicated by your instructor.

Have you ever had papers spread out all over your desk? Eventually there would be so many items scattered in so many different places that your work space would become an unusable mess. Eventually you would need a file cabinet to keep all your papers neat and organized so you could retrieve them quickly later. In a basic sense, a computer's hard disk is like a filing cabinet. And, like a filing cabinet with folders and papers in those folders, the information on the hard disk is organized into folders and files. A **folder** is a "container" in which you store documents, like a manila folder in a filing cabinet. Folders are the basic organizational building blocks of any computer system. Like in a filing cabinet, folders keep things orderly and tidy and make retrieval of documents easy. Without folders, it would be virtually impossible to keep track of all the data contained on even the smallest system. Folders store computer data, called **files**. A file is a block of information stored in a folder. It can be a document, or it can be a spreadsheet, a picture, a song, or a video. Even the software components of the computer itself are called files, and those files are maintained in folders on the computer. All the folders, and those folders nested within them (called subfolders), form a hierarchy on the computer called the **directory tree**. The directory tree is a virtual container on the computer system in which groups of folders and files can be kept and organized, as shown in Figure 2.4.

To open a folder, double-click its icon. When you open the folder, the contents of the folder are displayed. When you double-click a file, that item opens along with the program that is capable of displaying it. For example, when you open a Word document, MS Word will open so you can view the document.

If your classroom does not use a document-management program and your instructor does not specify a particular method for saving your work, you will need to create a file management system to save your work in an organized fashion. Save and store your document files on a blank CD to make storage and retrieval of your work fast and easy.

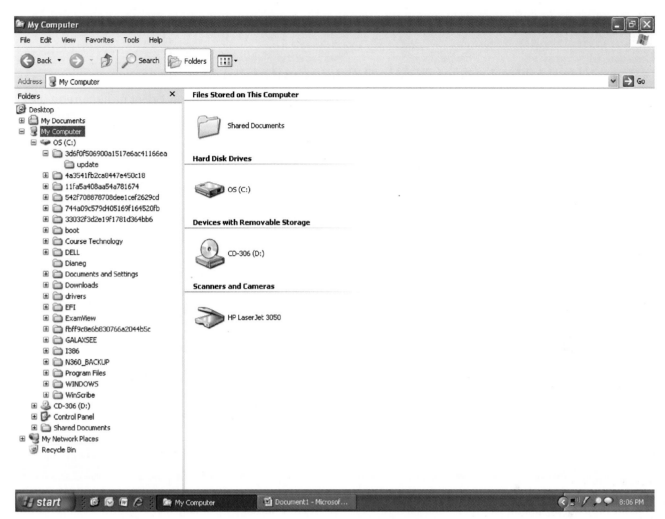

FIGURE 2.4. **Directory Tree.** A directory tree keeps folders and files organized on the computer.

Creating Folders and Organizing Files

One way to organize your files in this course is by chapter. When you begin a new chapter, you can create a central folder for all of the documents in that chapter by chapter number (for example, CHAPTER 10). Another way to organize files is to delineate them by document type and placing all work from the chapter into folders according to the type of document created (for example, LETTERS, CLINIC NOTES, DISCHARGE SUMMARIES, etc.).

Once you have devised a strategy for managing your files for this course, create folders and organize files within them as you progress thorough each chapter. To create a folder, do the following:

Access the CD drive of the computer, which is usually drive D: or E:. Select *File*, *New*, and then *Folder* from the drop-down menu on the top tool bar, or move your mouse pointer and click on the folder button positioned on the tool bar. (This command is the same for Word 2007.) A boxed icon and the highlighted words, *New Folder*, will appear on the screen. Key in the desired name of the folder (either a chap-

ter number or a document type) and press *Enter*. You now have a new folder where you can store your completed documents. For each completed document you want to save, locate the folder where you want to store the file. Then save the document in the selected folder.

CHAPTER SUMMARY

The standard of medical transcription demands that a document be correctly formatted and free of spelling and grammar errors. The transcribed dictation becomes a legal document, as well as a medical record on which diagnosis and treatment of a patient is based; there is simply no room for error. Medical transcription is typically a quantity-driven business, but unless a document is accurate in content and neatly prepared, speed is worthless. A medical transcriptionist who is viable today must adapt to the ever-changing tools and technology of the trade to always remain relevant and to work smarter as well as faster.

·I·N·S·I·G·H·T·

The Cost of Medical Documentation Mistakes

Tens of thousands of deaths are caused each year by mistakes in medical documentation. Latent medical transcription errors—the careless transcription of misinformation into a patient's medical record because of sloppy listening or typing skills—is a major threat to the safety of patients.

An error in transcription may appear to be minor, but even something as benign as an error in typing a patient's height and weight could result in an anesthesiologist administering too little—or too much—medication. Transcription errors that compromise patient safety also include confusing two drugs with similar names, mistyping zeros and decimal points, or misunderstanding abbreviations dictated by physicians. Although the Joint Commission discourages the use of abbreviations, many physicians still dictate them; and a medical transcriptionist must be careful to distinguish between, for example, such abbreviations as "q.h.s.," which means "at bedtime," and "q.h.," every hour.

Transcription errors also may result in a patient being denied insurance coverage. If an entry such as an adverse condition is inserted inadvertently into a patient's medical record because a medical transcriptionist was not listening closely enough to the dictation, an insurance company may have no choice but to refuse to cover treatment for an individual. Erroneous information in patient records could even compromise research projects where the protocol demands that all information on patients be comparable.

Although continuing advances in computerizing medical information are eliminating most errors caused by inaudible or sloppy dictation, it is the obligation of both healthcare information managers and medical transcriptionists to ensure that inaccuracies in medical records are kept to a minimum and do not become the underlying cause of errors that threaten the health of patients.

ABBREVIATIONS

Abbreviation	Meaning	Abbreviation	Meaning
CD	compact disk	LAN	local area network
CD-R	compact disk—recordable	LCD	liquid crystal display
CD-ROM	compact disk—read-only memory	SRT	speech-recognition technology
CD-RW	compact disk—rewritable	URL	Uniform Resource Locator
CPU	central processing unit	USB	universal serial bus
CRT	cathode-ray tube	VPN	virtual private network
FDA	Food and Drug Administration	VR	voice recognition
FTP	file transfer protocol	WWW	World Wide Web
IT	information technology		

Add Your Own Abbreviations Here:

_____

_____

_____

_____

_____

TERMINOLOGY

Term	Meaning
applications	Sets of instructions that enable the computer to perform a variety of tasks.
applications software	Also called "computer programs," sets of instructions that enable the computer to perform a specific work task.
back-end SRT	A process by which a physician dictates into a speech-recognition system and the recognized draft document is routed along with the dictated voice file to the transcriptionist, who verifies the accuracy of the draft and finalizes the report.
cathode-ray tube (CRT)	A computer monitor that displays images using an electron beam.
central processing unit (CPU)	A small but very advanced microprocessor chip that sits on the motherboard and processes data entered into the computer.
client/server architecture	A framework by which a remote file server computer system can provide files and services to the client user's local computer.
compact disk (CD)	A metallic disk coated with a special dye that allows data to be recorded onto it by a laser.
Compact Disk-Read Only Memory (CD-ROM) drive	A storage drive that reads data from CDs that can hold large amounts of information.
Compact Disk-Recordable (CD-R)	A type of CD that allows data to be read from it but to be recorded onto it only one time.
Compact Disk-Rewritable (CD-RW)	A type of CD that has the capability of both reading data and saving it to the disk multiple times.
data	A collective term that encompasses facts and information.
desktop	The view on the computer screen when Windows starts.
digital dictation	A method of recording information using the computer and Internet as opposed to tapes or other media.
directory tree	A virtual container on the computer system in which groups of folders and files can be kept and organized.
disk drives	Devices that store information in the computer.
earphones, syn. headset	A device that plugs into a transcriber or computer, allowing dictation to be heard.
e-mail	The way in which messages can be sent over the Internet.
encryption	A process whereby transmitted information is converted into a special coded computer language when transferring data over the Internet.
file	A block of information stored in a folder on the computer.
file server	The main hub computer that connects individual computers to a system.
file transfer protocol (FTP)	The method by which files are transferred from one computer to another over the Internet.
flash drive	A small, solid-state, portable drive that can hold a large amount of data.
folder	A place on the computer in which you store documents and other data, like a manila folder in a filing cabinet.
foot pedal	A device which allows the transcriptionist to keep both hands on the keyboard to type while controlling the flow of dictation played back.
footer	Text printed at the bottom of every page of a document.
front-end SRT	A process by which text is generated on-screen from dictation in real-time, allowing physicians to edit and correct the final document themselves.

Term	Meaning
function keys	Special keys found on the top of a computer keyboard that provide different functions depending on the software being used.
hard disk drive	A storage device that is fixed inside the computer and stores large volumes of data that can be accessed and retrieved quickly.
hardware	The term used to describe the equipment that makes up the computer system.
header	Text printed at the top of each page of a document.
icons	The name given to Windows graphic images.
information technology (IT)	A general term that refers to the processing, storage, and/or transfer of information.
keyboard	The device used for typing text into the computer.
liquid crystal display (LCD)	A computer monitor that displays images using a liquid crystal solution.
local area network (LAN)	A network system that is capable of serving a vast number of users at the same time.
macro	A series of commands that is recorded in a single command so it can be played back later.
monitor	The device that displays viewable images generated by the computer.
motherboard	A large circuit board with connections for other components of the computer.
mouse	A small device used to point to and select items on the computer screen.
navigation keys	Special keys on the computer keyboard used to reposition the cursor quickly.
numeric keypad	Special keys on the computer that allow for numbers to be entered quickly.
ports	Specific openings typically located on the back of the computer case.
shortcuts	The icons on the computer desktop that "point" to a real file on the hard drive.
software	One or more computer programs that provide instructions to the computer to perform a particular task.
speech-recognition technology (SRT), syn. voice recognition (VR)	A system that allows computers with a source of sound input, such as a microphone or hand-held dictation device, to interpret human speech, word for word, for transcription of medical documents.
spyware, syn. adware	Programs unknowingly installed on a computer that spy on a user's computer activity for advertising purposes.
stand-alone system	A computer that is not connected to any other computer in the office.
Start button and menu	The central launching point on the computer desktop for applications and tasks.
storage	The term used to describe the devices that are used to store and transfer data.
style book	A manual that provides information on medical transcription styles, forms, and grammar and usage specific to medical terms.
System tray	The small bar in the lower right corner of the computer desktop that contains miniature icons for easy access to system functions.
systems software	The computer program that coordinates all the data received by the computer and instructs the computer on how to process that data.
Task bar	The part of the computer desktop that displays software programs which are open and running simultaneously.
tower	The part of the computer that contains the circuitry needed for the computer to operate.
transcriber	A machine that makes it possible to listen to dictated recordings in order to transcribe them into written documents.

Term	Meaning
transcription platform	A type of digital dictation software that enables medical transcriptionists to retrieve, transcribe, and return reports directly from a central computer networking system.
tunnels	Encrypted connections between two locations, used to bypass insecure public networks found on the Internet.
Uniform Resource Locator	An address of a web site on the Internet.
universal serial bus (USB)	A standard connector that allows all types of devices to be plugged into the computer quickly and easily.
virtual private network (VPN)	A computer network that uses a public telecommunication infrastructure, such as the Internet, to provide remote offices or individual users with secure access to their organization's network.
widow/orphan control	A word-processing program feature that prevents a paragraph from being broken in such a way that a single line appears at the top or bottom of a page.
Windows	The operating system software used by most computers.
workstations	Individual computers connected to a local area network (LAN).
World Wide Web (WWW)	A term that refers to all the web pages and web sites on the Internet that contain some form of information.
zip drive	A kind of disk drive that uses special disks that can hold a lot of data.
zip files	The name given to files placed on a zip drive.

Add Your Own Terms and Definitions Here:

_____

_____

_____

_____

_____

_____

REVIEW QUESTIONS

1. What is the difference between a single computer workstation and a stand-alone system?
2. Explain the advantages and disadvantages of producing medical reports using speech-recognition technology.
3. What is the purpose of encryption?
4. What is a style book?
5. What does a file server do?
6. What is digital dictation?
7. Name three computer software program functions that can automate a medical office.
8. When or under what circumstances is Internet medical research better than using an on-site medical library?
9. What are Windows platforms?
10. How are word books different from medical dictionaries?

CHAPTER ACTIVITIES

Matching

Match the term in the left column with its definition in the right column.

A. tunnels   _____ A computer network that uses a public telecommunication infrastructure to provide remote offices or individual users with secure access to the company's computer network.

B. workstations   _____ Special coded computer language used to transmit information over the Internet.

C. VPN   _____ A machine that makes it possible to listen to dictated recordings.

D. CPU   _____ The main computer that stores centrally shared data and programs.

E. digital dictation _____ Individual computers that are connected to a network.

F. LAN   _____ Speech-recognition technology.

G. SRT   _____ A document with preset formatting and settings.

H. encryption   _____ The recording and storing of dictation in a digital format on a chip, disk or computer's hard drive instead of a tape or similar media.

I. file server   _____ A computer that is not connected to any other computer in the office.

J. template   _____ The part of the computer that contains processing cards and circuitry.

K. transcriber   _____ Local area network.

L. stand-alone system _____ Secure, encrypted connections between two locations on a network.

Research Activity

Using a pharmaceutical word book, locate the following brand-name drugs and indicate the generic name of the drug. Some drugs are a combination of one or more drugs. In that instance, list all of the combining drugs. If a pharmaceutical word book is not available, research this information using the Internet under the brand name.

1. Lorcet _____
2. Sustiva _____
3. Vytorin _____
4. Xanax _____
5. Plavix _____
6. Dilantin _____
7. Ceclor _____
8. Coumadin _____
9. Septra _____
10. Folgard _____

Fill-in-the-Blanks

Complete the following sentences with the missing word.

1. All components of a computer connect to the _____.
2. E-mails and other transmissions over the Internet use _____ that bypass insecure public networks.
3. _____ is an operating system software manufactured by Microsoft.
4. An individual computer connected to a network is called a _____.
5. A _____ is a required to control the flow of dictation while keeping both hands on the keyboard.
6. You would use a _____ to store a series of commands to play back later.
7. _____ a small, stick-shaped memory drive.
8. Windows uses _____, or graphic images, to click with a mouse.
9. Another name for speech recognition technology is _____.
10. MS Word is a kind of _____ used for word processing.

3

THE BASICS OF MEDICAL TERMINOLOGY

OBJECTIVES

After completing this chapter, you will be able to:

- Identify the basic component parts of medical terms.
- Identify common homonyms and soundalike words that are heard frequently in the dictation of medical reports, recognize and correctly pronounce words with unusual pronunciations, and explain how these word-confusion problems can lead to inaccuracies in medical transcription.
- Explain the difference between "slang" and "jargon" and be able to identify each.
- Use proper anatomic terms to describe the anatomic position, body planes, cavities, regions, and quadrants.

INTRODUCTION

Different professions use different "languages." The work of a medical transcriptionist involves the preparation of clear, accurate records using a language not found in everyday speech. This chapter illustrates the fundamentals of medical word-building skills, using prefixes, combined word forms, and suffixes to determine the proper spelling and meaning of medical words, and provides tips on working with the unique slang and jargon terms encountered in medical dictation. This chapter also discusses terms used to describe body direction and position when documenting where one part of the body is in relation to another. Although a thorough understanding of medical terminology is an essential component of an aspiring medical transcriptionist's education, please note that this chapter provides only an overview of these topics; it is not intended to take the place of a more comprehensive medical terminology course.

MEDICAL WORD BUILDING

The words that are used by the medical profession to describe the human body in health and illness are collectively referred to as **medical terminology**. Like every other language, medical terminology has changed considerably over time, but the majority of the terms are derived from Latin or Greek.

At first glance, medical language seems confusing and almost impossible to understand, but it makes sense once a word is analyzed and broken down into its component parts. Most people use medical terminology without even thinking about it: Words like *diarrhea*, *cardiac*, and *bronchitis* have become part of our everyday

QUICK CHECK 3.1

Identify the root word(s) in the following medical terms.

Term	Root Word(s)
hypercalcemia	_____
cardiology	_____
otolaryngology	_____
lithotomy	_____
esophagogastroduodenoscopy	_____

language and do not seem foreign because we understand their meanings.

English-language medical terms are commonly derived from Latin and Greek. As with all words, most medical terms are made up of one or more word parts. There are four basic parts, and any given medical term may contain one, some, or all of these parts:

- Prefixes
- Root words
- Suffixes
- Combining vowels that link root words and suffixes to form new words, called **combining forms**

Prefixes

A **prefix** is a syllable or group of letters at the beginning of a word that modifies the root and changes its meaning. The prefix is not a full word itself, but rather comes before the root word. See the prefix in the following words:

Word	Prefix
readdress	re
unmask	un
precursor	pre

Table 3.1 illustrates some common medical prefixes and their meanings.

Root Words

The **root word** is the foundation of a word. See the root word in the following words:

Word	Root Word
reading, reader, reads	read
shopper, shopping, shopped	shop
marking, marker, marks	mark

The root word establishes the basic meaning of a word. Every word has at least one root word, but some medical words have two, three, or even four roots. Some root

words are words that can stand alone other root words are simply the basic form of words, such as the word *duct*.

Any word containing more than one root word is known as a **compound word**. The English language has many compound words that are used every day, such as *storefront*, *sidewalk*, and *longstanding*. In theory, both root words that are contained in a compound word can stand alone as words. Many medical words are the same. For example, the word *lymphadenopathy* contains two words, *lymph* and *adenopathy*.

Suffixes

A **suffix** is a group of letters added to the end of a word that changes its meaning. You can see the suffix in the following words:

Word	Suffix
examining	ing
marker	er
testing	ing

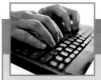

TRANSCRIPTION TIP:

Know the difference between *inter* and *intra*, prefixes that sound alike when dictated. A good way to remember the difference is to think of inter as something occurring between two items, whereas *intra* is something occurring within one item. For example, *interstate* highways cross between two (or more) states. If the dictator is using one of these prefixes when talking about one item (like a spleen), the word would be *intrasplenic*, referring to elements within the one spleen, not *intersplenic*, or two spleens. It might be helpful, also, to coin the phrase, "intra- is the opposite of extra-," in trying to remember the difference between the two.

TABLE 3.1   Common Medical Prefixes

Prefix	Refers To	Prefix	Refers To
ab-	away from, outside of, beyond	intra-	inside
ad-	toward, near to	macro-	big
ante-, pre-	before	meso-	middle
an-, anti-	against, opposed, without	meta-	beyond
bi-	two	micro-	small
brady-	abnormally slow rate	mono, uni-	one
con-, sym-, syn-	with	neo-	new
contra-	against	oligo-	a few
dia-	across, through	pan-	everywhere
dys-	bad, difficult	peri-	around
ed-, ecto-	outside	poly-	many, much
en-, endo-	inside	post-	after
ex-, exo-	outside	pre-	before, in front of
extra-	beyond	quadri-	four
hemi-, semi-	half	retro-	backward, behind
hyper-	above, beyond normal	sub-	below; less than; underneath
hypo-	below, below normal	tachy-	abnormally high rate
infra-	outside or below	tri-	three
inter-	between		

Reprinted with permission from A Short Course in Medical Terminology, by C. Edward Collins, Lippincott, Williams & Wilkins, 2006.

Table 3.2 lists some common medical suffixes and their meanings.

Combining Forms

What are combining forms? You can think of them as the LEGOs of language. As the name indicates, a **combining form** is a linguistic atom that occurs only in combination with some other word form. In medicine, a combining form contains a root word and a combining vowel. The root word contains the medical meaning of the word, and a **combining vowel** is a vowel that aids in the pronunciation of a word, used to combine a root and suffix or two root words. A combining vowel is usually an *o*, but it can also be an *i*, or an *a*. A combining vowel is used to join two medical words and make the resulting word easier to pronounce. The vowel is the link to other word parts and is essential to medical word building.

Together a combining form and a combining vowel form the foundation of a medical word. The root word is separated from the combining vowel by a forward slash. The combining vowel is at the end of the combining form. See Table 3.3 for a list of common combining forms used to make medical words.

Putting Word Parts Together

The following is an example of a medical word form using a root word, a combining vowel, and a suffix:

Word: *leukocyte*
Root word: leuk
Combining form: leuk/o
Suffix: -cyte

The combining vowel bridges the two parts of the word. In the preceding example, the combining vowel, *o*, is needed to create the word *leukocyte*. It would otherwise be difficult to pronounce the word *leukocyte* without a vowel to separate the root word and the suffix.

There are many variations in creating medical words using combining vowels. For example, if a suffix begins with a vowel, the combining vowel would not be used:

Word: *bronchitis*

There is no vowel necessary to combine the root word, *bronch*, with the suffix, *itis*, because the suffix, *itis*, begins with a vowel. Therefore:

Word: *bronchitis*
Root word: bronch
Combining form: (none)
Suffix: -itis

TABLE 3.2   Common Medical Suffixes

Suffix	Meaning	Suffix	Meaning
-ac, -al, -aneous, -ar, -eous, -iatric, -ic, -oid, -otic, -ous, -ular	converts a root or a noun term to an adjective	-meter	device for measuring
		-metry	act of measuring
		-oma	tumor
-cele	protrusion, hernia	-opsy	visual examination
-entesis	surgical puncture	-osis	condition
-cyte	cell	-pathy	disease
-desis	surgical binding	-penia	reduction of the size or quantity
-dynia	pain	-pexy	surgical fixation
-ectasis, ectasia	expansion or dilation	-phobia	a word meaning fear, often appearing as a suffix
-ectomy	surgical removal		
-edema	excessive fluid in intracellular tissues	-plasia	abnormal formation
		-plasty	surgical repair
-emesis	vomiting	-plegia	paralysis
-emia	blood	-poiesis	producing
-gen, -genic, -genesis	origin, producing	-ptosis	downward displacement
-globin	the protein of hemoglobin	-rrhage	flowing forth
-gram	written or pictorial record	-rrhaphy	suture
-graph	device for graphic or pictorial recording	-rrhea	discharge
		-rrhexis	rupture
-graphy	act of graphic or pictorial recording	-sclerosis	a word meaning "hard" that some-
-ian, -iatrics, -iatrist, -iatry, -ics, -ist, -logist, -logy	specialty of, study of, practice of		times combines with other roots as a suffix to indicate a condition of hard- ness
-iasis	a suffix used to convert a verb to a noun indicating a condition	-scope	device for viewing
		-scopy	act of viewing
-ism	a noun-forming suffix indicating a practice or a doctrine	-sis	condition
		-spasm	muscular contraction
-itis	inflammation	-stasis	level, unchanging
-lith	a stone, calculus, or calcification	-stenosis	narrowed, blocked
-lysis	disintegration	-stomy	permanent opening
-malacia	softening	-tome	instrument for cutting
-mania	a morbid impulse toward a specific object or thought	-tomy	incision
		-tripsy	crushing
-megaly	enlargement		

Reprinted with Permission from A Short Course in Medical Terminology, by C. Edward Collins, Lippincott, Williams & Wilkins, 2006.

If a suffix does not begin with a vowel, a combining vowel must be added:

Word: *arthroscopy*

The suffix, *-scopy*, does not begin with a vowel. The resulting word without a combining vowel would be *arthscopy*, which is not a word. The combining vowel, *o*, separates the root word, *arthr* (meaning *joint*), from the suffix, *-scopy*. Therefore:

Word: *arthroscopy*
Root word: arth

Combining form: arthr/o
Suffix: -scopy

If the root word ends in a vowel and the suffix begins with the same vowel, the final vowel is dropped and no combining vowel is used:

Word: *carditis*
Root word: cardi
Combining form: cardi/o
Suffix: -itis
Cardi/o + itis is spelled *carditis*, not *cardioitis*.

TABLE 3.3   Common Combining Forms

Root Word and Combining Vowel	Meaning	Root Word and Combining Vowel	Meaning
angi/o	vessel	laryng/o	larynx
appendic/o	appendix	leuk/o	white
arteri/o	artery	lith/o	stone; calculus
arthr/o	joint	my/o	muscle
bronch/o	bronchus	nephr/or	kidney
calc/o	calcium	ocul/o	eye
carcin/o	cancer	oste/o	bone
cardi/o	heart	pachy/o	thick
chol/o, chol/e	bile	path/o	disease
cyan/o	blue	pneum/o	lung; air
derm/o, dermat/o	skin	pseud/o	false
duoden/o	duodenum	psych/o	mind
enter/o	intestines	rhin/o, nas/o	nose
erythr/o	red	splen/o	spleen
esophag/o	esophagus	steth/o	chest
gastr/o	stomach	stomat/o	mouth
hem/o, hemat/o	blood	therm/o	heat
hepat/o	liver	trache/o	trachea (windpipe)
hyster/o	uterus	ur/o, urin/o	urine
iatr/o	medicine; physician	uter/o	uterus
lapar/o	abdomen		

Adapted from Medical Terminology: A Programmed Learning Approach to the Language of Health Care *by Marjorie Canfield Willis, Lippincott, Williams & Wilkins, 2003.*

When combining two roots and the second root begins with a vowel, the combining vowel is retained:

Word: *gastroenteritis*

The combining vowel is necessary to join the first root word, *gastr*, with the second root, *enter*. Therefore:

Word: *gastroenteritis*
Root words: gastr and enter
Combining form: gastr/o
Suffix: -itis

Of course, there are exceptions to every rule. Some common terms that are not combined, even though they may sound that way when dictated, include the following:

Dorsal lithotomy, not dorsolithotomy.
Jugular venous distention, not jugulovenous distention.
Brachial plexus, not brachioplexus.
Atrial septal defect, not atrioseptal defect.

Plural Endings

Most medical words have English plural endings. However, many words, mainly derived from Greek and Latin, have plural endings that do not always follow the common English-language rule of adding an *s* to the end of a word, as shown in Table 3.4. Sometimes physicians dictate plural forms that do not sound the way they are spelled. Here are a few general rules for making medical terms plural:

- When a word ends in *um*, change the *um* to *a*. Example: bacterium becomes bacteria.
- When a word ends in *ex*, change the *ex* to *ices*. Example: index becomes indices.
- When a word ends in *on*, change the *on* to *a*. Example: criterion becomes criteria.
- When a word ends in *en*, change the *en* to *ina*. Example: foramen becomes foramina.
- When a word ends in *ma*, change the *ma* to *mata*. Example: angioma becomes angiomata.
- When a word ends in *a*, change the *a* to *ae*. Example: sclera becomes sclerae.

There are other ways to make medical words plural. You will need to remember these variations, and check plural forms of words that are dictated but unfamiliar to you.

Singular	Plural	Singular Word	Plural Word
TABLE 3.4 Plural Endings Found in Medical Words			
-a	-ae	conjunctiva	conjunctivae
-ex	-ices	index	indices
-en	-ina	foramen	foramina
-is	-es	thrombosis	thromboses
-ix	-ices	appendix	appendices
-on	-a	ganglion	ganglia
-ma	-mata	stigma	stigmata
-nx	-ges	phalanx	phalanges
-um	-a	bacterium	bacteria
-us	-i	bronchus	bronchi

Analyzing Terms

A medical word is broken down by analyzing the prefix, root word (or combining form), and suffix of the word to determine its meaning. For example, the term *pericarditis* can be divided into three parts: *peri-card-itis*. Once divided into its essential parts, pericarditis can be translated into ordinary English as follows:

The prefix *peri-* translates as surrounding (as in *perimeter*).
The combining form *card/i* translates to heart (as in *cardiology*).
The suffix *-itis* translates to inflammation.

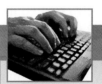

TRANSCRIPTION TIP:

When transcribing ophthalmologic reports, physicians often dictate the words *sclera* and *conjunctiva*, the singular forms of the words, when referring to both eyes. Identify if the dictator is talking about one eye or both eyes and use the proper forms of these terms—*sclerae* and *conjunctivae* if plural.

QUICK CHECK 3.2 ✓

Circle the letter corresponding to the best answer for the following questions.

1. Which prefix means under, beneath, or deficient?
   A. hyper-
   B. extra-
   C. hypo-
   D. endo-

2. Which prefix means middle?
   A. dia-
   B. meta-
   C. bi-
   D. meso-

3. Which prefix means inside?
   A. semi-
   B. micro-
   C. tri-
   D. intra-

4. Which prefix means new?
   A. neo-
   B. contra-
   C. meta-
   D. mega-

5. Which prefix means half?
   A. post-
   B. ab-
   C. hemi-
   D. pan-

QUICK CHECK 3.3

Match the following suffixes with their meanings.

_____ 1. -dynia   A. rupture

_____ 2. -rrhea   B. surgical crushing

_____ 3. -rrhexis   C. pain

_____ 4. -tripsy   D. surgical removal

_____ 5. -ectomy   E. discharge

A helpful way to analyze a medical term is to first go to the end of the word and locate the suffix. In the previous example, *-itis* is the suffix. Then go back to the beginning of the word and proceed in order of prefix and root(s) or combining forms. In the previous example, by locating the prefix, *peri-*, meaning surrounding, and the combining form, *card/i*, meaning the heart, you may conclude that the term pericarditis means *inflammation of the heart*, or more specifically, an inflammation of the outer layer of the heart.

By adding a new prefix or suffix to a root word, new terms are created. For example, if the combining form *my/o*, which means muscle, is added to the combining form *card/i* above, referring to the heart, a new word is created with *myocarditis*, meaning *inflammation of the muscles of the heart*.

WORD-CONFUSION PROBLEMS

One challenge faced by medical transcriptionists is the confusion of two words or terms that may sound similar when dictated. It is important to avoid a mistranscription when these terms are encountered in dictation. The most common word-confusion problems involve homonyms, soundalike words, and words with unusual punctuation.

Homonyms

A recurrent problem in medical transcription is the use of a word that is incorrect in the context of the report, even when it sounds like the one that belongs there. Words that sound *identical* but have different spellings and meanings, called **homonyms**, are a particular challenge. Many medical words sound identical to other words when dictated but, in reality, are completely unrelated, as shown in Table 3.5. For example, a common transcription error is typing the word *elicit*,

which means to call forth (as in, to elicit a response) for the word *illicit*, or contrary to law (as in, illicit drug use). These two terms sound identical when dictated but have completely different meanings. You should listen carefully to understand the context of the sentence to select the correct word.

Soundalike Words

Soundalike words are words that sound alike but have different spellings and meanings. Unlike homonyms, which sound identical, soundalikes have distinctly different pronunciations when listened to carefully, as shown in Table 3.6. For example, *Zantac*, the gastrointestinal drug, is not the same as *Xanax*, the anxiolytic; yet both words sound similar if not dictated clearly. It would be a crucial mistake to type the wrong medication into a medical report. Therefore, it is important to listen and understand the context of the dictation to discern between soundalike words. In the previous example, if the physician was dictating a clinic note about a patient with a stomach problem, the word in question would probably be *Zantac*, not *Xanax*.

See more homonyms and soundalike words pertaining to body systems in the chapters of this book.

Unusual Word Pronunciations

The English alphabet is composed of 26 letters, but these 26 letters make up 44 sounds. Some letters can have several sounds. In addition, letters combined with other letters can produce completely different sounds. For example the letter *n* makes a sound as in the word *no*, but the letters *p* and *n* together also make the identical sound, such as in *pneumonia*. These 44 sounds of English are called **phonemes**. A phoneme is a sound that can be represented by different combinations of letters. In medical terminology, silent letters and unusual punctuation that are a part of phonemes

TABLE 3.5   Common Homonyms

Word	Common Pronunciation	Homonym
accept: receive willingly, something given or offered.	ek-'sept	**except**: to prevent from being included or considered or accepted.
aide: someone who acts as an assistant.	'ād	**aid**: to provide help or assistance.
bare: lacking a natural, usual or appropriate covering.	bār'	**bear**: to support a weight or strain.
canker: a common term for a small ulcer on a mucous membrane.	kang'ker	**chancre**: a primary lesion of syphilis.
coarse: having large-grained or rough texture.	'koors	**course**: a mode of action.
complement: something added to complete or make perfect.	kom'plĕ-ment	**compliment**: a remark (or act) expressing praise and admiration.
discrete: separate; distinct.	dis-krēt'	**discreet**: having or showing good judgment in conduct.
elicit: to call forth (as in a response).	i-'li-sit	**illicit**: contrary to law.
fourth: the number after third.	'fōrth	**forth**: forward in time or order or degree.
mucus: viscid secretion produced by mucous membranes (a noun).	mūkŭs	**mucous**: pertaining to mucus; also, secreting mucus, as "mucous membranes" (an adjective).
plain: unadorned, as in x-ray.	plān	**plane**: a two-dimensional flat surface.
radical: designed to remove the root of a disease or all diseased tissue.	rad'i-kăl	**radicle**: a rootlet or structure resembling one, as a vein, a minute veinlet joining with others to form a vein, a nerve fiber that joins others to form a nerve.
sight: the range of vision.	sīt	**site**: physical position in relation to the surroundings. **cite**: to refer to for illustration or proof.
viscus: a main organ that is situated inside the body.	vis'kŭs	**viscous**: having a relatively high resistance to flow (like glue).

can make it difficult to ascertain the correct spelling of a word, as shown in Table 3.7. When you encounter a term in dictation that may be difficult to identify, try searching your resource materials for the word using different phonemes; this may make identification easier.

SLANG AND MEDICAL JARGON

By definition, **slang** is a type of language deliberately used in place of standard terms by a particular group. The language of medicine is full of slang, and all physicians use it when dictating. You must be able to recognize slang terms and be able to decide which expressions to transcribe verbatim, which ones to transcribe in formal terms, and which ones to not transcribe at all or to mark for review.

Most medical slang is derived from longer words that have been shortened in order to be dictated quickly. Some words have lost their beginnings, such as *crit* for hematocrit, or *scope* for bronchoscope; other words have

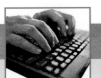

TRANSCRIPTION TIP:

Be aware of adjectives that cross over from general English usage into medicine—their meanings do not always remain the same. For example, a person described as *indolent* in general conversation may be lazy or dislike exertion, but in medical terminology, the same term means causing little pain (as in indolent sinusitis) or growing slowly (as in an indolent tumor).

TABLE 3.6   Common Soundalike Words

Word	Word Pronunciation	Soundalike	Soundalike Pronunciation
access: admittance; "access to."	ak′ses	**axis**: a real or imaginary straight line going through a structure around which it revolves, or would turn if it could revolve.	ak′sis
affect: to influence.	af′fekt	**effect**: result or a cause.	ef ′fekt
afferent: inflowing; conducting toward a center.	af′ĕ-rĕnt	**efferent**: conducting (fluid or a nerve impulse) outward from a given organ or part thereof.	efĕr-ent
apposition: the setting of one thing beside the other, as in suturing wounds.	ap-ō-zish′ŭn	**opposition**: the act of being opposite.	op-ō-zish′ŭn
bolus: a single, large quantity of a substance, such as a bolus dose of a drug injected intravenously.	bō′lŭs	**bullous**: relating to a fluid-filled blister.	bul′ŭs
canalization: the formation of canals or channels in a tissue.	kan-ăl-ĭ-zā′shŭn	**cannulization**: insertion of a cannula, or tube.	kan-ŭ-lĭ-zā′shŭn
enervation: failure of nerve force.	en-ĕr-vā′shŭn	**innervation**: the supply of nerve fibers functionally connected with a part.	in-ĕr-vā′shŭn
facial (with a long *a* sound): referring to the face.	fā′shăl	**fascial** (with a short *a* sound): relating to any fascia, which is the fibrous tissue that envelops the body beneath the skin.	fash′ē-ăl
gauge: a standard measure, as in surgical wire.	gāj	**gouge**: a hollow chisel used for cutting or removing.	gowj
homogeneous: of uniform structure or composition throughout.	hō-mō-jē′nē-ŭs	**homogenous**: having a structural similarity because of descent from a common ancestor.	hō-moj′ĕ-nŭs
perfusion: the pumping of a liquid into an organ or tissue.	pĕr-fyū′zhŭn	**profusion**: the property of being extremely abundant.	prō-fyū′zhŭn
phoresis: a biologic association in which one organism is transported by another.	fōr′ē-sis	**pheresis**: a procedure in which blood is removed from a donor, separated, and a portion retained, with the remainder returned to the donor.	fe-rē′sis
perfuse: to flow or spread, such as blood.	pĕr-fyŭs′	**profuse**: lavish, extravagant, bountiful.	prō-fyŭs′
regime: government or social system, often mispronounced in medicine for the word *regimen*.	rā-zhēm′	**regimen**: a systematic course of diet, therapy, or exercise.	rej′i-mĕn
tract: a system of organs, such as the gastrointestinal tract. Also, an abnormal passage through tissue, such as a sinus tract or fistulous tract. Most *tracts* are located *inside* the body.	trakt	**track**: a pathway. Most *tracks* are located *outside* of the body.	trak

TABLE 3.7   Phonemes

Letter(s)	Sounds Like	Example	Definition
ch	k	cheilitis	an inflammation of the lips
eu	u	euosmia	relating to a pleasant odor
gn	n	gnashing	the grinding together of teeth
j	y	johnin	a sterile solution used as an allergen to for testing cattle for Johne's disease
mn	n	mnemonics	a system for improving memory
ph	f	phalanx	one of the long bones of the digits of the hand or foot
pn	n	pneumonia	an inflammation of the lungs
ps	s	pseudo-	prefix for *false*
pt	t	ptosis	a sinking down or prolapse of an organ
rh	r	rheumatism	a disorder of muscles and joints
x	z	xanthoma	a yellow nodule on the skin

lost their endings, such as *consult* for consultation or *chemo* for chemotherapy; still other words have lost both their beginnings and endings, such as *flu* for influenza and *scrip* for prescription.

Some slang comes from letter abbreviations for words, where the initials of words are used instead of the full phrase. For example, *H&H* stands for *hemoglobin and hematocrit*, and *DC* can mean *discharge* or *discontinue*.

Jargon is a term used to describe the special language of a profession or an area of expertise, such as medicine or law. Often called "shop talk," this language is used by practitioners of certain trades, such as doctors, to discuss their activities or their equipment and its uses.

The use of slang and jargon is part of the "gear and tackle" of various trades. It is a tool that helps experts communicate with other experts in the same field. Many times slang and jargon become so integrated into our day-to-day language that they are often hard to recognize. However, *The Book of Style for Medical Transcription, 3rd ed.*, clearly states, "Edit inappropriate slang words and phrases, keeping in mind that many words start out as coined or slang terms but later evolve through usage to eventually become acceptable words in the American medical lexicon." Table 3.8 illustrates some common slang and jargon terms and the correct way to transcribe them.

MEDICAL ABBREVIATIONS

In patient care there is a lot of repetition of the same diseases, syndromes, body parts, symptoms, and diagnostic tests. In addition, doctors commonly use a variety of abbreviations to rapidly and succinctly record information about their patients. As a result, many of these terms and phrases have come to be known by their respective abbreviations. Unfortunately, abbreviations often sound confusing when dictated fast or mumbled into dictation equipment. For example, an *s* may sound deceptively like an *f*, or a *v* like a *d*. Therefore, you should be familiar with common abbreviations in order to be accurate and more productive.

Generally, abbreviations may be used in the body of a report if dictated by a physician, unless the healthcare facility for which you work specifies otherwise. Laboratory values often include abbreviations that should be transcribed as such, as should abbreviations that are rarely used in unabbreviated forms, such as *CT scan*, *Pap smear*, or *PPD test*.

Some preferred formats for commonly used abbreviations include the following:

Blood gas values: pH, PO_2, PaO_2, PCO_2, $PaCO_2$
EKG leads (including augmented limb and precordial leads):
    lead I, lead II, lead III
    aVR, aVL, aVF
    V1, V2, V3, V4, V5, V6, V7, V8, V9
    or V_1, V_2, V_3, V_4, V_5, V_6, V_7, V_8, V_9
    or sometimes dictated as sequential leads: V1 through V9 (V_1 through V_9)

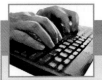

TRANSCRIPTION TIP:

Physicians often create an acronym out of an abbreviation. For example, the postanesthesia care unit (PACU) is a new designation for the recovery room after surgery. Surgeons will dictate this area as the "PAK-yoo." The surgical intensive care unit (SICU) is often pronounced as "SICK-yoo."

TABLE 3.8   Common Slang and Jargon

Slang/Jargon Word	Proper Transcription	Slang/Jargon Word	Proper Transcription
accels	accelerations	hep	hepatitis (A, B, or C)
afib	atrial fibrillation	kilos	kilograms
alk phos	alkaline phosphatase	lap chole	laparoscopic cholecystectomy
amp	ampicillin (also refers to ampule or ampere)	lap pads	laparotomy pads
appy	appendectomy	lymphos	lymphocytes
basos	basophils	lytes	electrolytes
bicarb	bicarbonate	mag ox	magnesium oxide (note there is a brand name drug called Mag-Ox)
bili	bilirubin	meds	medications
C diff	*C difficile* or *Clostridium difficile*	mets	metastasis or metastases
CA	cancer or carcinoma	mig per kig	milligrams per kilogram or mg/kg
cap	capsule	mikes	micrograms
cap refill	capillary refill	monos	monocytes
cath	catheter or catheterization	nebs	nebulizers
cathed	catheterized	neuro	neurologic or neurology
chemo	chemotherapy	preop	preoperative
clinda	clindamycin	pro time	prothrombin time or ProTime
crit	hematocrit	regurg	regurgitation
cysto	cystoscopy	sat	saturation
D-C	discontinued or discharged	sed rate	sedimentation rate
decels	decelerations	segs	segmented neutrophils
derm	dermatology, dermatologic	staph	staphylococcus
diff	differential	strep	streptococcus
echo	echocardoigram (also refers to echoencephalogram; unless you are sure of the expanded term, you should transcribe as is)	T-bili	total bilirubin
		tachy	tachycardia or tachycardic
		toco	tocolysis
		tox	toxicology
eos	eosinophils	trach	tracheotomy or tracheostomy
epi	epinephrine	triple a	abdominal aortic aneurysm
fem-pop	femoral-popliteal	utox	urine toxicology
flex sig	flexible sigmoidoscopy	vanc	vancomycin
gent	gentamicin	v-tach	ventricular tachycardia

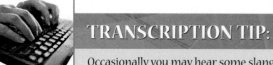

TRANSCRIPTION TIP:

Occasionally you may hear some slang or jargon that can be profane or defamatory. Flip, offensive language is out of place in a medical report. Flag such items as *hoagie* (a premature infant who is swaddled in an aluminum-type wrap to prevent hypothermia), *FLK* (a funny-looking kid) or *gomer* (a tiresome, difficult, or hypochondriacal patient) when they are dictated.

not V1 through 5 or V_1 through $_5$ (even if dictated)
not V1-5 or V_{1-5}
Immunoglobulins: IgA, IgD, IgE, IgG, and IgM
Blood pressure: mmHg

As a medical transcriptionist, you should transcribe abbreviations as they are heard. Some facilities do not allow certain abbreviations to be used in medical records, however. If that is the case, you should insert the full meaning of the abbreviation into the document. If an abbreviation has more than one meaning, it is up to you to determine the correct meaning. One way to do this is to look up the abbreviation in an abbreviation word book or style guide to view all available meanings of the abbreviation and determine the correct one according to the surrounding text or topic discussed. If you are still not sure of which meaning to use, or if there a chance that a meaning could be misconstrued, you should type the abbreviation without expanding it, or flag the item for review by a supervisor.

The **Joint Commission** is an independent, not-for-profit organization, established more than 50 years ago. The Joint Commission is a board of individuals comprising physicians, nurses, and consumers, and sets the standards by which healthcare quality is measured in America and around the world. To earn and maintain accreditation, organizations must have an extensive on-site review by a team of Joint Commission healthcare professionals at least once every three years in order to evaluate the organization's performance in areas that affect patient care.

One of the indicators assessed by The Joint Commission is compliance with patient safety goals. To help reduce the numbers of medical errors related to incorrect use of terminology, The Joint Commission issued a list of abbreviations that should no longer be used in charting, orders, and other clinical documentation. In addition, the **Institute for Safe Medication Practices** (ISMP), a nonprofit organization that partners with healthcare practitioners to improve medical error prevention and safe medication use, has issued a list of frequently misinterpreted and harmful medication errors. See Appendix 1 for the ISMP's List of Error-Prone Abbreviations, Symbols, and Dose Designations, which also includes The Joint Commission's "do not use" abbreviations. Healthcare facilities have implemented these lists, which apply not only to medication orders but to all clinical documentation, including physician orders, progress notes, consultation reports, and operative reports. Refer to these lists when transcribing to avoid typing abbreviations that are not acceptable.

ANATOMIC TERMS

Because anatomy is a descriptive science, it is vital to know the meaning of certain terms that describe body parts and positions. Physicians and clinicians have developed a set of terms, each of which has a precise meaning to describe the anatomy of the body.

Anatomic Position

The **anatomic position** is an arbitrary position used as a reference when describing parts of the body in relation to each other. When used with other terms relating to direction or movement, the anatomic position allows a standard way of documenting where one part of the body is in relation to another, regardless of whether the body is standing up, lying down, or in any other position. For example, a patient's eyes are always

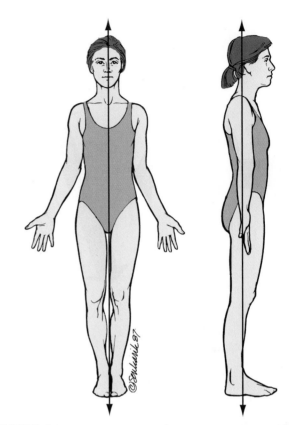

FIGURE 3.1. Anatomic Position. The anatomic position provides a standard way of documenting where one part of the body is in relation to another. Reprinted from Moore KL and Agur A. *Essential Clinical Anatomy,* 2nd Ed. Philadelphia: Lippincott Williams & Wilkins, 2002.

superior to the mouth, whether the patient is lying down or standing on his or her head.

Figure 3.1 illustrates the anatomic position of the human body: standing erect with eyes looking forward, arms at the sides, palms facing forward, and soles of the feet flat on the ground. No matter what position a body is in, surfaces are referred to as if the individual is standing erect in the anatomic position. For example, when a physician dictates the directions left or right, it is always from the point of view of the patient. Visualize this upright position when listening to the dictator describing locations in the body.

Directional Terms

Directional terms are used to discuss body parts in relation to one another, as shown in Figure 3.2. The **midline** is an imaginary vertical line that divides the body into equal right and left sides. The following terms refer to direction of the body:

- Anterior (ventral): Toward the front of the body.
- Posterior (dorsal): Toward the back of the body or "behind."
- Anteroposterior (AP): Direction or view going through the patient from anterior to posterior. The *AP view* is used when transcribing x-ray reports.

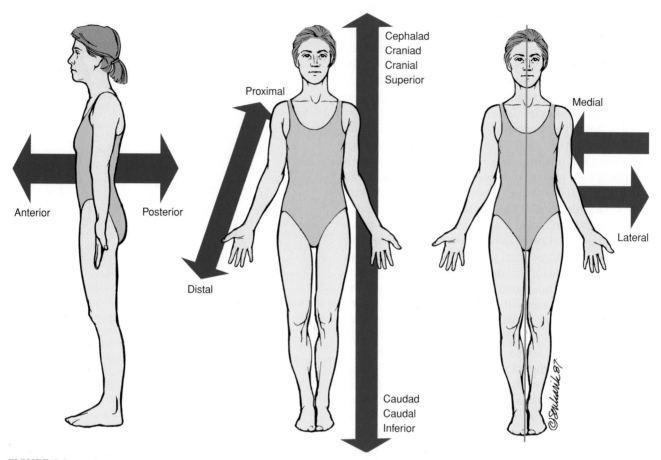

FIGURE 3.2. Body Directions. Directional terms are used to discuss body parts in relation to one another. Reprinted with permission from *Stedman's Medical Dictionary,* 27th ed. Baltimore: Lippincott Williams & Wilkins 2000.

- Medial: Toward the midline of the body.
- Lateral: Toward the side of the body, or away from the midline.
- Ipsilateral: On the same side of the body.
- Contralateral: On the opposite side of the body.
- Proximal: Nearest to the trunk or point of origin.
- Distal: Farther from the center of the body or point of origin.
- Superior (cranial): Above, or pertaining to or toward the skull.
- Inferior: Away from the head or toward the lower part of a body or structure; opposite of superior.
- Caudad: Situated farther from the head in relation to a specific reference point; opposite of craniad.
- Cephalad: Toward the head or upper part of a structure.
- Caudal: Pertaining to the tail.
- Craniad: Situated nearer to the head in relation to a specific reference point; opposite of caudad.
- Superficial (external): Pertaining to or nearer to the surface of the body.
- Deep (internal): Closer to the center of the body.
- Palmar: On or toward the palm of the hand.
- Plantar: On or toward the sole of the foot.

- Dorsum: On the upper or posterior surface of any body part.

Anatomic Planes

Medical professionals often refer to sections of the body in terms of **anatomic planes**, or flat surfaces. These planes are imaginary lines—vertical and horizontal—drawn through an upright body, as shown in Figure 3.3. Each anatomic plane divides the body into certain sections:

- Frontal plane: A vertical plane running from side to side that divides the body or organ into anterior and posterior sections.
- Sagittal plane: A vertical plane running from front to back that divides the body into right and left sides.
- Transverse plane: A horizontal plane that divides the body into upper and lower parts.

X-ray Positioning

When performing an x-ray or other radiologic procedure, the radiographer positions the patient based on

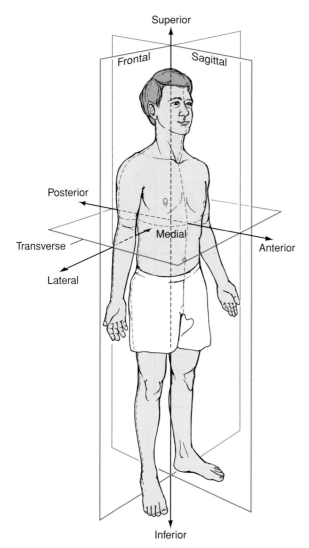

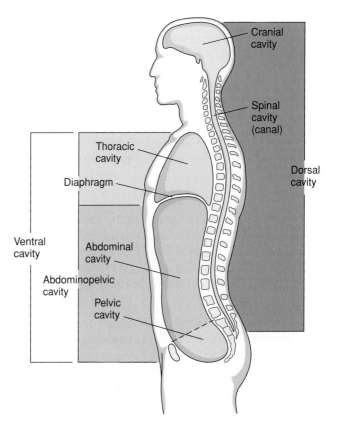

- Left lateral decubitus: The view with patient lying on the left side.
- Oblique: A view that is slanted or at an angle.
- Lordotic: The view with the patient leaning back while standing.

Body Cavities

Many organs and organ systems in the body are housed in compartments called **body cavities**. These confined spaces within the body serve to separate, support, and protect the internal organs from the daily wear of everyday movement. Body cavities also permit organs such as the lungs, the bladder, and the stomach to expand and contract while remaining securely supported.

The human body cavities are separated into ventral and dorsal cavities, as illustrated in Figure 3.4. These cavities are further subdivided into specific body cavities that house and protect internal organs:

- The cranial cavity, which encases the brain.
- The spinal cavity, which surrounds the spinal cord.
- The thoracic cavity, which contains the heart, esophagus, and organs of the respiratory system—the lungs, trachea, and bronchi.

FIGURE 3.3. Anatomic Planes. Body planes are imaginary reference lines—vertical and horizontal—drawn through an upright body. Reprinted with permission from Oatis CA. *Kinesiology: The Mechanics and Pathomechanics of Human Movement.* Baltimore: Lippincott Williams & Wilkins 2003.

the body part to be imaged, suspected defect or disease, and condition of the patient. Since many body parts overlay other internal structures, the radiographer positions the body part as well as the x-ray equipment to obtain the clearest image possible. X-ray exams usually consist of two or more radiographs. Some common positions used in radiologic studies include:

- Anteroposterior (AP): The view going through the patient from anterior to posterior.
- Posteroanterior (PA): The view going through the patient from posterior to anterior.
- Lateral: The view from the side of the patient or structure being imaged.
- Right lateral decubitus: The view with patient lying on the right side.

FIGURE 3.4. Body Cavities. Body cavities separate, support, and protect the organs from the daily wear of everyday movement. Reprinted with permission from Cohen BJ, Wood DL. *Memmler's The Human Body in Health and Disease,* 9th Ed. Philadelphia: Lippincott Williams & Wilkins, 2000.

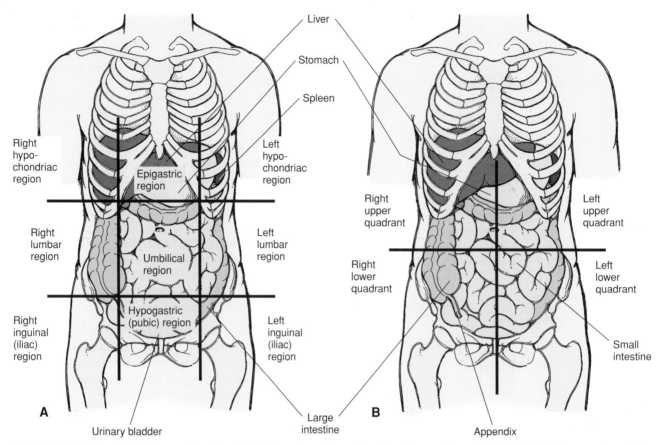

FIGURE 3.5. Abdominal Regions and Quadrants. Physicians refer to nine regions (**A**) and four quadrants (**B**) of the abdominal cavity to describe the location of abdominal organs, pains, or disorders. Reprinted with permission from *Stedman's Medical Dictionary*, 27th ed. Baltimore: Lippincott Williams & Wilkins, 2000.

- The abdominopelvic cavity, which contains the organs of the digestive, reproductive, and excretory systems.

The thoracic and abdominal cavities are separated by the **diaphragm**, a wall of muscle which aids in breathing.

Body Regions and Quadrants

Physicians refer to nine regions of the abdominal cavity to describe the location of abdominal organs, pains, or disorders, as shown in Figure 3.5(A). The nine regions are delineated by four planes: Two sagittal (vertical) and two transverse (horizontal) planes, and divided as follows:

- Midline sections (3): The epigastric (above the stomach); umbilical (at the umbilicus or navel), and hypogastric (below the stomach).
- Lateral sections (2): The right and left hypochondriac regions, positioned near the ribs.
- Right and left lumbar sections (2): Positioned near the small of the back, or lumbar region.
- Right and left iliac sections (2): Named for the upper bone of the hip (ilium) and also called the inguinal region, which refers to the groin.

In addition, physicians use imaginary quadrants to indicate locations of body structures for diagnostic and surgical procedures. These quadrants are a result of projecting two imaginary lines, one vertically along the body's midline and the other horizontally through the umbilicus, as illustrated in Figure 3.5(B). These lines separate the abdomen into four equal sections: the left upper quadrant, the right upper quadrant, the left lower quadrant, and the right lower quadrant.

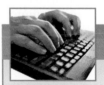

TRANSCRIPTION TIP:

The term **hypochondriac** literally means "beneath cartilage," referring to the cartilages of the ribs. The term is applied to a person who exhibits abnormal anxiety about his or her health because the hypochondriac region, especially the spleen, was thought to be the seat of this disorder.

QUICK CHECK 3.4

Complete the following sentences.

1. The _____ divides the body into right and left sides.

2. The anatomic term that describes a structure toward the front of the body is _____ .

3. The _____ separates the thoracic and abdominal cavities.

4. The term _____ refers to a structure toward the sole of the foot.

5. The brain and spinal cord are located in the _____.

CLOCK BODY POSITIONS

Another method of describing a location in a diagnostic or surgical procedure is by use of an imaginary analog clock face envisioned over the object, with 12 o'clock being at the top of the object and 6 o'clock at the bottom. When medical providers describe a location using this method, they will refer to it as "the 12 o'clock position" or "the 7 o'clock position." In describing more than one location, physicians may dictate the locations, for example, as "the 3-, 5-, and 7-o'clock positions." Sometimes to be more specific, a physician may use a half-hour notation, which is transcribed as, for example, "the 3:30 position."

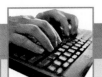

TRANSCRIPTION TIP:

When an anatomic position is described in terms of a clock face orientation as seen by the viewer, use the word *o'clock* unless the position is subdivided. For example, 3-o'clock position, or 3:30 position, but not 3:30-o'clock position.

CHAPTER SUMMARY

Learning medical terminology is the most difficult and extensive part of medical transcription. Basic familiarity with the fundamentals of body direction and position, as well as a thorough understanding of medical word building, will hone your ability to recognize unfamiliar terms when they are dictated and ascertain their meanings while you are transcribing.

As with learning any new language, you should read aloud when you can to familiarize yourself with the pronunciation of each medical term and practice using new terms as much as possible. When transcribing dictation that is difficult to understand, slang, or words that are unfamiliar to you, remember that you are creating not only a medical document that must be understood clearly, but also a legal document in which language cannot be ambiguous. Healthcare professionals must balance the time saved using slang or nonstandard language with the possibility that this choice of words might result in a transcription error. A clear, unambiguous statement is essential. Keep in mind that even with the auditory challenges you will face, accuracy and clarity must always be the main goals in creating medical reports.

· I · N · S · I · G · H · T ·

The Unique Language of Medicine

Although medical language derived from Greek and Latin origins, today English serves as the base of language used by medical doctors when they communicate with each other.

The oldest written sources of Western medicine are the Hippocratic writings from the 5th and 4th centuries BC, which cover all aspects of medicine at that time and which contain numerous medical terms. This was the beginning of the Greek era of the language of medicine, which lasted even after the Roman conquest, since the Romans, who had no similar medical tradition, advanced the study and practice of medicine using Greek terminology. They named numerous anatomic structures and diseases in Latin as well as Greek, and these words remain a part of medical language today.

Today, however, it would appear that medical doctors around the world have chosen English as the single language for international communication. All the most influential medical journals are written in English, and English has become the language of choice at international medical conferences. Many terms are derived from English and translated to the language of the user. For example, the Russians use the term *shuntirovanie*, which is a term derived from the English word, *shunt*, and the Danish use the verbs *screene* and *skanne*, for naturalized English words *screen* and *scan*, respectively. Whereas in former times new medical terms were derived from classical Greek or Latin roots, now they are often, partly, or wholly composed of words borrowed from ordinary English. For example, terms such as *bypass* operation, *screening*, and *scanning* are all commonly used even by doctors from non-English-speaking countries. The term *bypass* is accepted in German, Dutch, Scandinavian, Italian, and Romanian. English acronyms such as AIDS, CT, and MRI are universally accepted terms and nouns in their own right.

Linguists find the language of medicine fascinating for the flow of concepts and words from one tongue to another. For medical transcriptionists, an appreciation of the history and original meaning of words offers a new dimension to the language of their profession.

TERMINOLOGY

Term	Meaning
anatomic planes	Imaginary lines—vertical and horizontal—drawn through an upright body.
anatomic position	An arbitrary position used as a reference when describing parts of the body in relation to each other.
body cavities	Confined spaces in the body that house major organs.
combining form	A word containing the root word plus the combining vowel.
combining vowel	A vowel that aids in the pronunciation of a word, used to combine a root word and suffix or two roots.
compound word	A word that contains more than one root word.
diaphragm	A wall of muscle that aids in breathing.
homonym	Two or more identical-sounding words that have different spellings and meanings.
hypochondriac	A term applied to a person with abnormal anxiety about his or her health.
Institute for Safe Medication Practices (ISMP)	A nonprofit organization that partners with healthcare practitioners toward improvements in drug distribution naming, packaging, labeling, and delivery system design.
jargon	Often called "shop talk," the technical terminology used in a special field or profession, such as medicine or law.
The Joint Commission	An independent, not-for-profit organization that sets the standards by which health-care quality is measured in America and around the world.
medical terminology	The words that make up the language of medicine.
midline	An imaginary vertical line that divides the body into equal right and left sides.
phonemes	The 44 sounds of the English alphabet.
prefix	A syllable or group of letters at the beginning of a word that modifies the root word and changes its meaning.
root word	The foundation, or basic part, of a word.
slang	A type of language deliberately used in place of standard terms by a particular group.
soundalike words	Words that sound alike but have different spellings and meanings.
suffix	A group of letters added to the end of a word to change its meaning.

Add Your Own Terms and Definitions Here:

_____

_____

_____

_____

_____

_____

_____

REVIEW QUESTIONS

1. What is the difference between a homonym and a soundalike word?
2. Is it acceptable to use slang and jargon in medical reports? Why or why not?
3. What is the difference between a prefix and a suffix?
4. What is the term used to describe words that sound identical but have different meanings?
5. From what languages are medical terms commonly derived?
6. Why is the anatomic position referred to when using terms to describe the body?
7. What is the purpose of the Joint Commission's "dangerous abbreviations" list?
8. What are body cavities?
9. From what is slang derived?
10. What is the purpose of a combining vowel?

CHAPTER ACTIVITIES

Multiple Choice

Circle the letter corresponding to the best answer for the following questions.

1. The term "medial" refers to
    A. a direction toward the midline of the body.
    B. an anatomic position.
    C. a direction toward the foot of the body.
    D. a kind of soundalike word.

2. In the anatomic position, the hands are
    A. faced backward.
    B. in a fist.
    C. turned in.
    D. faced forward.

3. A transverse plane divides the body into _____ segments.
    A. 5
    B. 2
    C. 4
    D. 6

4. Words that make up the language of medicine are collectively referred to as
    A. medical terminology.
    B. medical ethics.
    C. slang and jargon.
    D. homonyms.

5. A compound word contains
    A. more than one root word.
    B. at least two prefixes.
    C. no root word.
    D. three word parts.

6. What is the plural form of bacterium?
    A. Bacteriae
    B. Bacteriums
    C. Bacteries
    D. Bacteria

7. _____ sound nearly alike but have different spellings and meanings.
   A. Soundalikes
   B. Homonyms
   C. Synonyms
   D. Slang terms

8. The imaginary vertical line that divides the body into equal right and left sides is known as the
   A. anatomic line.
   B. lateral division.
   C. midline.
   D. dorsal plane.

9. Words that sound identical but have different spellings and meanings are called
   A. soundalikes.
   B. jargon.
   C. synonyms.
   D. homonyms.

10. The _____ is found in the cranial cavity.
    A. diaphragm
    B. lungs
    C. spinal cord
    D. brain

Matching

Using a medical dictionary or other medical resource, look up the meaning of each soundalike term on the left and then match it to its corresponding definition on the right.

Term

Definition

1. _____ illicit
2. _____ elicit
3. _____ ACE
4. _____ Ace
5. _____ ace
6. _____ perineal
7. _____ peroneal
8. _____ ileum
9. _____ ilium
10. _____ dysphagia
11. _____ dysphasia
12. _____ regimen
13. _____ regime
14. _____ track
15. _____ tract

A. The area referring to the fibula or outer side of the leg.

B. Illegal.

C. Difficulty swallowing.

D. A systematic course of diet, therapy, or exercise.

E. The term referring to the area between the scrotum and anus in a male or vulva and anus in a female.

F. To call forth, as in a response.

G. The third portion of the small intestine.

H. A system of organs.

I. An impairment in the production of speech.

J. A brand name for bandages and wraps.

K. Broad, flaring portion of the hip bone.

L. A playing card or supreme achiever.

M. A government or social system.

N. Acronym for angiotensin-converting enzyme.

O. A pathway.

Soundalike Multiple Choice

Choose the correct term to complete each sentence.

1. She presented to the mental health clinic with a flat _____.
   - A. affect
   - B. effect

2. The patient was started on a new medical _____.
   - A. regime
   - B. regimen

3. The child's _____ membranes were pink and moist.
   - A. mucus
   - B. mucous

4. We turned our attention to the _____ of the inflamed appendix.
   - A. site
   - B. sight

5. The CT scan showed a _____ mass in the left lung.
   - A. discreet
   - B. discrete

6. The patient had no history of smoking, drinking, or _____ drug use.
   - A. elicit
   - B. illicit

7. After the surgery, she was given a _____ of IV gentamicin for her infection.
   - A. bullous
   - B. bolus

8. We could not _____ a response from the patient to any questions we asked.
   - A. elicit
   - B. illicit

9. The doctor ordered _____ x-ray films of the lumbar spine.
   - A. plain
   - B. plane

10. The patient works as a home health _____.
    - A. aid
    - B. aide

Word Definitions

Using a medical dictionary or other medical resource, look up and analyze the following terms. Indicate the prefix, the root word (or combining form), and suffix, as well as the definition of each term.

1. tachycardia
   prefix: _____
   root (combining form): _____
   suffix: _____
   definition: _____

2. hematopoiesis
   prefix: _____
   root (combining form): _____
   suffix: _____
   definition: _____

3. hemicolectomy
   prefix: _____
   root (combining form): _____
   suffix: _____
   definition: _____

4. gynecomastia
   prefix: _____
   root (combining form): _____
   suffix: _____
   definition: _____

5. polydipsia
   prefix: _____
   root (combining form): _____
   suffix: _____
   definition: _____

6. hypothermia
   prefix: _____
   root (combining form): _____
   suffix: _____
   definition: _____

7. esophagogastrostomy
   prefix: _____
   root (combining form): _____
   suffix: _____
   definition: _____

8. pneumonia
   prefix: _____
   root (combining form): _____
   suffix: _____
   definition: _____

9. euthermic
   prefix: _____
   root (combining form): _____
   suffix: _____
   definition: _____

10. subpleural
    prefix: _____
    root (combining form): _____
    suffix: _____
    definition: _____

Anatomic Terms Quiz

Fill in the blank with the correct term.

1. The knee is _____ to the ankle.

2. The heart is _____ to the lungs.

3. The nose is _____ to the chin.

4. The sagittal plane divides the body into _____ and _____ segments.

5. The stomach is in the _____ cavity.

6. The skin is _____ to the muscles.

7. The _____ section divides the body or an organ into anterior and posterior parts.

8. The _____ plane runs through the midline.

9. The arms are _____ to the trunk.

10. The _____ plane runs front to back.

Creating Medical Words

Consider the meaning of the combining form from which the medical term is made and write the meaning of the medical term. (You have not yet learned many of these terms but can build their meaning from the word parts.)

Combining form	Meaning	Medical Term	Meaning of Term
adenoid/o	adenoids	adenoidectomy	1. _____
laryng/o	larynx	laryngoplasty	2. _____
hepat/o	liver	hepatomegaly	3. _____
hyster/o	uterus	hysterectomy	4. _____
lith/o	stone, calculus	lithotripsy	5. _____
leuk/o	white	leukopenia	6. _____
nephr/o	kidney	nephrology	7. _____
cyan/o	blue	cyanosis	8. _____
pneum/o	lung; air	pneumonitis	9. _____
path/o	disease	pathologist	10. _____
rhin/o	nose	rhinorrhea	11. _____
arthr/o	joint	arthralgia	12. _____
gastr/o	stomach	gastritis	13. _____
cardi/o	heart	cardiology	14. _____
dermat/o	skin	dermatology	15. _____

Fill in the Blanks

Fill in the correct term for the definition listed. You have not yet learned many of these terms, but you can build them from the word parts that make up each word.

cardiac   hematemesis   bronchial
hemiplegia   thoracic   endometrial
myopathy   hemorrhage   uterine
appendicitis   cholangiogram   dermatitis

Definition	Term
1. pertaining to the thorax	_____
2. relating to the bronchus	_____
3. inflammation of the skin	_____
4. vomiting of blood	_____
5. paralysis of one side of the body	_____
6. pertaining to the endometrium	_____
7. inflammation of the appendix	_____
8. pertaining to the heart	_____
9. flowing of blood through vessel walls	_____
10. disease or abnormality of muscular tissue	_____
11. written record of the bile ducts	_____
12. pertaining to the uterus	_____

TRANSCRIPTION PRACTICE

Open your word processing software. Insert the student CD-ROM disk and locate the dictation for this chapter. Listen to the dictation number and transcribe the 10 sentences dictated on the CD. Be sure to listen carefully to each sentence before transcribing it. Use a medical dictionary or other medical references to assist you in finding the correct spelling of the words in each sentence. When finished, print one copy for your instructor and save a copy to your student disk.

MEDICAL CORRESPONDENCE AND REPORTS

4

OBJECTIVES

After completing this chapter, you will be able to:

- List the elements of a standard business letter.
- Describe the general formatting guidelines of medical reports.
- Identify different types of medical reports and explain how and when each is used.
- Describe the transcription process and strategies to succeed at transcribing reports, including organization of files and folders on the computer.
- Understand the transcription instructions for this course.

INTRODUCTION

The work performed by a medical transcriptionist involves the preparation of medical documents, correspondence, and other paperwork relating to various patient matters. These documents provide a means of communication among physicians, nurses, and allied health professionals who plan and conduct the care and treatment of the individual patient. They also create a legal record that benefits the patient and his or her healthcare providers. Therefore, these documents must be consistent in form and appearance and easy to read. This chapter describes the types of correspondence, medical forms, reports, and documents typically encountered when documenting patient care and outlines the general rules governing format and style in the preparation of those documents.

STANDARD BUSINESS LETTERS

Written communication is an essential part of a physician's interaction with patients and others. Letters and e-mails are routinely sent to patients, other medical providers, insurance companies, and even representatives of the court in matters involving litigation. Even if a physician is not particularly skilled in dictating correspondence, a medical transcriptionist must be able to transcribe the dictated material accurately and produce a neatly printed document. Part of this ability lies in the transcriptionist's familiarity with the rules of formatting written communication. It is important to be familiar with the structural components of a standard business letter and the ways in which they contribute to the overall design of the letter, as shown in Figure 4.1.

The **full-block letter style** is the easiest to use with word-processing and Windows software because tabs,

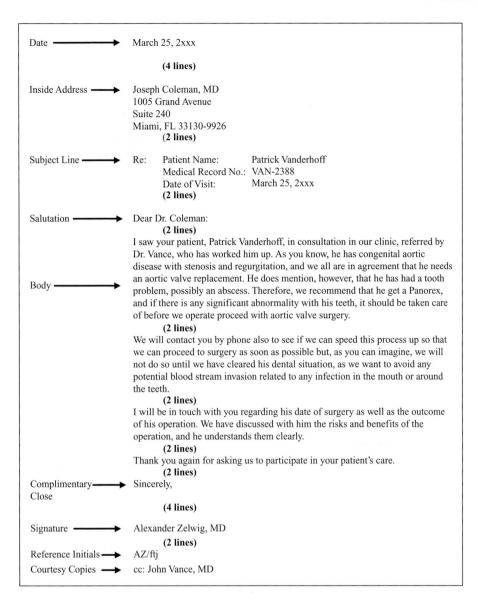

Date ──────▶	March 25, 2xxx
	(4 lines)
Inside Address ──────▶	Joseph Coleman, MD
	1005 Grand Avenue
	Suite 240
	Miami, FL 33130-9926
	(2 lines)

Subject Line ──────▶ Re: Patient Name: Patrick Vanderhoff
              Medical Record No.: VAN-2388
              Date of Visit: March 25, 2xxx
(2 lines)

Salutation ──────▶ Dear Dr. Coleman:
(2 lines)

Body ──────▶ I saw your patient, Patrick Vanderhoff, in consultation in our clinic, referred by Dr. Vance, who has worked him up. As you know, he has congenital aortic disease with stenosis and regurgitation, and we all are in agreement that he needs an aortic valve replacement. He does mention, however, that he has had a tooth problem, possibly an abscess. Therefore, we recommend that he get a Panorex, and if there is any significant abnormality with his teeth, it should be taken care of before we operate proceed with aortic valve surgery.

(2 lines)

We will contact you by phone also to see if we can speed this process up so that we can proceed to surgery as soon as possible but, as you can imagine, we will not do so until we have cleared his dental situation, as we want to avoid any potential blood stream invasion related to any infection in the mouth or around the teeth.

(2 lines)

I will be in touch with you regarding his date of surgery as well as the outcome of his operation. We have discussed with him the risks and benefits of the operation, and he understands them clearly.

(2 lines)

Thank you again for asking us to participate in your patient's care.

(2 lines)

Complimentary ──────▶ Sincerely,
Close
(4 lines)

Signature ──────▶ Alexander Zelwig, MD
(2 lines)
Reference Initials ──────▶ AZ/ftj
Courtesy Copies ──────▶ cc: John Vance, MD

FIGURE 4.1. **Full-Block Letter Style.** This style is the easiest to type because all structural parts of the letter begin at the left margin.

centering, and other formatting commands are omitted. All structural parts of the letter begin at the left margin. This is the style most commonly used in medical correspondence, and it is very popular because it takes the least amount of time to create and is the easiest to read.

In medical correspondence, physicians sometimes include headings similar to those found in medical reports to delineate their findings. This text is typed at the left margin in full-block style, followed by a colon and one or two spaces before the text begins. The amount of character spaces after a colon in text is largely dependent upon the policies of the facility or company for which you work. *The Book of Style for Medical Transcription, 3rd ed.,* advocates the use of a single space following a period or a colon. Numbered items are enumerated at the left margin, with the number followed by one space and the text. Each numbered item is single-spaced under the one before it, unless the items are long and single spacing would be too cumbersome to read.

If a letter requires a second page, carry at least two lines of text over to page 2. The second page should have a header at the top of the page that includes the recipient's name, the patient's name, the date of the letter, and the page number:

Sanjay M. Chakra, MD
Re: Patient's Name
October 12, 20xx
Page 2

The **complimentary close** is the term, expression, or phrase that immediately precedes the signature on a letter. It is placed two lines beneath the last line of the body. Only the first word of the complimentary close is capitalized, and the last word is followed by a comma. Closings include such standard phrases as:

Sincerely,
Very truly yours,
With kind regards,

The signature and title lines follow the closing. The writer's name is typed four lines below the complimentary close in order to leave ample space for the signature. The affiliation of the writer may be added on the next lines:

Sincerely,
John J. Morrison, MD
Thoracic Surgery Division

Because medical records are created and transmitted electronically, "original" documents, including letters, are viewed and signed by the physician via computer. The **Electronic Signatures in Global and National Commerce Act (E-Sign Act)**, enacted into law in 2000 by President Clinton, provides that an electronic signature on a document has the same legal effect as a handwritten signature on a document. This applies to all documents transmitted electronically in all areas of business. By definition, an **electronic signature** is an electronic symbol or process attached to or associated with a record by a person with the intent to sign the record. Physicians typically sign their reports electronically as entries in a patient's medical record. The physician **authenticates**, or signs, the report by entering a unique code or password that verifies the identity of the signer, thereby creating an individual "signature" on the document. The electronic signature then appears as typed text on the document. Signature lines generated in this manner are usually prefaced by a statement such as "Electronically signed by John Doe, MD, on (date and time)." Other information such as the physician's title may also be included in the signature block.

At the end of the letter, it is standard business practice to place reference initials and/or transcriptionist's initials or identification number two lines below the signature or title. This information can be entered into the document manually or electronically and serves to record who dictated the letter and who transcribed it. This practice can be particularly useful if the letter was produced in a large facility such as a hospital where documents are typed by a number of transcriptionists on a computer network server. The dictator's initials are typed in capital letters, followed by a slash, followed by the transcriptionist's initials in lowercase letters, or identification number:

JJM/mlg
or
JJM/394

Some computer systems omit the use of the writer's initials if the name is already typed in the signature block. Only the initials or identification number of the person who typed the document would appear, either in capital or lowercase letters:

/394
or
/mlg

MEDICAL REPORTS

A patient's medical record, whether in the hospital or in the clinic setting, is composed of several types of reports, notes, and other documents. The purpose of these records is to ensure that patients are adequately informed about their treatment options and to ensure that the information regarding a patient's history is complete and is readily available to any practitioner involved in the patient's care.

General Formatting Guidelines

Most hospitals and healthcare providers have specific guidelines concerning the format and style of the documents they produce as well as built-in templates for their digital platforms. Be sure to conform to the office or hospital policy when transcribing documents. Styles do vary, however, and while one method is probably no more "correct" than another, it is important to be aware of how the formatting or placement of various portions of text affects the document's effectiveness as a whole. All of the medical document illustrations in this chapter contain the basic elements outlined below, and these guidelines should prove acceptable in the most common medical transcription situations.

Page Numbering

Pages of a document are numbered consecutively. The page numbering can appear in a variety of positions on the page, and numbering styles can differ, depending on the preferences of the facility. Generally, the first page of a document is not numbered. The number can be part of the document text, or it may appear in the document's footer. Alternatively, the page number can be placed in the header at the top of each page, as many providers use headers to place reference information about the patient and current page number of each page of the report.

Headings

Section headings are used to document the evaluation and management of a patient in a logical fashion. Information may be set out in separate headings, or may be included in the history section of the report. Headings, if and when used, should follow the style and font required by the physician or facility. Some facilities use initial caps for headings whereas others use all caps and bold, and you should follow the preferences of your employer. However, be aware that an effort is underway in healthcare delivery toward standardization of report formats to facilitate meaningful data exchange in the electronic health record that will enable national, and even global, exchange of health data. The standardized format includes the following features:

- Major section headings use all capital letters.
- Subheadings use initial capital letters.
- The chief complaint, diagnoses, preoperative diagnoses, postoperative diagnoses, names of operations and similar entries are listed vertically.
- The word "diagnosis" is changed to "diagnoses" when more than one diagnosis is provided.
- Obvious headings that are not dictated may be inserted, but this is not required.
- Major sections of reports are separated by a double space.
- Subheadings are listed vertically at the left margin to assist the reader in identifying particular subsections.
- Abbreviations and brief forms of words are not used in headings except for such widely used and readily recognizable abbreviations such as HEENT, if dictated.

A typical medical report contains most or all of the following section headings, or a variation of them, which outline the patient's history, diagnosis, and plan of care.

- Chief Complaint. The chief complaint states the specific reason the patient sought medical care. It is stated in a short, concise statement, or sometimes stated using the patient's own words:

CHIEF COMPLAINT
Possible left foot fracture.
CHIEF COMPLAINT
"I fell on the ice and my knee hurts."

- History of Present Illness. The history of present illness (HPI) includes the complete story of why the patient is seeking medical attention. It includes all of the information pertinent to the chief complaint, both positive and negative. It is usually arranged in chronological order beginning with the earliest relevant facts and proceeding to the point where the patient was admitted. Sometimes a physician will dictate all positive historical findings related to the present illness, regardless of where the information normally would be placed. For example, a family history of sickle cell anemia may be mentioned in the history of a patient admitted for anemia, even though it may also be repeated in the family history farther down in the body of the report.
- Past Medical History. This section includes information about previous illnesses, injuries, or

chronic conditions a patient has or may have had. When dictating a past medical history of an infant or small child, items such as prenatal history, feeding history, growth and development, and immunizations may also be discussed in this section.

- Past Surgical History. This section contains information about past surgical procedures the patient has undergone.
- Medications. This section contains details about the medications that the patient is currently taking and the dosages of each medication.
- Allergies. This section lists a patient's allergies. Some physicians also dictate sensitivities to foods or other items here, such as rashes that may result from seafood or latex. Many facilities prefer that allergy information appear more prominently in the report, specifying that it be typed in all capital letters, underlined, or bolded.
- Family History. This section outlines information about any hereditary or family illnesses and provides evidence for considering those diseases as well as infections or contagious illnesses to which the patient may be exposed.
- Social History. This section includes a patient's marital status, and work and living situations. Additional information, including lifestyle habits such as smoking history, alcohol use, or illicit drug use may also be included.
- Review of Systems. This section contains a brief overall review of the medical condition of the patient's body organs systems at the time of the encounter, which may or may not be relevant to the HPI or the reason for admission. The systems review may be contained in one paragraph or may be subdivided into separate categories (such as pulmonary, cardiovascular, gastrointestinal, genitourinary, musculoskeletal, lymphatic, skin, hematologic, neurologic, and/or psychiatric). When all systems are negative, a brief phrase or sentence will be used, such as "noncontributory" or "All systems were reviewed and are negative."
- Physical Examination. The physical examination section of the report outlines the physician's thorough examination of the patient, including observations and findings, laid out in subheadings. The subheadings are addressed in a standard order from head to toe. They can appear in paragraph form underneath the main heading or as subheadings flush left under the main heading in a standardized format. These subheadings may include the following:
  - Vital Signs. This is usually first in the physical exam findings and indicates the patient's vital signs such as temperature, blood pressure, pulse, respirations, height, and weight. Extra

items such as body mass index (BMI) or oxygen saturation might also be indicated here.

- General Appearance. This section indicates the general appearance of the patient, such as personal hygiene and mood.
- HEENT (head, eyes, ears, nose, and throat).
- Neck.
- Chest.
- Lungs.
- Heart.
- Abdomen.
- Extremities.
- Neurologic Exam.
- Other headings may be included, such as a pelvic examination or rectal examination, when indicated.

- Laboratory Data. The laboratory data section includes information about laboratory and diagnostic testing results, such as initial blood work, x-rays, or urinalysis.
- Assessment and Plan. As in a clinic note, the assessment and plan detail the physician's findings and diagnoses based on the information already presented and, in order of problem presented, outlines a treatment plan, including procedures and their rationale, and plans for following the course of the patient's illness. The assessment and plan may appear together as one heading or be divided into two separate headings.

Text

All medical reports include the **demographic information** of the patient, which is a collective term encompassing the patient's statistical data. This information includes the patient's full name, date of birth, any internal record number, and the date of the encounter. If the note continues on a second page, a header containing the same or additional information appears at the top of all subsequent pages. The report also includes a place for the signature (either manually or electronic) for the person who dictated the report. In most reports, the text is typed single-spaced, in block style, with all lines flush left. All word-processing programs and digital platforms provide default margin settings for the top, bottom, right, and left sides of the page.

A paragraph that continues from one page to the next should have at least two lines of text on each page. A three-line paragraph should not be divided. Some facilities require that an entire paragraph be moved from the previous page in order to keep it from being divided by a page break. Most facilities prefer the signature line of the document to appear with at least two lines of text on the last page if not entered electronically by the proprietary software used.

In all medical reports, dictators often use abbreviations and short, clipped phrases in order to condense information as much as possible or to dictate findings as quickly as possible. When transcribing reports, you must type all abbreviations correctly so that no confusion may arise as to their exact meanings. For example, a physician who dictates the abbreviation *PVC* may be referring to a "premature ventricular contraction" or "pulmonary venous congestion." If you are not sure of the exact meaning of the abbreviation, you should follow the facility's or company's policy regarding the transcription of abbreviations. Some mandate that all abbreviations should be spelled out; in that instance, if you are not sure of the abbreviation's meaning, you should transcribe the abbreviation and flag the report to verify its meaning with the dictator. Other facilities wish all abbreviations to be transcribed as dictated. Many organizations have an approved list of abbreviations with clearly defined definitions that are acceptable for medical reports; follow those guidelines when encountering abbreviations in dictation.

Short phrases and incomplete sentences, even though they may omit a subject or verb needed for correct sentence structure, are acceptable and should be transcribed as dictated. For example:

REVIEW OF SYSTEMS
No nausea or vomiting.
ALLERGIES
None known.
OBJECTIVE
Neck supple. Oral cavity clear. Abdomen soft and nontender. Extremities without edema.

In addition, physicians may indicate headings for each section or simply dictate the narrative without indicating headings at all. You should be familiar with the type of information contained under each heading of a medical report in order to identify each section as it is being dictated and separate paragraphs accordingly.

In the review of systems and physical examination sections, formats may vary but commonly subheadings may appear flush with the left margin underneath the section heading. The information continues on the same line, using a colon after each subheading:

REVIEW OF SYSTEMS
CONSTITUTIONAL: No problems noted.
HEENT: Eyes appear jaundiced. Throat is clear.
CARDIOVASCULAR: No problems noted.
RESPIRATORY: No problems noted.
GASTROINTESTINAL: See details in the history of present illness.
GENITOURINARY: No problems noted.
MUSCULOSKELETAL: No problems noted.
INTEGUMENTARY: No problems noted.
NEUROLOGICAL: No problems noted.

PHYSICAL EXAMINATION

VITAL SIGNS: Blood pressure 140/90, pulse 72, respirations 16, temperature 98.7.

GENERAL: Patient alert and cooperative with exam. No apparent distress.

HEENT: Sclerae are anicteric. Conjunctivae are normal. Nares patent. No lymphadenopathy.

NECK: Supple, no masses, thyroid not enlarged.

HEART: Regular rate and rhythm. No murmurs.

LUNGS: Clear to auscultation bilaterally.

ABDOMEN: Soft, nontender, no masses or hepatomegaly. No rebound, rigidity, or guarding.

EXTREMITIES: No clubbing, cyanosis, or edema. Pulses are 2+. There is full range of motion.

NEUROLOGIC: Cranial nerves intact. Sensory and motor intact.

SKIN: No rashes noted on exam.

Signature

All medical reports contain at least one signature line, entered manually or electronically, for the physician who will sign it, as well as additional lines for dictating physicians, if required. If you are creating a signature line manually, begin at the left margin, or at a point designated by the facility, and type the desired number of spaces with the underline key depressed to reach the desired length of the line. Sufficient space should be allotted so that the handwriting of the signer does not overlap the line. Underneath the signature line, type the name of the person whose signature will be on the line. The physician may require the use of a descriptive title under the signature line as well. If there is more than one signature line on the document, allow three or four lines of space between individual signature lines. It is common practice to include the dictator's and transcriptionist's initials underneath the signature line, as well as the dates of the dictation and transcription of the report.

Time and Date Stamp

The date and time of dictation and transcription is typically indicated below the signature at the end of each report. It may be written as "D" and "T" or "Dictated" and "Transcribed" and is followed by a colon and the appropriate information. Most digital platforms enter this information electronically, but if entered manually, enter the date and time flush left below the initials of the dictator and transcriptionist, following the format as outlined by the facility.

Types of Medical Reports

Patients are assessed continuously throughout their care by different medical providers. This assessment and reassessment process is documented in different types

---

QUICK CHECK 4.1 ✓

Circle the letter corresponding to the best answer to the following questions.

1. The collective term that encompasses the patient's data in a report is the
   A. medical record number.
   B. demographic information.
   C. footer.
   D. none of the above.

2. A paragraph that continues from one page to the next should have at least _____ lines of text on each page.
   A. three
   B. one
   C. four
   D. two

3. A page number placed at the bottom of a page is said to appear in the _____ of the document.
   A. footer
   B. header
   C. title page
   D. signature line

4. The process of entering a unique code to verify the identity of a person signing a document transmitted electronically is called
   A. a full-block signature.
   B. authentication.
   C. the electronic marking.
   D. none of the above.

5. In most reports, the text is
   A. triple-spaced.
   B. double-spaced.
   C. single-spaced.
   D. spaced according to the transcriptionist's choice.

of reports, including clinic notes, history and physical examinations, operative reports, consultation reports, and discharge summaries.

Clinic Note

A physician dictates a note into a patient's chart after each and every encounter with the patient, either by phone or in person. Also referred to as a **chart note**, a **clinic note** documenting a typical patient visit includes a chief complaint or reason for the visit, the supporting information about the illness and patient, the findings on physical examination, and a plan of treatment. The clinic note is usually short (only a few paragraphs), but some may carry over into subsequent pages.

Clinic Note

PATIENT NAME: Alan Deloja

MEDICAL RECORD NO.:   55-84711

DATE OF SERVICE: 04/21/xxxx

ATTENDING PHYSICIAN: Eric T. Barmena, MD

CLINIC NOTE

REASON FOR VISIT
The patient presents to our office for a scar on his nasal bridge that has been present for several months.

HISTORY OF PRESENT ILLNESS
The patient is a 35-year-old male who reportedly sustained a sunburn last summer while boating on the lake. Soon after, he noticed a blister on his nose that progressed to an open wound. This healed rapidly, leaving the subsequent deformity.

PAST MEDICAL HISTORY
He sustained a left elbow fracture 10 years ago while playing football.

PAST SURGICAL HISTORY
Open reduction and internal fixation of the left elbow fracture, as mentioned above. Tonsillectomy and adenoidectomy at age 8.

MEDICATIONS
None.

ALLERGIES
No known drug allergies.

SOCIAL HISTORY
He smokes 2 packs per day. No alcohol and no illicit drug use.

REVIEW OF SYSTEMS
A 10-point review of systems was performed and was negative.

PHYSICAL EXAMINATION
Vital Signs: Temperature 98.7, blood pressure 120/85, pulse 65, respirations 16, and weight 225 pounds. The patient is a well-developed, pleasant gentleman in no acute distress. Focused examination of the nasal deformity reveals a scar measuring 1.2 cm vertically and 8 mm horizontally. It is hyperpigmented. It is an atrophic scar. The surrounding nasal skin demonstrates much more thickness than average with adherence in almost all the nasal zones. There is really no significant skin immobility that there usually is in the upper half of the nasal bridge.

ASSESSMENT
Atrophic scar of the nasal bridge of significant size in the upper half of the nasal skin envelope with surrounding strong tissue adherence to the underlying skeleton.

PLAN
After the discussion above and after understanding all the risks, benefits, and alternatives, the patient agreed to proceed to surgery for adjacent tissue rearrangement and excision of the overlying scar. He will be placed on the operative schedule for next month and come in approximately a week prior to that time for preoperative clearance.

_____

Electronically signed by Eric T. Barmena, MD

ETB/xx
D: 04/21/xxxx
T: 04/21/xxxx

Some clinic notes follow a formatting style called **SOAP**, which is an acronym for $\underline{S}$ubjective, $\underline{O}$bjective, $\underline{A}$ssessment, and $\underline{P}$lan. A clinic note using the SOAP format is similar in appearance to that of other notes, except that the headings used in the note are simply *Subjective, Objective, Assessment,* and *Plan.* Each heading is described as follows:

- The *Subjective* section details the reason for the visit and the immediate history behind the patient's visit.
- The *Objective* section sets out the physical examination findings and results of laboratory or other diagnostic tests performed with regard to the patient's problem.

- The *Assessment* follows the presentation of the history and physical examination and contains the physician's discussion of the diagnosis based on the information presented.
- Finally, the *Plan* indicates the treatment plan developed by the physician, given the patient's diagnostic assessment in the report, and plans for further followup, if applicable.

Most chart or clinic notes loosely follow the SOAP format for conveying information. Some notes, while following the SOAP format, use additional subheadingsfor a patient's past history, medications, and allergies, as well as additional headings for laboratory and diagnostic testing results.

SOAP Note

PATIENT NAME:	Roshaunda Brown
MEDICAL RECORD NO.:	00-2468
DATE OF SERVICE:	08/01/xx
ATTENDING PHYSICIAN:	John Smith, MD

SUBJECTIVE

This is a 16-month-old African American girl, a regular patient of mine, who is here today for a physical for preschool and tuberculin skin testing. Mom says the child has been doing fine. She was last seen by me several months ago and all her immunizations are current. Lead level was obtained at that time which was within normal limits.

OBJECTIVE
Temperature 97.8, head circumference 47 cm, weight 24 pounds, height 31 inches. General: Alert, active, and well nourished. HEENT: Unremarkable. Heart: Regular rate and rhythm. No heart murmurs. Lungs: Clear to auscultation bilaterally. Abdomen: Soft and depressible. Normoactive bowel sounds. No masses palpable. The rest of the exam was unremarkable.

ASSESSMENT
Well child normal physical exam. Mom was given reassurance. Immunizations are current.

PLAN
Tuberculin skin test was placed to be read within the next 2–3 days, and child is to return to clinic in 2 months for her next regular checkup. Mom voiced understanding and agrees to follow up accordingly.

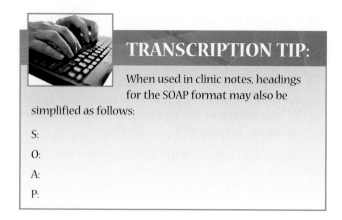

TRANSCRIPTION TIP:

When used in clinic notes, headings for the SOAP format may also be simplified as follows:

S:

O:

A:

P:

History and Physical Examination

A **history and physical examination** (also called an H&P) is dictated by a physician when a patient is admitted to the hospital. Obtaining an accurate history is the critical first step in determining the cause of a patient's problem and is the foundation of the patient's hospital record. It is usually a priority item because it is a summary of the patient's information known at the time of admission and is referred to when making plans for treatment during the hospital stay. The H&P follows a standard format of approaching the patient's complaint, including an assessment of the problem and a plan of care.

Operative Report

The **operative report** (also referred to as an **op note**) is dictated by the operating physician or assistant immediately after completion of surgery. It contains a detailed narrative of the operative procedure, including the preoperative and postoperative diagnoses, the type of surgery or surgeries that were performed, the name(s) of the surgeon(s) and attending nursing staff, the type of anesthesia and the name of the anesthesiologist, estimated blood loss (EBL), complications encountered, operative findings, and a detailed description of the operative procedure itself. Often the report will end with disposition or the location to which the patient was transferred after leaving the operating room (usually the recovery room) and the condition of the patient at the time of transfer. An example of an operative report is provided.

History and Physical Examination

PATIENT NAME: Ella Mae Jones

MEDICAL RECORD NO.:   4599900

DATE OF ADMISSION: 07/15/xxxx

ATTENDING PHYSICIAN: Frederick M. Frazier, MD

HISTORY AND PHYSICAL EXAMINATION

CHIEF COMPLAINT
Shortness of breath.

HISTORY OF PRESENT ILLNESS
The patient is a 79-year-old female with longstanding end-stage renal disease due to hypertensive nephropathy who was admitted today to the medicine service. She complains of 3 weeks of right-sided parasternal chest pain that radiated around to her back as well as worsening dyspnea on exertion. She also has malaise, dry cough, vague abdominal pain, and worsening orthopnea and PND.

PAST MEDICAL HISTORY
Extensive stage, newly diagnosed small-cell lung cancer. End-stage renal disease, on dialysis.

MEDICATIONS
1. Lipitor 80 mg p.o. at bedtime.
2. Renagel 800 mg p.o. before meals.
3. Lisinopril 20 mg p.o. daily.
4. Nephro-Vite 1 tablet p.o. daily.

ALLERGIES
No known drug allergies.

SOCIAL HISTORY
She is a previous smoker, about a 20-pack-year history. No alcohol or drugs. She used to work as a school teacher.

FAMILY HISTORY
Her father died of an MI at age 72. Mother died in her early 70s of renal failure and hypertension. She has 5 sisters, and some family members with diabetes.

PHYSICAL EXAMINATION
The patient looks well and in no acute distress. HEENT: Normocephalic and atraumatic. Pupils equal, round, and reactive to light. Oropharynx is clear. Neck is supple without lymphadenopathy. Chest is clear to auscultation except for decreased breath sounds on the right side at the right base. The left lung is clear. Cardiovascular exam is regular rate and rhythm, normal S1 and S2, no murmurs, rubs, or gallops. Abdomen exam shows normal bowel sounds, nontender, nondistended, no hepatosplenomegaly. Extremities show no clubbing, cyanosis, or edema. Neurologic exam shows she is alert and oriented. She ambulates without difficulty.

DIAGNOSTIC STUDIES
Sodium 138, potassium 4.9, chloride 95, bicarbonate 24, BUN 40, creatinine 8.3, glucose 100, calcium 10.3. White count 13,000, hematocrit 35.2, and her platelet count is 336.

ASSESSMENT
Newly diagnosed lung cancer. With the pleural fluid that is positive for carcinoma, she has obviously quite locally advanced disease, and of course, there is the issue of the adrenal nodules and adenopathy, so I would consider an extensive-stage small-cell lung cancer.

PLAN
We will admit the patient for cisplatin and etoposide. She will continue to have dialysis through the chemotherapy. We will continue her on hemodialysis and the renal team will follow with us.

_____

Electronically signed by Frederick M. Frazier, MD

FMF/xx
T: 07/15/xxxx
D: 07/15/xxxx

Operative Report

PATIENT NAME:	Sandra Wilkinson
MEDICAL RECORD NO.:	8442-3355
DATE OF ADMISSION:	03/02/xxxx
ATTENDING PHYSICIAN:	Jonathan K. Burton, MD

OPERATIVE REPORT

PREOPERATIVE DIAGNOSIS
Abdominal pannus secondary to weight loss.

POSTOPERATIVE DIAGNOSIS
Abdominal pannus secondary to weight loss.

OPERATION
Abdominal panniculectomy.

SURGEON
Eugene Z. Hodges, MD

ASSISTANT
Richard W. McNeal, MD

ANESTHESIA
General.

DRAINS
Three 10 mm Jackson-Pratt drains connected to bulb suction.

COMPLICATIONS
None.

INDICATIONS FOR PROCEDURE
This is a 42-year-old Hispanic female who is status post gastric bypass surgery last year. She lost over 100 pounds, going from 280 to 160 pounds. Since losing weight, she has developed excessive skin and subcutaneous tissue in the lower abdomen with an overhanging pannus. She is an excellent patient for abdominal panniculectomy.

PROCEDURE
After informed consent was obtained, the patient was taken to the operating room and laid supine on the operating room table. General anesthesia was induced and the abdomen was prepped and draped in the usual sterile fashion. A transverse incision was made in the suprapubic region extending to the flanks past the anterosuperior iliac spines bilaterally. This incision was then made and carried down through the subcutaneous tissue to the abdominal fascia. Cautery was used to control bleeders. Next, a circumferential incision was made around the umbilicus. The umbilicus was dissected down to the fascia, preserving a healthy stalk. The abdominal wall apron was dissected superiorly in the plane above the rectus fascia to the costal margins and xiphoid process. Next, traction was applied to the apron and the apron was pulled downward. The excess skin and subcutaneous tissue was excised. The wound was approximated with staples and hash marks were made to line up the closure. The staples were removed and a final check for hemostasis was performed. Three 10 mm Jackson-Pratt drains were placed and brought out through the suprapubic region. These were secured with 2-0 nylon drain sutures. Closure was performed with interrupted 2-0 Polysorb for the Scarpa layer, 3-0 Polysorb for the deep dermal layer, and a 4-0 Monocryl subcuticular for the skin. The umbilicus was brought out through a new incision in the midline by cutting out a new vertically oriented ellipse of skin. The umbilicus was secured with interrupted 4-0 Polysorb for the deep dermal layer and interrupted 4-0 nylon for the skin. Dry dressings were placed. The drains were attached to bulb suction. An abdominal binder was placed. The patient was awakened from anesthesia and transferred to recovery room in stable condition. The patient tolerated the procedure well. All instrument and sponge counts were correct at the end of the case.

Electronically signed by Eugene Z. Hodges, MD

EZH/xx
D: 03/02/xxxx
T: 03/02/xxxx

Other information may be dictated in the description of an operative procedure, including the following items:

- Materials, such as screws, wires, pins, or other objects are often left in the patient as part of the surgical procedure. Listen for brand names, sizes, and location of such objects in the dictation. The names of these materials can be found in a surgical word book, medical equipment word book, or online by entering a search into Google or other Internet search engine. The Internet can be helpful, especially if the material is a brand name of a new product not yet included in printed references.
- Types of closure. Types and brands of sutures (stitches) and other closure devices are described when closing each layer of the body cut during surgery. The tissues may be closed with stitches with such names as Vicryl, chromic, catgut, Prolene, Maxon, etc. Know which type of suture is capitalized as well as the method of closure. Listen for terms such as mattress, pursestring, horizontal, and transverse to describe suture closure. The skin may be closed with clips, adhesive strips (also called Steri-Strips), or tape. Wounds are covered with sterile gauze with names such as Adaptic, Kling, Xeroform, and 4 × 4's (dictated as "four by fours"), as well as dressings, or slings. Again, brand names, specific sizes, and types are dictated and can be located in medical references specializing in surgical words and equipment.
- Sponge, needle, and instrument counts. In order to avoid having foreign materials or objects inadvertently left inside the patient, many hospitals require that an accurate count of sponges, needles, and instruments used during the operation be conducted and dictated into the record. You may hear the dictator say, "Sponge, needle, and instrument counts were correct times 2," meaning that the count was performed twice for greater security.

Consultation Report

When a patient's physician desires a second opinion about a patient's condition or diagnosis, he or she may request a consulting physician to evaluate the patient. A **consultation report** is dictated by this consulting physician to provide his or her evaluation of the patient, assessment of findings, and recommendations for treatment. The consultation may be dictated in a letter format to the attending physician or it can be dictated as a medical report and look similar in appearance and formatting as other reports. Both styles can contain subheadings such as History of Present Illness, Past History, Physical Examination, Impression, and Recommendations for Treatment. Illustrations of both styles are provided.

Consultation—Letter Style

July 1, 20xx

_____

_____

_____

Jon Peter Williams, MD
5400 Memorial Avenue
Dover, DE 19901

RE: *Name of Patient:*   Virginia Larson
     Medical Record No.:   0083368
     Date of Visit: June 15, 20xx

Dear Dr. Williams:

Thank you for referring your patient, Virginia Larson, to our office for consultation. Her history dates back to a year ago when she developed worsening bilateral leg edema. Workup revealed enlarged retroperitoneal and mesenteric lymph nodes, right axillary lymph node involvement, and bilateral intrapulmonary parenchymal masses, a 3.5 cm left upper lobe lesion and a 1.5 cm right upper lobe lesion. The patient received 6 cycles of CHOP and Rituxan, which she tolerated well. Her hypoproteinemia has completely resolved. Her most recent protein studies revealed a total protein of 6.3 and an albumin of 4.2, and the patient has had complete resolution of her lymphadenopathy and her pulmonary lesions by CT scan.

Past Medical History: Two cesarean sections and an abdominoplasty.

Current Medications: Aspirin 81 mg daily and Coumadin 2 mg daily.

Allergies: Penicillin causes a rash.

Social History: She is an administrative assistant. She is single. She does not smoke. She drinks alcohol socially.

Physical Examination: The patient is a well-developed, well-nourished female in no acute distress. Vital signs show weight 165.1 kg, height 157 cm, temperature 36.3 degrees C., pulse 71 and regular, respirations 16 and regular, blood pressure 130/80. Skin, head, ears, eyes, nose, and throat are unremarkable. Neck is supple and nontender. Lungs are clear to auscultation and percussion. Heart shows a regular rate and rhythm without murmurs or gallops. Abdomen is soft and nontender with normal bowel sounds and no organomegaly. Extremities are without cyanosis, clubbing, or edema.

Impression and Plan: Follicular small-cleave-cell lymphoma. The patient has had an excellent response to CHOP and Rituxan. However, her presentation is atypical with pulmonary intraparenchymal lesions, which would be uncommon for follicular lymphoma. I will ask our hematopathologists to look at the biopsy and see if there is any evidence of transformation. If there is, we should consider bone marrow transplant.

Thank you for allowing me to participate in the care of this interesting patient.

Sincerely,

_____

_____

_____

Fuller B. Bryant, MD

FBB/xx
D: 06/15/xxxx
T: 06/15/xxxx

PATIENT NAME: Margarita Sanchez

MEDICAL RECORD NO.:   77-2258

DATE OF SERVICE: 05/05/xxxx

ATTENDING PHYSICIAN: Luis Castillo, MD

CONSULTATION REPORT

CONSULTING PHYSICIAN
Cristina Fiore, MD

REASON FOR CONSULTATION
The patient is a 70-year-old pleasant Hispanic female with a history of SLE.

HISTORY OF PRESENT ILLNESS
The patient's problems started 5 years ago with a fall in the x-ray suite where she worked as a technician, with an apparent injury to her left wrist. Over time she developed severe diffuse musculoskeletal pain with myalgias along with fevers, sweats, dysphagia, and around a 40-pound weight loss, with poor sleep. Her symptoms have caused her total functional disability and she has relied on her husband for her care since that time.

Currently she complains of increasing fatigue, leg pains, and diffuse arthralgias since the last month. She denies any skin rash. She has had minimal hair loss lately, and she also denies any mucositis. She has intermittently noted discoloration and coldness of her fingers and toes with any cold exposure, and she continues to have dry mouth.

PAST MEDICAL HISTORY
SLE with secondary fibromyalgia, GERD, and irritable bowel syndrome.

MEDICATIONS
1. Prednisone 2.5 mg every evening.
2. Plaquenil 200 mg every evening.
3. Synthroid 0.5 mcg daily.
4. Nexium 40 mg daily.

REVIEW OF SYSTEMS
GENERAL: She has problems with sleep.
SKIN: She denies any skin rashes or psoriasis.
HEENT: She does complain of having dry eyes and dry mouth.
PULMONARY: She denies any history of pleurisy.
CARDIAC: She denies any history of pericarditis.
GASTROINTESTINAL: She has a history of irritable bowel and denies any problems with swallowing.
GYNECOLOGIC: She denies any vaginal discharge or bleeding.
EXTREMITIES: She has noted intermittent swelling of her extremities in the past and detailed musculoskeletal review is as per History of Present Illness.

PHYSICAL EXAMINATION
VITAL SIGNS: Weight 131 pounds, temperature 97.2, blood pressure 136/69, pain rated 8/10.
SKIN: Livido reticularis; however, there is no other skin rash.
HEENT: Head and neck exam reveals no thrush or ulcers.
LUNGS: Clear to auscultation bilaterally.
HEART: Regular rate and rhythm.
ABDOMEN: Soft and nontender. Bowel sounds are present.
EXTREMITIES: No pedal edema and nontender calves. There is crepitus in bilateral knees. There are positive fibromyalgia tender points.
NEUROLOGIC: No focal deficits.

IMPRESSION
Systemic lupus erythematosus.

RECOMMENDATION
I recommend she start on Plaquenil at a total dose of 400 mg daily. However, she will continue with her current prednisone dosage.

_____

Electronically signed by Christina Fiore, MD

CF/xx
D: 05/05/xxxx
T: 05/06/xxxx

Progress Note

A **progress note** documents a patient's day-to-day care while in the hospital. The attending physician dictates the progress note after meeting and examining the patient. A progress note is usually short and outlines any new findings since the patient's last examination, physical findings, any updated laboratory results, and the immediate plan of care based on the findings. A sample progress note is provided.

Progress Note

PATIENT NAME: Steve Burns

MEDICAL RECORD NO.:   OS-10088

DATE OF ADMISSION: 04/23/xxxx

ATTENDING PHYSICIAN: Harold B. Miller, MD

DAILY PROGRESS REPORT

PATIENT IDENTIFICATION
The patient is a 65-year-old male admitted with complications secondary to his non-Hodgkin lymphoma.

INTERVAL HOSPITAL COURSE
The patient received his methotrexate and rituximab without major complications. He is ambulating and he is eating. He is afebrile. We will continue with supportive care and close followup as well as his leucovorin.

_____

Electronically signed by Harold B. Miller, MD

HBM/xx
D: 04/23/xxxx
T: 04/23/xxxx

Discharge Summary

A **discharge summary** is dictated for each patient who is discharged from the hospital. It provides a chronological summary of the events that occurred during the patient's stay, including tests and other workups performed, and pertinent physical findings throughout the course of the hospital stay. The report concludes with a list of medications the patient was discharged on as well as any discharge instructions and followup information for the patient.

Discharge Summary

PATIENT NAME:	Roger A. Winfield, Jr.
MEDICAL RECORD NO.:	37762-0
DATE OF ADMISSION:	12/10/xxxx
DATE OF DISCHARGE:	12/13/xxxx
ATTENDING PHYSICIAN:	Kimberly Britton, MD

DISCHARGE SUMMARY

ADMITTING DIAGNOSIS
Abscess, right elbow, with right arm cellulitis.

PROCEDURES PERFORMED
1. Irrigation and debridement of right elbow abscess (done at patient's bedside in the emergency room).
2. Occupational therapy consultation.

BRIEF HISTORY
This is a 39-year-old male who noticed a blister over his right lateral epicondyle 2 weeks prior to admission. The patient attempted to lance the blister with a pin, which resulted in the spreading of redness and increase in pain and swelling. Patient initially tried at-home warm soaks and peroxide but it continued to progress. Patient denied any fever or chills on admission and reported to the emergency room for evaluation.

HOSPITAL COURSE
Patient was seen and evaluated and was found to have an erythematous and fluctuant area over his right lateral epicondyle/elbow. He had irrigation and debridement of this area done at the bedside under local sedation. Patient tolerated this without difficulty. He will be discharged after 24 hours of IV antibiotics and will follow up in a week's time.

CONDITION ON DISCHARGE
Stable and improved.

DISCHARGE MEDICATIONS
1. Colace 100 mg twice per day.
2. Oxycodone 5 mg, 1–2 tablets p.o. every 4–6 hours.
3. Keflex 500 mg 4 times per day for 7 days.

DISCHARGE INSTRUCTIONS
1. Regular diet.
2. Activity as tolerated to the right upper extremity.

FOLLOWUP INSTRUCTIONS
Patient is to follow up in a week's time.

_____

Electronically signed by Kimberly Britton, MD

KB/xx
D: 12/13/xxxx
T: 12/14/xxxx

QUICK CHECK 4.2 ✓

Match the following situations on the left to the type of medical document used on the right.

1. _____ A second opinion is needed.

2. _____ Documents a surgery done in the hospital.

3. _____ Summarizes a patient's hospital stay.

4. _____ The first document generated upon admission to the hospital.

5. _____ Generated during a visit in the outpatient setting.

A. Discharge Summary

B. History and Physical Exam

C. Consultation Report

D. Clinic Note

E. Operative Report

THE TRANSCRIPTION PROCESS

When learning any new skill, it is helpful to become familiar with the steps in the process. Transcription requires coordinating your eyes, ears, fingers, and foot (when using a foot pedal). Whatever the advances of technology and equipment, transcription will always require the production of neat, accurate medical documents from dictation; and this is best accomplished in an orderly, concise manner:

1. Prepare your workstation. Remove everything from your work space except the information and materials you need.
2. Access your word-processing software or company's digital platform.
3. Plug the headset into the speakers of the computer or dictating machine and put them on. Adjust your posture to enable your foot to reach the foot pedal comfortably.
4. Access the audio file.
5. Listen and transcribe the dictation. Make adjustments to the volume, speed, and tone as necessary. Replay the dictation to listen to a group of words again if needed. Stop as often as necessary to look up new or unfamiliar words for spelling and meaning.

TRANSCRIPTION TIP:

Depending on the discharge type, the discharge summary may have a different name. If the patient is being discharged to another facility (such as a nursing home or rehabilitation center), the dictator may refer to the note as a "transfer summary." If the patient dies while an inpatient, the dictator will refer to the note as a "death summary." A death summary must contain the date and time of death as well as the cause of death.

6. Proofread the document carefully and make corrections.
7. Save the document and submit it according to your employer's instructions regarding the transmission of completed documents.

STRATEGIES FOR SUCCESS

In transcription there is a lot of repetition. People generally seek medical care for the same chronic diseases and syndromes, have the same symptoms, and receive the same treatment. As a result, words and phrases describing illnesses and treatments will become familiar to you as you transcribe, making it easier to prepare medical reports as time goes on. However, following certain practices, as outlined below, will help you to increase speed and perform more efficiently, even when you are a novice in the field.

1. Keep your work environment quiet. Experienced medical transcriptionists know how important it is to have their surroundings as quiet as possible. Sometimes extraneous noise is unavoidable, such as the sounds of small children when working from home, or the sound of people coming and going and talking when working around others in a healthcare facility. In addition, the dictation itself may contain background noise (crying children, staff conversations, sirens, ringing telephones, etc.).

   Although it is possible to transcribe with background noise, speed and accuracy are almost always adversely affected. Make every effort to keep noise in your work space to a minimum. If you are working in a transcription pool, try to make sure people walking through the area are kept away from your work space. At home, it might be a good idea to work in the evening or through the night when children are sleeping and the house is quiet.

2. Listen closely. Pay attention to soundalike words and small words and syllables that may not be heard easily or might be interchanged. For example,

the word *now* can sound like *not*, or the dictated word *cheerful* can actually be *tearful*. The articles *a* and *the* can convey important meaning, yet sometimes these tiny words are dropped because they are easily missed. Some words may be small and seemingly insignificant but can play a vital role in the meaning of a sentence.

Words that sound alike are often easily confused, especially when they are spoken quickly or mumbled. Sounds become extremely difficult to differentiate when heard over background noise or bad audio. For example, an *S* sound may sound like *F*, or a *D* sound may sound like *T*, making it difficult to ascertain the exact word being spoken. When you hear an unfamiliar word, try to phonate the sounds out loud a few times to familiarize yourself with them. Then try looking up the word by using possible spelling variations of the sounds. For example, the word *steatohepatitis* can sound a lot like *stereo hepatitis* (which is not even a valid medical term). Pronounce the unfamiliar word out loud a few times, and then use your transcription resources to try to locate the word by using phonemes and other possible spelling variations for the sounds you hear.

3. Focus on the topic of the dictation and the story being told rather than just listening for words. One of the factors that contribute to transcription errors is the mistranscription of words in a report that may sound similar but have nothing to do with the subject of discussion. Transcription of a sentence such as "Head was turned to the right eye," when the actual statement dictated was "Attention was turned to the right eye," makes the company and transcriptionist appear unprofessional. In addition, distractions faced by clinicians when they dictate their notes in a hospital environment may lead to sentence cut-offs and repeated portions of dictation. For example, if a dictator states the reason for visit is "pain in the left ear," the physical exam would likely discuss abnormal findings regarding the one perforated tympanic membrane of the ear in question, not both ears. Be sure to focus on the information being conveyed to make sure the text makes sense with regard to tense, number (*is* versus *are*), and words that may be dictated but not heard clearly.

4. Watch for formatting and speaking errors. Physicians are generally terrible spellers and often miscount numbered items. Never trust a dictator's spelling of a term or medication. When in doubt, look up the word; or if you are not sure, leave a blank. Make sure numbered items are enumerated correctly.

Doctors may insert punctuation inappropriately in text. Some dictators with foreign or unfamiliar accents say words like "full stop" when indicating the period at the end of a sentence, or say "semicolon" when they mean to use a comma. When transcribing, you should be alert to a dictator's punctuation style and make sure it complies with known style mechanics for punctuation, such as those indicated in *The Book of Style for Medical Transcription, 3rd ed.*, and lightly edit accordingly.

Be especially vigilant with difficult dictators or dictators with foreign accents. Difficult dictators may dictate fast or mumble. Dictators with unfamiliar accents may pronounce words differently or place accents on the wrong syllables, making them sound unfamiliar.

5. *Do not guess* at the words being dictated! If, after researching the word or phrase, you are not sure of what is being said, leave it blank. Everything you transcribe should be accurate and verifiable. If you are in doubt, ask—because if the problem dictation involves drug names, drug dosages, patient-described symptoms, among others, guessing incorrectly could have life-threatening implications if your error goes through the healthcare system unnoticed.

6. Strive to avoid mistranscriptions. A mistranscription occurs when the word is clearly dictated but a substantive error occurs when transcribing it to

---

QUICK CHECK 4.3

Indicate whether the following statements are true (T) or false (F).

1. If you cannot hear the dictation clearly, it is acceptable to type what you think you hear.   T   F

2. Always proofread a document before returning it.   T   F

3. A dictator's spelling of a word is always correct and should be used.   T   F

4. If you are to work effectively, your work area should be quiet.   T   F

5. Text-expander entries should not be identical to "real" English words.   T   F

paper; for example, typing the word *arthritis* (a form of inflammation of the body's joints) instead of *arteritis* (an inflammation of an artery).

Text expanders can create problems with mis-transcriptions. As discussed previously, sometimes when using a text expander, it is easy to hit the wrong shortcut and accidentally insert the wrong word into a document. For example, *hyc* may be expanded to "hydrocortisone" when you meant to type the word "hydrocodone," a totally different drug.

7. Remember to proofread your document for errors before returning it to the facility. A badly proofed document reflects on you personally and professionally and can be potentially dangerous to the patient about whose record it appears. When proofreading, look for spelling errors not caught by the spell checker, typographical errors in the text, and errors in punctuation and grammar.

TRANSCRIPTION INSTRUCTIONS

You will transcribe medical reports and other documents from audio files on a CD. Your goal is to produce documents with as few errors as possible. Unless otherwise specified by your instructor, review and follow these guidelines for transcribing these medical reports:

1. Become familiar with the content and format of the sample forms illustrated in this chapter. The respective templates you will use to transcribe the reports are provided for you on the student CD, as listed in Table 4.1.

2. Open MS Word. Insert the student CD-ROM and locate the audio file of the report to be transcribed. For each transcription activity in the textbook, there is a list of items in the "listen for these terms" list. As an extra activity to reinforce your knowledge of medical terminology, your instructor may ask you to look up each item in the list and write down a brief definition of the term on a separate sheet of paper. Submit this list of definitions along with your transcribed document.

3. Locate and open the template of the report to be transcribed. The template contains all of the margins, formatting, styles, and headings that are typically used for that report.

4. Listen to the dictation file and transcribe the dictation into the template form. Listen to as much of the dictation as you can retain in memory at one time, pause the dictation, and type the words. Type the report verbatim, or word for word, although light editing is acceptable to correct grammatical errors or errors in context. Rewind the audio file to listen again if there are any words you cannot understand. If you encounter a word you cannot understand, use the reference resources available to you (e.g., medical dictionary, word books, the Internet) to try and find the word. If you still cannot understand the word after reasonable research, leave a blank of seven spaces using the underline key (_____) in that portion of the dictation and flag that portion of the report, briefly explaining why you left a blank, noting what the dictation sounds like, and asking for feedback for future reference. A **flag** is a notation by the medical transcriptionist to the originator of a report, drawing attention to missing data, unclear dictation, errors in dictation, inconsistent dictation, equipment problems, potentially inflammatory remarks, etc. Flags contribute to risk management by calling attention to information in the report that may be contradictory or compromise patient care. Place a flag in the report using boldface type. Place an opening bracket and indicate the inconsistency or problem, followed by a closing bracket, as follows: **[Dictator refers to male patient being status post a cesarean section]**.

The text inside the brackets may reflect additional details such as what an unintelligible word sounds like or the text of the inconsistency and asking for clarification, for example, **[s/l "lortine"]**. Similarly, flag medication inconsistencies you are not sure of, for example, **[Physician dictates allergy to morphine, then prescribes morphine in discharge medications]**. Flagging inconsistencies ensures the report will be reviewed, in your class by your instructor and on the job by the facility, for correction and/or accuracy.

5. You may use abbreviations in the body of the report as dictated by the physician. Do not use an abbreviation in a preoperative or postoperative diagnosis in an operative note or in the admitting or discharge diagnosis of a discharge summary. Do not expand an abbreviation unless you are absolutely sure of its meaning.

6. Refer to the Joint Commission's and the ISMP's lists of abbreviations, acronyms, symbols, and medication dosages that should not be used in reports due

TABLE 4.1	Templates on Student CD
CN-tem	Clinic Note
SOAP-tem	Note in SOAP Format
HP-tem	History and Physical Examination
OP-tem	Operative Note
CONS-tem	Consultation Note
CONSLTR-tem	Consultation Letter
PN-tem	Inpatient Progress Note
DS-tem	Discharge Summary
IMAGE-tem	Diagnostic Imaging (x-ray, MRI, etc.)

to the potential for them to be misread or misunderstood (see Appendix 1). For the reports in this textbook, make the appropriate term or medication dosage substitution when you hear one of these terms dictated.

7. Transcribe the text as dictated into the appropriate headings, in paragraph form, according to the samples in this chapter. If additional headings are dictated, they should be typed with the same formatting and capitalization as the rest of the headings in the report. Change the word "DIAGNOSIS" in headings to the plural form if there are multiple diagnoses. Delete any unused headings.

8. If the physician dictates the word "same" for a postoperative diagnosis in an operative report (indicating it is the same text as the preoperative diagnosis), do not type the word "same." Instead, type the same text as in the preoperative diagnosis.

9. When typing dates, use numeric dates with four digits for the year (01/01/xxxx) for the dictation and transcription dates at the bottom of the report and in the demographic and header information. In the body of the report, write out the date (January 1, 20xx). Do not type the word *of* between the month and the year, even if the physician dictates it.

10. If the report consists of more than one page, complete the header that will appear at the top of each succeeding page by filling in the name of the patient and the medical record number; the page number will number automatically.

11. For items in a numbered list, start the list directly below the heading. Type the number, then hit the TAB key, and type the text. Do not double space between numbered items. If the physician dictates only one item, it should not be numbered or indented but typed on the line beneath the heading.

12. For the purposes of this course, listen for inconsistencies you may encounter in the dictation, such as numbered items dictated out of order, mispronounced words, and other possible dictation errors. These inconsistencies have been intentionally dictated into some reports to give you practice in listening

closely to details. If the inconsistency can be resolved confidently and competently (such as number items in correct chronological order, or knowing the patient, Mary, is female and not male), then edit the report accordingly. However, if the discrepancy cannot be resolved with certainty, the item should be flagged in the manner outlined above so it may be brought to the attention of your instructor for clarification.

13. At the end of each report, indicate the physician's signature by typing, "Electronically signed by . . ." and the name of the physician. Skip and line, then type the reference initials of the dictator and your initials as transcriptionist. On the next line, fill in the date the report was dictated (D:) and on the next line, the date the report was transcribed (T:). See the samples in this chapter for formatting of this information.

14. When you are finished with a report, print one copy for your instructor and submit it along with your list of definitions. Save the completed document to your disk in the method outlined by your instructor for saving documents on your CD.

CHAPTER SUMMARY

The correspondence and reports you transcribe provide chronological documentation of health care and medical treatment provided to a patient by the professional members of his or her healthcare team. Each of these documents exist to ensure that the information regarding a patient's history is complete and is readily available to any practitioner involved in the patient's care. An accomplished medical transcriptionist has a working knowledge of the type of document being produced, is familiar with the mechanics of producing the document, and knows the types of headings and other information unique to a particular document. If you are well versed in the appearance and specifications of each type of document generated in patient care, you will be able to prepare reports properly and competently without excessive supervision.

· I · N · S · I · G · H · T ·

Medical Transcription and Risk Management

When transcribing medical reports, medical transcriptionists often face decisions that have moral and ethical implications. Therefore, they must have a working knowledge of their legal and ethical responsibilities concerning the creation and handling of medical records as laid out by HIPAA, discussed in Chapter 1. Standards or procedures that are used to determine, minimize, and prevent adverse effects on a business are collectively referred to as **risk management**.

A competent transcriptionist can weed out dictated imperfections before they have a chance to perpetuate throughout a patient's medical record. A medical transcriptionist should be alert for such an instance; for example, hearing that a patient is allergic to a medication and then hearing that same medication prescribed to the patient later in the report.

The Association for Healthcare Documentation Integrity (AHDI) offers guidelines for responsible behavior and resolving ethical dilemmas in its Code of Ethics, as follows: "Instances may arise when members' and certificants' ethical obligations may appear to conflict with relevant laws and regulations. When such conflicts occur, members and certificants must make a responsible effort to resolve the conflict in a manner that is consistent with the values, principles, and standards expressed in this Code of Ethics."

This means that you should be alert to situations that raise questions about a potential legal risk to the patient or medical providers as you transcribe medical reports. For example, a physician may ask you to sign a medical report for him without his even reviewing it. Or, an office manager may ask you to forward copies of a patient's discharge summary to another individual who has no legitimate need to know this information. In situations such as these, you should not guess what to do or attempt to take care of the matter yourself; instead, flag the item or bring it to the attention of the appropriate personnel.

ABBREVIATIONS

Abbreviation	Meaning	Abbreviation	Meaning
BMI	body mass index	HEENT	head, eyes, ears, nose, and throat
EBL	estimated blood loss	HPI	history of present illness
H&P	history and physical	SOAP	subjective, objective, assessment, and plan

Add Your Own Abbreviations Here:

_____

_____

_____

_____

_____

_____

TERMINOLOGY

Term	Meaning
authentication	The process of "signing" a document electronically by entering a unique code or password that verifies the identity of the signer and creates an individual signature on the document.
clinic note, *syn.* chart note	A short report entered into a patient's chart to document his or her visit with the physician.
complimentary close	The term, expression, or phrase that precedes the signature on a letter.
consultation report	A report dictated by a consulting physician to a case that discusses his or her evaluation of the patient, assessment of findings, and recommendations for treatment.
demographic information	A collective term encompassing the patient's statistical data.
discharge summary	A report that gives a chronological summary of the events that occurred during the patient's stay, including tests and other workup performed and pertinent events that occurred throughout the hospital course.
electronic signature	An electronic symbol or process attached to or associated with a record by a person with the intent to sign the record.
Electronic Signatures in Global and National Commerce Act (E-Sign Act)	A law enacted in 2000 that provides that an electronic signature on a document as the same legal effect as a handwritten signature on a document.
flag	A mark or notation by the medical transcriptionist to the originator of a report, drawing attention to missing data, unclear dictation, errors in dictation, or other inconsistencies requiring attention by the originator.
full-block letter style	A letter style that places all structural parts of the letter at the left margin.
history and physical examination (H&P)	A report dictated by a physician when a patient is admitted to the hospital utlining the patient's history, admitting diagnosis, and plan of care.
operative report	A detailed narrative of a patient's operative procedure.
progress note	A report that documents a patient's day-to-day care while in the hospital.
risk management	Standards or procedures that are used to determine, minimize, and prevent adverse effects on a business.
SOAP format	A note format using the headings Subjective, Objective, Assessment, and Plan.

Add Your Own Terms and Definitions Here:

_____

_____

_____

_____

_____

_____

REVIEW QUESTIONS

1. What does the acronym SOAP stand for in medical reports?
2. When would a physician dictate information about a patient's family history in the History of Present Illness section of a report?
3. What two additional items are indicated in a death summary as opposed to a discharge summary?
4. What are the structural components of a business letter?
5. What is the purpose of a history and physical exam report?
6. Where is the signature line placed in a medical document?
7. Name two reasons that a patient's family history would be important to the medical record.
8. In a letter, how many blank lines are left between the complimentary close and the writer's name?
9. Name three methods of suture closure found in an operative report.
10. What items are usually included in the demographic information section of a medical report?

CHAPTER ACTIVITIES

SOAP Exercise

Indicate the section of a note's SOAP format (subjective, objective, assessment, or plan) in which the following sentences may be found:

1. "The patient does not drink or smoke."   _____

2. "Abdomen: Soft, nontender, and nondistended."   _____

3. "The patient presents with a cough and fever for the past 3 days."   _____

4. "The patient will return to clinic in 4 weeks for followup."   _____

5. "With regard to this right-sided abdominal pain, obviously there is a concern for biliary colic."   _____

6. "His only deficit at this time includes changes in sensation on the left side of his body, mainly related to temperature."   _____

7. "She brought with her today the most recent MRI, which I reviewed in detail."   _____

8. "I believe this is a lesion that would benefit from surgery, seeing that this cavernoma has hemorrhaged before."   _____

9. "The patient had sinus surgery approximately 5 years ago with no relief."   _____

10. "We will defer the details of the surgery until the patient returns to clinic after his sleep study next month."   _____

Multiple Choice

Circle the letter corresponding to the best answer to the following questions.

1. In a SOAP clinic note, the sentence, "Extremities have no clubbing, cyanosis, or edema" would be found in the
   A. Assessment.
   B. Plan.
   C. Objective.
   D. Subjective.

2. Fora history and physical exam report, in which section would the findings of CT scan be found?
   A. Review of Systems
   B. Social History
   C. Chief Complaint
   D. Laboratory Data

3. For a SOAP clinic note, in which section would information about the patient's returning to the clinic be found?
   A. Plan
   B. Subjective
   C. Objective
   D. Assessment

4. Which heading is *not* part of an operative note?
   A. Surgeon
   B. Complications
   C. Objective
   D. Anesthesia

5. If a patient is moved to another facility upon discharge, the note dictated is often referred to as a
   A. transfer summary.
   B. assessment and plan.
   C. death summary.
   D. consultation note.

6. Progress notes are typically dictated while the patient is
   A. an outpatient.
   B. not admitted yet.
   C. an inpatient.
   D. going home.

7. What is *not* included in the laboratory data section of a report?
   A. blood work
   B. the patient's vital signs
   C. x-ray findings
   D. MRI studies

8. The time and date of a patient's death are required in a
   A. history and physical exam.
   B. consultation note.
   C. discharge summary.
   D. death summary.

9. The letter *S* in the SOAP format stands for
    A. saturation.
    B. surgeon.
    C. special notes.
    D. subjective.

10. In a SOAP clinic note, the patient's laboratory workup would be found in which section?
    A. Objective
    B. Subjective
    C. Plan
    D. Assessment

11. A report generated by another physician rendering a second opinion about a patient is called a(n)
    A. Operative Report.
    B. History and Physical Exam.
    C. Consultation Report.
    D. Progress Note.

12. The dictated sentence, "Tympanic membranes are clear bilaterally" would be found under which topic?
    A. Extremities
    B. HEENT
    C. Chest
    D. Neck

13. In a clinic note, the dictated sentence, "This is a 9-year-old boy who is seen today for followup on habitual toe walking," would be found under which heading?
    A. History of Present Illness
    B. Chief Complaint
    C. Assessment
    D. Plan

14. In a SOAP clinic note, the sentence, "There do not appear to be any neurological deficits on examination," would be found under which heading?
    A. Objective
    B. Subjective
    C. Plan
    D. Assessment

15. "Estimated Blood Loss: 500 mL" would typically be found in
    A. a history and physical exam.
    B. a clinic note.
    C. a consultation.
    D. an operative note.

Terminology Mixup

Unscramble the following terms found in medical reports.

BIEOCEVTJ __ __ __ __ __ __ __ __ __

LISHCPAY __ __ __ __ __ __ __ __ __

RIEVAPTEO __ __ __ __ __ __ __ __ __

PCDEGMAHROI __ __ __ __ __ __ __ __ __ __ __

NULNOICOATTS __ __ __ __ __ __ __ __ __ __ __

TAESMNESSS __ __ __ __ __ __ __ __ __ __

JUCTIVESEB __ __ __ __ __ __ __ __ __ __

COBLK __ __ __ __ __ __ __ __ __

NALP __ __ __ __ __ __ __ __ __

XMEA __ __ __ __ __ __ __ __ __

Proofreading Practice

Read and identify the errors in the SOAP note provided by circling them. After you have proofread it, retype it in the correct form. When finished, print one copy and save the corrected report as CHAPTER-4-SOAP.

SUBJECTIVE
This is a 4-yer-old african American girl patient of our clinic who came here today four tuberculosis test reading. The patient had a TB test placed previously and to day, 48 hours later, shows a positive reaction. TeeBee test was presented in the left forearm and there is an area of erythema and induration corresponding to about 20 mm. This was measured by the nurse and verified for me.

   Mom denies child being exposed to any one with tuberculosis. She had been test a couple of times during the past year but mom never come in for the reading. She said there was no reaction to it on ether occasion accept this won time. She also says that she is only around the family and the kids in school: She is not aware of anyone being diagnosed with tuberculosis and child has been completely fin, alert, active, and feeding well with no problems.

OBJECTIVE
Temperature 98.8, blood pressure 80/60, weight 32 ponds, heart rate 80. General: Alert, active, well nourished, African American girl. Neck: supple, no lymphadenopathy. Heart: Regular rate and rhythm. No heart murmurs. Lungs, Clear to auscultation bilaterally. No rhonchi, crackles, or wheezing.

ASESSMENT
An African American girl with positive tuberculin skin teste.

PLAN
I ordered chest x-rays to rule out active tuberculosis. The patient very likely has latent BB and mom was explained that she would be a good candidate for INH prophylaxis. The patient is to return to clinic in the next cople of weeks. Mom voiced understanding and agrees to follow up accordingly.

TRANSCRIPTION PRACTICE

Open your word-processing software. Insert the student CD-ROM and locate the dictation for this chapter. For each of the words in the "listen for these terms" list for each report, look up and write down a brief definition of the term on a separate sheet of paper to attach with your work. Then listen to the dictation and transcribe each report. Proofread your work, print one copy for your instructor along with your term definitions, and save the completed report to your student disk.

Report #T4.1: Outpatient Clinic Note
Patient Name: Carl Ewing
Medical Record No.: 5477211
Physician: Sabrina Scott, MD

Listen for these terms:
sciatica
Vicodin
trapezius
Lexapro
glabellar
tinnitus
saw palmetto
EKG

Report #T4.2: Inpatient Progress Note
Patient Name: Lois A. Summers
Medical Record No.: 0800453
Physician: Michael Josephs, MD

Listen for these terms:
biopsy
cocci
neutrophil
ciprofloxacin

Report #T4.3: History and Physical Exam
Patient Name: Lynette Collins
Medical Record No.: 723-93-441
Physician: Andrea Biggs, MD

Listen for these terms:
ulcerative colitis
hemicolectomy
parastomal
ileostomy
hernia
ostomy
NPO

5

MECHANICS OF EDITING

INTRODUCTION

English is the second most commonly spoken language in the world (Mandarin is the first) and the base of the language used by medical doctors when they communicate with each other, yet thought by many to be one of the most difficult languages to learn. Although we may feel comfortable with the misuse of grammar in our everyday conversation, improper use of punctuation and grammar is not only a distraction to the reader, but it can also change the meaning of a sentence.

This chapter provides an easy reference for many of the grammar and punctuation questions you may encounter when transcribing dictation. This chapter also discusses document revision through proofreading, which involves more than just scanning the document quickly for misspelled words. A carelessly proofread medical document not only makes a bad impression, but, in the case of medical reports, might endanger a patient's health.

Most grammar, punctuation, and proofreading rules are based on well-established, commonly used conventions of style. Although this chapter provides an easy reference for many of the problems you may encounter on the job, this is only a review. For a complete guide to the rules of grammar, punctuation, and document revision used in medical transcription, you should have a comprehensive writing handbook or *The Book of Style for Medical Transcription, 3rd, ed.*, on hand as part of your reference library.

GRAMMAR REVIEW

Have you ever read a letter or other document that contained a grammatical error? If so, what was your first impression about the person who drafted it? You probably immediately thought that the person was unprofessional or uneducated. Although slips in grammar often are made in speech, errors in writing are simply unacceptable. It is essential to have a working knowledge of basic grammar, including sentence structure, to create an effective and unambiguous business document.

Sentence Structure

Imagine a house where the front door opens into a closet. To get to the kitchen, you have to go through the attic, and windows are placed in every corner. That would not make sense! In order to be functional, a house must have certain elements organized in a logical way, just like a sentence.

You probably haven't thought about sentence structure since you were in grade school, but sentences are the building blocks of writing, and you should have a thorough understanding of how to structure sentences correctly. A change in the order of the words and phrases that construct a sentence can change the meaning of that statement. Not only might a poorly structured sentence alter patient care, it also looks unprofessional. You should purchase a basic grammar book as part of your resource library to keep these rules at hand. In order to get a better idea of how sentences are put together, Table 5.1 lists the basic parts of speech that help form sentences. Although it is no substitute for a grammar handbook, this list of terms will help you recognize and identify various parts

of speech in order to follow the rules of grammar and punctuation outlined below.

Putting Sentences Together

An **independent clause** can function as a complete sentence; it consists of a subject (s) and a verb (v) and expresses a complete thought.

The <u>patient</u> <u>left</u> the clinic.
    (s)   (v)

Many sentences contain multiple subjects and verbs, as well as a **helping verb** (hv), a verb which modifies the main verb:

The patient's <u>bloodwork</u> <u>was</u> <u>completed</u>, and <u>he</u> <u>left</u> the clinic for home. (s)   (hv)   (v)   (s) (v)

At the core of the sentence, however, is still the subject and verb. Without both of them, a group of words is not a sentence.

Many sentences contain more than one subject or more than one verb:

The <u>patient</u> and his <u>mother</u> <u>left</u> the clinic.
   (s)   (s)   (v)

TABLE 5.1	Basic Parts of Speech
Term	*Meaning*
Noun	A word that names a person, place or thing. A **proper noun** is a noun that begins with a capital letter because it is the name of a *specific* or *particular* person, place, or thing. A **pronoun** is a word that takes the place of a noun for subject, object, or possessive case. Objects and subjects in sentences are nouns.
Verb	A word used to show action or a state of being.
Preposition	A word such as *in, on, at, after,* or *with* that defines the relationships between other words in a sentence: "I put my book <u>in</u> the closet." A **prepositional phrase** is a group of words that consists of a preposition, a noun, or a pronoun that serves as the object of the preposition, and any words that modify the object: "The nurse <u>with the red hair</u> <u>in a ponytail</u> answered the phone."
Conjunction	A word such as *and, but, for, or, nor, yet,* or *so* that joins words, phrases, or clauses, thereby indicating their relationship. A **subordinating conjunction** (while, where, since, after, yet, so) connects two unequal parts, for example, a dependent and independent clause.
Adverb	A word used to describe or modify a verb, adjective, clause, or another adverb and typically answer the questions "When?" (adverbs of time), "Where?" (adverbs of place), and "How?" (adverbs of manner) something happens or happened. A **conjunctive adverb** is a word, such as *subsequently, consequently, finally,* and *thus,* that connects two independent clauses.
Adjective	A word that describes a noun. A **compound adjective** is two or more words used together as a single modifier of a noun.
Object	The person or thing (noun) affected by the action described in the verb. A verb may be followed by an object that completes the verb's meaning. A **direct object** is a noun or pronoun that receives the action of a verb in an active sentence or shows the result of the action. It answers the question "What?" or "Whom?" after an action verb. An **indirect object** is a word that precedes the direct object and receives the action of the verb.
Subject	A noun that shows *who* or *what* a sentence is about.
Predicate	The "completer" of a sentence that contains the verb.

The <u>radiologist</u> <u>read</u> and <u>interpreted</u> the x-ray results.
    (s)   (v)   (v)

As indicated above, many verbs can contain both a **main verb** (mv), which is the main action word in a sentence, and a helping verb:

The physician <u>has</u> <u>read</u> the preliminary report.
         (hv) (v)

The patient <u>will</u> <u>consider</u> the alternatives to surgery.
       (hv)   (v)

Some sentences can be very short, with only two or three words expressing a complete thought, like this:

Lungs clear.
Pupils equal and reactive.
All systems negative.

The above examples illustrate complete sentences, but the verb is silent. Although complete sentences are the grammatical rule, physicians often dictate short, clipped sentences, omitting some basic parts of the sentence as dictated, yet they still express a complete thought. These silent-verb sentences are particularly common in the *physical examination*, *laboratory results*, and *review of systems* sections of reports, even when complete sentences are used in the same sections or other parts of the report.

Sentence Fragments

A **sentence fragment** is a group of words that is only part of a sentence and does not express a complete thought. Some fragments are incomplete because they lack either a subject or a verb, or both:

at the site of the injury. (What is?)
return next week. (Who will return?)

To fix a sentence fragment, remember the basics: subject, verb, and complete thought. There are two ways to fix a sentence fragment:

1. Attach the sentence fragment to another sentence. That other sentence could be before or after the sentence fragment.
   <u>There was swelling present</u> at the site of the injury.
2. Add a subject, verb, or both to make the sentence complete.
   <u>The patient will</u> return next week.

Subject-Verb Agreement

One of the biggest errors transcriptionists make is transcribing sentences that are incorrect in terms of subject-verb agreement. Even if dictated that way, it is a glaring grammatical error. **Subject-verb agreement** means that subjects must agree with their verbs in

TRANSCRIPTION TIP:

Many companies accept and often prefer sentence fragments to be transcribed as dictated rather than edited to create complete sentences, and this is acceptable practice when the phrases convey the idea of the sentence without loss of clarity.

terms of number (singular or plural) and person (first, second, or third).

I pretend
You pretend
He/she/it pretend<u>s</u>
We pretend
They pretend

Identify the subject in a sentence to determine the correct form of the verb. Match the verb to the subject, whether it is single or plural:

The <u>chart</u> **needs** to be filed. (singular subject and verb)
The <u>charts</u> **need** to be filed. (plural subject and verb)

If the subjects (whether singular or plural) are joined by the word *and*, the verb is plural:

The <u>president</u> *and* <u>his cabinet members</u> are on vacation this week.

However, if the multiple subjects work as a single unit, then the verb should be singular:

<u>Spaghetti and meatballs</u> is my favorite dish.

If the multiple subjects are preceded by *each* or *every*, then the verb should be singular:

Every <u>nurse</u> and <u>nursing student</u> is required to attend the meeting.

TRANSCRIPTION TIP:

The verb "be" is irregular in form and must agree in both the present and past tenses:

I am (was)

You are (were)

he/she/it (is, was)

we (are/were)

you (are/were)

they (are/were)

If the subjects are joined by *or* or *nor*, the verb should agree with the subject that is closest to the verb:

Neither the <u>president</u> nor his <u>cabinet members</u> are in town this week.

Neither the <u>cabinet members</u> nor the <u>president</u> is in town this week.

The basic order of a sentence is subject, then verb, but sometimes other words separate them. These **interrupters** can include prepositional phrases and modifiers:

Carlos, <u>in fact</u>, will be the best man at my wedding. (prepositional phrase interrupter)

Carlos, <u>who is my cousin</u>, will be the best man at my wedding. (noun clause modifying Carlos interrupter)

Eliminate the interrupters to make sure your subjects and verbs agree:

The <u>painting</u>, [~~to the surprise~~] [~~of millions~~], <u>was</u> stolen in broad daylight from a museum in Norway.

The <u>painting</u>, [~~which is~~, [~~by far~~], ~~the most famous painting~~] [~~by any of the impressionists~~], <u>was</u> stolen in broad daylight from a museum in Norway.

Most of the time physicians dictate the correct form of verb for the subject, but not always. Problems occur most commonly in the following situations:

1. When subject and verb are separated. Make sure the verb agrees with the correct noun in the sentence.

   Incorrect: The review of systems are negative. (The subject is *review*, not *systems*. By eliminating the prepositional phrase, *of systems*, the subject of the sentence can be determined more easily.)
   Correct: The review of systems is negative.

2. When subject and verb are reversed.

   Incorrect: There has been several scans showing masses in the breast. (The subject is *scans*.)
   Correct: There have been several scans showing masses in the breast.

3. With **collective nouns**. Collective nouns are nouns that refer to groups of people or things: company, management, or group. Usually these words are singular.

   The company is going bankrupt (not, *are going*).
   XYZ Hospital Systems has opened a new facility downtown (not *have opened*).

4. With indefinite pronouns. Many indefinite pronouns are singular.

   Each of the nurses has a cell phone.
   None was found in the supply cabinet.
   Everybody is getting a tour of the new lab.

When used as subjects, the indefinite pronouns listed below are always singular and, therefore, always take singular verbs.

Indefinite Pronouns

another	anybody	anyone	anything	each
either	every	everybody	everything	much
neither	nobody	no one	nothing	one
something	someone			

Transitional words are conjunctive adverbs that join two related independent clauses and help the reader transition from the idea of the first sentence to the idea expressed in the second sentence. Examples of transitional words include *however* and *therefore*. When the transitional word introduces the second clause, use a semicolon preceding and comma following the conjunctive adverb to separate the transitional word from the rest of the sentence.

The child had watery eyes; therefore, he was brought into the clinic.

Use a comma to set off the transitional word when it occurs within a sentence.

The diagnosis of kidney disease did not explain the patient's symptoms, however.

The diagnosis of kidney disease, however, did not explain the patient's symptoms.

However, the diagnosis of kidney disease did not explain the patient's symptoms.

Below are some other common transitional words used in medical reports:

also	furthermore	likewise	otherwise
anyhow	hence	meanwhile	similarly
anyway	however	moreover	still
besides	incidentally	nevertheless	then
consequently	indeed	next	therefore
finally	instead	nonetheless	thus

PUNCTUATION REVIEW

Punctuation marks are an important part of language. They make written text easier to understand, help reduce ambiguity, and emphasize major points. When we speak English, things such as stress, intonation, rhythm, and even pauses make our meaning clear. In writing, however, the meaning that might be expressed by vocal devices must be handled almost entirely by punctuation. Therefore, it is important to master the conventional system of punctuation for written English in order to convey meaning clearly.

Following the basic conventions of punctuation will result in reports that are both easy to understand and accurate in the meaning conveyed.

Period

A **period** (.) is placed at the end of a sentence that makes a statement. A period is used to indicate the end

QUICK CHECK 5.1

Match the term in the left column with its definition in the right column.

A. helping verb   _____ Adverbs that join two independent clauses with a semicolon before and a comma after.

B. sentence fragment   _____ A sentence consisting of a subject and verb that expresses a complete thought.

C. independent clause   _____ A verb that modifies a main verb.

D. transitional words   _____ Independent clauses that are connected to each other with commas.

E. subject-verb agreement   _____ Subjects must agree with their verbs.

---

of most sentences and to mark many abbreviations. There is no space between the last letter and the period. There is typically one space between the period and the beginning of the next sentence, although you should find out the preference of your employer. The period can be dictated specifically as "period" or "full stop."

1. A period is placed at the end of a sentence that makes a statement.

   The hospital was founded in 1722.
   She left for her appointment this morning.

2. Use a period at the end of a polite request or command. Use a period to end this kind of sentence if you expect your reader to respond by *acting* rather than by giving you a yes or no answer.

   Would you please send the patient's laboratory results to my attention.
   May I suggest you change your forms to be HIPAA compliant in the future.

3. A period is used at the end of a sentence that states a question indirectly.

   I wonder if my text-expander program is working correctly.

4. A period is used in some abbreviations, such as *Dr.* or *Mr.*, and some medical abbreviations, such as *p.r.n.*

   Dr. Johanssen is in town for the convention.
   The patient is to take aspirin p.r.n.

   Note: While the use of periods in abbreviated personal and courtesy titles is still acceptable, there continues to be a strong trend toward dropping them, and their omis-

sion is now preferred. However, you should always defer to the facility's preference.

5. A period is used in instances of time, courtesy titles, and lower-case drug-related abbreviations.

   10 a.m.
   p.r.n.
   q.a.m.

6. Separate values of unrelated tests by periods.

   White blood cell count was 5.9, hemoglobin 12, and hematocrit 42. Total cholesterol was 210.

7. If a sentence ends with an abbreviation or some other word that ends in a period, do not add another period to end the sentence.

   Incorrect: The lab closes at 4 p.m..
   Correct: The lab closes at 4 p.m.

8. Do not use periods within or at the end of most abbreviations, including abbreviated units of measure, and brief forms.

   Michael Johanssen, MD
   mg
   CMT
   subcu

Question Mark

A **question mark** (?) is placed at the end of a sentence that asks a direct question.

When is the operating room available?
Who told you that?

1. If the question is a direct quotation, repeating the speaker's exact words, place the question mark inside the quotation marks.

   "When is the operating room available?" the doctor asked.
   "Who told you that?" inquired her instructor.

2. Place a question mark outside the quotation marks if the quoted matter itself is not a question but is placed within an interrogative sentence.

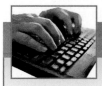

TRANSCRIPTION TIP:

Avoid the frequent mistranscriptions *alot, often times, moreso,* and *adlib.* The correct terms are *a lot, oftentimes, more so,* and *ad lib.*

What did he mean when he said, "I am allergic to doctors"?

3. Sometimes a question mark may be placed before a statement to show that something is uncertain. It can be placed either before or after the questionable material, but not both before and after. Note, there is no space after the question mark.

The patient is currently taking lisinopril ?20 mg.
DIAGNOSIS
?Hypertension.

Comma

A **comma** (,) usually is used to indicate a break in thought, to set off material, or to introduce a new but connected thought. A comma separates the structural elements of a sentence into manageable segments.

1. Use commas to separate two or more adjectives if each modifies the same noun.

The patient is an elderly, obese, Hispanic female.

Use a comma to separate two or more items in a simple series in which none of the items contain internal commas. Do not use a comma if all the items are joined by the conjunctions *and* or *or*. Always use a serial comma before the conjunction preceding the final item the series.

No abdominal tenderness, distention, or enlargement of the liver (final comma required).
The external ears, auditory canals, and tympanic membranes are normal.

Use commas to set off an adjective or adjectival phrase directly following the noun it modifies.

She had debilitating arthritis, left knee, with pain on ambulation.

2. Use a comma before coordinating conjunctions *and, but, for, or, nor, yet,* or *so* when they join an independent clause, as each represents a complete thought that is capable of standing alone.

The patient spoke no English, so an interpreter was summoned.
He was seen in the emergency room, but he was not admitted.
She was brought to the operating room, and she was sterilely prepped and draped.

3. Do not use a comma when an independent clause is followed by a **dependent clause**. A dependent clause has a subject and a verb, but it cannot stand alone.

Dependent clause: *after John fell off his new bicycle.*
Jimmy's mother called for an ambulance after John fell off his new bicycle.

If the dependent clause *precedes* the independent clause, then a comma is required.
After John fell off his new bicycle, Jimmy's mother called for an ambulance.

4. Use a comma to set off an **introductory clause**, which is a dependent clause that provides background information or introduces the main part of the sentence (the independent clause).

After you get the CT scan, we will perform lab work. Despite having a high fever, the patient elected to go home.

5. Use a comma after conjunctive adverbs, or words that connect two independent clauses, such as *however, furthermore, thus, finally, then, therefore,* and *subsequently.* If the conjunctive adverb connects two independent clauses, it is preceded by a semicolon and followed by a comma.

Therefore, it is imperative that you take immediate action.
He reported feeling better; therefore, he was discharged home.

6. Do not use a comma before a coordinating conjunction that links two subjects or two verbs.

She completed the clinical trial and immediately signed up for another one.
Her knee was swollen but not tender.

7. Do not use a comma or other punctuation between units of the same dimension.

The infant weighed 7 pounds 14 ounces.
The patient's height is 5 feet 2 inches.

8. Use a comma to set off the year when the month, day, and year are given in sequence.

She was first seen on January 15, 20xx, and returned on March 1, 20xx.
Do not use commas when the month and year are given without the day.
She was first seen in January 20xx and returned in March 20xx.

9. An **appositive** is a word or phrase placed before or after a noun that explains, identifies, or restates it. Appositive are often used as context clues for determining or refining the meaning of the word(s) to which they refer. Use commas to set off appositives or to set off words and phrases not essential to the meaning of the sentence.

John, Ms. Parker's oldest son, crashed his motorcycle into a tree and broke his arm.
We have commas around *Ms. Parker's oldest son* because this is an appositive for *John*. John is Ms. Parker's oldest son.

Note that nonessential words or phrases are not necessarily appositives. They could simply be parenthetical. (*Hint*: If you can remove the words from the sentence without changing the meaning, then the word or phrase is parenthetical and commas are required.)

John, whose helmet was too big for his head, crashed his motorcycle into a tree.

You can remove "whose helmet was too big for his head" without changing the basic meaning of the sentence: John crashed his motorcycle into a tree.

Do not use commas to set off essential, or defining, appositives, or to set off those words and phrases essential to the meaning of the sentence:

Ms. Parker's son John crashed his motorcycle into a tree. (Ms. Parker has more than one son.)

10. Use a comma after Latin abbreviations and their English translations (such as *e.g., i.e., et al.,* or *viz a viz*) when they are used as parenthetical expressions within a sentence.

He only gets the epigastric pain after eating certain foods, for example, spicy burritos.
She refused to take her pain medication, i.e., the Vicodin that was prescribed.

When two independent clauses appear in a sentence without any punctuation between them, it is referred to as a **run-on sentence**. A **comma splice** is a type of run-on sentence and occurs when independent clauses are connected to each other with commas. In this type of sentence, the independent clauses should be linked by a coordinating conjunction or by some other form of punctuation to delineate them as separate sentences.

Run-on sentence: The child had watery eyes he was brought into the clinic.
Comma splice: The child had watery eyes, he was brought into the clinic.

Revision with a comma and coordinating conjunction: The child had watery eyes, and he was brought into the clinic.
Revision with a period: The child had watery eyes. He was brought into the clinic.
Revision with a semicolon: The child had watery eyes; he was brought into the clinic.
Revision with a dependent and independent clause: Since the child had watery eyes, he was brought into the clinic.
Revision with a conjunctive adverb: The child had watery eyes; therefore, he was brought into the clinic.

Semicolon

A **semicolon** (;) indicates a weaker break in a sentence than a period but a stronger break than a comma. A semicolon is extremely useful when writing about complex ideas, constructing extensive lists of items, and connecting thoughts together without having to make two distinct sentences.

1. Use a semicolon to join two independent clauses that are closely related in meaning when no connecting word (such as *or, and, but,* or *nor*) is used. Although the independent clauses could be written as separate sentences, keep in mind that the semi-colon demonstrates a relationship or link between the independent clauses that a period does not.

Dr. Eller is my cardiologist; Nancy is his nurse practitioner.
This room is the sonography suite; that room contains the x-ray machine.

2. Use a semicolon to separate items in a list when any of the listed items contains internal commas.

The unit manager congratulated Yang Ling, nursing supervisor; Jeremy Daily, floor nurse; and Nicole Redman, nursing assistant.

3. Use a semicolon between closely related independent clauses joined by conjunctive adverbs words such as *however, also, in fact, therefore,* or *hence.* Note the comma that follows the conjunctive adverb.

I think he is right; however, it is difficult to know for sure.

Colon

A **colon** (:) usually introduces and/or highlights the words that follow it. Use either one space or two spaces following the colon, depending on your employer's preference. Be consistent.

1. Use a colon to introduce a list or an explanation directly related to something just mentioned.

The surgical staff went on strike for three reasons: better pay, shorter working hours, and more stylish scrubs.
HEENT: Pupils were equal and reactive.

2. Use a colon after salutations in business letters.

Dear Dr. Smith:
Dear Sir/Madam:

3. Do not use a colon to introduce words that fit properly into the grammatical structure of a sentence without the colon.

HEENT: Pupils were equal and reactive.
or HEENT shows pupils were equal and reactive.
not HEENT shows: Pupils were equal and reactive.

4. Use a colon to express a ratio.

The solution was diluted 1:100,000.
The patient's E:A ratio was adequate.

5. Use a colon to separate hours and minutes of time.

Her appointment was scheduled for 10:30 a.m.
Do not use a colon to separate hours and minutes when using military time. (Note, if the word *hours* is not dictated, it may be added for clarity, but this is not absolutely necessary).

1400 hours
0930 hours

6. Capitalize the word following the colon if it is normally capitalized, if it follows a section or subsection

TRANSCRIPTION TIP:

Military time identifies the day's 24 hours using arabic numbers 0100 through 2400, with 0100 through 1200 consistent with morning hours 1 a.m. through noon and 1300 through 2400 corresponding to hours 1 p.m. through midnight, as shown in Figure 5.1. When transcribing military time, always use four numerals, using zeros if necessary, and do not use a.m. or p.m.

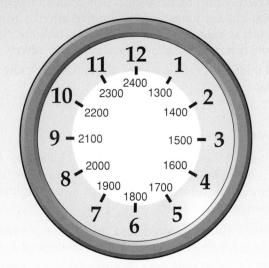

FIGURE 5.1. Military Time. Arabic numbers 0100 through 2400, with 0100 through 1200 consistent with morning hours 1 a.m. through noon and 1300 through 2400 corresponding to hours 1 p.m. through midnight. Reprinted with permission from Willis MC, CMA-AC. *Medical Terminology: A Programmed Learning Approach to the Language of Health Care.* Baltimore: Lippincott Williams & Wilkins, 2002.

heading, or if the list or series that follows the colon includes one or more complete sentences. Do not capitalize the word following the colon if the items are separated by commas.

The patient takes the following medications: Lasix, metoprolol, and Xanax.
PAST HISTORY: Negative.

Chest x-ray revealed the following: No cardiomegaly. No pulmonary infiltrates. Normal cardiac silhouette.

Apostrophe

An **apostrophe** (') is used to indicate the possessive case of nouns, to form some plurals of words, or to denote omitted letters or numbers in contractions.

1. Use an apostrophe at the end of a noun or indefinite pronoun to indicate possession, whether singular ('s) or plural (s'). Note most nouns ending in an *s* sound form the possessive with *'s*.

The patient's records were delivered by her son, John.
I will review everybody's files.
She is Dr. Harris's patient.

However, when the possessive form sounds awkward when not only the last but also the next-to-last syllable ends in an *s* sound, a simple apostrophe may be more correct.

physicians' orders
the nurses' paychecks

2. Use apostrophes to show possession of units of time.

She will follow up in one week's time.
He will follow up in two weeks' time.

3. Use apostrophes to show plurals of letters, symbols, lowercase abbreviations, and single-digit numbers or terms.

ab's
rbc's
4 × 4's
serial 7's

4. Do not use apostrophes with uppercase abbreviations.

RBCs
EKGs
PVCs

5. Know the difference between the words *its* and *it's*. The word *it's* always denotes the contraction (it is), while *its* denotes possession.

It's not my turn to work.
I placed the x-ray back into its jacket.

Hyphen

A **hyphen** (-) is typically used in numbers and compound words. Generally, a space is not used before or after a hyphen, with a few exceptions. Check appropriate English and medical dictionaries for guidance on particular terms.

1. Use a hyphen to join compound adjectives. A **compound adjective** is two or more words used together as a single modifier of a noun. When the compound adjective comes before the noun, join the words with a hyphen.

a well-developed, well-nourished female
a well-known physician
a high-risk patient
over-the-counter medication

However, when the compound adjective follows the noun, the words are not hyphenated.

The patient was well nourished and well developed.
The patient is considered to be high risk.
The physician was well known.

TRANSCRIPTION TIP:

Although apostrophes are used to form contractions (*don't, can't,* etc.), contractions are generally not used in medical writing. If you hear a contraction during dictation, unless it is a direct quote, write out the words.

2. Single-space after a **suspensive hyphen**, or a hyphen that is used to connect a series of compound modifiers with the same base term.

    She used 3- and 4-inch bandages on her wound.
    She suffered from second- and third-degree burns.

3. Hyphens may be used in words that contain repetitive vowels or consonants for easier readability.

    ileo-ascending colostomy
    salpingo-oophorectomy
    anti-inflammatory

    Note: There are many words with consecutive double letters, and industry resources cite both the hyphenated and nonhyphenated forms. Both are acceptable, but when in doubt, you should defer to the preference of your employer as to whether to hyphenate these words.

4. Use a hyphen to join the component parts of a compound noun that contain a number or single letter.

    Chem-7
    C-section
    x-ray

5. Use a hyphen to show suture sizes.

    4-0 Vicryl
    2-0 nylon

6. Use a hyphen with mixed fractions.

    A 3-1/2-year-old girl
    7-11/12 weeks
    10-1/4

7. Hyphenate fractions, whether spelled out as simple fractions less than one or written with numerals.

    The bottle was found to be two-thirds full.
    She was given one-half normal saline.
    2-1/2 inches
    3-3/4 hours

8. Use a hyphen when indicating gauges, catheters, sounds, and other instruments.

    A 20-gauge needle
    5-French catheter

9. Use a hyphen with adjectives.

    The patient is a 33-year-old woman.
    1-month course

one-half normal saline
heme-negative stool
a 20-pack-year history of smoking

10. Use a hyphen with other numbers and letters.

    ST-T segment abnormality
    beta-2 globulin
    non-A, non-B hepatitis
    CIN-1

    Some words with a single letter or symbol followed by a word are hyphenated; others are not. Check appropriate references for guidance and consider the use of hyphens in such terms as optional if you are unable to document. *Generally, even if such terms are unhyphenated in their noun form, they should be hyphenated in their adjective form.*

    B complex   B-complex vitamins
    T wave   T-wave abnormality

11. Hyphens are not used in adverb-adjective modifiers where the adverb ends in –*ly*.

    a mildly firm mass
    a neurologically alert patient

    If the adverb precedes a compound modifier, a hyphen is not used in the compound modifier.

    a significantly well documented chart
    a reasonably well distinct lesion

12. A hyphen is not used with compound modifiers in names of diseases.

    air space disease
    small cell lymphoma
    graft versus host disease

13. Do not use a hyphen joining *most* prefixes, including the prefix "non" (although there are exceptions).

    Nonweightbearing, preoperative, postoperative, lightheadedness, outpatient, nontender, noncontributory, noncompliant, midline, extraocular, nearsighted, and bimanual.

14. Do not use a hyphen for specific vertebrae of the spine.

    L5, S1, C1, T11

15. Do not use a hyphen with tumor cell markers.

    CD4, CD38

    However, there are a few exceptions. Check a medical word book or dictionary for clarification.

    CA19-9
    CA15-3

16. Use a hyphen to join adjectives that are equal, complimentary, or contrasting when they precede or follow the noun they modify.

    doctor-patient relationship
    a false-positive result
    a happy-sad affect

Dash

Although not used often in medical transcription, a **dash** (—) draws attention to nonessential material and highlights it. If your word-processing program does not have an **em dash** (a dash that is the width of a capital M) in its special character set, use two hyphens (--) to make a dash. There is no space between or on either side of the dash itself.

1. Use dashes to mark off a parenthetical element that represents an abrupt break in thought.

   The patient's speedy recovery—he suffered from sepsis, renal failure, and liver abnormalities—was nothing short of a miracle.

2. Use dashes to emphasize examples.

   This is one of our ads—for Mercy Hospital—that appeared in the national bulletin.

3. Use dashes to highlight parenthetical information.

   Three of our nursing supervisors—Mary, Annie, and Tyler—are from the south.
   Coordinating conjunctions—*and*, *but*, *or*, *nor*, *yet*, *so*—are usually preceded by a comma.

Quotation Marks

Quotation marks, also called "quotes," are punctuation marks used in pairs to set off speech, a quotation, or a phrase.

1. Quotation marks are used in pairs to set off direct quotations and titles. A direct quote begins with a capital letter.

   "My arm has been hurting," the patient stated.
   Dr. Hanson wrote the article, "New Tests for Diabetes," which appeared in the latest issue of *Medicine Today*.

   Note: Typically titles of articles appear in quotations, while names of books are underlined or italicized.

2. Do not use a capital letter to begin incomplete quotations.

   The patient stated she became sick after eating some "bad food" at a picnic.

3. Commas and periods go inside closing quotation marks; semicolons and colons go outside the closing quotation marks. The placement of a question mark in relationship to an ending quotation depends on the meaning of the sentence.

   "Money is no object," Peter responded to the doctor's question.
   The pathologist announced, "I have made my final diagnosis"; then he left the room.
   Why did you say, "John is an atheist"?
   Bill asked, "Is John an atheist?"

Parentheses

Parentheses are punctuation marks used in pairs to enclose or surround textual material.

1. Parentheses are used in pairs to refer to enclose words, phrases, or complete sentences that digress, amplify, or explain.

   In MS Word, when the *Overtype* feature is on (indicated by the letters OVR appearing in the status bar at the bottom of the screen), you will replace characters with newly typed characters.

2. Parenthetical text that appears within another sentence need not begin with a capital or end with a period.

   The patient's sister (who arrived late to the meeting) disagreed with the team's findings.

3. A comma may follow the closing parenthesis (if needed) but one should never precede the opening parenthesis.

   The patient received his antibiotics today (without major complications), and he will see his doctor tomorrow morning.

CAPITALIZATION

The following section reviews both general rules of capitalization as well as those used specifically in medical transcription.

1. Capitalize the first word of a sentence and, in a letter, the first word of a salutation and of a complimentary close.

   The patient is feeling much better today.
   Dear Dr. Nelson:
   Sincerely yours,

2. Capitalize the first word following the first set of opening quotation marks in directly-quoted speech.

   The patient said, "My throat is hurting."
   "I have chest tightness every day," the patient reported.

3. Do not capitalize the second part of an interrupted sentence in a quotation:

   "The patient will be transferred to the operating room," said Dr. Jones, "after she has a consultation with Anesthesia."

4. Capitalize the first word of a sentence in parentheses and end it with closing punctuation inside the closing parentheses. Do not capitalize the first word of text in parentheses if it comes inside another sentence.

   I have reviewed the lab results. (They are markedly elevated.)
   as opposed to:
   I have reviewed the lab results (which are markedly elevated).

QUICK CHECK 5.2 ✓

Indicate whether the following sentences are true (T) or false (F).

1. Dashes are used with compound words.   T   F

2. A appositive is a word or phrase that restates or modifies an immediately preceding subject.   T   F

3. An apostrophe indicates the possessive case of nouns.   T   F

4. Do not use a colon to separate hours and minutes when using military time.   T   F

5. Hyphens are used with antigens.   T   F

5. Capitalize proper nouns. Proper nouns include such things as names of individuals, countries, continents, states, counties, cities, regions, languages, races, companies, product brands, days of the week, months of the year, and holidays.

 The nursing staff applied a Band-Aid to the wound.
 The patient is a Hispanic female.
 The patient is a Catholic nun.
 Caucasian female.
 African American male.
 The patient is of Ashkenazi Jewish descent.

6. Do not capitalize skin color.

 white female
 black male

7. Do not capitalize terms that follow a person's name that are not actually proper titles.

 Sam McDonald, the hospital administrator, will be retiring this year.

8. Capitalize credentials and academic degrees that are abbreviated such as MD, RN, CMT, RHIT, BA, etc.. According to *The Book of Style for Medical Transcription, 3rd ed.*, the *preferred* style of academic titles is without periods. However, if periods are used, do not space within the abbreviation. Do not capitalize titles after a name except for high-ranking officials.

 Jerry Drake, MD, performed the colonoscopy.
 Rosemary Chang, attorney at law, spoke at the conference.

9. Capitalize the major words in the titles of movies, songs, books, magazines, and articles. Do not capitalize *a, an, the*, short prepositions, or conjunctions unless they are the first word of the title.
 The information can be found in the latest issue of the *Journal of the American Medical Association.*

10. Capitalize the names of a specific academic course, but do not capitalize academic subject areas unless they contain a proper noun.

 I took *Medical Terminology 101* as part of my academic training.

I also am taking keyboarding and accounting courses at night.

11. Capitalize the names of specially designated rooms but not common nouns designating rooms that are generic and can be applied to all similar rooms.

 The patient will be seen next week in the Sarah Jones Cardiology Clinic.
 He was seen in the emergency room.
 She was admitted to the intensive care unit.

12. Do not capitalize common nouns designating department names. Use capital letters for proper nouns or adjectives or when part of a government agency name.

 She works in the surgery department.
 The patient arrived at the emergency department by ambulance.
 Social Security Administration

 However, do capitalize a department name that is referred to as an entity.
 The x-rays were read by Radiology.
 The specimen was sent to Pathology for analysis.
 She will be seen by Anesthesia preoperatively.

13. Capitalize brand names of drugs.

 Xanax
 Lipitor
 Tylenol
 Nexium

14. Do not capitalize generic forms of drugs.

 alprazolam (Xanax)
 atorvastatin (Lipitor)
 acetaminophen (Tylenol)
 esomeprazole (Nexium)

15. Do not capitalize medical specialties.

 The patient was seen by the medicine service.
 A cardiology consultation was called.

16. Do not capitalize specific hospital rooms.

 The patient was taken to the operating room.
 The patient's test was performed in the endoscopy suite.

The patient left the emergency room against medical advice.

17. Do not capitalize the *p* in *pH*. The term *pH* is used to designate alkalinity or acidity. If it is dictated first in a sentence, the word *the* should precede it.

    The pH was 7.42 (*not*, "pH was 7.42.")

18. Capitalize the genus but not the species name for bacteria. If the genus is abbreviated, capitalize the one-letter abbreviation. The use of a period after the genus name abbreviation is acceptable, but both AHDI and the American Medical Association (AMA) recommend dropping it.

    Staphylococcus aureus
    E coli
    Clostridium difficile
    H influenzae

19. Genus names of bacteria can be transcribed in lowercase letters when they are in common use, used as an adjective, or stand alone without a species name.

    staph
    staph infection
    strep throat
    staphylococcal infection
    streptococcus

20. Do not capitalize words that indicate classification or categories except those containing a proper noun.

    grade 1
    stage III
    Dukes class A
    New York Heart Association class 2

21. Do not capitalize the words *gravida* or *para*. The abbreviated form *ab* (abortion) may be in all uppercase or lowercase letters.

    gravida 1, para 1, ab 2

22. Some preferred capitalization formats for commonly used lab values include the following:

Blood gas:	pH, pCO2, PaCO2, PO2, PaO2
EKG leads:	I, II, III, aVF, aVR, V1 through V6
Immunoglobulins:	IgA, IgD, IgE, IgG, and IgM
Blood pressure:	mmHg

NUMBERS

A **number** is an abstract entity that represents a count or measurement. There are several different types of numbers and numbering systems used in medical reports. **Ordinal numbers** are numbers that denote the position in an ordered sequence (*1st, 2nd, 3rd,* etc.). **Cardinal numbers**, also called **arabic numbers** or **figures**, are used to indicate "how many," (*1, 2, 3,* etc.). **Roman numerals** derive from a numbering system used in

ancient Rome that is based on certain letters that are given values as numerals (*I, II, III,* etc.).

Most numerals used in medicine are expressed as arabic numerals, with a few exceptions.

She was taken to the hospital 1 hour after the accident. The baby weighed less than 5 pounds.

1. When two numbers appear consecutively, spell out one of them to avoid confusion.

   He was to take two 75 mg tablets of Zantac daily. The surgeon used 15 two-inch pins.

2. Arabic numbers are used to indicate quantity. Numeric values less than one should have a zero preceding the decimal point.

   "Premarin point six-two-five," as dictated, would be typed as Premarin 0.625.

3. Neither a whole number nor a decimal number should have a zero after it unless specifically dictated to emphasize the preciseness of a measurement such as a pathology specimen or laboratory value.

   A potassium level dictated as "4.0" should be typed simply as 4 unless specifically dictated.

4. Use numbers for obstetric history data.

   The patient is a G1, P1-0-0-1.

5. Ordinal numbers (1st, 2nd, 3rd, etc.) are used to indicate position in a series. Ordinals are commonly spelled out, especially when the series goes no higher than 10 items; however, according to *The Book of Style for Medical Transcription, 3rd ed.*, numerals are recommended: 1st, 2nd, 3rd, etc.

   9th rib (or ninth)
   5th finger (or fifth)
   4th cranial nerve
   The clinic is open on the 10th and 25th of the month.

6. Common or accepted usage may dictate that a word be spelled out. For example, do not use a numeral when its placement may imply a precise quantity where none is intended.

   His symptoms went from one extreme to the other. I was the one chosen for the position.

7. Stage, type, and fracture classifications use roman numerals with subdivisions using capital letters and arabic numbers, without commas or spaces.

   stage III
   stage IIIA
   type II open fracture

8. Arabic numbers are used for grades.

   grade 1
   grade 2/6 systolic ejection murmur
   CIN grade 3

9. For level, phase, and class, use arabic numbers or roman numerals according to the system being referenced.

She entered a Phase III trial.
Haggitt level 4 colorectal adenocarcinoma

10. Use a comma to separate groups of three numerals in numbers greater than 10,000, but a comma is optional in numbers below 10,000. A comma is not used with decimals.

greater than 100,000 colonies of bacteria.
a white blood cell count of 9500 *or* 9,500.
4.123456
98765.43

For cranial nerves, either arabic numbers or roman numerals can be used.
cranial nerves I–XII
cranial nerves 1–12

Generally, there is a trend away from the use of roman numerals in favor of arabic numbers, as roman numeral II could be misread as the arabic number 11. Most numbers in medicine are expressed in the arabic format. Therefore, arabic numbers should be used unless there is strong documentation that the preferred form is roman (for example, to indicate cancer staging).

SYMBOLS

A **symbol** is a written or printed sign that stands for another word. There are many symbols used in medical texts, but in medical reports, they should only be used when they have been approved by the transcription service provider or physician. Generally, symbols are used when they occur along with arabic numbers.

Examples:

alert and oriented x3 (not x3 or x *three*; dictated as "times 3"), but not: 3x (dictated as "three times")
blood pressure 120/60 (dictated as 120 over 60)
lidocaine with epinephrine, 1:100,000 (dictated as "1 to 100,000)
pulses are 2+ (not *2 plus*; dictated as "two plus")
muscle strength is 5/5 or −4/5 (dictated as "5 over 5"or "minus 4 over 5")
3 × 2 mm mass (dictated as "3 by 2")
Vicodin 5/500 (dictated as "Vicodin 5, 500")
#3-0 nylon sutures (dictated as "number 3-oh")
vision is 20/20 (dictated as "20 20")
C&S test (dictated as "C and S")
3 + 3 = 6 carcinoma (dictated as "3 plus 3 equals 6")
99 °F (dictated as "99 degrees Fahrenheit")
mg/kg (dictated as "milligram per kilogram")

1. When using the abbreviation for *number* (No.), use an uppercase initial letter and an ending period, followed by a space and the figure. When the number symbol is used (#), the numeral follows with no space between.

No. 10 blade
#10 blade

2. Temperature degrees are typed with numerals except for zero.

zero degrees
98 degrees
36 °C
98 °F or 98 degrees Fahrenheit

Type the temperature scale name (Celsius, Fahrenheit, or Kelvin) only if dictated. If using the degree sign (°), it is immediately followed by the abbreviation for the temperature scale without a space. If the degree sign is not available, write out the word *degrees* followed by the temperature scale, if dictated. Do not type the temperature scale name if it is not dictated.

3. Exponents are usually superscripted, but if superscripting is not available, use appropriate abbreviations instead.

10^5 would be typed 10 to the 5th.
4 cm^2 would be 4 sq cm (*not* cm2).
8 mm^3 would be 8 cu mm (*not* mm3).

Do not place the numeral on the line with the abbreviation for easier readability (for example, *not* 4 cm2).

4. When designating a percentage value, the percent sign (%) should be used. Do not write the word *percent*. When two percentages are indicated, the percent symbol is repeated.

Her progesterone receptor was positive with staining in less than or equal to 5% of cells.
His oxygen saturation was 97% to 98% on room air.

EPONYMS

An **eponym** is a word or phrase formed from, or including, the name of a person. In the past, many anatomic structures and diseases derived their name from the person who first described it. Eponyms are often used in describing names of diseases. There are thousands of such names used in medical language; and separate medical references that specifically address such entities, including brief biographical information on the person, associated terms, and the definition of the disease or item named for that person, are available.

1. Do not use the possessive form of an eponym.

Hodgkin lymphoma
Parkinson disease
Tinel sign

However, in awkward constructions, such as when the noun following the eponym is omitted, the possessive form is preferred.

The patient's wife suffers from Alzheimer's.

Statistically, Hodgkin's is an uncommon form of lymphoma.

2. When typing terms using eponyms, capitalize the eponym but not the common nouns, adjectives, and prefixes that accompany them.

Cushing syndrome
tetralogy of Fallot

3. Do not capitalize words derived from eponyms.
cushingoid facies

parkinsonian symptoms

TABLE 5.2	Physician Acronyms
Dictated As	**Transcribed As**
"mick-you"	MICU (medical intensive care unit)
"nick-you"	NICU (neonatal intensive care unit OR neurosurgical intensive care unit)
"sick-you"	SICU (surgical intensive care unit)
"pack-you"	PACU (postanesthesia care unit)
"pick-you"	PICU (pediatric intensive care unit)

ACRONYMS

An **acronym** is a word that is formed by combining some parts (usually selected letters) of other words. In everyday speech, the term is also used to refer to **initialisms**, which are combinations of letters representing a longer phrase. The difference is that an acronym is pronounced as if it were a word, even when the speaker knows that the individual letters stand for other words. For example HIPAA (pronounced *"HIP-ah"*), the federal legislation affecting the healthcare industry, is the acronym derived from The Health Insurance Portability and Accountability Act of 1996 and is pronounced as if it were a word. Some acronyms have been used in language for so long that they have actually become regular words that follow the capitalization rules for capitalizing proper and common nouns:

- laser—Light Amplification by Stimulated Emission of Radiation
- radar—RAdio Detecting And Ranging
- scuba—Self-Contained Underwater Breathing Apparatus

Many medical illnesses have so many features or such a long name that it becomes helpful to use a single word or phrase. Other times it's simply a shortcut or timesaving way to jog the memory. But more often than not, it's simply the name that stuck, perhaps because it is "user-friendly" and easy to remember. For example, in *LASIK* (laser-assisted in situ keratomileusis) surgery, the cornea is reshaped while in its normal location with the help of lasers; "in situ" means "in the normal location" and "keratomileusis" means "to shape the cornea." The term LASIK becomes easier to understand and remember.

TRANSCRIPTION TIP:

Physicians use acronyms when referring to specialty units in the hospital, as shown in Table 5.2.

PROOFREADING TECHNIQUES

The proofreading and editing processes are the most crucial steps of creating a medical report. They ensure that the text is accurate and presentable and does not contain any errors that will distract the reader.

Verbatim Transcription versus Light Editing

Theoretically, medical transcriptionists are to transcribe dictation **verbatim**, which means typing the same words dictated, word for word. Different companies may define "verbatim" in different ways, but generally, a verbatim account will require reports to be transcribed exactly as dictated regardless of whether the text is grammatically or factually incorrect, whether a dictator from another country does not speak English correctly, or whether one sentence is three paragraphs long. In practice, however, it is often necessary to edit and correct obvious errors in grammar, punctuation, or spelling in the dictation itself, as few people speak in a manner that allows what they say to be converted into printed form without at least minor editing. This is called **light editing**, and there are times when it will be necessary to lightly edit text as you work to make the dictated words accurate and/or comprehensible. For example, a dictator can make obvious grammatical mistakes in his or her dictation, such as mistakes in subject-verb agreement or verb tense. The physician may be dictating about a patient's diagnostic studies and say, "The patient's medications include a white count of . . . ," in which case the transcriptionist can assume the dictator meant "lab values" or "laboratory results" rather than "medications." Physicians also may make simple errors in internal consistency, such as "he" for "she" or "left" for "right." In these instances, you should make the correction, but not otherwise change or delete the medical content.

Light editing may mean simply reorganizing a sentence so that it is grammatically correct. For example, the dictated sentence, "There were evidence of changes on the patient's bone scan," can be corrected to, "There was evidence of changes on the patient's bone scan." An

QUICK CHECK 5.3 ✓

Circle the letter corresponding to the best answer for the following questions.

1. A (An) _____ is used to indicate "how many."

   A. arabic number
   B. whole number
   C. roman numeral
   D. lowercase letter

2. A word or phrase formed from, or including, the name of a person, is called a(an)

   A. abbreviation.
   B. proper noun.
   C. acronym.
   D. eponym.

3. What are *not* considered to be proper nouns?

   A. names of individuals
   B. cities
   C. run-on sentences
   D. months of the year

4. Which of the following are always capitalized?

   A. academic degrees
   B. specific clinics
   C. song titles
   D. all of the above

5. Another term for *initialism* is

   A. capitalization.
   B. acronym.
   C. eponym.
   D. symbol.

---

awkwardly constructed sentence such as, "We will defer treatment to his neurosurgeon, *which he has a followup appointment to him*," could be recast to, "We will defer treatment to his neurosurgeon, *with whom he has a followup appointment*," for clarity.

Occasionally a dictator may use a phrase that you know to be wrong. For example, a dictator may say, "The placement of a rod in the femur was indicative of a prior colonoscopy." Unless you are completely certain that you know you can ascertain the word by the context of the sentence, you should leave a blank or make a notation about the error.

In situations like this, medical transcriptionists are expected to recognize minor dictation errors in internal consistency or verbiage and correct them. Light editing requires good judgment and the ability to make sound, professional decisions. It is important, however, *never* to delete, change, alter, or otherwise manipulate the medical content. The meaning of the sentence should remain unchanged after you make minor corrections to a physician's dictation error.

As a medical transcriptionist, it is not your job to substitute more creative words to make the text sound more eloquent or entertaining simply for the sake of providing literary prose, nor is it your job to make assumptions about a dictator's intentions based on what is being said. However, it is your responsibility to prepare reports that are as correct, clear, consistent, and complete as can be reasonably expected in order to facilitate reading and understanding of the report. When performing light editing as you transcribe, focus on grammar, punctuation, spelling, and similar dictation errors as necessary in order to simply achieve clarity.

Light editing may also may be necessary in the following situations:

1. The dictator is factually wrong and you are absolutely sure of it, such as dictating "he" for "she" or "right" for "left."

2. Words in the sentence are in an order that do not make sense.

3. Subject and verb do not agree.

4. The dictator spells a word that you know is misspelled or numbers items incorrectly.

5. When transcribing medication quantities, which always take a single verb.

   Dictated (incorrect): Valium 10 mg were given to the patient for sedation.
   Transcribed (correct): Valium 10 mg was given to the patient for sedation.

6. When verbs start a sentence.

   Dictated (incorrect): CHEST: Was clear to auscultation and percussion.
   Transcribed (correct): CHEST: Clear to auscultation and percussion.

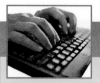

TRANSCRIPTION TIP:

Medical transcriptionists often mistype the term *followup* in medical reports. Use the words *follow up, follow-up,* and *followup* correctly according to context. Use *followup* or *follow-up* for the noun and adjectival forms. Use *follow up* as two words only when the word is used as a verb.

As a noun or adjective:

The patient will return for a *followup* visit (or *follow-up*).

The patient will return for *followup*.

As a verb:

The patient will *follow up* next week.

7. When transcribing the phrase *off of*, which is often dictated but not grammatically correct.

Dictated (incorrect): The patient was taken off of the respirator.

Transcribed (correct): The patient was taken off the respirator.

8. Transcribing the word *reoccur*. There is no such word as *reoccur*, although many dictators use it. Edit to *recur*.

Dictated (incorrect): The mother felt the patient's seizures were reoccurring.

Transcribed (correct): The mother felt the patient's seizures were recurring.

9. When sentences begin with numbers. Sentences that are dictated as such should be recast to add the words *then*, *the*, or *a*.

Dictated (incorrect): 6-0 bridle suture was placed near the limbus.

Transcribed (correct): A 6-0 bridle suture was placed near the limbus.

Light editing skills are developed over time, and eventually you will find yourself correcting these types of errors as they occur. Meanwhile, if you are

uncertain about exactly what is being dictated, you should bring it to the attention of the dictator or supervisor.

Proofreading Guidelines

Proofreading, the process of reviewing a document for errors is the final step in the production of a medical document and involves more than just scanning a report quickly for obvious spelling errors. Typographical errors and careless formatting mistakes make both the medical transcriptionist and the physician look unprofessional. The difference between a mediocre medical transcriptionist and a top-notch one lies in the way each handles the smallest of details. Effective proofreading requires both diligence and objectivity and, of course, tireless attention to detail. The most important work you do on a medical report—work that could make the difference between a "fair" product and an "outstanding" product—may take place in the proofreading stage, because it is in this stage that you can review what you have done and make improvements to ensure that your work is concise, complete, and correct.

Items that are typically missed during proofreading, which a spell check will not catch, include those as seen in Table 5.3.

Proofread all of your work before you send it to your employer. Use the following steps to evaluate your reports as you complete them:

1. Run a spell check on the document. Identifying misspellings is one of the biggest parts of proofreading. Each and every word in a medical document—both medical and otherwise—must be spelled correctly.

2. Print one copy of the report and look it over for the first time as a draft. Read the document slowly, looking for spelling errors not picked up by the spell checker, punctuation errors, missing words, incorrect words, run-on sentences, and grammatical errors. Look for errors in areas that frequently give

TABLE 5.3 Typical Items Missed During Proofreading	
Type of Error	*Example*
Missing letters	"no" for "now"; "though" for "thought"
Missing words	"The patient (had) undergone …"
Mistranscribed letters	"be" for "he"; "that" for "than"; "not" for "now"
Garbage punctuation	periods in the middle of sentences; extra punctuation at the end of sentences
Extraneous spaces (around words or punctuation)	"this" for "this"; more than one space between words
Mistakes involving homonyms or soundalike words	"plural" instead of "pleural"; "elicit" instead of "illicit"
Goose eggs, or completely unrelated words in a sentence	"The patient had severe shaking and *wagers* (instead of rigors)"

QUICK CHECK 5.4 ✓

Fill in the blank for the following sentences.

1. _____ means transcribing "word for word."

2. The word HIPAA is an example of a (an) _____.

3. A word or phrase formed from, or including, the name of a person is called a (an) _____.

4. You should edit the word *reoccur* to the word _____.

5. _____ is the process of reviewing a document for errors.

you trouble. For example, if you know you make errors in sentence punctuation involving the use of commas, check all sentences where commas would be required, and check all sentences in which you have used commas.

3. After first reading the document as a draft, go back and read the document more slowly. This time, look at it in an artificial way. For example, you might try reading the report backwards word by word or sentence by sentence; or try reading it aloud. These methods of distancing yourself from your words enable you to see or hear things you might miss if you were reading normally.

4. While you are proofreading, mark any mistakes with a red pen. Then make the changes you have noted. As you make them, check them off the hard copy. After you have finished correcting the mistakes, glance over the report to make sure all your changes have been checked.

5. Transmit the final, proofread report to your employer.

CHAPTER SUMMARY

A "finished" report always takes effort, but the best reports are those that are presentable and accurate and free of grammatical and punctuation errors. However, keep in mind that the ongoing changes in medical knowledge and advances in technology may result in periodic changes in transcription styles, forms, and practices. Strive to keep up with new and changing procedures. Mastering the essential skills of grammar, punctuation, and proofreading will enable you to produce accurate medical reports and demonstrate to employers that you are enthusiastic about your work and willing to invest time in making a positive contribution to a patient's medical record.

·I·N·S·I·G·H·T·

Little Dark Dots

Even "little dark dots" like periods or decimal points can wreak havoc in the medical system if they are used incorrectly.

Physicians and other healthcare providers write notes in a patient's medical record, describing the type of treatment provided. Medical coders convert these notes into alphanumerical codes, which insurance providers use to compensate the healthcare provider.

To correctly file a claim for each third-party payor, the coder has to choose combinations from a complex standard coding system consisting of over 10,000 numeric codes and key the right code for accurate billing. Medical billing problems are all too common. Errors in coding these bills can lead to problems for the patient as well as for the insurance company. For example, a medical coder who places a decimal point in the wrong place in a code could inadvertently bill an insurance company for a procedure that was never done or enter an incorrect diagnosis, resulting in rejection of the claim by the insurance company. Or, even if the claim is paid, the error could find its way into a patient's permanent medical record without the patient even being aware of it.

Something as miniscule as a misplaced period can lead to complications, frustrations, and possibly even legal issues for the provider. Therefore, careful attention to even the smallest of details plays a key role in keeping medical mistakes to a minimum.

TERMINOLOGY

Term	Meaning
acronym	A word that is formed by combining first letters of some other terms.
apostrophe	A punctuation mark used to indicate the possessive case of nouns, to form some plurals of words, or to denote omitted letters or numbers in contractions.
appositive	A word or phrase placed before or after a noun that explains or identifies it.
arabic numbers	Another name for *cardinal numbers*.
cardinal numbers	Numbers that are used to indicate "how many" (one, two three, etc.).
collective nouns	Nouns that refer to groups of people or things.
colon	A punctuation mark that usually introduces and/or highlights the words that follows it.
comma	A punctuation mark that separates the structural elements of a sentence into manageable segments.
comma splice	A situation that occurs when independent clauses are connected to each other with commas.
compound adjective	Two or more words used together as a single modifier of a noun.
conjunctive adverbs	Another name for *transitional words*.
dash	A punctuation mark that draws attention to nonessential material and highlights it.
dependent clause	A sentence that has a subject and verb but cannot stand alone.
em dash	A dash that is the width of a capital M.
eponym	A name or phrase formed from, or including, the name of a person.
figures	Another name for *cardinal numbers*.
helping verb	A verb that modifies the main verb.
hyphen	A punctuation mark typically used in numbers and compound words.
independent clause	A complete sentence consisting of a subject and verb and expressing a complete thought.
initialisms	A combination of letters representing a longer phrase.
light editing	The process of editing and correcting mistakes of obvious grammatical, punctuation, or spelling errors in dictation.
main verb	The main action word in a sentence.
number	An abstract entity that represents a count or measurement.
ordinal numbers	Numbers that denote position in an ordered sequence (first, second, third, etc.).
parentheses	Punctuation marks used in pairs to enclose or surround textual material.
period	A punctuation mark placed at the end of a sentence that makes a statement.
proofreader's marks	A combination of symbols and short notations used to mark up draft documents.
proofreading	The process of reviewing a document for errors.
question mark	A punctuation mark placed at the end of a sentence that asks a direct question.
quotation marks	Punctuation marks used in pairs to set off speech, a quotation, or a phrase.
roman numerals	A numbering system derived from ancient Rome based on certain letters that are given values as numerals (I, II, III, etc.).
run-on sentence	A situation that occurs when two independent clauses appear in a sentence without any punctuation between them.

Term	Meaning
semicolon	A mark that indicates a weaker break in a sentence than a period but a stronger break than a comma.
sentence fragment	A group of words that is only part of a sentence and does not express a complete thought.
subject-verb agreement	Subjects must agree in number with verbs in a sentence.
suspensive hyphen	A hyphen used to connect a series of compound modifiers with the same base term.
transitional words	Adverbs that join two independent clauses with a semicolon before and a comma after.
verbatim	Transcribing "word for word," or in precisely the same words used by the dictator.

Add Your Own Terms and Definitions Here:

_____

_____

_____

_____

_____

_____

_____

_____

REVIEW QUESTIONS

1. What is the difference between typing verbatim and light editing?
2. Where are sentence fragments frequently found in medical reports?
3. How many spaces are typed after a period at the end of a sentence?
4. How are the genus and species name of bacteria capitalized?
5. When is an eponym not capitalized?
6. What are the necessary parts of every sentence?
7. What is a compound adjective?
8. What is the purpose of proofreaders' marks?
9. What should be done with sentences that begin with a number?
10. When are dashes used?

CHAPTER ACTIVITIES

Numbers and Symbols

Study the phonetic pronunciations of numbers and symbols on the left and write the correct formatting of the term on the right.

1. *three-oh* Vicryl   _____
2. *one hundred one point two degrees fahrenheit*   _____
3. *won on won* discussion   _____
4. a *number fifteen french* blade.   _____
5. *gravida one para one zero zero one*   _____
6. *ten milligrams per kilogram* per day   _____
7. Premarin *zero point six two five milligrams*   _____
8. *seventy five to eighty percent* healed   _____
9. *six millimeters squared*   _____
10. Tylenol *number 3*   _____

Comma or Semicolon?

Each of the following sentences needs either a comma or a semicolon. Choose the correct punctuation mark and place it in the blank provided.

1. She did not want to proceed with any further radiation ___ however ___ she states that she feels like the radiation ___ as well as chemotherapy ___ has benefited her.
2. His option would be neutron radiotherapy ___ which was not offered here ___ and the patient at that point was not able to travel.
3. She ran into the driveway ___ and then she ran across the street.
4. The patient remained on cyclosporine for two years ___ however___ secondary to the side effects of cyclosporine toxicity, it was eventually discontinued.
5. Her jugular venous pulse was somewhat difficult to assess ___ it was because of the width of her neck.
6. The CT scan of the left nasal cavity first showed mild inferior turbinate hypertrophy ___ and then it was clear.
7. The patient can go back to school ___ and he is not to play baseball for a week.
8. At this time, patient is doing well status post surgery ___ but he still complains of nausea.

9. He ambulates with crutches ___ and he has no tenderness on palpation of his legs.

10. The surgery was thoroughly discussed with the patient ___ subsequently the patient agreed with the plan.

Subject-Verb Agreement

Circle the correct word to complete each sentence.

1. There (is/are) no otorrhea, drainage, or hearing loss in the right ear.
2. Evaluation of the patient's x-rays (shows/show) a left-sided rib fracture.
3. Sclerae (is/are) not injected.
4. There (is/are) also bilateral pathological nodes, one more prominent on the right side of the neck.
5. The hot flashes, according to the patient, (occur/occurs) every day.
6. He did have some mild disequilibrium for 2–3 days postoperatively, which (has/have) since resolved.
7. Her 12-organ review of systems (is/are) otherwise negative.
8. The area of stiffness, redness, and swelling (is/are) of concern to me.
9. The symptoms the patient felt, I believe, (is/are) related to her previous treatment.
10. There (was/were) no findings of a stone or other obvious abnormality in the diagnostic testing.
11. No facial asymmetry or weakness (was/were) observed on exam.
12. Findings at cardiac catheterization (include/includes) a severely occluded right coronary artery.
13. CT scan of the neck done today (shows/show) soft tissue masses within the right medial masticator space.
14. Labs done today (shows/show) a white blood cell count of 6600, hemoglobin 10.9, and hematocrit 32.9.
15. He uses Larry's Solution as needed and oxycodone, from which he (get/gets) good relief.

Capitalization Practice

Capitalize the words where indicated in the following sentences by underlining the word to be capitalized.

1. her medications include amoxicillin, zantac, ibuprofen, and tylenol for pain.
2. then six 3-0 vicryl sutures were used to close the wound, followed by bacitracin ointment.
3. he also used zofran twice per day as well as compazine for nausea.
4. the anticoagulant warfarin is the generic name for coumadin.
5. the patient complained, "the medications are not working."
6. the patient is a 33-year-old hispanic female who presented to the cardiology clinic after having studies done in radiology.
7. this white female of ashkenazi jewish descent underwent chemotherapy with taxol and carboplatin last year.
8. Dr. miller, the president of the american nurses association, spoke at our dinner last night.
9. allison grey, md, autographed her best-selling book, all doctors on call in central america.
10. the patient is a gravida 1, para 1 female with a blood pressure of 138/90 mmhg.

Matching Acronyms

Match the acronym in the first column with the clue in the second column. Then in the third column, indicate the definition of the acronym. You may use a medical dictionary or a book of acronyms to look up the ones you do not know. The first one is completed for you.

Acronym	Clue	Definition
A. THR	__H__ A disorder characterized by changes to the ovaries such that multiple follicles accumulate in the ovaries without ovulation.	Polycystic ovarian syndrome
B. BNP		
C. AAA	_____ The presence of low-grade abnormal, precancerous cells on the surface of the cervix or its canal.	_____
D. PTCA		
E. MOM	_____ A type of diabetes not requiring insulin.	_____
F. DNR	_____ A total replacement of the hip joint.	_____
G. NASH	_____ A procedure where the prostate is shaved from inside the urethra to provide a better urinary stream.	_____
H. PCOS		
I. AIDS	_____ A scoring system to quantify consciousness after a trauma.	_____
J. TURP	_____ In cardiology, an operation for enlarging a narrowed vascular lumen.	_____
K. BMP		
L. LGSIL	_____ A mixture of magnesium hydroxide used as an antacid.	_____
M. SIADH		
N. PEG	_____ A surgical procedure for placing a feeding tube without having to perform an open operation on the abdomen.	_____
O. NIDDM	_____ Part of a physical exam pertaining to the head, eyes, ears, nose, and throat.	_____
P. MRSA		
Q. BKA	_____ A nonresuscitation order placed on a patient's chart.	_____
R. OCD	_____ The inability of the body to excrete dilute urine.	_____
S. HEENT	_____ An amputation of the lower extremity.	_____
T. GCS	_____ In cardiology, a natriuretic peptide.	_____

_____ A serious disease of the immune system.   _____

_____ An anxiety disorder characterized by intense, recurrent, unwanted thoughts and rituals.   _____

_____ A dilation of a portion of the aorta in the abdomen.   _____

_____ A group of blood tests that monitor the status of the kidneys, electrolytes, blood sugar, and calcium levels.   _____

_____ A bacteria that is resistant to the antibiotic methicillin.   _____

_____ A liver disease that occurs in people who drink little or no alcohol.   _____

Proofreading Exercise 1

Read the following paragraphs and determine which punctuation marks do not belong in the clinic report. Then retype the report using corrected punctuation. When finished, print one copy and save the corrected report as **CHAPTER-5-NOTE1.**

HISTORY OF PRESENT ILLNESS: This is a 55-year-old? male, who presented to the ENT clinic several weeks ago after being beaten up with brass-knuckles. At that time, it was determined he had a left tripod fracture—and he was taken to the operating room on December 8, -20xx?, for repair. In the operating room, it was found that he had several-fractures, which included a tripod-fracture involving the root of his left zygomatic arch as well as the lateral orbital rim and, a fracture extending down the anterior table of the maxilla. through the infraorbital foramina. The fractures' were reduced and he was plated in the O.R.

On the day, of his discharge, he was set for discharge and prescriptions, were written, but patient left the hospital before picking up these prescriptions. and before checking out. Therefore, he had no antibiotics, or pain coverage, but he says the pain has been minimal and he has not had any other complications-He also left before obtaining followup and showed up to clinic today to have sutures removed.

Proofreading Exercise 2

Proofread the following text. Circle the punctuation, capitalization, grammar, and formatting errors you find.

Then retype the document in correct form. When finished, print one copy of the paragraph and save the completed document as **CHAPTER-5-TX1.**

Over time our profession has faced calls that a new electronic gadget would replace medical transcriptionists we have survived them all. Computers replaced typewriters, and were still here. Then the "global village economy send many transcription jobs oversees and we survived that. The no. 3 idea called Voice Recognition claimed it could "do all the work of an MT', and indeed medical transcriptionists are still here. More ideas arrive to challenge us to re-think the ways in wich medical transcriptionist perform there job duties.

we as medical transcriptionists should always be mindful of the changes occurring in are field and move forward with progress instead of away from it. We are living in a rapidly changing world where tecnology is constantly involving and creating new ways to do our werk. we must keep current with these changes so that they can be more competitive and valuable employees. won way we can achieve this goal is by taking advantage of educational oportunities that become available so that we may stay current with the happenings in the medical field. well always encounter new ideas as we carry on our journey in our special field of health care. Change will always be in the air by embracing these changes we can make great things happen as we lern new waves to farther our scope and place in the health care profeshun.

Special Message Word Search

First find the listed words hidden in the rows and columns of letters. After all the words are found, a hidden message will be spelled out by the unused letters. Read the message from left to right, top row to bottom.

```
M  I  S  L  A  N  O  I  T  I  S  N  A  R  T  T
H  E  L  P  I  N  G  V  E  R  B  A  K  E  S  K
S  I  N  E  D  I  T  A  I  N  G  A  N  M  R  D
K  P  R  O  O  F  R  D  C  E  A  D  Y  A  I  N
R  S  G  C  A  N  B  O  E  R  N  N  M  O  A  T
A  O  E  N  L  Y  F  I  R  U  O  N  S  P  T  R
M  C  O  M  M  A  A  R  T  P  O  N  O  I  M  N
N  G  T  O  I  T  H  E  E  I  E  S  Y  A  R  E
O  A  D  E  R  C  B  P  T  U  T  T  I  M  C  V
I  C  O  S  T  L  O  S  H  R  Y  N  T  O  T  E
T  O  H  E  P  A  E  L  O  S  V  T  I  E  N  R
A  L  T  X  F  U  M  P  O  E  A  T  R  L  N  B
T  O  X  L  Q  X  H  Q  R  N  R  D  L  Y  L  A
O  N  P  P  T  E  T  B  L  N  E  H  P  Y  H  T
U  G  N  I  D  A  E  R  F  O  O  R  P  P  Z  I
Q  N  P  A  R  E  N  T  H  E  S  E  S  X  M  M
```

www.WordSearchMaker.com

ACRONYM	PARENTHESES
APOSTROPHE	PERIOD
COLON	PROOFREADING
COMMA	QUESTION MARK
DASH	QUOTATION MARKS
EPONYM	SEMICOLON
HELPING VERB	TRANSITIONAL
HYPHEN	VERBATIM
MAIN VERB	

Hidden Message: _____

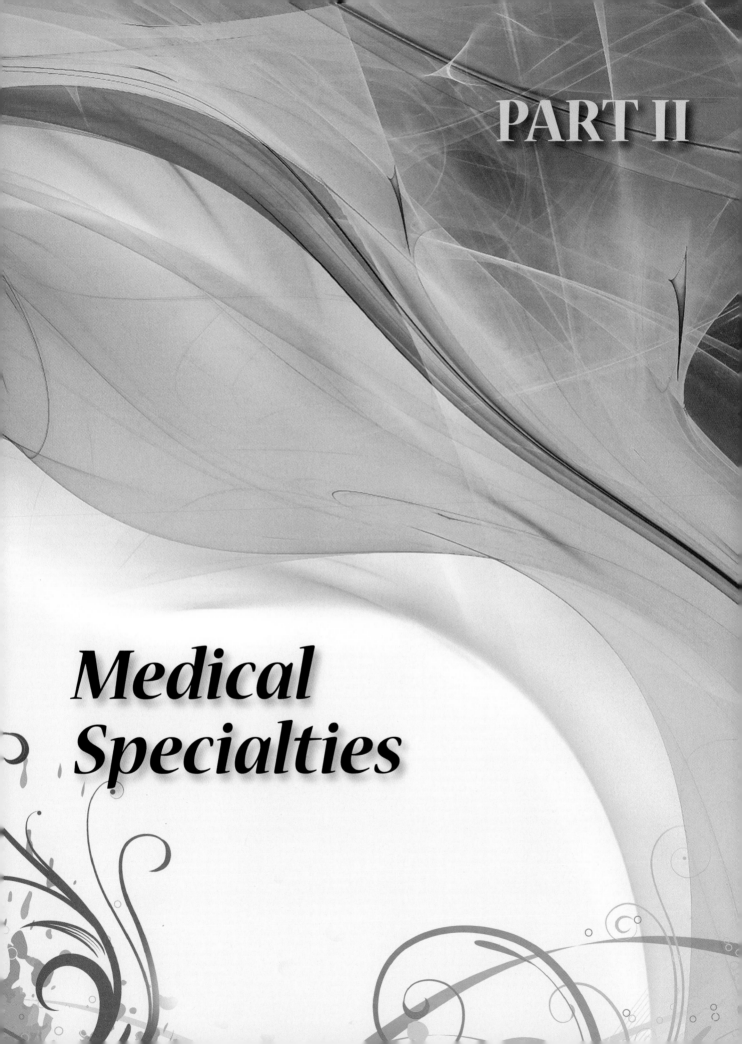

PART II

Medical Specialties

SURGERY

OBJECTIVES

After completing this chapter, you will be able to:

- Discuss the general concepts involved in surgery, including various types of surgical procedures and the differences between each.
- List the component parts of the surgical process.
- Define common terminology used to describe surgical procedures.
- Identify common prefixes, suffixes, and combining word forms used to describe surgical procedures.

INTRODUCTION

The safe delivery of surgical care affects the lives of millions of people every year. About 234 million major operations are performed worldwide annually. The accurate and grammatically correct preparation of the documentation of surgical procedures is one of the most challenging tasks encountered by transcriptionists. Understanding the terminology used in such surgical procedures is an integral part of creating accurate operative reports. This chapter introduces concepts of surgery along with terms typically encountered by a medical transcriptionist in operative reports. It also covers the terminology used to describe the surgical process and the tools and equipment used at each phase of an operation. Familiarity with these terms and concepts will help the transcriptionist prepare accurate reports in the demanding specialty of surgery.

GENERAL SURGERY CONCEPTS

Surgery is the medical specialty that treats diseases and disorders through physical intervention, such as cutting, removing, or changing parts of the body in some way, in a procedure called an **operation** or **surgical procedure**. The term is derived from the Latin word *chirurgiae*, meaning "hand work." A physician who specializes in performing procedures in an operating room or surgical center is known as a **surgeon**.

The term *surgery* is used in different ways to describe procedures. As a general rule, a surgical procedure involves the cutting of a patient's tissues or the closure of a previously sustained wound. However, other procedures that do not involve cutting but do involve common elements associated with surgical procedures—such as the use of a sterile environment, anesthesia, typical surgical instruments, and closing or suturing of wounds—may also be called "surgery." For example, an **endoscopy** is the examination of the interior of the body with the use of a special flexible lighted instrument called an **endoscope**. Endoscopy does not require

119

cutting into the body but is performed using sterile conditions and, sometimes, conscious sedation to help alleviate patient discomfort during the procedure.

Generally, surgical procedures are categorized by the type of procedure, body system involved, and instruments used. Common types of procedures include:

- Invasive procedures. These procedures involve cutting into an organ or body tissue. The cut is called an **incision**. These types of procedures end in the suffix –*tomy*, meaning "cut into or incision." A **cholecystectomy** is the surgical removal of the gallbladder by cutting through the abdominal wall to gain access to the gallbladder. A **tonsillectomy** is the surgical removal of the tonsils.
- Minimally invasive procedures. This type of surgery involves making small incisions into the body through which a special scope or other instruments are inserted. These types of procedures end in the suffix –*scopy*, meaning visual examination. For example, a **laparoscopy** is the visual examination of the abdomen using a special instrument called a laparoscope, which is inserted through small incisions made into the body.
- Noninvasive surgery. This usually refers to an excision that does not penetrate the body or structure being excised, such as the removal of a mole on the skin or the correction of vision using laser methods.
- Elective surgery. This type of procedure is performed to correct a non-life-threatening condition and is carried out at the patient's request, such as a tubal ligation or plastic surgery.
- Emergency surgery. Emergency surgery is an operation that must be done quickly in order to save the patient's life or to restore functional capacity. An example of this type of surgery can include an emergency appendectomy or cesarean section.
- Exploratory surgery. This is a procedure performed to aid or confirm a diagnosis, such as a laparoscopy or a colonoscopy. A **colonoscopy** is a visual examination of the colon with a visual tube called a colonoscope.
- Therapeutic surgery. Therapeutic surgery treats a previously diagnosed problem or condition. **Mastectomy,** which is the surgical removal of one or both breasts in order to treat serious breast disease, such as breast cancer, is an example of therapeutic surgery.
- Reconstructive surgery. This type of procedure involves the reconstruction of an injured, mutilated, or deformed part of the body. These procedures end in the suffix –*plasty*, meaning surgical repair. A **rhinoplasty** is the surgical reconstruction of the nose.
- Transplant surgery. Transplant surgery involves the replacement of an organ or body part by insertion of another part from a different person or animal into the patient, such as a heart or liver transplant.
- Cosmetic surgery. This is a procedure performed to improve the appearance of an otherwise normal body part or structure. An example of this type of surgery would be breast augmentation surgery to enhance the appearance of the breasts.
- Ostomy surgery. This is an operation that is performed to create a permanent or semi-permanent opening in the body, ends in –*stomy*, meaning artificial opening. A **tracheostomy** is a surgical opening made in the trachea in order to facilitate breathing.

Surgical procedures may also be categorized by organ system or structure. For example, cardiac surgery is performed on the heart, gastrointestinal surgery is performed on the digestive tract and accessory organs, and gynecologic surgery is performed on the female reproductive organs.

THE SURGICAL PROCESS

Typically inpatient surgery is performed in a hospital's operating room, while outpatient procedures are performed in surgery centers or, sometimes, a doctor's office. Prior to the surgery, the patient is given a medical examination and preoperative laboratory and/or imaging test to ensure he/she is a viable candidate for the surgical procedure. If there is no contraindication to the patient receiving the surgery, he/she signs an **informed consent**, which is the written permission given by the patient to undergo the surgical procedure. Informed consent is obtained once the patient understands all the risks, benefits, and alternatives involved. The patient is usually asked to abstain from food or drink after midnight on the night prior to the procedure to minimize the risk of aspiration if the patient vomits during or after the procedure because of an adverse reaction to preoperative or postoperative medications. This order is referred to in the record as the patient being **n.p.o.**, the Latin abbreviation for *nothing by mouth.*

On the day of surgery, the patient is taken to the preoperative area where he/she is placed on a gurney and vital signs are taken. Among the procedures performed prior to surgery is the placement or insertion of peripheral intravenous lines through which preoperative medication (such as antibiotics and sedatives, etc.) is given. If hair is present at the surgical site, it is shaved off to provide a clear operating field. **Drapes** are pieces of cloth used to cover all of the patient's body except for the surgical site and the patient's head. The drapes are attached to a pair of poles near the head of the bed to form a screen to separate the anesthesiologist's working area, which is unsterile, from the surgical site, which is sterile.

Patients often do not think about who actually will be in the operating room during their surgery, but anyone present during the procedure must be noted in the medical record. A medical transcriptionist will often transcribe the names and titles of at least some of these individuals in the formal operative report. These may include:

- The primary surgeon, who is the physician performing the surgery and who is responsible for the patient's overall care.
- The second surgeon or assistant, who assists the primary surgeon.
- The anesthesiologist, who is responsible for the patient's medical care while he/she is under anesthesia.

When the patient is taken to the operating room, an anesthesia agent is administered and the patient may be intubated to help facilitate breathing while the patient is sedated and paralyzed. **Intubation** is a procedure that involves the placement of a flexible plastic tube into the trachea (the wind pipe) to protect the patient's airway and provide a means of mechanical ventilation. The most common tracheal intubation is **orotracheal intubation**, where the tube is passed through the mouth, larynx, and vocal cords, into the trachea. A bulb is then inflated near the distal tip of the tube to help secure it in place and protect the airway from blood, vomit, and secretions.

At this point, an incision is made to access the surgical site and work to correct the problem in the body proceeds. This work may involve any of the following procedures:

- **Excision**, which is the complete surgical removal of an organ, tumor, or other tissue.
- **Resection**, which is the partial removal of an organ, tumor, or other tissue.

- **Ligation**, which is the tying off a duct or a blood vessel with a ligature to prevent further bleeding or leakage of fluid.
- **Grafting**, which is taking healthy tissue from one part of the body and transplanting it to another part of the body.
- **Anastomosis**, which is the surgical connection made between two blood vessels or other tubular structures.
- **Debridement**, which is the removal of dead, damaged, or diseased tissue from a part of the body.
- **Suturing**, which is the procedure used to close a wound by stitching edges together with thread or other material.
- **Dressing**, which is applying a sterile bandage over the wound to prevent infection and facilitate healing.

Blood or blood products may be administered to compensate for blood lost during surgery due to trauma or disease. To decrease the risk of infection and immunologic complications during this process, most hospitals and surgery centers offer a preoperative blood donation program where the patient donates blood for his/her own use, if needed, prior to the surgery. This is called an **autologous blood donation**. If blood needs to be replaced during the surgery, it can be returned to the patient via a **cell saver**, which is an intraoperative cell salvage machine whose purpose is to replace blood lost during a surgical procedure with the patient's own donated blood collected before the procedure.

Once the incision is closed, anesthesia is stopped or reversed, the patient is taken off mechanical ventilation, and the orotracheal tube, if used, is removed, called **extubation**. The patient is then taken to the recovery room or post-anesthesia recovery unit and monitored for any postsurgical complications. When the patient is determined to have recovered from anesthesia, he/she is transferred either to the recovery floor of the hospital, or discharged to home for followup care and recovery.

QUICK CHECK 6.1 ✓

Fill in the blanks with the correct answers.

1. Surgery used to treat a previously diagnosed problem or condition is called _____ .

2. The suffix –*stomy* means _____ .

3. Generally, the cutting of a patient's tissues or the closure of a previously sustained wound is known as a _____ .

4. The person who assists the primary surgeon in an operation is called the _____ .

5. The surgical removal of an organ, tumor, or other tissue is called _____ .

COMMON SURGICAL TERMINOLOGY

An operative procedure often follows certain steps and procedures, many of which are documented using common terms and definitions.

Patient Positioning

Before the surgery begins, the patient is positioned on the operating table to allow for adequate access to the surgical site and to prevent the patient from falling or injuring soft tissues or bony prominences. The position of the patient is usually dictated in the first paragraph of the operative report. Some common positions used in patient positioning include the following, as illustrated in Figure 6.1.

- Supine: Lying on the back, face up.
- Prone: Lying face down.
- Dorsal lithotomy position: A supine position with the patient's buttocks at the end of the operating room table, hips and knees up and apart and feet strapped in metal supports.
- Dorsal recumbent position: A reclining position with the patient's knees bent, hips rotated outward, and feet flat.

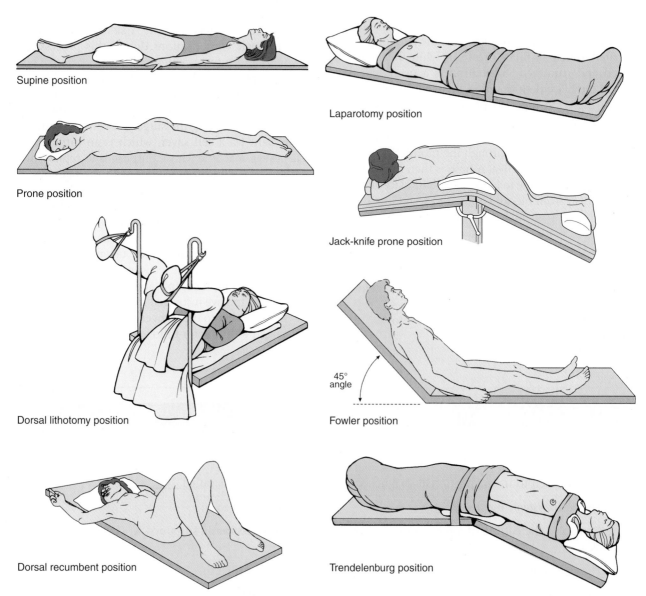

FIGURE 6.1. **Body Positions**. The surgeon determines the position of the patient by considering the surgical approach, the physical condition of the patient, and the physical condition of the patient, among other factors. Reprinted with permission from *Stedman's Medical Dictionary for the Health Professions and Nursing, Fifth Edition*, 2005.

- Laparotomy position: A supine position with only the upper torso exposed
- Jack-knife prone position: A prone position with the buttocks raised
- Fowler position: A recumbent position in which the head of the bed is elevated 45–60 degrees above level
- Trendelenburg position: A supine position on the operating table, which is inclined at varying angles so that the pelvis is higher than the head; used during and after operations in the pelvis or for shock

Anesthesia Administration

By definition, **anesthesia** is the loss of normal sensation or feeling. Anesthesiologists use drugs to produce this loss of feeling or awareness. Properly administered anesthesia prevents the patient from feeling pain during the procedure, and they often have no memory of the proceedings. The anesthesia care team consists of an anesthesiologist and a nurse anesthetist. An **anesthesiologist** is a physician who has completed medical school plus additional training in medicine and anesthesia. A certified **registered nurse anesthetist** is a registered nurse who has received additional education in anesthesia. The nurse anesthetist assists the anesthesiologist during the entire surgery to make sure that no complications occur during the procedure.

The type of anesthesia used depends on the type of surgery being performed. Typical types of anesthesia include:

- Infiltration, which is a local anesthetic that is injected directly into the tissue where the surgery will take place. Patients may encounter this technique in the emergency department when a doctor injects local anesthetic before sewing up a cut or during minor procedures performed in the operating room. Although the injections may be performed by the surgeon, an anesthesiologist is often needed to monitor the patient and to give sedation or other medications that may be required during the operation.

- Regional anesthesia, also called *local anesthesia*, is the application of an anesthetic agent to a major nerve bundle around a particular region or part of the body (such as a limb), providing a loss of sensation in that region and all the nerves supplying it. Unlike general anesthesia, the patient remains awake during the procedure, reducing side effects of the anesthesia and enabling the patient to respond to the surgeon during the procedure. There are two types of regional anesthesia: peripheral nerve blocks, which involve a relatively small part of the body, such as an arm or a foot; and spinals and epidurals, which can involve the entire lower portion of the body. Epidural anesthesia medication is placed in the epidural space, or the outermost part of the spinal canal of the back, with a catheter. This method is often used in childbirth and gynecological surgery. Spinal anesthesia is injected through a needle directly into the fluid that bathes the spinal nerves. In each case, the result is a loss of sensation in the abdominal and genital and pelvic areas.

- Sedation is a medical procedure involving the administration of tranquilizing drugs to produce a state of reduced excitement or anxiety during surgery. It is used in smaller operations or less invasive procedures. Sedation can range from a light to deep state of unconsciousness. During light sedation, the patient can be easily aroused and can breathe without help, whereas at deeper levels of sedation the patient may need to be aroused with stimulation and may need some assistance with breathing.

- General anesthesia is the type of anesthesia familiar to most people, in which the patient is unconscious and paralyzed during surgery. In practice, general anesthesia ranges from the relatively light levels used during minor surgery to the deepest levels used in major operations. Unlike regional anesthesia, general anesthesia acts primarily on the brain rather than on the nerves leading to the brain. The patient is usually intubated and placed on a mechanical ventilator to assist with breathing.

Table 6.1 shows the different types of anesthesia agents used during surgery.

Fluids and Medications

Prior to surgery, an intravenous catheter is placed in a vein in the patient's arm to deliver fluids, medications, or blood during surgery. The intravenous line is used to administer various fluids that help maintain hydration, maintain blood pressure, and in the event of an adverse reaction during the procedure (such as sudden, uncontrolled bleeding), to allow for instant access to bloodstream with possibly life-saving medications. Table 6.2 illustrates some of the common fluids and medications

TABLE 6.1   Anesthesia Agents Used During Surgery

Name	*Description*
bupivacaine (brand name Marcaine); Marcaine plain	A local anesthetic used in regional analgesia.
Hurricaine spray	Brand name for a spray-type anesthetic
lidocaine (brand name Xylocaine); lidocaine without epinephrine	A regional anesthetic agent that can be used locally or in IV form.
lidocaine with epinephrine	Lidocaine with added epinephrine for vasoconstriction, decreased bleeding, and prolongs the duration of the anesthetic effect.
Marcaine with epinephrine	Bupivacaine with added epinephrine for vasoconstriction.
Mepivacaine (Carbocaine)	Used as an emergency wound anesthetic.
nitrous oxide	A gaseous anesthetic used in combination with other anesthetic agents; also called "laughing gas."
tetracaine	A local anesthetic used in spinal injection and topical anesthesia.

used during surgery that may be transcribed in an operative report.

Tools and Instruments

A variety of instruments and tools are used in the operating room in order to perform specific actions like removing or modifying body tissue or structures or to provide access for viewing them. Some tools have multiple purposes and can be used to perform similar tasks in various types of surgeries, while others are designed for a specific procedure only. The names of surgical instruments follow patterns, such as a description of the action an instrument performs, the name of its inventor, or a compound scientific name related to

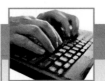

TRANSCRIPTION TIP:

Sometimes it is difficult to tell whether a dictator is saying *effusion* or *infusion*. **Effusion** refers to the escape of fluid into a tissue or body part. **Infusion** is the therapeutic introduction of fluid (not blood) into a vein by means of gravity.

the kind of surgery in which it is used. Commonly used instruments for a particular type of surgery are usually grouped together on an **instrument tray** in the operating room for use by the surgeon, as shown in Figure 6.2.

TABLE 6.2   Medications and Fluids Commonly Used in Surgery

Antibiotics	
Ancef	Brand name for type of injectable cephalosporin antibiotic.
bacitracin	A multifunctional antibacterial ointment.
Betadine scrub, solution, or paint	Topical antiseptic widely used in presurgical preparation and cleansing.
gentamicin ointment	Antibiotic used against gram-positive and gram-negative pathogens.
Maxitrol ointment	Antibiotic used against gram-positive and gram-negative pathogens.
Polysporin ointment	Brand name for an antibacterial ointment.
Anticoagulant	
heparin	An anticoagulant that prevents or retards the clotting of blood.
Fluids	
crystalloid	A solution that passes through membranes.
lactated Ringer solution	Also called simply "lactated Ringer's," an intravenous fluid used to replenish electrolytes.
saline solution	An isotonic aqueous solution of sodium chloride.
sorbitol	A solution used as an irrigating fluid in prostatic or transurethral surgeries.

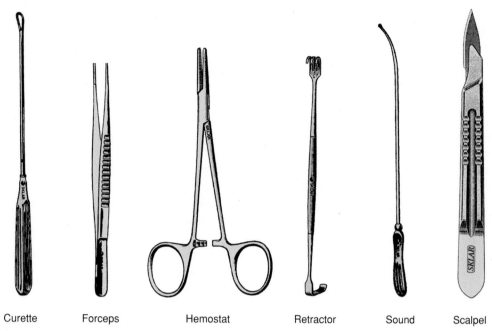

| Curette | Forceps | Hemostat | Retractor | Sound | Scalpel |

FIGURE 6.2. Surgical Instruments. Many types of instruments are used to perform specific tasks during surgery. Reprinted with permission from Cohen BJ. *Medical Terminology.* 4th Ed. Philadelphia: Lippincott Williams & Wilkins, 2003.

An ever-increasing number and variety of surgical tools and instruments have been invented or refined as a result of the technological advances in the operating room. Many traditional instruments have been replaced with more precise and efficient energy-based instruments like electrocauteries, laser technology, ultrasound, electric scalpels, and robotics. Table 6.3 describes some of the common tools used in general surgery and the purpose of each.

Wound Closures and Coverings

Wound healing is a natural and spontaneous phenomenon. When tissue has been disrupted so severely that it cannot heal naturally (without complications or possible disfiguration), dead tissue and foreign bodies must be removed and infection treated, and the tissue must be held together or held in **apposition**, until the healing process provides the wound with sufficient strength to withstand stress without outside support. A wound may be closed with sutures, staples, clips, skin closure strips, or topical adhesives. Coverings include dressings, bandages, and gauze pads.

Sutures

A **suture** is a strand of material used to **ligate**, or tie, blood vessels or to **approximate**, or bring close together, tissues. Sutures are used to close wounds by sewing the edges of the wound together with a needle to form a seam.

Sutures were used by both the Egyptians and Syrians as far back as 2,000 B.C. Through the centuries, a wide variety of materials—strands of silk, linen, cotton, horsehair, animal tendons and intestines, and wire made of precious metals—have been used as sutures. Some of these are still in use today. Today sutures can be designed for specific surgical procedures, but suturing a wound still involves the same basic procedure used by physicians to the Roman emperors. The surgeon still uses a surgical needle to penetrate body tissue and advance a suture strand to its desired location.

Suture size is indicated by the diameter of the suture material. Suture size is stated numerically; as the number of zeros in the suture size increases, the diameter of the strand decreases. For example, size 5-0 (which is transcribed as 5-0 but dictated as "five-oh"), or 00000, is smaller in diameter than size 4-0, or 0000.

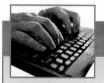

TRANSCRIPTION TIP:

Listen carefully to hear the difference between Duval and Davol. There are several types of Duval forceps and clamps used in intestinal and lung surgeries. There are Davol catheters, tubes, drains, tunnelers, dermatomes, forceps, and other tools.

TABLE 6.3   Common Tools and Instruments Used in General Surgery

Tool	Purpose
cautery instrument	A device that uses high-frequency electric current to a specific area of the body in order to remove unwanted tissue, seal off blood vessels, or create a surgical incision.
clamps	Used as an occluder for blood vessels and other organs.
scalpels, blades, rasps, scissors, trocars	Cutting tools that incise.
dilator or speculum	Device used to allow for access to narrow passages in the body.
drills and dermatomes	Powered devices used to make or enlarge a hole in a bone.
elevators	Used for prying up a sunken body part or organ, or elevating tissues attached to bone.
evacuators	Used to remove fluid or materials from a body cavity.
forceps	Used to grasp objects.
laser	A device used to concentrate light into a narrow beam to remove diseased tissue or treat bleeding blood vessels by heating the targeted cells until they "burst."
needles	Used for puncturing tissues, closing wounds, injection, aspiration, biopsy, or to guide introduction of a catheter into a vessel or other space.
pins, screws, wires, plates	Fixation devices used to fasten objects together and hold them in place.
plug	Used to fill a hole or close an orifice.
retractors	Used to draw aside edges of a wound or for holding back structures adjacent to the operative field.
rongeur	A strong biting forceps for nipping away bone.
rulers and calipers	Used to measure.
saw	A metal operating instrument having an edge of sharp, tooth-like projections for dividing bone, cartilage, or plaster.
scopes and probes	Instruments used to visually examine an organ or structure.
stereotactic device	A mechanical device with head-holding clamps and bars which puts the head of the patient in a fixed position in order to allow experimental and surgical intervention in deep-seated structures of the brain.
suction tips and tubes	Vacuum-type devices used to remove body fluids.
surgical stapler	A device used to seal or close an opening in the body.

Sutures are further classified according to the number of strands of which they are comprised. **Monofilament sutures** are made of a single strand of material. **Multifilament sutures** consist of several strands of material that are twisted or braided together, which afford greater strength and flexibility. Sutures also are classified according to their ability to degrade in the body. Sutures that degrade rapidly and eventually dissolve in the body are called **absorbable** sutures. Sutures that maintain their strength and must be manually removed from the body are called **nonabsorbable** sutures.

Table 6.4 illustrates suture types and materials commonly used in operative reports.

Dressings and Bandages

Dressings and bandages are used in wound management. The purpose of bandages and dressings is to protect the wound, promote healing, and retain or remove moisture from the wound. A **dressing** is a material applied directly to a wound to promote healing or prevent further harm. Although, by definition, a dressing is an adjunct to a wound covering, the word is often used to encompass both the dressing and bandage as one unit. Dressings can consist of a wide range of materials, including gels, foams, transparent film, or other materials. Some dressings contain medication to facilitate wound healing as they are placed directly against the wound. A **bandage**, also called **gauze**, is a piece of cloth

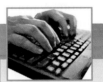

TRANSCRIPTION TIP:

The *LigaSure* is a brand-name tissue closing system that uses a combination of pressure and energy tools to permanently fuse vessels during surgery. Do not confuse this with the soundalike word *ligature*, which is a thread, wire, or other material that is tied tightly around a vessel or other structure to constrict it.

TABLE 6.4   Common Suture Types

Suture	Type	Absorption
chromic	chromic	absorbable
Ethibond	braided	nonabsorbable
Ethilon	monofilament	nonabsorbable
Monocryl	monofilament	absorbable
Nurolon	braided	nonabsorbable
nylon	monofilament	nonabsorbable
PDS	monofilament	absorbable
Prolene	monofilament	nonabsorbable
silk	braided	nonabsorbable
surgical gut (also called "cat gut")	plain	absorbable
Vicryl	monofilament	absorbable

TABLE 6.5   Common Surgical Wound Coverings

Ace bandages (also called Ace wraps)	A brand name for a woven elastic bandage placed around the wound.
Adaptic dressing	Band name for a nonstick bandage infused with petrolatum.
CELOX gauze	Brand name of a gauze-type material used for wound packing and bandaging.
Coban	Brand name for an elastic bandage material that sticks only to itself with no additional adhesive necessary.
compression garment	Apparel worn surgically that keeps the wound under pressure while healing and to avoid swelling.
compressive dressing	A form of bandage that not only covers the wound but also forces the edges together.
FloSeal	Brand name of a gelatinous material used for packing and bandaging.
Gelfoam	Brand name of a gelatinous material used for packing and bandaging.
Kerlix gauze bandage	A brand name for a woven gauze dressing designed to cushion and protect the wound area.
QuikClot gauze	Brand name of a gauze-type material used for wound packing and bandaging.
Steri-Strips	Brand name for a type of self-adhesive bandage used for closure of shallow wound that do not require actual stitches.
Xeroform gauze dressing (or packs)	A bandage impregnated with Xeroform and petrolatum.

or other material used to bind or wrap a diseased or injured part of the body. Bandages are either placed directly against the wound or used to bind a dressing to the wound. Bandages can be used to hold dressings in place, to relieve pain, and to generally make the patient comfortable. Table 6.5 illustrates common types of bandages used in surgery.

SURGICAL PREFIXES, SUFFIXES, AND COMBINING FORMS

Operative reports that describe surgical procedures contain terminology composed of many prefixes, suffixes, and combining forms. Over time, you will come to understand many of the recurrent terms and components used in operative notes, enabling you to determine their meanings. A summary list of common operative prefixes, suffixes, and combining forms are presented in Table 6.6.

QUICK CHECK 6.2

Match the word part in the first column with the definition in the second column.

Word Part	Definition
1. _____ -logy	A. around
2. _____ lith/o	B. study of
3. _____ peri-	C. cold
4. _____ cry/o	D. middle, mean
5. _____ mes/o	E. stone, calculus, calcification

TABLE 6.6   Common Prefixes, Suffixes and Combining Forms Used in Operative Procedures

Term	Meaning	Term	Meaning
-al, -ic	pertaining to	-lysis	dissolution
angi/o, vas/o, vascul/o	vessel	mes-, mes/o	middle, mean
cardi/o	heart	-opsy	excision or removal of
-centesis	puncture	oste/o	bone
circum-	around, circular, circular movement	ox/o	oxygen
cry-, cry/o	cold	para-	alongside of (or abnormal)
-desis	binding, stabilizing	peri-	around
-ectomy	excision or removal	-pexy	surgical fixation
electr/o	electric; electricity	-plasty	surgical repair of a defect
enter/o	small intestine	-rrhaphy	surgical suturing
esophag/o	esophagus	-rrhexis	rupture
-esthesia	perception, feeling, sensitivity	-scope	instrument for viewing
gastr/o	stomach	-stasis	stop, stand
hem/o, hemat/o	blood	-stomy	creation of an opening
hyper-	above or excessive	sym-, syn-	together, with, joined
hypo-	below or deficient	-tome	a cutting instrument
-itis	inflammation	-tomy	surgical incision
lip/o	fat	trans-	across, through, beyond
lith-, lith/o	stone, calculus, calcification	-tripsy	rubbing, crushing
-logy	study of		

CHAPTER SUMMARY

Methods of conducting a surgical procedure may differ from hospital to hospital or in different sections of the country, but the fundamentals that ensure a positive outcome for the patient remain the same. For years, the medical community has expressed the need for transcriptionists with exceptional skills in creating accurate operative reports. The demand for well-trained transcriptionists who can produce accurate operative reports will continue to grow as surgical intervention is increasingly viewed as the answer to the problems of epidemics, infections, heart disease, cancer, and trauma. The terms presented in this chapter will serve as a foundation upon which to build your knowledge of this special area of medicine.

· I · N · S · I · G · H · T ·

Robots in the Operating Room

Robots were first used in the operating room in the 1980s to perform relatively simple tasks, such as controlling cameras that view the inside of the body. Today, robotic technology is used for more intricate surgical maneuvers. The robots respond by manual or voice-activated commands to maneuver mechanical arms or cameras and allow the surgeon to view the operating field much more closely than human vision would allow. This results in extreme precision, for example, in removing cancerous tumors and thus, perhaps, affords a better chance to excise the entire growth, resulting in a better surgical outcome. A robotic arm can provide improved access using smaller incisions for many procedures. It can also provide improved dexterity, reducing any tremor effect from the surgeon's hand.

At present, it is not practical for robots to perform entire operative procedures. Issues regarding malpractice, credentialing and training, research, and cost efficiency in the use of surgical robots are still the topics of debate. However, it is anticipated that in the future, the benefits of the enhanced precision and effectiveness afforded by robotic technology will help to secure robots a more active role in improving surgical procedures and minimizing trauma to the patient.

TERMINOLOGY

Term	Meaning
absorbable sutures	Sutures that degrade rapidly and eventually dissolve in the body.
anastomosis	The surgical connection made between two blood vessels or other tubular structures.
anesthesia	The loss of normal sensation or feeling.
anesthesiologist	A physician who has undergone additional training in medicine and anesthesia.
apposition	The act of putting two items side by side.
approximate	To bring together.
autologous blood donation	Blood that is donated by a person for their own use prior to surgery.
bandage (syn. gauze)	A piece of cloth or other material used to bind or wrap a diseased or injured part of the body.
cell saver	An intraoperative cell salvage machine that replaces blood lost during a surgical procedure with the patient's own donated blood collected before the procedure.
cholecystectomy	The surgical removal of the gallbladder.
colonoscopy	A visual examination of the colon using a visual tube called a colonoscope.
debridement	The removal of dead, damaged, or diseased tissue from a part of the body.
drapes	Pieces of cloth used to cover all of the patient's body except the surgical site and the patient's head.
dressing	A material applied directly to a wound to promote healing and prevent further harm.
effusion	A term that refers to the escape of fluid into a tissue or body part.
endoscope	A special lighted instrument used to examine the interior of the body.
endoscopy	The visual examination of the interior of the body using a special flexible lighted instrument.
excision	The surgical removal of an organ, tumor, or other tissue.
extubation	The process of removing the previously placed tube into the patient's trachea.
grafting	The taking of healthy tissue from one part of the body and transplanting it to another part of the body.
incision	A cut; a surgical wound; a division of the soft parts made with a knife.
informed consent	The written permission given by the patient to undergo a surgical procedure.
infusion	A term that refers to the therapeutic introduction of fluid (not blood) into a vein by means of gravity.
instrument tray	A tray holding instruments that are commonly used together for a particular type of surgery.
intubation	A procedure that involves the placement of a flexible plastic tube into the trachea to protect the patient's airway and provide a means of mechanical ventilation.
laparoscope	A special lighted instrument used to examine the inside of the abdomen.
laparoscopy	The visual examination of the abdomen using a special lighted instrument called a laparoscope.
ligate	To tie.
ligation	The tying off of a duct or blood vessel with a ligature to prevent further bleeding.
mastectomy	The surgical removal of one or both breasts in order to treat serious breast disease, such as breast cancer.

Term	Meaning
monofilament sutures	Sutures that are made of a single strand of material.
multifilament sutures	Sutures that consist of several strands of material that are twisted or braided together.
n.p.o.	The Latin abbreviation for *nothing by mouth*.
nonabsorbable sutures	Sutures that maintain their strength and must be manually removed from the body.
operation (syn., surgical procedure)	A procedure performed by a surgeon in an operating room or surgical center.
orotracheal intubation	The most common form of tracheal intubation where the tube is passed through the mouth, larynx, and vocal cords, into the trachea.
prone	Face down.
registered nurse anesthetist	A nurse who has undergone additional training in anesthesia.
resection	The partial removal of an organ, tumor or other tissue.
rhinoplasty	The surgical reconstruction of the nose.
supine	Face up.
surgeon	A physician who specializes in performing operative procedures.
surgery	The specialty of medicine that treats diseases and disorders by physical intervention to tissues, such as cutting, removing, or changing the body in some way in a surgical procedure.
suture	A strand of material used to ligate.
suturing	The procedure used to close a wound by stitching parts together with thread or other material.
tonsillectomy	The surgical removal of the tonsils.
tracheostomy	A surgical opening made in the trachea in order to facilitate breathing.

Add Your Own Terms and Definitions Here:

_____

_____

_____

_____

_____

_____

REVIEW QUESTIONS

1. What is the difference between absorbable and nonabsorbable suture material?
2. What kind of surgery does not invade the body?
3. What is the purpose of placing an intravenous line?
4. What is the name of the document used to obtain a patient's permission to perform an operation?
5. Explain the difference between the dorsal lithotomy position and the dorsal recumbent position.
6. What type of surgical process would best be used to reattach two sections of colon during surgery?
7. What type of surgical process would be used to thoroughly clean a wound?
8. What type of surgery is used to confirm or aid in a diagnosis?
9. Name the Latin abbreviation used to indicate that the patient has no food or drink after midnight on the night prior to a surgical procedure.
10. Which individual in the operating room is responsible for the patient's overall care?

CHAPTER ACTIVITIES

Matching

Match the brand name in the left column with the type of tool or instrument in the right column.

1. _____ Kerrison   A. scissors
2. _____ Mayo   B. catheter
3. _____ Ferris-Smith   C. forceps (clamps)
4. _____ Freer   D. rongeur
5. _____ Heaney   E. retractor
6. _____ Kocher   F. elevator
7. _____ biting
8. _____ Barbie
9. _____ Allis
10. _____ Cobb
11. _____ Yasargil
12. _____ Optiva
13. _____ Balfour
14. _____ Metzenbaum
15. _____ pigtail

Understanding Terms

Break the given surgical term into its word parts and define each part. Then define the medical term.

For example:

arthritis   *word parts:*   arthr/o itis
                   meanings: joint / inflammation of
                   term meaning: inflammation of the joints

1. tracheostomy   *word parts:*   _____ / _____
                   meanings: _____ / _____
                   term meaning: _____

2. anesthesia
   word parts: _____/_____
   meanings: _____/_____
   term meaning: _____

3. colposcopy
   word parts: _____/_____/_____
   meanings: _____/_____/_____
   term meaning: _____

4. uterotomy
   word parts: _____/_____
   meanings: _____/_____
   term meaning: _____

5. endoscopy
   word parts: _____/_____
   meanings: _____/_____
   term meaning: _____

6. rhinoplasty
   word parts: _____/_____
   meanings: _____/_____
   term meaning: _____

7. oophorectomy
   word parts: _____/_____
   meanings: _____/_____
   term meaning: _____

8. nephrectomy
   word parts: _____/_____/_____
   meanings: _____/_____/_____
   term meaning: _____

9. laparotomy
   word parts: _____/_____/_____
   meanings: _____/_____/_____
   term meaning: _____

10. herniorrhaphy
   word parts: _____/_____
   meanings: _____/_____
   term meaning: _____

Fill-In-The-Blank

Fill in the blank with the correct term.

1. In _____ anesthesia, the patient remains awake during the procedure.
2. The term _____ means *face down.*
3. _____ is another word for tying off a duct or vessel to prevent further bleeding.
4. _____ is a type of surgery that involves making small incisions into the body.
5. The _____ assists the primary surgeon in the operating room.

6. In the _____, the patient is inclined to approximately 45 degrees.

7. _____ is a method where local anesthetic is injected directly into the tissue where the surgery will take place.

8. _____ are used to cover the patient's body before surgery.

9. _____ are used to draw aside the edges of a wound.

10. _____ is a kind of plain, absorbable suture.

True or False

Read each statement and indicate whether it is true or false. If false, rewrite the sentence in the Correction column to make the statement true.

Statement	True (T) or False (F)	Correction, if False
1. Absorbable sutures degrade rapidly and eventually dissolve in the body.	____	_____
2. Emergency surgery is an operation that must be done quickly in order to save the patient's life.	____	_____
3. The Trendelenburg position is a supine position with only the upper torso exposed.	____	_____
4. A retractor is an example of a fixation device.	____	_____
5. Heparin is an anticoagulant.	____	_____
6. *Resection* means to close the wound.	____	_____
7. Hurricaine spray is also known as "laughing gas."	____	_____
8. The anesthesiologist is responsible for the patient's medical care while he/she is under anesthesia.	____	_____
9. Maxitrol is widely used in presurgical preparation and cleansing.	____	_____
10. Elevators are used to remove fluid or materials from a body cavity.	____	_____

7

PHARMACOLOGY

OBJECTIVES

After completing this chapter, you will be able to:

- Recount the history of pharmacology.
- Describe the process of developing and regulating a new drug.
- Understand the different forms of administration of drugs, including the terminology related to the types, dose, and dosage frequency.
- Define controlled substances and how they are categorized.
- Understand the nomenclature required for the transcription of drugs in medical reports.

INTRODUCTION

A **drug**, or **medicine**, is defined by U.S. law as any substance (other than a food or device) intended for use in the diagnosis, cure, relief, treatment, or prevention of disease, or intended to affect the structure or function of the body (such as an oral contraceptive). **Pharmacology** is the study of all drugs, legal or illegal, and their actions on living organisms. Pharmacology is a multifaceted medical discipline that affects many people's lives. In the U.S., over 3 million prescriptions are written annually, a 61 percent increase over the past decade. This chapter explores the history, regulation, and development of drugs, and the terminology used in medical reports to indicate drug forms, types, and routes of administration that are transcribed regularly by medical transcriptionists.

OVERVIEW OF PHARMACOLOGY

The word *pharmacology* derives from the Greek words *pharmacon*, meaning "medicine," and the suffix *–ology* meaning "the study of." The term *drug* comes from the Dutch word *droog*, which means dry, and refers to the use of dried herbs and plants as the first medicines used to treat disease. The word *medicine* is derived from the Latin word *medicina*. These words are used interchangeably, but a drug or medicine can be thought of as simply any nonfood chemical substance that affects the mind or body. Pharmacology is not synonymous with *pharmacy*, which is the name used for a profession, though the two terms are confused at times in common usage. Pharmacology deals with the ways in which drugs interact within biological systems to affect function. It is the study of drugs, of the body's reaction to drugs, and the sources, nature, and properties of drugs. In contrast, **pharmacy** is a medical science concerned with the safe and effective use of medicines.

Subspecialty fields of pharmacology include:

- **Pharmacotherapeutics**: The study of the use of drugs to treat disorders, or *drug therapy* in its simplest terms.
- **Pharmacoepidemiology**: The study of the effect of drugs on populations of people.
- **Pharmacoeconomics**: The study of the cost effectiveness of drug treatments.
- **Pharmacokinetics**: The study of how the body absorbs, distributes, metabolizes, and excretes drugs.

Drugs are divided into two categories: prescription drugs and nonprescription, or over-the-counter, medications. **Prescription drugs** are drugs that may be dispensed only with a prescription, or a written order, from a licensed medical professional and which are regulated by the government. **Nonprescription drugs** are those drugs considered to be safe for use without medical supervision and sold over the counter. In the United States, the **Food and Drug Administration (FDA)** is the government agency responsible for deciding which drugs require a prescription and which do not.

Knowledge of drug names is crucial when transcribing medical reports. Every drug has at least three names: a chemical name, a generic (nonproprietary) name, and a trade (proprietary or brand) name. The **chemical name** describes the chemical or molecular structure of the drug, which is usually too complex for common use. Therefore, the drug is given a generic name. The **generic name** is the established, official name for the drug. In the United States, the generic name is created by the U.S. Adopted Names (USAN) Council. International drug names are coordinated by the World Health Organization (WHO). The **trade name** is the name chosen by the pharmaceutical company that manufactures and markets the drug. It may suggest a use or indication, and it often incorporates the manufacturer's name.

The difference between a generic drug and a trade name drug is that the generic drug is produced and distributed without patent protection. A **patent** is a grant by the government that gives the company that developed a new drug an exclusive right to sell the drug as long as the patent is in effect, usually approximately 15–20 years. Most of the profits that a company earns from marking a drug will occur while the drug is under patent and there is no competition from other manufacturers. By this time, the company has already spent substantial money on research, development, marketing, and promotion of the new drug, and the time during which the drug is under patent allows the company to recover most of those expenses.

Generic drugs only become available when the original manufacturer's patent expires. Once the patent expires, other drug companies can make their own versions of the drug, driving its price down and resulting in the original drug company making much less money on that drug. Generic drugs are less expensive because those manufacturers do not incur the cost of drug

discovery and instead are able to engineer known drug compounds to allow them to manufacture bioequivalent versions. Generic manufacturers also do not bear the burden of proving the safety and efficacy of the drugs through clinical trials, since these trials have already been conducted by the brand name company. Companies incur fewer costs in creating the generic drug, and are, therefore, able to market the drug at a lower price to consumers.

HISTORY OF PHARMACOLOGY

Pharmacology is one of the oldest branches of medical knowledge. Since the dawn of humankind, mixtures of animal parts, plants, and minerals have been used to treat wounds, sores, and ailments. Treatments have evolved from the rudimentary to the sophisticated. In fact, many substances historically used for murder, magic, and folk medicine are currently clinically acceptable drugs. For example, the leaves of the purple foxglove, *Digitalis purpurea*, an herb used to treat dropsy in 18th century England, provide the cardiac medication digitalis, a drug currently used to treat heart failure. Prehistoric humans believed evil spirits were the cause of disease and developed various rituals they felt were essential for prevention and cure. Over time, while foraging for food, they discovered that various roots, berries, leaves, and barks could help treat wounds and broken bones. Medicine men used these substances in "magic" rituals. Prehistoric humans also learned, through trial and error, the toxic effects of these substances as well.

Records of the medicinal use of plant and animal substances have been discovered in early Indian, Egyptian, Chinese, and Greek cultures. By the 5th century BC, the Greek physician Hippocrates believed that disease came from natural rather than spiritual causes and laid the foundation for the development of a more rational approach to medicine. He believed that people had the natural ability to overcome disease and that physicians should find ways to assist the body's natural healing process. Over time, more sophisticated views of illness evolved, accompanied by an increasingly scientific approach to the isolation of drugs from natural products. These concepts, in addition to advances in the field of chemistry and physiology, led to the birth of modern pharmacology. In 1897, Felix Hoffman, a research chemist employed by Bayer and Co., synthesized acetylsalicylic acid, or aspirin, which became a trademark name for the drug two years later.

During the 20th century, many new drugs were developed to treat disease and improve people's quality of life. Key discoveries of the 1920s and 1930s, such as insulin and penicillin, became mass-manufactured and distributed; and legislation was enacted to test and approve drugs and to require appropriate labeling. Prescription and nonprescription drugs became legally distinguished from one another as the pharmaceutical industry matured. There has been a tremendous increase in new discoveries, new technology, and the development of preventative and maintenance medications in recent years. Disorders such as microbial infections, diabetes, hypertension, depression, and even AIDS, all of which once caused people to die prematurely or suffer needlessly, are now successfully treated. The pharmaceutical industry is changing rapidly and continues to develop and evolve at an ever-increasing pace.

DRUG REGULATION AND DEVELOPMENT

Each year many new prescription drugs are approved by the FDA, but the approval process is not a speedy one. Medicine is one of the most highly regulated products in the world. Data demonstrating safety and efficacy must be filed with government agencies in order to move a potential drug through clinical development and obtain approval to sell it. This approval process takes approximately 10 years. A medical transcriptionist may be involved in this process, transcribing the results of such testing of new drug products, so it is important to understand the process of developing and bringing new drugs to market.

The first step, a preclinical phase, is finding a promising agent or substance after extensive medical research (see Figure 7.1). This requires an understanding of disease, pharmacology, computer science, and chemistry. The next step before attempting a clinical trial in humans is to test the drug in living animals, usually rodents. The FDA requires that certain animal tests be

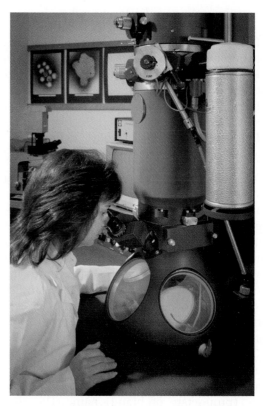

FIGURE 7.1. A Medical Researcher Using an Electron Microscope. Reprinted with permission from James Gathany and the Centers for Disease Control and Prevention.

conducted before humans are exposed to a new molecular entity. If the FDA is satisfied with the documentation, the stage is set for a clinical trial of the drug. A **clinical trial** is a research study that tests how well a new medical treatment works in people. Patients who take part in these studies are called **participants**.

Clinical trials help to move the setting for basic scientific research about a drug or condition from the laboratory into the patient's treatment room. They are the final step in a long research process required to make a new drug or treatment modality available to the public. Government agencies, such as the National Institutes of Health (NIH), sponsor and conduct clinical trials. In addition, medical organizations such as hospitals, foundations, or pharmaceutical companies also sponsor clinical trials. The name of the trial may have a simple title (such as the STAR trial, an actual NIH-sponsored study comparing breast cancer treatment drugs) or use a combination of letters and numbers that indicate a particular name or property of the drug being studied, such as RTOG-0522.

A clinical trial typically takes place in four main phases, each designed to answer different research questions.

- Phase I looks at the safety of a new substance or treatment in patients. This part of the trial studies the best way to give patients the new agent (for

QUICK CHECK 7.1

Indicate whether the following sentences are true (T) or false (F).

1. Clinical trials are open to only women.   T   F

2. Pharmacotherapeutics is "drug therapy" in its simplest from.   T   F

3. Pharmacy is the medical science concerned with the cost effectiveness of drug treatments.   T   F

4. Insulin and penicillin were discovered in the 1920s and 1930s.   T   F

5. Tribal medicine men believed that diseases were the result of natural causes.   T   F

example, by pill or injection), how often it should be given, what the safest dose is, and whether the new agent is of benefit.

- Phase II continues to test the safety of the new agent and begins to evaluate how well it works against a specific type of disease. Participation in phase II trials is often restricted based on the previous treatment received; that is, participants in these trials have been treated with other treatment modalities, but the treatment has not been effective.

- Phase III compares a new treatment to the standard, or most widely accepted, treatment for a disease. Researchers investigate whether the new treatment is better than, the same as, or worse than the standard treatment. These studies are called **randomized clinical trials**, as participants are randomly assigned to one of two or more treatment groups in the trial. Most randomized trials have at least two groups, called **arms**, but some have three or more, depending on the treatments being compared. The participants are placed into one of the arms of the study at random, via a computer program or table of random numbers. Randomization ensures that unknown factors, such as human choices, beliefs about which treatment they think is best, or other factors, do not influence the trial results. Participants have an equal chance of being assigned to a group of patients who are receiving the standard treatment or to the group that is getting the new treatment.

- Phase IV continues to further evaluate the long-term safety and effectiveness of the new treatment. These trials usually take place after the new treatment has been approved by the U.S. Food and Drug Administration (FDA) for standard use.

If a drug survives the clinical trials, it is submitted to the FDA for approval for use in the general population. After receiving all of the data and research surrounding the new drug or treatment, the FDA completes an independent review and makes recommendations as to its approval. If the drug is not approved, the applicant is given the reasons why and advised as to what information could be provided to make the application acceptable. Sometimes the FDA makes a tentative approval recommendation, requesting that a minor deficiency or labeling issue be corrected before final approval. Once a drug is approved, it can be marketed. Phase IV continues the study of the drug post marketing to delineate additional information about the drug's risks, benefits, and optimal use.

DRUG ADMINISTRATION

Physicians commonly dictate which medications were prescribed for a patient and in what form as well as how the medication is administered. A medical transcriptionist must always take care to transcribe drug names, dosages, and forms correctly and never, ever guess on this information. Drug names that sound alike or are spelled alike have different uses. For example, Xanax, the antianxiety drug, can be easily confused with Zantac, the antacid used to treat some gastrointestinal disorders. The antidepressant Paxil could easily be mistaken for Doxil, a drug used in cancer chemotherapy. In addition, drug dosages can sound deceptively similar, such as 15 mg versus 50 mg. One careless mistranscription could, at best, change the course of patient care—or at worst, harm the patient. The ISMP provides a list of confused drug names, which includes sound-alike and look-alike pairs, on their website, www.ismp.org.

TRANSCRIPTION TIP:

If the dictator does not expand a form of a drug, it is not expanded when transcribed. Example: "The patient was told to take Zantac 75 mg 2 <u>tabs</u> nightly."

Drug Forms

Medicines come in a variety of forms:

- Tablets. Tablets can be **scored**, or have a line across the middle so they can be broken in half. **Enteric** tablets are covered with a special coating to prevent stomach irritation. Slow-release or long-acting tablets release equal amounts of a drug into the body over a period of time, and may be indicated with the abbreviations SR (*slow-release*) or LA (*long-acting*) after the name of the drug, such as Entex LA. Short-acting or immediate-release (IR) tablets, as the name implies, dissolve quickly in the body and are designed for fast pain relief.
- Capsules. A capsule can come in the form of a gel coating with liquid inside or with a hard covering that can be broken so that the solid contents can be removed.
- Liquid. A **solution** is a liquid form of a drug, with each part of the solution containing the same amount of drug. A **suspension** is a water-based drug in which the medicine is suspended in liquid, and it must be shaken before administration. **Elixirs** are medicines that dissolve in alcoholic solutions. A **syrup** is a solution that contains sugar, water, and flavorings but no alcohol.
- Suppositories. This form of drug is contained in glycerin or cocoa butter and administered rectally or vaginally.
- Transdermal. The term **transdermal** means *through the unbroken skin*. This type of drug is applied directly to the skin (such as a cream or ointment) or in time-release form (such as a skin patch).
- Pellets or beads. These forms of drugs are implanted under the skin and slowly released into the body.

Drug Dosage Forms

Drugs may be administered in different ways, some of which are illustrated in Figure 7.2.

TRANSCRIPTION TIP:

According to The Joint Commission's "dangerous abbreviations" list of abbreviations, acronyms, and symbols that should no longer be used in clinical documentation (as discussed in Chapter 3), the abbreviation *cc* for liquid measures (not mass) should not be used. When you hear this abbreviation dictated, use the metric abbreviation *mL* instead.

- Oral or under the tongue (**sublingually**). The oral route is most popular and least expensive route of administration.
- **Parenterally**, which is by some other means than through the gastrointestinal tract. A drug can be injected into a vein (**intravenously**), into a muscle (**intramuscularly**), into the space around the spinal cord (**intrathecally**), or beneath the skin (**subcutaneously**).
- Inhalational, which is inhaled through the nose or mouth.
- Topical (**transdermally**), or applied to the surface of the skin.

Drug Dosages and Frequency

In medicine, precise measurements are necessary to evaluate health or make a diagnosis. The metric system, derived from the International System Units adopted in 1960, is used to measure mass, volume, and length. Drugs are often measured in metric units, although in reality, in any given patient record, references to American units (pounds, teaspoons, tablespoons) can be found in the same report as metric units (mg, cm, mL) when quantifying drugs. Doctors may measure a patient's

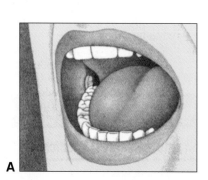

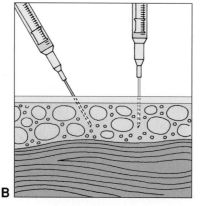

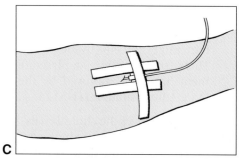

FIGURE 7.2. Common Dosage Forms. The (**A**) sublingual, (**B**) subcutaneous, and (**C**) intravenous routes are common forms of medication administration. Reprinted with permission from *Nursing Procedures*, 4th Edition. Ambler: Lippincott Williams & Wilkins, 2004.

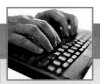

TRANSCRIPTION TIP:

Use the decimal form of metric units of measure even when dictated as fractions, unless they are not easily converted. For example, 4.5 mm, not 4-1/2 mm, but 4-1/3 mm (not easily converted).

weight in pounds or kilograms to compute a dosage of medicine administered in grams or milliliters.

The metric units of measure most commonly used in medical reports when describing medication dosages are indicated in Table 7.1.

Nonmetric units of measure that express weight, depth, distance, height, length, and width are generally spelled out:

pounds
ounces
teaspoons
tablespoons
inches

Dosage Frequency

Drugs are measured not only in terms of the amount of the dosage but also in terms of the frequency of the dosage. Latin abbreviations are often used to indicate dosages, as shown in Table 7.2. Transcribe these abbreviations in lowercase with periods.

TABLE 7.1	Metric Drug Measurements
Metric Measure	**Meaning**
cm	centimeter
dB	decibel
dL	deciliter
g	gram
Hz	hertz
L	liter
mcg	microgram
mEq	milliequivalent
mg	milligram
mL	milliliter
mm	millimeter
mmHg	millimeters of mercury
mmol	millimole
msec, ms	millisecond

TABLE 7.2	Latin Abbreviations of Frequency of Drug Dosages	
Abbreviation	**Latin Translation**	**English Translation**
a.c.	ante cibum	before meals
ad lib.	ad libitum	as needed
b.i.d.	bis in die	twice a day
n.p.o.	nil per os	nothing by mouth
p.c.	post cibum	after meals
p.r.n.	pro re nata	as needed
q.h.	quaque hora	every hour
q.i.d.	quarter in die	four times a day
t.i.d.	ter in die	three times a day

TYPES OF DRUGS

There are many different types of drugs, both legal and illegal. All can be grouped into about 30 primary classifications and hundreds of subclassifications. Drugs are grouped according to similar action and chemical structure. Table 7.3 lists types of drugs commonly encountered by an MT during transcription and how they are used. Familiarize yourself with this list so that you are able to recognize the types of drugs when dictated and transcribe them accurately.

CONTROLLED SUBSTANCES

A **controlled substance** is generally a drug or chemical whose manufacture, possession, and use are regulated or outlawed by the government because of the potential for abuse or addiction. The **Drug Enforcement Administration (DEA)** is responsible for regulating the manufacturing and dispensing of these drugs by enforcing the Controlled Substances Act, established in 1970. These substances are classified according to schedules and include **narcotics**, which are drugs with potent analgesic effects associated with significant alteration of mood and behavior and which are potentially addictive. The schedules also include

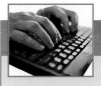

TRANSCRIPTION TIP:

As a medical transcriptionist, you may hear the term **half-life** when a drug's metabolism in the body is being discussed. A drug's half-life is defined as the time required for the body to metabolize half of the drug. This concept helps physicians determine how long a drug will remain in the body when prescribing a drug dosage and frequency.

QUICK CHECK 7.2 ✓

Match the following drug characteristic with the type of drug.

_____ 1. Applied to the surface of the skin.   A. Pellets/beads

_____ 2. A suspension.   B. Parenteral

_____ 3. Inserted into the rectum or vaginal.   C. Transdermal

_____ 4. A drug injected into the body.   D. Liquid

_____ 5. Implanted under the skin.   E. Suppository

stimulants, depressants, hallucinogens, and cannabis. Providers refer to these drugs in dictation collectively as _schedule drugs_ or _controlled substances_.

For the sake of regulation, controlled substances are classified into five groups, called schedules, based on whether they have an accepted medical use, their relative potential for abuse, and the degree of dependence that may be caused by abuse of the drug. The following characteristics apply to the schedules:

Schedule I:
(a) The drug or other substance has a high potential for abuse.
(b) The drug or other substance has no currently accepted medical use in treatment in the United States.
(c) There is a lack of accepted safety for use of the drug or other substance under medical supervision.
Examples include PCP, heroin, marijuana, mescaline, and peyote.

TABLE 7.3   Common Types of Drugs

Type of Drug	Purpose
analgesic	A drug used to relieve pain.
antibiotic	A drug used to treat infection by killing or inhibiting the growth of bacteria.
anticholinergic	A drug that opposes or blocks the action of acetylcholine, a substance found in nerve cells that helps them communicate with other nerve cells in the brain, glands, and involuntary muscles.
antidepressant	A medication used to treat mood disorders.
antiemetic	A drug that prevents or alleviates nausea and vomiting.
antifungal	An agent that destroys or prevents the growth of fungi.
antihistamine	A medication that is used to treat allergies or allergic reactions by blocking the effects of histamine, which is a chemical released by the body following exposure to a substance that causes an allergic reaction.
antihypertensive	A drug that reduces high blood pressure.
antineoplastic	A drug used in chemotherapy to kill cancer cells.
antipruritic	A medication that relieves or prevents itching.
antiseptic	A drug that inhibits the growth and reproduction of microorganisms but does not kill them.
antispasmodic	A drug used to relieve or prevent muscular spasms.
antitussive	A medicine used to suppress or relieve coughing.
antiviral	A drug that inhibits or stops the growth and reproduction of viruses.
bronchodilator	A drug that relaxes and dilates the bronchial passageways in order to improve the passage of air into the lungs.
corticosteroid	A drug that decreases severe inflammation or itching by suppressing the response of the immune system.
diuretic	A drug that increases the flow of urine, which causes the body to excrete excess water.
mydriatic	A drug that causes the pupil of the eye to dilate.
placebo	An inactive substance that may be used in medical studies which compares the effects of a given treatment with no treatment.
vasodilator	A drug that causes dilation of blood vessels.
vasopressor	A drug that constricts blood vessels in order to increase blood pressure.

Schedule II:

(a) The drug or other substance has a high potential for abuse.

(b) The drug or other substance has a currently accepted medical use in treatment in the United States or a currently accepted use with severe restrictions.

(c) Abuse of the drug or other substance may lead to severe psychological or physical dependence.

Examples include Fentanyl, methadone, hydromorphone, cocaine, Dilaudid, MS Contin (morphine), Demerol, and Ritalin.

Schedule III:

(a) The drug or other substance has a potential for abuse less than the drugs or other substances in Schedules I and II.

(b) The drug or other substance has a currently accepted medical use in treatment in the United States.

(c) Abuse of the drug or other substance may lead to moderate or low physical dependence or high psychological dependence.

Examples include anabolic steroids (*body building* drugs), Paregoric, Lortab, Vicodin, and Tussionex.

Schedule IV:

(a) The drug or other substance has a low potential for abuse relative to the drugs or other substances in Schedule III.

(b) The drug or other substance has a currently accepted medical use in treatment in the United States.

(c) Abuse of the drug or other substance may lead to limited physical dependence or psychological dependence relative to the drugs or other substances in Schedule III.

Examples include Xanax, Valium, Darvocet, Klonopin, Librium, Restoril, Ativan, Talwin, and Ambien.

Schedule V:

(a) The drug or other substance has a low potential for abuse relative to the drugs or other substances in Schedule IV.

(b) The drug or other substance has a currently accepted medical use in treatment in the United States.

(c) Abuse of the drug or other substance may lead to limited physical dependence or psychological dependence relative to the drugs or other substances in Schedule IV.

Examples include Guiatussin with codeine, Lomotil, cough syrups with codeine, Phenergan with codeine, and Tylenol with Codeine.

TRANSCRIBING DRUG NOMENCLATURE

When transcribing drug names and dosages in medical reports, do not use commas to separate drug names from doses and instructions. In a series of drugs for each of which the dose and/or instructions are given, use commas to separate each complete entry, except when entries in a series of medications have internal commas, in which case semicolons or periods may be used. Medications may also be placed in a vertical list. For example:

The patient was discharged on doxycycline 100 mg daily for 10 days.

The patient is to resume her following previous medications, including Neurontin 300 mg p.o. t.i.d., Flovent 1 puff daily, and albuterol inhaler.

The patient was discharged on insulin, 3 units 40 minutes after breakfast, lunch, and dinner and 5 units at bedtime; Losartan 50 mg per day; and Coumadin 7.5 mg daily.

Discharge Medications
1. Benazepril 40 mg p.o. daily.
2. Norvasc 10 mg p.o. daily.
3. Protonix 40 mg p.o. daily.
4 Aspirin 81 mg p.o. daily.

Some drug names contain a percentage of active drug contained in the medication. When transcribing, use the percent symbol (%) and indicate the percentage after the drug name. For example:

D: The patient was discharged on gentamicin sulfate solution zero point three percent.
T: The patient was discharged on gentamicin sulfate solution, 0.3%.

CHAPTER SUMMARY

Drugs are an important part of modern medicine and patient treatment. Once a diagnosis has been made and medical treatment is deemed necessary for a patient, safe and effective medications are selected by the medical provider. The provider chooses the drug by name, the administration, the dosage, and the frequency. If the details of the prescribed medication are not transcribed accurately, very serious consequences can occur. The human brain is amazing in that even when words are misspelled, it will subconsciously rearrange letters in order to comprehend the message as being correct. Careless or casual work in transcribing or proofreading the details of drug names and dosages selected for patient use can be harmful or even deadly to the patient. Therefore, it is vital to pay careful attention when listening to drug names and dosages and to be precise and correct when transcribing them.

·I·N·S·I·G·H·T·

Pharmacy Automation with E-Prescriptions

Every year, countless medication errors occur as a result of miscommunication of the details of prescriptions or mis-interpretation of illegible handwritten prescriptions. Because of this and changes in the Medicare law, pharmacies are using technology to advance toward safer and more efficient operations. Electronic transcribing of prescriptions, commonly termed **e-prescribing**, currently accounts for roughly 5% to 7% of physicians' prescriptions. However, changes in U.S. Centers for Medicare and Medicaid Services (CMS) requirements finalized in 2009 set into motion the process of e-prescribing prescriptions for tens of millions of Medicare Part D clients.

In a medical e-prescription system, the physician's office computer is linked to a central computer server provided by an e-prescribing vendor that contains insurance formularies, drug interaction files, and a drug-information database. The system allows physicians to access information and to write prescriptions from data that includes the patient's insurance plan, as well as the ability to check for allergies and drug interactions against the list of the patient's previously prescribed drugs. The drug dose, quantity, directions, and/or refill information is selected; the prescription is digitally signed; and it is sent electronically to the patient's pharmacy.

The advantages of this type of system are that it allows the physician to address insurance eligibility issues for the medication, keep a database of previously prescribed medications online, and avoid the problems involved with misreading handwriting and phone calls to the pharmacy to verify the details of the prescription. In terms of efficiency, an e-prescription refill can take seconds with the push of a few buttons as opposed to several minutes to pull a chart and review the prescription previously written. The most important benefit to e-prescribing is the increased safety that comes from the automated screenings for allergies and interactions provided by the e-prescription software program.

However, some physicians still believe that computers are too cumbersome to use, and software systems are usually perceived as too expensive. In addition, some have concerns about the compatibility of their current systems with these newer systems and are apprehensive about the lack of system standards. And, of course, a few physicians believe that they can write a prescription faster than they can generate one on a computer terminal or hand-held device.

As e-prescribing technologies become easier to use and less expensive, it is likely that the number of physicians adopting it will increase. Managed care plans will eventually start demanding these electronic capabilities from their network physicians and pharmacists, so e-prescriptions are likely to be the wave of the future.

ABBREVIATIONS

Abbreviation	Meaning	Abbreviation	Meaning
CMS	U.S. Centers for Medicare and Medicaid Services	LA	long-acting
		NIH	National Institutes of Health
DEA	Drug Enforcement Administration	SR	sustained-release
FDA	Food and Drug Administration	USAN	U.S. Adopted Names Council
IR	immediate-release	WHO	World Health Organization

Add Your Own Abbreviations Here:

_____

_____

_____

_____

TERMINOLOGY

Term	Meaning
arm	A branch or part of a clinical study.
chemical name	The name of a drug that describes the chemical or molecular structure of the drug, which is usually too complex for common use.
clinical trial	A research study that tests how well a new medical treatment works in people.
controlled substance	A drug or chemical whose manufacture, possession, and use are regulated or outlawed by the government because of their potential for abuse or addiction.
Drug Enforcement Administration (DEA)	The government agency responsible for regulating the manufacturing and dispensing of controlled substances.
drug, *syn.* medication	Any substance (other than a food or device) intended for use in the diagnosis, cure, relief, treatment, or prevention of disease or intended to affect the structure or function of the body.
elixir	A medicine that dissolves in an alcoholic solution.
enteric (tablet)	A tablet that has a special coating to prevent stomach irritation.
Food and Drug Administration (FSA)	The government agency responsible for deciding which drugs require a prescription and which ones do not.
generic name	The established, official name of a drug.
half-life	The time required for the body to metabolize half of an administered drug.
intramuscularly	The process of injecting a drug into a muscle.
intrathecally	The process of injecting a drug into the space around the spinal cord.
intravenously	The process of injecting a drug into a vein.
narcotic	A drug with potent analgesic effects associated with both alteration of mood and behavior, which is potentially addictive.
nonprescription drugs	Those drugs considered to be safe for use without medical supervision and are sold over the counter.
parenterally	The process of administering a drug by some other means than through the gastrointestinal tract.
participants	The name given to patients who take part in a clinical trial.
patent	A grant by the government that gives the company that developed a new drug an exclusive right to sell the drug for as long as the patent is in effect.
pharmacoepidemiology	The study of the effect of drugs on populations of people.
pharmacokinetics	The study of how the body absorbs, distributes, metabolizes, and excretes drugs.
pharmacology	The study of all drugs, legal or illegal, and their actions on living organisms.
pharmacotherapeutics	The study of the use of drugs to treat disorders.
pharmacy	A medical science concerned with the safe and effective use of medications.
prescription drugs	Drugs that may be dispensed only with a prescription, or a written order, from a licensed medical professional and are regulated by the government.
randomized clinical trial	A clinical trial in which participants are placed in one of the parts (arms) of the study at random, determined by computer or table of random numbers.
scored (tablet)	A tablet that has a line across the middle so it can be broken in half.
solution	A liquid form of a drug, with each part of the solution containing the same amount of drug.

Term	Meaning
subcutaneously	The process of injecting a drug beneath the skin.
sublingually	The process of administering a drug under the tongue.
suspension	A water-based drug in which the medicine is suspended in a liquid that must be shaken before administration.
syrup	A solution that contains sugar, water, and flavorings but no alcohol.
trade name, *syn.* brand name	The name of a drug chosen by the pharmaceutical company that manufactures and markets the drug.
transdermally	The process of applying a drug to the surface of the skin.

Add Your Own Terms and Definitions Here:

_____

_____

_____

_____

_____

_____

_____

REVIEW QUESTIONS

1. Name three ways that drugs can be administered.
2. What is the difference between the studies of pharmacology and pharmacy?
3. What is a drug's chemical name?
4. What is the purpose of a clinical trial?
5. What type of drug is implanted in the skin and slowly released into the body?
6. How are nonmetric measures that express weight, depth, distance, height, length, and width transcribed?
7. How are Latin abbreviations transcribed?
8. What does mmHg mean?
9. What is the English translation for q.i.d.?
10. Who believed that disease came from natural causes and not from spiritual causes?

CHAPTER ACTIVITIES

Multiple Choice

Circle the letter corresponding to the best answer for each of the following questions.

1. What is the generic name for Tylenol?
   A. acetaminophen
   B. acetazolamide
   C. acetic acid
   D. acetohexamide

2. What is the brand name of warfarin?
   A. Latisse
   B. Lantus
   C. Lasix
   D. Coumadin

3. What is the normal dosage range for Nexium?
   A. 100, 200, 300 mg
   B. 20, 40 mg
   C. 0.5, 1.5 mg
   D. 0.12%, 0.25%

4. What is the drug lisinopril used for?
   A. Nasal congestion
   B. Peptic ulcer disease
   C. Congestive heart failure
   D. Any one of the above

5. What is the generic name for Imitrex?
   A. sumatriptan
   B. digoxin
   C. almotriptan
   D. zolmitriptan

6. The generic name for Hismanal is:
   A. cetirizine.
   B. astemizole.
   C. terconazole.
   D. terfenadine.

7. A drug commonly prescribed to treat ringworm of the body is:
    A. diphenhydramine.
    B. Percocet.
    C. ampicillin.
    D. griseofulvin.

8. Alendronate sodium is used to treat:
    A. inflammatory muscle conditions.
    B. muscle spasm.
    C. joint pain.
    D. osteoporosis.

9. What is the normal dosage range for Imdur?
    A. 30, 60, 120 mg.
    B. 250, 500, 750 mg.
    C. 0.1, 0.2, 0.5 mg.
    D. None of the above.

10. Which drug is misspelled?
    A. Atenolol.
    B. Linezalid.
    C. Norvasc.
    D. Humulin.

Fill in the Blanks

Fill in the generic name for the following brand name drugs. The first one has been filled in for you.

1. Bactrim   <u>trimethoprim; sulfamethoxazole</u>
2. Procardia   _____
3. Claritin   _____
4. Xanax   _____
5. Prilosec   _____
6. Foltx   _____
7. Remeron   _____
8. Coumadin   _____
9. Lovenox   _____
10. Dyazide   _____
11. Aldactone   _____
12. Lortab   _____
13. Advil   _____
14. Abelcet   _____
15. Zocor   _____
16. Lipitor   _____
17. Phenergan   _____
18. Clinoril   _____
19. Keflex   _____
20. Keppra   _____

Matching

Using your book or other medical reference, match the following controlled substances to the schedule category to which they belong.

_____ 1. Lomotil   A. Schedule I

_____ 2. MS Contin   B. Schedule II

_____ 3. Marijuana   C. Schedule III

_____ 4. Xanax   D. Schedule IV

_____ 5. Darvocet   E. Schedule V

_____ 6. Lortab

_____ 7. Ambien

_____ 8. Dilaudid

_____ 9. Vicodin

_____ 10. Valium

8

LABORATORY STUDIES AND MEDICAL IMAGING

OBJECTIVES

After completing this chapter, you will be able to:

- Explain the basic concept of pathology and the processes that pathologists use to diagnose a given condition.
- Describe common laboratory tests and discuss the common components of each.
- Differentiate between radiologic imaging techniques used in hospitals and clinics and explain under what circumstances each is used.

INTRODUCTION

Medical tests play a variety of roles in patient care. Screening tests check for disease in people before they show symptoms in order to treat a potential problem as early as possible or prevent it entirely. Diagnostic tests confirm the presence of a disease when there is already suspicion or evidence of an illness to determine the extent of disease and monitor how well a patient responds to treatment. Some tests gather information about a potential disease and treat it at the same time.

These tests are a part of nearly every report transcribed by a medical transcriptionist. The terminology can be very descriptive and specific. You may not type a lot of actual pathology reports or reports of radiographic examinations, but you will enter the descriptions, findings, and comments about such studies into a patient's medical record. This chapter reviews common laboratory and imaging methods used by physicians to diagnose and treat illness. Where applicable, specific tests and radiology subtypes, along with the correct transcription of laboratory values and abbreviations, are discussed.

UNDERSTANDING PATHOLOGY

Pathology, considered to be the most scientific branch of medicine, is the study of structural and functional changes in cells that cause disease or harmful abnormalities, such as cancer. A **pathologist** is a medical doctor with additional training in the study of pathology. A pathologist does not see patients, but studies specimens taken from autopsies, biopsies, or other types of excisions where the specific diagnosis or cause of an illness is sought. Pathologists are experts at interpreting microscopic views of body tissues.

Although pathologists do perform autopsies, such procedures represent less than 10% of the workload of a typical modern pathologist. The larger portion of a pathologist's workday is devoted to laboratory work done on a patient's behalf. In addition to the diagnosis of disease and the administration of medical laboratories, pathologists often teach classes to medical students and conduct research that involves human body tissue. Pathology attempts to explain the "whys" and "wherefores" of the signs and symptoms manifested by patients and helps to provide a foundation for the patient's treatment. The primary work of a pathologist involves four main aspects of diagnosing disease:

- Identifying the cause of a disease
- Identifying the mechanism by which certain factors cause disease
- Identifying the structural changes that occur in cells, tissues, and organs
- Identifying the clinical consequences of those changes

Some of the techniques used by a pathologist in the study of a specimen include:

- **Gross pathology**, which is the recognition of a disease based on examination of a tissue or specimen with the naked eye or by direct observation at autopsy.
- **Histopathology**, which is the diagnosis of disease based on the microscopic study of abnormal tissue (**histology** is the microscopic study of tissues). Tissue can be obtained through a variety of methods. In a **fine-needle aspiration** (FNA), a very thin needle on a syringe is inserted into a lesion to remove some of the cells for examination. In a **biopsy**, a small part of a lesion is removed and examined in order to make a diagnosis. In an **excisional biopsy**, an entire lesion is removed and sliced up into thin sections and examined.
- **Cytology**, which is the microscopic examination of cells from tissue fluid for early signs of disease. Two common cytology tests are the cervical smear test (Pap smear) and sputum analysis for lung cancer cells.
- **Tissue chemistry**, which is the chemical properties of the specimen.
- **Flow cytometry** (sometimes referred to as simply "flow" in dictation), which is a procedure that uses a laser-powered instrument to measure the fluorescence from stained cells in a specimen for DNA. This technique is used to evaluate the risk for recurrence of some diseases, such as cancer.
- Culture and sensitivity, which is a procedure whereby an organism is grown in a nutrient medium (called a **culture**) and then tested for sensitivity to certain antibiotics. In this procedure, a moist area of the body is swabbed with a sterile cotton tip, which is placed into a **Petri dish**. The dish was named after its inventor, German bacteriologist Julius Richard Petri, and is a flat dish with a cover, made of plastic or glass, that is used primarily to grow bacteria. The dish is then placed into an incubator to see if bacteria will grow from the swab. Once the bacteria have grown, they can be identified under the microscope and tested for sensitivity to certain antibiotics. This is known as the **culture and sensitivity test**.

A pathologist studies the cells and renders an opinion in the form of a **pathology report** addressed to the doctor requesting it, as shown below:

DATE:	12/06/xxxx
PATHOLOGY NO.:	M02-3551
REG. NO.:	000038
PATIENT NAME:	Sally M. Goodwin
MEDICAL RECORD NO.	70783220
DATE OF BIRTH	03/04/xxxx
SEX:	Female
RACE:	White

HISTORY: Multiple transurethral resections of bladder for grade II transitional cell carcinoma; multiple tumors.

GROSS DESCRIPTION: The specimen is received in two parts. They are labeled #1, "biopsy bladder tumor," and #2, "scalene node, left." Part #1 consists of multiple fragments of gray-brown tissue that appear slightly hemorrhagic. They are submitted in their entirety for processing. Part #2 consists of multiple fragments of fatty yellow tissue that range in size from 0.2 to 1 cm in diameter. They are submitted in their entirety for processing.

MICROSCOPIC DESCRIPTION: Section of bladder contains areas of transitional cell carcinoma. No area of invasion can be identified. A marked acute and chronic inflammatory reaction with eosinophils is noted together with some necrosis. Sections are examined at six levels. Section of lymph node contains normal node with reactive germinal centers.

DIAGNOSES:
1. Papillary transitional cell carcinoma, grade II, bladder biopsy.
2. Acute and chronic inflammation, most consistent with recent biopsy procedure.
3. Scalene lymph node, left, no pathologic diagnosis.

COMMENT: This transitional cell carcinoma is well differentiated. Tissue has been sent for immunohisto-chemical studies. These results will be issued as an addendum. The results of this case were discussed with Dr. Matthew Brenner on 12/06/20xx at 0830 hours.

_____

Kim J. Nguyen, MD

Pathologist

QUICK CHECK 8.1 ✓

Match the definitions on the left with the terms on the right.

1. _____ A procedure that uses a laser-powered instrument to measure the fluorescence from stained cells.

2. _____ The diagnosis of disease based on the microscopic study of abnormal tissues.

3. _____ The study of cells.

4. _____ A small part of a lesion that is removed and examined.

5. _____ The result of growing a microorganism in a nutrient medium.

A. histopathology

B. culture

C. flow cytometry

D. cytology

E. biopsy

A pathology report is typically divided into several basic sections:

- The date of the report. The date usually coincides with the date on which the slides were read, or, if the specimen was taken during an operative procedure, the date corresponding to the operative report.
- The patient's demographic information and pathology department specimen-identifying information. The identifying data of the specimen itself, along with the statistical information of the patient, are indicated in the report.
- History. Some pathologists include a short clinical history of the patient, which describes the reasons why the tissue was removed for analysis.
- The gross description. This section describes the actual appearance of the specimen as viewed by the pathologist's naked eye.
- The microscopic description of the specimen. This describes the appearance of the specimen when viewed under a microscope.
- The diagnosis. This usually indicates the site of the body from which the specimen was removed, along with a final diagnosis.
- Comments. Some pathologists add a comment section to the report. Others may add comments in the diagnosis section. Comments are used to further clarify information about the diagnosis or to inform other physicians that other studies are pending.

TRANSCRIPTION TIP:

When transcribing descriptions of specimens obtained for pathology, you may hear that the specimen was placed in formalin. **Formalin** is a special chemical solution used as a disinfectant or to preserve biological specimens for pathologic review.

LABORATORY STUDIES

A **laboratory test** is a medical procedure in which a sample of blood, urine, or other tissues or substances in the body is analyzed for certain features or enzymes that would cause a certain chemical reaction to occur in the body. By definition, **enzymes** are proteins that facilitate chemical reactions. In the body, enzymes interact with other substances in the body to cause a certain process. For example, stomach enzymes help with the digestion of food and processing of fats in the intestines.

Physicians order laboratory tests to obtain information that cannot be discovered through a patient's history and physical examination. This information assists the physician in determining a patient's diagnosis, planning a course of treatment, and monitoring the course of treatment over time. The test results are usually interpreted based on their relation to a **reference range**, which reflects the results expected for 95% of a given population (or, what is considered "normal" for a given population). Normal range values are developed by each individual laboratory based on the instruments used to conduct the test, the method by which the test is performed, and the type of population being served. For example, children may not have the same reference ranges as adults; men may have different values than women.

Many medical tests are often grouped when they are reported. This is because a group of tests may give more information about a disease or body organ than one single test. Although any human tissue or substance can be tested for disease, the most common laboratory tests are performed on urine and blood.

Urine Tests

Urine, a waste product made by the kidneys, may contain various substances indicative of different types of disease. Physicians use urine testing as a diagnostic tool

TABLE 8.1   Urinalysis Report

PATIENT:	EDWARDS, VERNON	MED. REC. #:	M0011938888
		AGE/SX:	49/M
ADM PHYS:	Dillon, Douglas A.	DOB:	04/03/xxxx

SPEC #:	0112:CT:U00094R	COLL: 01/12/xxxx – 1630		STATUS: COMP
		REC'D: 01/12/xxxx – 1707		SUBM DR.: Dillon, Douglas A.
ENTERED:	01/12/xxxx – 1815			
ORDERED:	URINALYSIS			
COMMENTS:	Campus: Downtown			
	If UA is positive, does physician want culture? N			
	Hold order until collected? N			

Test	Result	Flag	Reference Range
URINALYSIS DIPSTICK:			
UA COLOR	YELLOW		YELLOW
UA APPEARANCE	CLEAR		CLEAR
UA SPEC GRAVITY	1.025		1.00–1.035
UA pH	5.0		5.0–9.0
UA LK ESTERASE	NEG		NEGATIVE
UA NITRITE	NEG		NEGATIVE
UA PROTEIN	NEG		NEGATIVE
UA GLUCOSE	NEG		NEGATIVE
UA KETONES	NEG		NEGATIVE
UA UROBILINOGEN	NORMAL		NORMAL
UA BILIRUBIN	NEG		NEGATIVE
UA BLOOD	**TRACE**	*	NEGATIVE
UA COMMENT	MICROSCOPIC NEEDED		NEGATIVE
MICROSCOPIC:			
UA RBC	0–2		0–2 /hpf
UA EPITHELIAL CELLS	0–2		0–2 /hpf
UA BACTERIA	TRACE		TR /hpf

to identify chemical reactions in the body that may signal a condition requiring further evaluation and treatment. An examination of a urine sample, called a **urinalysis** (UA), measures several different components of urine. A urinalysis breaks down the components of urine to check for the presence of drugs, blood, protein, and other substances, which may indicate another disease process in the body. For example, blood in the urine (**hematuria**) may be the result of a harmless condition but it can also indicate an infection or other problem. High levels of protein in the urine (**proteinuria**) may indicate a kidney or cardiovascular problem. A complete urinalysis includes physical, chemical, and microscopic examinations that screen for urinary tract infections, kidney disease, and diseases of other organs that result in the appearance of abnormal byproducts in

the urine. Table 8.1 illustrates a sample of a typical laboratory's urinalysis report.

The urine sample is collected in an unused disposable plastic cup with a tight-fitting lid. The best sample for analysis is collected in this sterile container in midstream after the external genitalia have been cleansed, called a **clean catch**. The sample is then examined using three methods of assessment: the macroscopic examination, the dipstick examination, and the microscopic examination.

The **macroscopic examination** is the observation of abnormalities in the urine using the naked eye. The urine's odor and appearance are first evaluated. Normal urine has a slight odor, and some laboratories will note strong or atypical odors on the urinalysis report. Normal urine appears as a clear, straw-colored liquid. Abnormal findings may show the urine as appearing hazy or **turbid**, or cloudy, indicating the presence of particles or sediments in the urine.

Many of the tests done on urine are performed using a urine **dipstick**, which is a chemically treated stick-pad that is dipped briefly into a urine sample. The technician then reads the colors of each test and compares them with a reference chart to indicate a positive or negative result.

A complete urinalysis simultaneously tests for several characteristics at once:

- **Specific gravity** is the ratio of a material to the density of another substance, such as water. In a urinalysis, specific gravity measures the amount of particles dissolved in the urine. It also indicates how well the kidneys are able to adjust the amount of water in urine. The higher the specific gravity, the more solid material is dissolved in the urine. For example, when the kidneys produce a greater-than-normal amount of dilute urine (such as when you drink a lot of fluid), the specific gravity is said to be low. When you drink very little liquid, the kidneys will produce only small amounts of concentrated urine, in which case the specific gravity is said to be elevated. Increased urine specific gravity may indicate dehydration, diarrhea, or the presence of glucose in the urine. Decreased urine specific gravity may indicate excessive fluid intake or the kidneys' failure to reabsorb water. The specific gravity value consists of four numbers but sometimes is dictated as a pair of numbers. For example, you may hear, *"the specific gravity was 10–20,"* or *"the specific gravity was one-oh-two-oh,"* but the value should be transcribed as the whole number 1 plus a decimal, followed by three digits, in this case, 1.020.
- The **potential of Hydrogen (pH)**, or the measurement of the acidity or alkalinity of urine.
- Protein, which is not normally found in urine. Protein can indicate kidney damage, blood in the urine, or an infection.
- **Glucose**, which is a simple sugar that is the main source of energy for the body. Glucose is not normally found in urine. A positive amount of sugar can indicate the presence of diabetes.
- **Ketones**, which are substances that are made when the body breaks down fat for energy. A finding of ketones in the urine indicates that the body is using fat as the major source of energy instead of glucose, which is abnormal.
- **Nitrites**. Bacteria that cause a urinary tract infection (or UTI, further discussed in Chapter 15, *Urology*) produce an enzyme that creates nitrites. A nitrite is a salt of nitrous acid. The presence of nitrites in urine indicates a UTI.
- Blood. Normally negative, the presence of blood can indicate an infection, kidney stones, trauma, or bleeding from a bladder or kidney tumor.

- **Bilirubin** and **urobilinogen**. Bilirubin is a breakdown product of hemoglobin, the substance in blood that carries oxygen, described below. Urobilinogen is a substance formed in the intestine from the breakdown of bilirubin. These products are cleared by the liver and normally not found in the urine. Detectable amounts of bilirubin in urine may indicate liver disease and, when combined with urobilinogen, may help identify disorders that can cause jaundice.
- **Leukocyte esterase**, which is an enzyme found in certain white blood cells. This value is normally negative. The presence of white blood cells in the urine suggests a urinary tract infection.

In the microscopic analysis, the urine is spun in a **centrifuge**, which is a device that uses centrifugal force to separate the solid materials referred to as **sediments** from the urine. The sediment is spread on a slide and examined under a microscope. Types of materials that may be found include:

- Red or white blood cells. Normally blood cells are not found in urine. Inflammation, disease, or injury to the urinary system can cause blood in urine. White blood cells can indicate infection, cancer, or kidney disease.
- Casts. Casts are plugs of material that are flushed into the urine from the kidneys. The type of cast (blood cells, protein, or other substances) can provide information about the type of kidney disease that may be present.
- **Crystals**. Crystals are a kind of mineral salt that form in the kidneys and can lead to the formation of kidney stones.
- Bacteria, yeast cells, or parasites, the presence of which can indicate an infection.

Hematologic Studies

Hematology is the study of the anatomy, physiology, pathology, symptomatology, and therapeutics related to the blood and blood-forming tissue. **Hematologic studies**, or blood tests, are another link between the patient's presentation of symptoms and the doctor's treatment for a particular condition or disease. A variety of blood tests are used to check the levels of substances

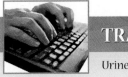

TRANSCRIPTION TIP:

Urine will show *nitrites*, but never *nitrates*. *Nitrates* are a type of cardiac medication. The word is often mispronounced by dictators.

TRANSCRIPTION TIP:

Sometimes a dictator will list two or more lab test names and then give the results later in the sentence. For example, "The hematocrit and hemoglobin were 38 and 15, respectively." The correct word in this context is *respectively*, not *respectfully*.

in the blood that indicate how healthy the body is and whether infection is present. Some tests can reveal elevated levels of waste products, indicating that the kidneys are not working properly. Other tests check the presence of chemical compounds that are critical to the body's healthy functioning. Blood studies can also determine how quickly blood clots. The results of these tests are used by the physician to pinpoint or to support a diagnosis, to monitor or determine treatment, or to screen for undiagnosed conditions.

Complete Blood Count with Differential

The **complete blood count** (CBC) measures the size, number, and maturity of the different blood cells in a specific volume of blood and is one of the most common tests performed. As shown in the report in Table 8.2, a CBC is actually a series of tests that include the following:

- The **white blood count** (WBC) is a count of the actual number of white blood cells per volume of blood. White blood cells fight infection; therefore, an increased number of white blood cells may indicate the presence of an infection.
- The **red blood count** (RBC), also called the **erythrocyte count**, is a count of the actual number of red blood cells per volume of blood. Red blood cells are important for carrying oxygen to the body's cells.
- The **hemoglobin** (Hgb) portion of the CBC measures the oxygen-carrying capacity of the red blood cells in a volume of blood.
- **Hematocrit** (Hct) measures the percentage of volume of red blood cells contained in the blood

TABLE 8.2   Complete Blood Count

PATIENT:	EDWARDS, VERNON	MED. REC. #:	M0011938888
		AGE/SX:	49/M
ADM PHYS:	Dillon, Douglas A.	DOB:	04/03/xxxx

SPEC #:	0112:CT:U0366R	COLL: 01/12/xxxx – 1630	STATUS: COMP
		REC'D: 01/12/xxxx – 1707	SUBM DR.: Dillon, Douglas A.
ENTERED:	01/12/xxxx – 1815		
ORDERED:	CBC W/DIFF		
COMMENTS:	Campus: Downtown		

Test	Result	Flag	Reference Range
CBC W/DIFF:			
WBC	7.9		3.8–10.8 K/mm³
RBC	5.34		4.40–5.80 M/mm³
HEMOGLOBIN	16.2		13.8–17. gm/dl
HEMATOCRIT	46.8		41.0–50.0%
MCV	87.6		80.0–100.0 fl
MCH	30.4		27.0–33.0 pg
MCHC	34.7		32.0–36.0 g/dl
RDW	12.8		11.5–14.5%
PLATELETS	224		150–450 K/cumm
RETIC COUNT	2.5		0.5–2.5 k
DIFFERENTIAL:			
NEUTROPHIL %	52.5		39–72%
LYMPH %	36.5		22–40%
MONO %	7.0		3–10%
EOS %	3.0		1–5%
BASOS %	1.0		0–2%

sample. For example, a hematocrit of 32 (or 32%) indicates that 32% of the blood's volume is composed of red blood cells.

- The **platelet count** (PLT) is the number of platelets that clot in order to prevent bleeding. **Platelets** are types of blood cells that prevent the body from bleeding and bruising easily. When platelet counts are low, it may take longer for blood to clot. When platelet counts are too high, unnecessary blood clots may occur.

The CBC then lists the **red blood cell indices**, which are a group of three measurements that describe the size, hemoglobin concentration, and hemoglobin weight in the red blood cell population:

- The **mean corpuscular volume** (MCV) is a measurement of the actual size of red blood cells. Larger red blood cells may indicate anemia due to vitamin B6 or folic acid deficiency; smaller red blood cells may indicate anemia due to iron deficiency.
- The **mean corpuscular hemoglobin** (MCH) shows the amount of oxygen-carrying hemoglobin inside red blood cells.
- The **mean corpuscular hemoglobin concentration** (MCHC) is a calculation of the concentration of hemoglobin inside red blood cells.
- The **red (blood cell) distribution width** (RDW) is a calculation of the variation in the size of red blood cells.
  - Reticulocyte count. **Reticulocytes** are immature red blood cells that are made by the bone marrow and then released into the bloodstream. The reticulocytes remain in the bloodstream for 24–48 hours while maturing. A reticulocyte count test measures how rapidly the reticulocytes mature; the results can be used to detect anemia or to monitor its progress.

The CBC also lists the white blood cell **differential**, often dictated as a slang expression, *diff*. This part of the

CBC is an estimate of the percentage of each white blood cell type making up the total white blood cell count in the sample. Each type of cell plays a different role in protecting the body. The numbers of each one of these types of white blood cells give important information about the immune system. They are often dictated in an abbreviated form and include **segmented neutrophils** (dictated as *segs*), which fight infection, **band neutrophils** (*bands*), which also fight infection; **lymphocytes** (*lymphs*), which produce antibodies and aid other immune system activities; **monocytes** (*monos*), which also fight infection; and **eosinophils** (*eos*) and **basophils** (*basos*), which are involved with identifying allergic or toxic reactions to certain medications or chemicals.

When transcribing the white blood cell differential, the values may be given as whole numbers or percentages. Type the terms out or use the abbreviated forms of the words according to your employer's preferences.

Example:
The CBC showed WBCs of 6500 with 60% segs, 8% bands, 21% lymphs, 7% monos, 2% eos, and 2% basos.
OR
The CBC showed a white blood count of 6500 with 60 neutrophils, 8 bands, 21 lymphocytes, 7 monocytes, 2 eosinophils, and 2 basophils.

Metabolic Panel

A **basic metabolic panel** (BMP), sometimes called a **chemistry panel**, is a group of specific tests that provide a physician with information about the current status of a patient's kidneys, electrolyte balance, blood sugar, and calcium levels. Significant changes in these values could result in kidney failure, insulin shock, respiratory distress, or abnormalities in heart rhythm. A physician may also order a **comprehensive metabolic panel** (CMP), which is a set of 14 tests that includes the BMP as well as liver function studies. Table 8.3 illustrates an example of a comprehensive metabolic panel report.

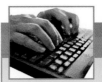

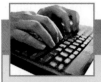

TRANSCRIPTION TIP:

Do not confuse the soundalike abbreviations BMP (basic metabolic panel) and BNP (B-type natriuretic peptide). BMP is a series, or panel, of blood tests. BNP is a single cardiac test that measures the amount of the BNP hormone, made by the heart, present in the blood. A helpful way to remember the correct abbreviation is to listen to the number of values indicated for the test. If several values are dictated, the test is a BMP; if only one value is dictated, it is BNP.

The CMP measures the following:

- **Electrolytes**, which are minerals that regulate the body's balance of fluids and help maintain normal functions, such as heart rhythm, muscle contractions, and brain function. These include sodium, potassium, chloride, and carbon dioxide (or bicarbonate), and are typically ordered together. These minerals help to maintain water distribution in tissues, maintain regular muscle function, and regulate body pH.
- Blood glucose, which indicates the status of carbohydrate metabolism and utilization.
- Kidney function, which includes testing for **blood urea nitrogen** (BUN) and **creatinine**. The BUN is a waste product in the blood from protein metabolism, and this test measures the amount of nitrogen in the blood that comes from the waste product **urea**. Urea is a substance formed in the intestines and liver when protein is broken down in the body and eliminated from the body through the kidneys. High levels of urea may mean that the kidneys are not excreting waste properly. Creatinine is a waste by-product formed by the breakdown of the substance creatine phosphate, which supplies energy to muscles. The creatinine is filtered out of the blood by the kidneys and then passed out of the body in urine. High levels of these substances, therefore, suggest that the kidneys

---

TABLE 8.3   Comprehensive Metabolic Panel (CMP)

PATIENT:	EDWARDS, VERNON	MED. REC. #:	M0011938888	
		AGE/SX:	49/M	
ADM PHYS:	Dillon, Douglas A.	DOB:	04/03/xxxx	

SPEC #:	0112:CT:U3569J	COLL: 01/12/xxxx – 1630		STATUS: COMP
		REC'D: 01/12/xxxx – 1707		SUBM DR.: Dillon, Douglas A.
ENTERED:	01/12/xxxx – 1613			
ORDERED:	CMP			
COMMENTS:	Campus: Downtown			

Test	Result	Flag	Reference Range
CMP:			
SODIUM	142		135–146 MEQ/L
POTASSIUM	3.7		3.5–5.3 MEQ/L
CHLORIDE	105		95–108 MEQ/L
CO_2	29		20–32 MEQ/L
GLUCOSE	90		70–115 mg/dL
BUN	15		7–25 mg/dL
CREATININE	1.1		0.7–1.4 mg/dL
BUN/CREAT RATIO	13.6		6–25 RATIO
TOTAL PROTEIN	7.2		6.0–8.5 GM/DL
ALBUMIN	4.5		3.2–5.0 GM/DL
CALCIUM	8.9		8.5–10.3 MG/DL
TOTAL BILIRUBIN	0.7		0.0–1.3 mg/dL
AST (SGOT)	28		0–60 INTERNATIONAL UNITS/L
ALT (SGPT)	73	High	0–60 INTERNATIONAL UNITS/L
ALK PHOS	106		20–225 INTERNATIONAL UNITS/L

may not be working properly. The **BUN-to-creatinine ratio** is the ratio between the BUN and creatinine. This ratio is used to help determine if kidney function is impaired due to damaged or diseased kidneys or another factor outside of the kidneys. If both BUN and creatinine are high, the ratio usually indicates damage to the kidneys. If BUN is high but creatinine is normal, then the kidney is generally not damaged but is not getting adequate blood supply due to another problem, such as dehydration or heart failure.

- **Liver function tests** (LFTs), also called a "liver panel," are a series of blood chemistry tests measuring enzymes excreted by the liver during abnormal functioning due to metastases, obstruction, or other conditions. These tests include alkaline phosphatase, total protein, albumin, globulin, **aspartate aminotransferase** (AST), **alanine aminotransferase** (ALT), and bilirubin. Sometimes dictators will say either the term AST or SGOT, which is an older term for aspartate aminotransferase, and ALT or SGPT, which is an older term for alanine aminotransferase. Whatever term is used should be transcribed as dictated.
- Bone health. A bone profile includes measurements of calcium, phosphorus, and uric acid.

Iron Studies

Humans require iron for every function of metabolism. Iron carries oxygen from the lungs through the bloodstream and releases it in the body where it is needed. It is also necessary in the production of **myoglobin**, the oxygen-carrying and storage protein of muscles, and for several other essential enzymes that help to detoxify poisons and to convert sugars into energy. Decreases in iron levels can lead to anemia, indicated by the presence of lower-than-normal numbers of red blood cells. Too much iron can damage the heart, liver, and pancreas as well as the joints. **Hemochromatosis** is an inherited disease that disrupts the way the body metabolizes iron. Normally the body will absorb the amount of iron it needs and expel any excess amount. In hemochromatosis, the body erroneously stores excess iron that should be expelled. Continuing unabated, the body continues to absorb iron and deposit it throughout the body. Left unchecked, this excess iron accumulation can cause damage to the joints, the major organs, and overall body chemistry, and ultimately lead to death.

Serum iron studies measure the following elements:

- Serum iron level, or the level of iron in the blood
- **Ferritin**, an iron-carrying protein, which measures the amount of stored iron in the body
- Total iron-binding capacity (TIBC), which measures the amount of **transferrin**, a protein that transports iron in the blood from the intestines to the cells that use it

Thyroid Function Tests

Thyroid function tests (TFTs) is a collective term for blood tests used to evaluate the function of the thyroid gland, which is located in the neck, just below the larynx. Thyroid hormones regulate the rate at which the body converts food into energy. The major thyroid hormone secreted by the thyroid gland is **thyroxine**, also called T4 because it contains four iodine atoms. This hormone along with a second hormone, **triiodothyronine** (T3), act together to regulate the body's metabolism. The production of these hormones and their release into the bloodstream is controlled by another hormone produced in the pituitary gland located at the base of the brain, called **thyroid stimulating hormone** (TSH). (For a more detailed discussion of the relationship between the thyroid gland and its related hormone function, see Chapter 19, *Immunology*, and Chapter 21, *Endocrinology*.)

The best way to initially test thyroid function is to measure the thyroid hormone levels in a blood sample. Abnormal TSH levels can indicate that the thyroid gland is either overactive or failing completely. The free T4 fraction is the most important to determine how the thyroid is functioning. Finally, T3 is evaluated to determine the severity of the thyroid malfunction.

Blood Clotting Studies

This group of tests, also called coagulation studies, measures the duration of bleeding time after a standardized skin incision (such as during surgery) before blood forms a clot to close the wound, called **coagulation**, and the effectiveness of blood-thinning drug therapy. Prolonged bleeding may indicate the presence of blood disorders or liver disease. The tests that measure blood coagulation time are prothrombin time (PT), partial thromboplastin time (PTT), and International Normalized Ratio (INR).

TRANSCRIPTION TIP:

The value for potassium is always measured in milliequivalents, or mEq. The same rule applies when transcribing medication values for potassium chloride, for example, *potassium chloride 20 mEq daily*, not 20 mg. In addition, many physicians will dictate the chemical abbreviation for potassium chloride, *KCl*. Note how this chemical is typed when transcribing the abbreviation for potassium chloride, for example, *KCl 20 mEq daily*. Be sure to use the correct measure of *mEq*, even if the dictator says *mg*.

TRANSCRIPTION TIP:

A physician may refer to coagulation tests together or separately, such as "the patient's PT-PTT" or "PT-INR." These values may be transcribed as PT, PTT, PT/PTT, or PT/INR. In most cases, dictators use the abbreviations "PT" "PTT" and "INR," not their expanded forms.

The test for PT (also dictated as *pro time*) measures the time it takes for a patient's blood to clot. It is often done before surgery to evaluate how likely the patient is to have a bleeding or clotting problem during or after a surgical procedure. The PTT test is performed to show the function of all clotting factors in the blood and to determine if blood-thinning drug agents are effective. The INR portion of the test is a standardizing measurement of PT to monitor the effectiveness of blood-thinning drugs.

Cultures

Cultures are used to locate the principal site and type of bacterium, fungus, or other microorganism involved in infection to treat the infection appropriately. To determine the site and organism, samples of body fluids or stool samples are placed in a culture medium in special sterile containers and incubated for up to several days. These cultures are examined to determine if bacteria or fungi are present in significant numbers. If they are present, the organisms can be identified and tested with several antibiotics to determine which antibiotic kills the organism. The two most common types of cultures are urine and blood.

TRANSCRIPTION TIP:

When transcribing blood tests, listen for "go-togethers," or terms that are often dictated very close to each other. For example:

Sodium, potassium (often dictated together)

BUN, creatinine (often dictated together)

Protein, albumin, bilirubin, AST, ALT, alkaline phosphatase (liver studies, often dictated together)

Calcium, phosphorus, uric acid (bone health studies, often dictated together)

PT, PTT, INR (coagulation studies, often dictated together)

Urine Culture

A **urine culture** is a test to detect and identify organisms (usually bacteria) that may be causing a urinary tract infection. With a urine culture, a small sample of a patient's urine is collected and sent to a laboratory for testing. In the laboratory, a portion of the urine sample is cultured and placed in an incubator at body temperature for 24 hours to determine if there is any growth of bacteria. If there is no growth at the end of that time, the culture is considered negative for significant number of microorganisms that could cause an infection. If bacteria are present, the total number of organisms are counted and identified.

Once an organism is identified, sensitivity (or susceptibility) testing is done to help determine the antibiotic that will be most effective against the specific types of bacteria infecting a person.

Blood Culture

A **blood culture** is done to detect the presence of microorganisms such as bacteria, mycobacteria, or fungi that may have spread from a specific site in the body into the bloodstream. As with a urine culture, a sample of blood is obtained and placed into a special laboratory preparation and incubated in a controlled environment for one to seven days. The culture is examined for the presence of microorganisms over that period. If organisms are present, further culturing may take place to identify the organisms. As with a urine culture, sensitivity testing may also be done to classify the organism so that antibiotic therapy can be started before final culture results are available.

The **Gram stain**, named after Hans Christian Gram, the Danish bacteriologist who originally devised it in 1882, is a staining technique used in the identification of bacteria. Microorganisms that are stained by the Gram stain method are commonly referred to as being gram-positive or gram-negative. Remember not to capitalize an eponym when used as an adjective.

RADIOLOGIC IMAGING

Radiology, or diagnostic imaging, is the branch of medicine that determines the nature of a patient's disease through studying radiation images of the human body. Radiology is sometimes referred to as **clinical radiology** because of the many uses of imaging techniques for diagnosis and treatment of an injury or disease. A **radiologist** is a physician who has taken additional training in the interpretation of medical images to specialize in radiology. This training usually takes five to six years after completing medical school.

Radiology uses radiation for different types of imaging, including x-rays. **Imaging** is the term used to

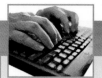

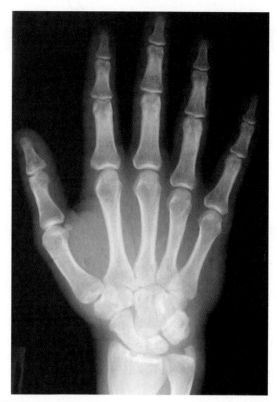

FIGURE 8.1. **X-ray of an Adult Human Hand.** Bones and tumors appear white or light on x-ray film, whereas muscles and tissues would appear darker on film. Reprinted with permission from Bucholz RW, MD and Heckman JD, MD. *Rockwood & Green's Fractures in Adults*, 5th ed. Lippincott, Williams & Wilkins, 2001.

describe the creation of an image of a dense object in the body with the use of radiant energy. The radiologist's reading of an image is called the "official" result, even if a patient's primary physician has reviewed the images and come to a conclusion before the radiologist's reading is rendered.

Although radiology began with the use of x-rays and simple flat sheets of photographic films, modern radiology now encompasses a variety of tools, utilizing different technologies for imaging living patients to diagnose disease and injury, sometimes before symptoms even appear. The following list includes the most common of these noninvasive, or minimally invasive, procedures.

X-ray

An **x-ray**, also called a radiograph, is an imaging study that uses radiation transmission to obtain pictures of bones and other body structures. The first x-ray image was created by German scientist Wilhelm Roentgen in 1895. At the time, he labeled the rays he discovered with the scientific symbol "X," meaning unknown, because he did not understand their makeup. Six years later, he was awarded the Nobel Prize in physics for his discovery. Once in a while you may even hear a dictator refer to an x-ray as a **roentgenogram**, in honor of this inventor.

Figure 8.1 shows an example of an x-ray image. X-rays are actually electromagnetic waves. When they are passed through a patient's body to a photographic film plate on the other side, they create a picture of internal body structures called a **radiograph**. Radiographs, which are the most common imaging tests, can reveal abnormalities in body organs (such as pneumonia, tumor, or fluid), and bones (such as broken or abnormal bones). The less dense a structure of the body is, the more radiation passes through it and reaches the film plate. The x-rays expose the film, changing its color to gray or black, much like light would darken photographic film. Therefore, less dense types of tissue such as watery secretions, blood, and fat leave a darkened area on the x-ray film. More dense items, such as muscle and connective tissues (ligaments, tendons, and cartilage) appear gray. Very dense items (bones) appear white. When structures appear light or white, they are said to be **radiolucent**. When structures appear black or dark, they are said to be **radiopaque**.

X-rays can be taken of the entire body. A chest x-ray can detect air in the pleural spaces of the lungs as well as broken ribs and sternal fractures; it can also rule out lung disease. In the abdomen and pelvis, x-rays can visualize hernias, gallstones, uterine fibroids, appendicitis, and foreign objects such as coins or bullets. In the extremities, x-rays locate bone fractures and signs of degenerative joint disease.

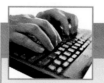

QUICK CHECK 8.2 ✓

Fill in the blanks with the correct terms.

1. Minerals that regulate bodily function are called _____.

2. The report of the percentages of the types of WBCs present is called the _____.

3. Plugs of material that are flushed into the urine from the kidneys are called _____.

4. Cells that clot to prevent bleeding are called _____.

5. A staining technique used in the identification of bacteria is called a _____.

After the film plates are developed, the images are reviewed and interpreted by a radiologist. The radiologist "reads" the image to pinpoint an injury to determine how serious the injury is or to help detect abnormalities such as tumors. The radiologist then issues a report of the findings to the requesting physician, as shown below:

PATIENT NAME: Zang, Jia

MEDICAL RECORD NO.: HW-49222L

DATE OF ADMISSION: 06/27/xxxx

ATTENDING PHYSICIAN: Dimaza Dilawaar, MD

DATE OF EVALUATION: June 28, 20xxxx

ORDERING PHYSICIAN: Dimaza Dilawaar, MD

TYPE OF TEST: X-ray evaluation.

INDICATION: Cardiac palpitations.

FINDINGS: The lungs show essentially mild increase in interstitial markings. The cardiac silhouette is enlarged. The costophrenic angles are clear. Hilar regions are within upper limits of normal in size.

IMPRESSION: Mildly increased interstitial markings in the lung fields that represent mild component of venous congestion. Follow-up examination is recommended.

The cardiac silhouette is within upper limits of normal in size.

_____

Kip Yeune, MD

Attending Radiologist

KY/gw

T: 06/28/xxxx

D: 06/28/xxxx

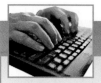

X-rays are ordered on a daily basis in hospitals and clinics all over the world. The most common views are the routine PA (posteroanterior) and lateral (sideways) chest films, dictated as "PA and lateral" or "PA and lat," where the patient is standing and the x-ray tube is behind the patient and the film is in front, and a lateral view is taken when the patient is standing sideways. Other x-rays can be taken at the bedside with a portable x-ray machine when the patient is bedridden, unconscious, or otherwise unable to stand. Other common terms used to describe positioning of the patient in order to obtain a radiologic image include:

- Anteroposterior (AP): The view going through the patient from anterior to posterior.
- Posteroanterior (PA): The view going through the patient from posterior to anterior.
- Lateral: The view from the side of the patient or structure being imaged.
- Right lateral decubitus: The view with patient lying on the right side.
- Left lateral decubitus: The view with patient lying on the left side.

- Oblique: A view that is slanted or at an angle.
- Lordotic: The view with the patient leaning back while standing.

CT Scan

Unlike conventional x-rays, which take a single picture of a part of the body, a **computed tomography (CT) scan** is an imaging tool that generates hundreds of x-ray images in a single examination and produces a three-dimensional image from the pictures. A CT scanner is a special x-ray machine combined with a computer that produces cross-sectional images or "slices" of any part of the body, which enables images from the CT scan to be viewed on a three-dimensional plane. As a result, a physician can see the entire anatomy of a structure, as shown in Figure 8.2. To visualize the advantage of using CT, imagine the inside of a fruitcake, with a variety of objects inside that cannot be seen on the outside of the cake. Only when the cake is cut into slices can the depth and complexity of the separate ingredients of the cake be seen.

During the examination, an x-ray tube that surrounds the patient takes continuous pictures from many angles. The scanner's computer then processes the images in slices, or cross-sectional views, which makes it possible to display them in different ways for viewing on a display screen. When using a CT to visualize blood flow in arterial and venous vessels, the patient may be given a dose of contrast material. **Contrast** material, often dictated as just "contrast," is a substance that has an opacity different from that of soft tissue; this material is injected into the patient or swallowed by the patient in order to identify blood vessels and other

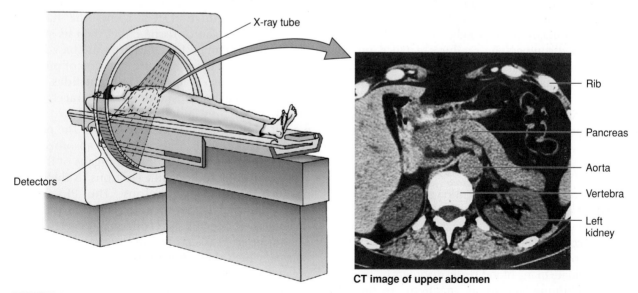

CT image of upper abdomen

FIGURE 8.2. **CT Scan of Upper Abdomen**. The x-ray tube rotates around the person in the CT scanner and sends hundreds of images to a computer, which then reconstructs them into one scanned image. The scan is oriented so it appears the way an examiner would view it when standing at the foot of the bed and looking toward a supine person's head. From Moore KL and Agur A. *Essential Clinical Anatomy*, 2nd Ed. Philadelphia: Lippincott Williams & Wilkins, 2002.

QUICK CHECK 8.3 ✓

Indicate whether the following sentences are true (T) or false (F).

1. X-rays are actually microwaves.   T   F

2. An MRI uses a large magnet in the imaging process.   T   F

3. A CT scan uses a transducer to take pictures of structures.   T   F

4. Bones appear dark on an x-ray image.   T   F

5. Doppler technology uses sound waves to evaluate structures.   T   F

---

objects during an imaging study. For example, patients undergoing CT scanning of the digestive tract may be asked to swallow the contrast material in a drink prior to the test to highlight certain structures in the intestines or colon.

CT is used in other areas as well. For example, a **CT angiogram** uses x-ray pictures to visualize blood flow in arterial and venous vessels throughout the body, from arteries serving the brain to those bringing blood to the lungs, kidneys, and arms and legs. Like a conventional CT, a CT angiogram uses beams of x-rays that are passed through the area of interest in the patient's body from several different angles to create cross-sectional images, which are then assembled by computer into a three-dimensional picture of the area being studied. CT angiography can be used, for example, to evaluate for obstructions in the pulmonary arteries, to visualize blood flow in the arteries supplying the kidneys to rule out kidney disorders, or to identify weak spots in the walls of the aorta or other major blood vessels.

Computed tomography produces detailed images that can reveal abnormalities conventional x-rays cannot pick up. This method of imaging is useful in checking the brain for tumors, aneurysms, and bleeding. It can also unveil tumors, cysts, and other problems in other organs of the body.

MRI/MRA

Magnetic resonance imaging (MRI) is another modality used for examining the structures of the body without surgery. An MRI is an imaging tool that uses a large magnet, a computer, and radio waves to look inside the body and to evaluate various body parts. It can also be used to evaluate many blood vessel disorders by using a similar technique known as **magnetic resonance angiography (MRA)**.

The MRI technique detects varying concentrations of hydrogen atoms (ions) from one tissue to another.

During an MRI scan, the patient lies on a table that slides into a tubular scanner. Inside the tube, a large magnet creates a magnetic field. Pulse radio waves are directed into the magnetic field and absorbed by the hydrogen atoms in the body. The machine's computer then creates an image of the body's internal structures and tissues by measuring the emission of energy from the movement of hydrogen atoms within the body. MRI technology is frequently used to detect cancers that would otherwise be difficult to diagnose. It can also evaluate various body parts, such as the brain, neck, and spine, and can be used to detect blood vessel disorders common in heart and vascular disease and stroke.

PET Scan

Positron emission tomography (PET) imaging is a diagnostic examination that shows the functional activity of an organ or tissue rather than its structure. The images obtained by a PET scan are based on the detection of radiation from the emission of **positrons**, tiny particles also known as **radionuclides** emitted from a radioactive substance called a **tracer** injected into the patient's bloodstream or inhaled by the patient in the form of a radioactive gas. The positron-emitting compounds of the tracer are absorbed in different amounts by the tissues and organs of the body. These positrons collide with electrons in the body to produce high-energy photons. The PET scanner records the signals that the tracer emits as it journeys through the body and as it collects in targeted organs. A computer reassembles the signals into actual images, which then show biological maps of normal organ function and failure of organ systems. PET scans are able to show areas of inadequate blood flow, such as areas of the brain damaged by stroke or those areas with high biochemical changes, such as with cancer.

Ultrasonography

Ultrasound, also called **ultrasonography**, uses sound waves to generate pictures of the body by bouncing sound waves off organs and other interior body structures. The pictures are created by applying a warm gel to the skin and then moving a wand, called a **transducer**, along the outside of the body over the body part being examined to gather data. The transducer sends out high-frequency sound waves, far above the range of human hearing. When the waves hit the body structure being studied, some are absorbed by the tissues and some are echoed back to the transducer. The machine measures the amount of sound reflected back and displays an image called a **sonogram** on a video screen, as shown in Figure 8.3.

A **Doppler ultrasound** is a procedure that uses the Doppler effect in ultrasound to detect movement of red blood cells by analyzing the change in frequency of the returning echoes to evaluate heart, blood vessels, and valves. This test helps doctors evaluate blood flow through the major arteries and veins of the arms, legs, and neck. It can show blocked or reduced blood flow through narrowing in the major arteries of the neck that could cause a stroke or reveal blood clots in leg veins.

During a Doppler ultrasound, the transducer is passed over the skin above a blood vessel. The transducer sends and receives sound waves that are amplified through a microphone. The sound waves bounce off solid objects, including blood cells. The movement of blood cells causes a change in pitch of the reflected sound waves (the "Doppler effect"). If there is no blood flow, the pitch does not change. Information from the reflected sound waves can be processed by a computer to provide graphs or pictures that represent the flow of blood through the blood vessels.

Ultrasonography can be used to discover multiple pregnancies and birth defects as well as to identify cysts, cancerous cells, and the cause of pelvic bleeding. Nearly every organ in the body can be examined by ultrasound, depending on the type of information required by the physician.

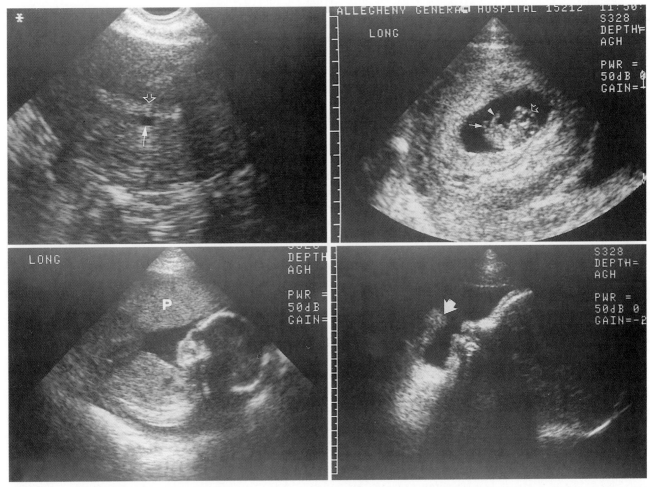

FIGURE 8.3. Ultrasound Imaging. These four ultrasound images reveal the progressive growth and development of a normal embryo, and later the fetus. Reprinted with permission from Daffner RH. *Clinical Radiology: The Essentials*, 2nd ed. Baltimore: Lippincott Williams & Wilkins, 1998.

CHAPTER SUMMARY

The results of laboratory tests and diagnostic imaging studies influence many clinical decisions that physicians make in patient care. Highly accurate laboratory studies and imaging tools enable physicians to pinpoint their diagnoses and to treat patients without jeopardizing their safety with invasive procedures.

Diagnostic testing plays a crucial role in medical decision-making, and each test has a set of terminology, abbreviations, and descriptions all its own. To ensure that information pertaining to these tests is accurately transcribed into a patient's medical record, a transcriptionist must have a thorough understanding of the purpose of each test, as well as the testing process and the terminology used to describe the results. As medical technology continues to grow at an exponential rate, it is important to keep abreast of new techniques used to diagnose and treat illness so that you will be able to understand the information being dictated and to transcribe that information accurately into the patient's medical record.

· I · N · S · I · G · H · T ·

"Feeling Tissue" with Imaging

Malignancies and other pathological processes are often characterized by marked changes in tissue properties. During a physical exam, physicians palpate, or feel, various parts of a patient's body to help locate abnormal or diseased tissue. In fact, many tumors of the thyroid, breast, and prostate are still first detected by this centuries-old diagnostic technique. Unfortunately, small or inaccessible lesions cannot be detected by touch. Moreover, it is a subjective technique that may not reveal the presence of disease until it is in its advanced stages.

Magnetic resonance elastography (MRE) is emerging as a practical and powerful technique for quantitatively assessing the properties of organs, tissues, cells, and other biomaterials by using harmonic low-frequency acoustic waves. Currently it is being used to help diagnose liver disease earlier than standard studies. For example, a liver damaged by alcohol feels much harder than a healthy liver, called *fibrosis*. The standard test to determine this damage is to insert a needle into the abdomen and remove a small piece of liver as a pathologic specimen, which is then examined under a microscope for abnormal cells. The procedure is invasive and poses potential risks for complications, such as bleeding and infection, not to mention being a painful procedure for the patient. In contrast, the MRE is a painless, noninvasive procedure.

In this procedure, the patient is placed in the MRI machine with a small pad resembling the head of a drum strapped to the abdomen. The "drum" vibrates in different ways as acoustic waves are delivered to the liver, powered by a remotely located audio speaker operating at very low, almost inaudible frequencies. The device is extremely sensitive to tissue motion and creates images of these audio waveforms. The waveform images are animated and displayed on a computer screen, which allows physicians to observe the motion and use a preset algorithm to calculate the stiffness of the tissue. The result is called an *elastogram*, which is a detailed map of tissue elasticity. If hardened tissue is found early enough, treatment may halt the disease before it causes irreversible liver damage. In recent studies, researchers found the MRE method to have a sensitivity for diagnosing liver fibrosis of 98% and an absence of false positives of 99%.

Many diseases cause the properties of tissue to change and would be likely candidates for diagnosis using MRE in the future. Currently studies are underway to evaluate whether this promising technology can distinguish between other types of tissue, such as benign and cancerous lumps in the breast. If successful, it can be used to noninvasively palpate many regions of the body that are beyond the reach of the physician's hand, offering a reliable method for diagnosing disease that is intrinsically safer, less expensive, and probably more accurate than a conventional biopsy.

Common Soundalike Words

Word	Word Pronunciation	Soundalike	Soundalike Pronunciation
plain (x-ray): a radiograph made without use of a contrast medium	plân	**plane**: an imaginary surface formed by extension through any axis or two definite points (as in "anatomic plane")	plân
axis: the central line of the body or any of its parts; also the vertebral column	ak'sis	**access**: a way of entering or leaving	ak'ses
anatomic: relating to anatomy	an'ă-tom'ik	**atomic**: relating to an atom	ă-tom'ik
contusion: an injury caused by a blow resulting in hemorrhage beneath unbroken skin (bruise)	kon-tū'zhŭn	**confusion**: a mistake that results from taking one thing to be another	kon-fū'zhŭn
corpus: the main part of an organ or other anatomic structure	kōr'pŭs	**copious**: large in number or quantity	'kō-pē-ŭs
foci: plural of *focus*; center points	fō'sī	**fossa**: a depression below the level of the surface of a part	fos'ă
denervation: loss of nerve supply	dē-něr-vā'shŭn	**innervation**: the supply of motor and sensory nerve fibers functionally connected with an organ or region	in-ěr-vā'shŭn
necrosis: pathologic death of one or more cells or of a portion of tissue or organ resulting from irreversible damage	ně-krō'sis	**narcosis**: unconsciousness induced by narcotics or anesthesia	nar-kō'sis
radical: denoting treatment by extreme, drastic, or innovative, as opposed to conservative, measures	rad'i-kăl	**radicle**: a nerve fiber that joins others to form a nerve	rad'i-kěl
viral: of, pertaining to, or caused by a virus	vī'răl	**virtual**: occurring or existing primarily online	ver'chū-ăl
perfuse: to flow or spread, such as blood	pěr-fyŭs'	**profuse**: lavish, extravagant, bountiful	prō-fyŭs'
contrast: an internally administered substance that is used to visualize parts of the body	kon'trast	**contract**: an explicit bilateral commitment by a physician and patient to a defined course of action	kon-trakt'

Combining Forms

Combining Form	Meaning	Combining Form	Meaning
anter/o	before; front part	iatr/o	physicians, medicine, treatment
axi/o	axis	kary/o	nucleus
blast/o	process of budding by cells or tissue	later/o	side
		magnet/o	magnet
chrom-, chromat/o, chrom/o	color	nucle/o	nucleus
		osm/o	osmosis
cin/e	movement	path/o	disease
cycl/o	cycle; circle	poster/o	back part
cyt/o	cell	project/o	throw forward
duc/o	bring or move	radi/o	radiation
ech/o	echo (sound wave)	roentgen/o	x-ray; radiation
electr/o	electricity	rotat/o	rotate
emiss/o	to send out	scint/i	point of light
fluor/o	fluorescence	son/o	sound
gen/o	being born, producing, coming to be	spir/o	coil
		tom/o	a cut, slice, or layer
hem/o, hemat/o, haem/a	blood	trac/o	visible path

Add Your Own Combining Forms Here:

_____

_____

_____

_____

_____

_____

ABBREVIATIONS

Abbreviation	Meaning	Abbreviation	Meaning
ALT	alanine aminotransferase	MCV	mean corpuscular volume
AST	aspartate aminotransferase	MRA	magnetic resonance angiography
BMP	basic metabolic panel	MRE	magnetic resonance elastography
BNP	B-type natriuretic peptide	MRI	magnetic resonance imaging
BUN	blood urea nitrogen	PA	posteroanterior
C&S	culture and sensitivity	PET	positron emission tomography
CBC	complete blood count	pH	potential of Hydrogen
CMP	comprehensive metabolic panel	PLT	platelets
CNS	central nervous system	PT	prothrombin time
CT	computed tomography	PTT	partial thromboplastin time
FNA	fine-needle aspiration	RBC	red blood count
Hct	hematocrit	RDW	red (cell) distribution width
Hgb	hemoglobin	T3	triiodothyronine
INR	International Normalized Ratio	T4	thyroxine
LFTs	liver function tests	TIBC	total iron binding capacity
MCH	mean corpuscular hemoglobin	TFTs	thyroid function tests
MCHC	mean corpuscular hemoglobin concentration	UA	urinalysis
		WBC	white blood count

Add Your Own Abbreviations Here:

_____

_____

_____

_____

_____

_____

TERMINOLOGY

Term	Meaning
alanine aminotransferase (ALT)	An enzyme produced by the liver and used elsewhere in the body.
aspartate aminotransferase (AST)	An enzyme produced by the liver and used elsewhere in the body.
band neutrophils (bands)	A type of white blood cell that fights infection.
basic metabolic panel, syn. chemistry panel	A group of specific tests that provides information about the status of a patient's kidneys, electrolytes, blood sugar, and calcium levels.
basophils (basos)	A type of white blood cell involved in identifying allergic or toxic reactions to certain medications or chemicals.
bilirubin	A breakdown product of hemoglobin.
biopsy	The procedure of removing a small part of a lesion for pathologic examination.
blood culture	A test used to detect the presence of microorganisms such as bacteria, mycobacteria, or fungi that may have spread from a specific site in the body into the bloodstream.
blood urea nitrogen (BUN)	A waste product in the blood from protein metabolism that comes from the waste product urea.
BUN-to-creatinine ratio	The ratio between the BUN and creatinine, which is used to help determine if kidney function is impaired due to a damaged or diseased kidneys or another factor outside of the kidneys.
casts	Plugs of material that are flushed into the urine from the kidneys.
centrifuge	A device that uses centrifugal force to separate solid materials from liquids.
clean catch	Urine collected in a sterile container in midstream after the external genitalia have been cleansed.
coagulation	The process by which blood forms a clot over an open wound.
complete blood count	A test that assesses the cells in the blood for infection and disorders.
comprehensive metabolic panel	A group of 14 tests that includes the basic metabolic panel (BMP) as well as liver function studies and a bone profile.
computed tomography (CT) scan	A type of imaging study that generates hundreds of x-ray images in a single examination to produce a three-dimensional image from the pictures.
contrast	A substance that has a different opacity from soft tissue that is injected into the patient or swallowed in order to identify blood vessels and other objects in an imaging study.
creatinine	A waste by-product formed by the breakdown of the substance creatine phosphate, which supplies energy to muscles. The creatinine is filtered out of the blood by the kidneys and then passed out of the body in urine.
crystals	A kind of mineral salts that form in the kidneys.
CT angiogram	A CT procedure that uses x-rays to visualize blood flow in arterial and venous vessels throughout the body.
culture	The result of growing a microorganism in a nutrient medium.
culture and sensitivity test	The process of identifying the species of bacteria under a microscope and testing it for sensitivity to certain antibiotics.
cytology	The study of cells under a microscope.
differential	An analysis of the percentages of the types of white blood cells.

Term	Meaning
dipstick	A chemically treated stick-pad that is briefly dipped into a urine sample and analyzed.
Doppler ultrasound	The procedure that uses the Doppler effect in ultrasound to detect movement of scatterers (usually red blood cells) by analyzing the change in frequency of the returning echoes to evaluate heart, blood vessels, and valves.
electrolytes	Minerals that regulate body function.
enzymes	Proteins that accelerate chemical reactions.
eosinophils (eos)	A type of white blood cell involved in identifying allergic or toxic reactions to certain medications or chemicals.
erythrocyte count	Another term for red blood cell count.
excisional biopsy	The process of removing an entire lesion for pathologic examination.
ferritin	An iron-carrying protein that measures the amount of stored iron in the body.
fine needle aspiration	A procedure of withdrawing cells from a lesion for examination with a fine needle on a syringe.
flow cytometry	A procedure that uses a laser-powered instrument to measure the fluorescence from stained cells in a specimen for DNA.
formalin	A 37% aqueous solution of formaldehyde used to transport specimens in for pathologic review.
glucose	A simple sugar which is the main energy source for the body.
Gram stain	A staining technique used to identify bacteria.
gross pathology	The recognition of a disease based on examination of a specimen with the naked eye or at autopsy.
hematocrit	The percentage of blood volume occupied by red blood cells.
hematologic studies, syn. blood tests	A variety of blood tests used to check the levels of substances in the blood that indicate how healthy the body is and whether infection is present.
hematology	The study of the anatomy, physiology, pathology, symptomatology, and therapeutics related to the blood and blood-forming tissue.
hematuria	Blood in the urine.
hemochromatosis	An inherited disease wherein the body stores excess iron that gradually accumulates, causing organ damage over many years.
hemoglobin	Oxygen-carrying protein in red blood cells.
histology	The microscopic study of tissues.
histopathology	The diagnosis of disease based on the microscopic study of abnormal tissues.
imaging	The creation of an image of a dense object in the body with the use of radiant energy.
International Normalized Ratio (INR)	A standardizing measurement of prothrombin time (PT) to monitor the effectiveness of blood-thinning drugs.
ketones	Substances that are made when the body breaks down fat for energy.
laboratory test	A medical procedure in which a sample of blood, urine, or other substances in the body is analyzed for certain features.
leukocyte esterase	An enzyme found in certain white blood cells.
liver function tests	A panel of tests that assesses the health of liver cells.
lymphocyte (lymph)	A type of white blood cell that produces antibodies and other immune system activities.

Term	*Meaning*
macroscopic exam	In a urinalysis, the observation of abnormalities in the urine using the naked eye.
magnetic resonance angiography (MRA)	An imaging tool that uses a large magnet, a computer, and radio waves to analyze blood vessels in the body.
magnetic resonance imaging (MRI)	An imaging tool that uses a large magnet, a computer, and radio waves to look inside the body and to evaluate various body parts.
mean corpuscular hemoglobin	Shows the amount of hemoglobin inside red blood cells.
mean corpuscular hemoglobin concentration	The calculation of concentration of hemoglobin inside red blood cells.
mean corpuscular volume	A measurement of the actual size of red blood cells.
microscopic exam	In a urinalysis, the process of observing the urine under a microscope for chemical and cellular properties not able to be observed with the naked eye.
monocytes (monos)	A type of white blood cell that fights infection.
myoglobin	The oxygen-carrying and storage protein of muscle.
nitrites	Chemicals created from bacteria that cause a urinary tract infection.
partial thromboplastin time (PTT)	A test that shows the function of all clotting factors in blood and determines if blood-thinning drug agents are effective.
pathologist	A medical doctor with additional training in the study of pathology.
pathology	The study of structural and functional changes in cells that cause disease or harmful abnormalities.
pathology report	The report of the description of cells and tissues made by a pathologist based on microscopic examination, as well as a diagnostic finding based on that examination.
Petri dish	A flat dish with a cover made of plastic or glass that is used primarily to grow bacteria.
platelet count	The number of platelet cells that clot in order to prevent bleeding.
platelets	One of the main components of blood that forms clots in order to close injuries and prevent hemorrhage.
positron emission tomography (PET) scan	A diagnostic examination that shows the functional activity of an organ or tissue rather than its structure.
positrons	Tiny particles emitted from a radioactive substance injected into the patient's body during a PET scan.
potential of Hydrogen (pH)	A measure of the acidity or alkalinity of a solution.
proteinuria	Protein in the urine.
prothrombin time (PT)	A measure of the time it takes for a patient's blood to clot.
radiograph	A picture of internal body structures created by an x-ray.
radiologist	A physician who has taken additional training in the interpretation of medical images to specialize in radiology.
radiology	The study of images of the human body.
radiolucent	The term given to structures that appear light or white on an x-ray image.
radionuclides	Tiny particles emitted from a radioactive substance injected into the patient's body during a PET scan.
radiopaque	The term given to structures that appear black or dark on an x-ray image.
red (blood cell) distribution width	A calculation of the variation in the size of the red blood cells.
red blood cell indices	A group of three measurements that describe the size, hemoglobin concentration, and hemoglobin weight in the red cell population.

Term	*Meaning*
red blood count	The actual number of red blood cells per volume of blood.
reference range	A range of laboratory results expected in 95% of a given population.
reticulocytes	Immature red blood cells that are made by the bone marrow and then released into the bloodstream.
sediments	Solid materials that are separated from liquid.
segmented neutrophils (segs)	A type of white blood cell that fights infection.
sonogram	The image produced during an ultrasound.
specific gravity	The measurement of how dilute urine is.
thyroid function tests (TFTs)	A collective term for blood tests used to evaluate the function of the thyroid.
thyroxine (T4)	The major thyroid hormone secreted by the thyroid gland.
tissue chemistry	In a pathologic examination, the chemical properties of a specimen.
tracer	A substance injected into the patient's bloodstream or inhaled by the patient in the form of a radioactive gas that emits radioactive energy and/or particles that allows for detection and management by imaging scanners.
transducer	A wand that, when moved over the body, transmits sound waves to create pictures during ultrasound testing.
transferrin	A protein that transports iron in the blood from the intestines to the cells that use it.
triiodothyronine (T3)	A thyroid hormone that, along with T4, works to regulate the body's metabolism.
turbid	Cloudy (in appearance).
ultrasonography	A method of using sound waves to generate pictures of the body.
urea	A waste product that is made in the intestines and liver when protein breaks down, which is then eliminated from the body in urine.
urinalysis	An examination of a urine sample.
urine	A waste product made by the kidneys.
urine culture	A test to detect and identify organisms that may be causing a urinary tract infection.
urobilinogen	A substance formed in the intestine from the breakdown of bilirubin.
white blood count	The actual number of white blood cells per volume of blood.
x-ray, syn. roentgenogram	An imaging study that uses electromagnetic waves to obtain pictures of body bones and structures.

Add Your Own Terms and Definitions Here:

_____

_____

_____

_____

_____

_____

REVIEW QUESTIONS

1. How is histopathology different from gross pathology?
2. When was the Gram stain developed and by whom?
3. What is a reference range?
4. Why is contrast used in some imaging studies?
5. What is the difference between an x-ray and a CT scan?
6. What is Doppler ultrasound?
7. What is the white blood differential?
8. What is a BMP?
9. What is the medium used to obtain images in ultrasonography?
10. What is a urine culture?

CHAPTER ACTIVITIES

Soundalike Word Choice

Circle the correct word in the following sentences.

1. The patient's (CBC/CDC) reflected a very high white blood cell count.

2. (Ferritin/ferrign) measures the amount of stored iron in the body.

3. Mr. Smith will be discharged if his urine (cumulus/culture) remains negative.

4. Her brain (MRO/MRI) showed a soft tissue brain abnormality.

5. She underwent a (CT/CD) scan, which showed progression of her disease.

6. The (PAP/PA) and lateral views of her right knee reveal a widened lateral joint space.

7. (Cytology/cytometology) is the study of cells.

8. The high concentration of (PLTs/PFTs) indicated that blood clots may occur.

9. The white blood cell differential included 62% (sigs/segs).

10. A complete metabolic panel also includes a (BMP/BNP).

Multiple Choice

Circle the letter corresponding to the best answer to the following questions.

1. The test that assesses cells in blood for such disorders as anemia, infection, and many other diseases is called a(n)
   A. BNP.
   B. CBC.
   C. CMP.
   D. UA.

2. What is *not* found in a microscopic analysis of sediments removed from urine?
   A. casts
   B. crystals
   C. red blood cells
   D. bilirubin

3. An MRI uses _____ to obtain images.
   A. sound waves
   B. radionuclides
   C. a large magnet
   D. x-rays

4. The measurement of the actual size of red blood cells in a CBC is called the
   A. mean corpuscular hematocrit.
   B. mean corpuscular hemoglobin.
   C. mean corpuscular volume.
   D. mean corpuscular concentration.

5. The term *segmented neutrophils* is often dictated as
   A. s. neutrophils.
   B. segs.
   C. seg. neut.
   D. s. neu's.

6. What is *not* included in a pathologist's report?
   A. the diagnosis
   B. the white blood cell differential
   C. the gross description
   D. the patient's name

7. The PET scan uses _____ to create images.
   A. a large magnet
   B. x-rays
   C. transducers
   D. positrons

8. A(n) _____ measures different components of urine.
   A. UN
   B. TIA
   C. UA
   D. UBC

9. _____ clot to prevent bleeding.
   A. Phagocytes
   B. Platelets
   C. White blood cells
   D. Neutrophils

10. The image produced in an ultrasound examination is called a(n)
    A. sonogram.
    B. Doppler.
    C. angiogram.
    D. roentgenogram.

Proofreading Exercise 1

Study the following imaging report below and circle the formatting, punctuation, and spelling errors you find. Look up words of which you are unsure. Then retype the corrected report using the same format on a blank document screen. When finished, print one copy and save the corrected report as **CHAPTER-6-IMAGE1.**

DATE OF EVALUATION:	April 7, 20xx
ORDERING PHYSICIAN:	Tong Lu, MD
TYPE OF TEST:	CD scan of abdomen: and pelvis.
INDICATIONS:	Possible renal colic?

FINDNGS

The visalized lung basses are clear. The heart size is—witin normal limits. The postoperative chnges are present in the stomach. There is no obvious masses in the abdomen or pelvis.

mild rite hydronephrosis and right hydroureter are noted from a 1 mm calcalous in the right ureterovesical junction. Non-obstructing renal calcula are present in the left kidney, 1 2-mm in size. Mild amount of left perinephric fluid is noted? There is none evidence for a leftsided hydronephrosis.

The visualized gi tract shows gastric bypas surgery. There is no focle or generalized bowl wall thickening sines of obstruction - ilios or perforation. Mild athrosclerotic calcifications are noted in the aorta and its branches. Mild degenerative change are present in the spine.

In the pelvis, there is a 1 mmm calculis of the right ureteropelvic junction seen on image number 106. The bladder wall is thickened likely related to its empty state. a amount mild of pelvic fre fluid is present.

Impresion—

Right renal hydronephrosis and hydroureter mild, related to a stone in the right pelviureteric junction.

Mild/left perinephric fluid is noted but without evidence for hydronephrosis. Non-obstructive calculi are present in the left kidney.

The patient is status-post gastric bypass and cholecystectomy.

Proofreading Exercise 2

Study the following report and circle the formatting and spelling errors you find. Look up words of which you are unsure. Then retype the corrected report using the same format on a blank document screen. When finished, print one copy and save the corrected report as **CHAPTER-6-REPORT1.**

REFERRING PHYSICIAN
Dr. Charles Jones department of Otolaryngology; head and Neck Surgery: Dr. Ding-Jen Wang, Department of radiation oncology; Dr. Daniel Snow, Department of Plastic Surgery; and Drs Levy, division of Plastic surgery?

REASON for EVALUATION
Management of a progressing adenoid cystic carcinoma of the head and neck.

HISTORY OF PRESENT ILLNESS
Ms. Spencer is a 65 year old woman who developed rite facial numness and pain a year ago. This did not respond to standard care and as such 6 months later she presented with dipopia. An mri reviewed apparently showed a mass and she was subsequently referred to the eye clinic. examination at that time revealed a right extra-ocular movement deficit in all directions with a slight right proptysis and a sensory defect in vee one, v2, and V3 of cranial nerve V.

The patient has been followed cereally by Drs. D.j. Lee and Jones. A most recent note by Dr. Lee suggested that the patient had procession of disease. She was seen by Dr. Jones more recently and underwent a CT scan which demonstrated markedly progression of disease including her mass filling the entire right orbit with marked proptosis. the mass was infiltrating the extraocular muscles and optic nerve. The patient was then referred to medical oncology for evaluation regarding paliative treatment.

review of systems; The patient reports that her mane issue is pain in the right obit and face extending down the bilateral neck. She is eating and swallowing without odontophagia and dysphagia but estimates that she has lost about twenty seven pounds in the recent past/ She previously had lower extremity edema and was on lasix and aldactone but these medicals are stopped and her edema is only slightly reocurred. She has no chest pain, no abdominal camping no numbness or tingling of the fingers or toes. She reports sleeping poorly at night.

PHYSICAL EXAMINATION
She is a somewat elderly- appearing woman accompanied by 2 of her daughters. She is complaining of pain behind the right eye going down the right side of the face. Her temperature is 979 with a pulse of 84, weight 135, and blood pressure 185-77. She has conjunctivae edema with unability to open the right eye. The left eye opens with normal extraocular movements and pupillary response. She is stable on her foot but somewhat slow and deliberate. The lungs were unremarkable. The cardiac exam was benine. The abdomen had no tenderness or masses. Her lower extremities has 1 plus edema at the ankle and she had some tenderness of the left ankle to palpitation. She had 1 plus distal pulses.

IMPRESSION
This is a 65-year-old man with locally advanced unresectable adenoid cystic carcinoma of the right maxillary sinus and orbit who presents for discussions regarding palliative therapy.

therapies for salivary type tumors could include doxorubicin and cisplatin, taxol, xeloda, and an Adriamycin/based regiment. I will discuss her case with my colleagues here.

I have arranged for the patient to go upstairs to the treatment area and receive IV morphine every fifteen minutes until pain is controlled at that point, I will convert her to longacting oral narcotics. The constipation will only worsen as we increase her narcotic dose. As such, we will start her on lactulose therapy.

TRANSCRIPTION PRACTICE

Open your word-processing software. Insert the student CD-ROM and locate the dictation for this chapter. For each of the words in the "listen for these terms" list for each report, use a medical dictionary or other resources to identify and write down a brief definition of the term on a separate sheet of paper to attach with your work. Then listen to the dictation and transcribe each report. Use the current date for each report. Insert a heading into the document if the text falls to a second page.

At the end of each report, indicate the name of the dictating physician under the signature line and insert reference initials. For date dictated and transcribed and date of admission, use the current date. Proofread your work, print one copy for your instructor along with your term definitions, and save the completed report to your student disk.

Use the imaging template for all of the dictation exercises in this chapter, which is located on the student CD under the file name *IMAGE-tem.*

Report #T8.1: Ultrasonography
Patient Name: Oleta Preston
Medical Record No.: 11808003
Attending/Ordering Physician: Gloria Davis, MD
Radiologist: Sabrina Scott, MD

Listen for these terms:
sonography
transverse
longitudinal
endometrial stripe
cul-de-sac

Report #T8.2: Chest X-ray
Patient Name: Luis Hernandez
Medical Record No.: 976-54441
Attending/Ordering Physician: Stuart Greenberg, MD
Radiologist: Andrea Biggs, MD

Listen for these terms:
interstitial markings
cardiac silhouette
costophrenic angle
hilar

Report #T8.3: CT scan
Patient Name: Dale Wix
Medical Record No.: 00077385
Attending/Ordering Physician: Mark Tokar, MD
Radiologist: Samuel Voorhees, MD

Listen for these terms:
pubic symphysis
hydronephrosis
hydroureter
ureterovesical junction
perinephric fluid
atherosclerotic
pelviureteric
cholecystectomy

9

DERMATOLOGY

OBJECTIVES

After completing this chapter, you will be able to:

- Describe the components of the integumentary system.
- Describe common conditions, diseases, and disorders that affect skin and the treatment options for each.
- Differentiate between types of skin cancer and the appropriate diagnostic procedures and treatments for each.
- Describe various diagnostic studies and procedures that evaluate skin conditions and explain how they differ from one another.

INTRODUCTION

The **skin** is the soft outer covering of the body and the site of the sense of touch. It is the largest organ in the body, weighing about six pounds and covering approximately 3,000 square inches on an average adult. The average square inch of skin contains 650 sweat glands, 20 blood vessels, 60,000 melanocytes, and more than a thousand nerve endings. The skin performs many functions to protect the body: It regulates body temperature; maintains water and electrolyte balance; and is the focal point of the body's sense of touch, pressure, temperature, and pain. Skin is an essential part of the body's defense against infection by invading organisms such as viruses, bacteria, fungi, and parasites; it also shields the body from the sun's harmful effects and protects the body's deeper tissues from injury. This chapter will explore the basic anatomy of the skin, common skin disorders, the procedures used to treat these disorders, and the tests used to diagnose them.

ANATOMY OF THE INTEGUMENTARY SYSTEM

When physicians dictate, they may refer to the skin collectively as **integument**. Medically speaking, the **integumentary system** consists of the skin; its accessory structures, such as hair and sweat glands; and the underlying tissue. **Cutaneous** describes something relating to the skin.

The skin covers the entire surface of the body and is composed of several different layers of tissue. Nerves, glands, hair follicles, and blood vessels are situated in these layers of tissue beneath the surface of the skin. Figure 9.1 shows a cross-section of the skin and its corresponding layers of tissue: epidermis, dermis, and subcutaneous.

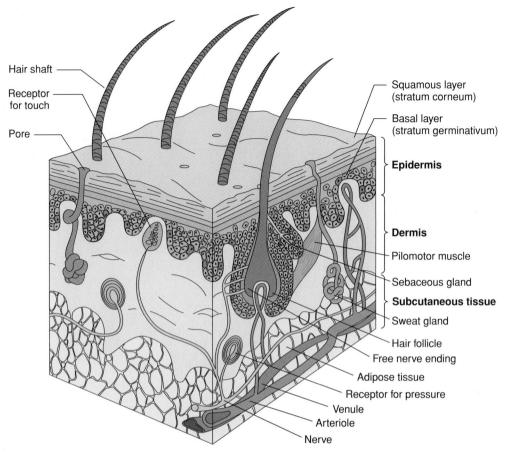

Hair shaft

Receptor for touch

Pore

Squamous layer (stratum corneum)

Basal layer (stratum germinativum)

Epidermis

Dermis

Pilomotor muscle

Sebaceous gland

Subcutaneous tissue

Sweat gland

Hair follicle

Free nerve ending

Adipose tissue

Receptor for pressure

Venule

Arteriole

Nerve

FIGURE 9.1. **A Cross-Section of the Skin.** Reprinted with permission from Willis MC. *Medical Terminology: The Language of Health Care,* 2nd ed. Baltimore, MD: Lippincott Williams & Wilkins, 2006.

Epidermis

The **epidermis** is the outermost, or superficial, layer of skin that is made up of stratified, or layered, tissue. It is the thinnest layer, and it is the first barrier of protection against most bacteria, viruses, and other foreign substances that may try to enter the body.

Keratinocytes are the principal cells of the epidermis. These cells are produced by constant mitosis in the deeper regions. **Mitosis** is the basic process of cell division in which two identical cells are reproduced from the parent cell. Thus, the cells are constantly dividing and producing new cells. With time the cells move up to the surface of the epidermis, die, and are worn away, to be replaced by the next wave of newly produced cells. This process of the continual replacement of cells from the deeper layers below is called **desquamation**. During desquamation, keratinocytes produce a tough, fibrous protein called **keratin** as they are pushed toward the surface of the skin. Keratin, which serves to toughen the skin, is also found in fingernails and hair. The life of a given keratinocyte is about 7 to 10 days from production to sloughing.

The epidermis is made up of five sublayers, each with its own type of cells and function:

- The **stratum germinativum,** or bottom epidermal layer, which is made up of **basal cells** and **melanocytes.** Basal cells are small, rounded cells found in the base of the epidermis. Melanocytes are cells that produce **melanin,** the pigment responsible for skin color. People with dark skin have melanocytes that produce greater amounts of melanin than light-skinned people. The activity of melanocytes is genetically regulated; therefore, skin color is inherited.
- The **stratum spinosum,** or spiny layer, which is made up of flattened cells with spiny projections.
- The **stratum granulosum,** or grainy layer, which is made up of keratinocytes.
- The **stratum lucidum,** or clear layer, which is made up of a clear pink band of tissue. This layer is particularly thick in areas subjected to heavy wear and tear, such as the palms of the hands and soles of the feet.
- The **stratum corneum,** or horny layer, which contains flattened cells called **squamous skin cells.** It is the uppermost layer of the epidermis. Most of the cells in this layer are dead; all that is left is their keratin. The stratum corneum functions as a barrier to prevent water from entering or leaving the body. It also provides the main barrier against skin infection.

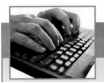

Dermis

The **dermis**, often called "true skin," is the inner layer of skin and is composed of fibrous tissue made from proteins called **collagen** and **fibrillin** that give elasticity, tone, and strength to the skin. This layer contains nerve endings, hair follicles, and blood vessels. The cells in this layer are also involved in defending the body against foreign invaders that pass through the epidermis.

The dermis and epidermis meet at the **papillary layer**. The papillary layer contains capillaries that nourish not only the dermis but also the overlying epidermis. The epidermis has no capillaries and depends on the blood supply provided by the papillary layer in the dermis for oxygen and nutrients. The folds of this layer contain the receptors that regulate the body's sensitivity to touch or pressure. This layer is also responsible for fingerprint patterns and the formation of wrinkles. The elastic fibers in the papillary layer provide skin tone. A young person has many more fibers than an elderly person and, therefore, as a rule, has fewer wrinkles.

Subcutaneous Layer

Below the dermis lies the **subcutaneous layer**, or fat layer. The word **subcutaneous** means *beneath the skin*. This layer serves to fasten the skin to the underlying body surface and is also the storage site of most body fat. This layer helps insulate the body from heat and cold, provides protective padding, and serves as an energy-storage area.

Specialized Structures

The specialized structures of the skin are located in the dermis. These structures consist of hair follicles, nails, glands, and nerve endings.

Hair

Hair is a fine, threadlike structure made up of dead cells composed of keratin, arranged in columns around a central core. These cells also contain varying amounts of melanin, which is responsible for the color of the hair. The hair shaft projects from the surface of the skin, whereas the root is embedded in the subcutaneous tissue. The root ends in an onion-shaped structure called a **bulb**, which is lodged in a pit in the skin called a **follicle**. Each living follicle gives rise to a single hair. Each follicle is surrounded by smooth muscle cells called **arrector pili muscles**. When the arrector pili muscles contract, such as from cold temperatures or fright, they flex and pull the hair into an upright position, causing skin dimples, or *goose bumps*.

The skin of the average adult contains about five million hairs. Hair covers nearly all parts of the body and has a protective function. Hair on the scalp protects the head from physical trauma, heat loss, and sunlight. Eyelashes and eyebrows shield the eyes from sunlight and other particles. Nose hairs keep dust and foreign particles out of the respiratory tract.

Nails

Nails develop from the epidermis and protect the sensitive tips of fingers and toes. Each nail is composed of a free edge at the outer tip of the finger or toe, the nail bed, the lunula, and the root. The **lunula** is the white half-moon shape located on top of the nail at the proximal end of the nail bed, or where the nail actually begins to grow. The root, also located at the proximal end but underneath the nail bed, is where nail growth takes place. Although the nail itself consists of dead keratinized cells, the nail bed beneath the nail is living tissue. The nail bed appears pink because of a rich blood supply to the underlying dermis.

Although most nail maladies are minor and heal easily, some can become lingering problems. For example, bites or tears to the skin at the side or base of a fingernail can cause a tender and swollen bacterial infection called a **paronychia**. A fungal infection in the nail, called **onychomycosis**, is more persistent and is likely to occur on a toe rather than a finger. Characterized by discolored, peeling, brittle nails, onychomycosis may cause the nail to separate from the nail bed and, eventually, may destroy the nail. The treatment for onychomycosis is an oral antifungal medication taken over several months.

Glands

Glands are a group of cells which work together to produce and secrete substances that have a function either at that site or another part of the body. There are two types of glands: **exocrine glands**, which drain their secretions through **ducts**, or tubes, to the surface of the body or other sites; and **endocrine glands**, which release their secretions directly into the bloodstream or tissue spaces for circulation to other parts of the body. The presence of the duct is what distinguishes exocrine glands from endocrine glands. In some types of exocrine glands, the cells release their secretion while retaining their cellular material, while in other types the cell becomes filled with the material to be secreted and is shed along with the secretion.

The exocrine glands of the skin have their secretory ducts in the dermis. The skin contains two types of exocrine glands: **sebaceous glands** and **sweat glands**. Sebaceous glands open into hair follicles and secrete an oily substance called sebum. **Sebum** softens and lubricates the skin to prevent drying and cracking, damage that can provide an entryway into the body for harmful bacteria. Sebum also helps control the growth of microorganisms such as bacteria and fungi on the skin. When a sebaceous gland becomes blocked, it may fill with fatty material, forming a **sebaceous cyst.** This type of cyst can be left alone or can be surgically removed if it becomes unsightly or infected.

Sweat glands secrete a salty, watery fluid called **sweat** in response to heat. Sweat is transported by ducts to the skin surface, where it can be evaporated by excess body heat, helping to control body temperature. Although mostly activated when the body becomes overheated, sweat glands are occasionally activated by emotions, such as fear, giving rise to the term **cold sweat.**

Mammary glands, found only in mammals, are structurally related to the skin in that they are a modified type of sweat gland but functionally related to the reproductive system because they produce breast milk for the nourishment of offspring. Breast milk is produced in the mammary glands after pregnancy and secreted through ducts that converge at the nipple. The sucking of the infant on the nipple stimulates the secretion of hormones, which leads to the release of milk (see Chapter 16, *Obstetrics and Gynecology*, for more information about the mammary glands).

Nerve Endings

The skin contains millions of specialized nerve endings, or **receptors**, all over the body. Receptors are located in the dermis. The sensitivity of an area of skin is determined by the amount of receptors present, which is why some areas of the skin are more sensitive than others. For example, the fingertips contain many more nerve receptors per square inch than the upper arm. When receptors detect changes (such as pain, heat, cold, pressure, and touch), they generate nerve impulses that travel to the brain. The brain interprets the impulses as a particular cutaneous sensation.

COMMON DERMATOLOGIC DISEASES AND TREATMENTS

The overall appearance of the skin can indicate specific skin disorders, but it can also indicate an injury to other body systems. Skin problems typically manifest themselves in the form of rashes and skin infections. A **rash**, also called **rubor**, is an inflammation of the skin

---

QUICK CHECK 9.1 ✓

Circle the letter corresponding to the best answer to the questions below.

1. Hair, nails, and glands are referred to as
   A. skin layers.
   B. dermal components.
   C. skin tissues.
   D. specialized structures.

2. The subcutaneous layer is also called the
   A. fat layer.
   B. dermal layer.
   C. glandular layer.
   D. follicle layer.

3. The gland that secretes a substance called sebum is the
   A. follicle gland.
   B. sebaceous gland.
   C. tissue gland.
   D. subdermal gland.

4. The epidermis is made up of _____ sub-layers.
   A. five
   B. four
   C. three
   D. seven

5. Collagen and fibrillin are found in the
   A. epidermis.
   B. subcutaneous layer.
   C. dermis.
   D. sebaceous glands.

TABLE 9.1 Common Terminology Used in Skin Appearance

Term	Description
atrophic skin	Skin that is paper-thin and wrinkled.
crust (scab)	Dried blood, pus, or skin fluids on the surface of the skin. A crust can form whenever skin is damaged.
erosion	Loss of part or all of the top surface of the skin due to skin damage.
excoriation	A hollowed-out or linear crusted area caused by scratching, rubbing, or picking at the skin.
lichenification	Thickened skin with accentuated skin folds or creases that appear as deep grooves and wrinkles, produced by prolonged scratching.
macule	A flat, discolored spot of any shape less than three-eighths inch in diameter. Freckles, flat moles, port-wine stains, or rashes are referred to in dictation as *macular*.
nodule	A solid bump, deeper and easier to feel than a papule, which may be raised. A large nodule is called a **tumor**. A tumor that is filled with fatty tissue is called a lipoma.
papule	A solid bump less than three-eighths inch in diameter. Warts, insect bites, and skin tags are examples of papules and are described as *papular* in dictation.
plaque	A flat, raised bump or group of bumps typically more than three-eighths inch in diameter.
pustule	A blister containing pus.
scales	Areas of heaped-up, dead epidermal cells, producing a flaky, dry patch. Examples include psoriasis, eczema, and other skin disorders.
scar	An area where normal skin has been replaced by fibrous (scar-forming) tissue.
telangiectasia	Dilated blood vessels within the skin that have a twisted appearance and that whiten with pressure.
ulcer	Like an erosion but deeper, penetrating at least part of the dermis.
vesicle	A small, fluid-filled spot less than one-eighth inch in diameter. Insect bites, chickenpox, burns, and irritations form vesicles and blisters. Physicians dictate descriptions of this type of spot as *vesicular*.
wheal (hive)	Swelling in the skin that produces an elevated, soft spongy area that appears suddenly and then disappears. Wheals often appear in allergic reactions and may be described as *wheal and flare* in dictation.

Adapted from The Merck Manual of Medical Information—Second Home Edition, *edited by Mark H. Beers. Copyright 2003 by Merck & Co., Inc., Whitehouse Station, N.J.*

that affects its appearance or texture. A rash may be localized to one specific area on the skin or it may affect the entire body. Rashes develop either because of an infection or because of a reaction by the body's nervous system. Symptoms of a rash include **erythema** (redness), **pruritus** (itching), **edema** (swelling), **urticaria** (hives), scaling, cracking, or blistering. Physicians use terminology such as that listed in Table 9.1 above to describe the characteristics and appearance of a rash or inflammation for inclusion in the medical record.

Dermatitis

Dermatitis is an inflammation of the upper layers of the skin that results in a rash. The causes of dermatitis vary widely and can include stress, weather extremes, allergens, and even some medical conditions. Although it is not contagious and is usually not life-threatening, dermatitis tends to recur and can become a chronic problem.

Seborrheic Dermatitis

Seborrheic dermatitis is an inflammation that causes scaly, flaky, itchy patches over the sebum-rich areas of skin of the scalp, face, and occasionally the trunk of the body. Dandruff and cradle cap are both forms of seborrheic dermatitis. Although the definitive cause is unknown, seborrheic dermatitis is thought to be

TRANSCRIPTION TIP:

Drug reactions and viral skin lesions may be described as **maculopapular**, consisting of both macules and papules. Do not transcribe this description as *macular papular or macular popular.*

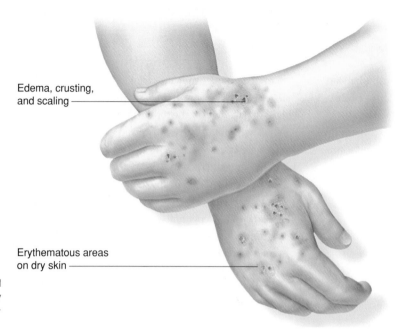

Edema, crusting,
and scaling

Erythematous areas
on dry skin

FIGURE 9.2. **Eczema.** This disorder is characterized by itching, scaling, thickening of the skin, and is usually located on the face, elbows, knees, and arms. Asset provided by Anatomical Chart Co.

caused by a fungal infection that, while thriving without incident in normally functioning individuals, can become inflamed in individuals with decreased immunity (a form of seborrheic dermatitis occurs in as many as 85% of people with acquired immunodeficiency syndrome, AIDS). In those cases, the body's epidermis responds unfavorably to the infection, becoming inflamed and shedding large scales of skin in a failed attempt to rid itself of the fungus.

The condition is usually chronic. Dandruff can be controlled by frequent shampooing with preparations containing selenium sulfide or an antifungal drug. Cradle cap is usually treated with ketoconazole, a broad-spectrum antifungal cream. Sometimes steroid creams are applied to the affected skin. In each case, treatment must be continued for several weeks.

Atopic Dermatitis (Eczema)

Atopic dermatitis, also known as **eczema**, is one of the most common skin diseases described as a chronic rash and dry, thickened skin. The cause of atopic dermatitis is unknown, but those who have it typically have other allergic disorders, even though atopic dermatitis is not an allergy to a particular substance. The disorder is characterized by itching, scaling, thickening of the skin, and is usually located on the face, elbows, knees, and arms. The itching associated with eczema leads to uncontrollable scratching, which can leave the skin vulnerable to infection by bacteria. Atopic dermatitis is identified by the physician according to the characteristics and pattern of the rash and often by whether the patient or other family members have allergies, as eczema appears to be a hereditary skin dis-

order. Figure 9.2 illustrates the typical appearance and symptoms of eczema.

There is no cure for atopic dermatitis, but itching can be controlled with oral drugs, such as antihistamines or antibiotics. Topical steroid creams help decrease the inflammation in the skin, thus decreasing the itching and swelling. **Phototherapy** (exposure to ultraviolet, or UV, light) is used to treat certain skin disorders like eczema. UV light alters the chemicals in skin cells and can kill certain cells that can be involved in skin disease. It is sometimes combined with the use of **psoralen**, which is a drug taken orally before treatment with UV light to lessen the side effects of UV therapy. The combination of psoralen and UV light is known as **PUVA therapy.** PUVA is an acronym for oral administration of *p*soralen and subsequent exposure to long-wavelength ultraviolet light (*uv-a*).

A class of drugs called **topical immunomodulators (TIMs)** has been developed for use in severe cases of eczema. TIMs inhibit inflammatory skin reactions, while producing fewer side effects than topical steroids. Two of these drugs, tacrolimus ointment (Protopic), and pimecrolimus topical cream (Elidel), have been found to be helpful in relieving the symptoms of atopic dermatitis.

Rosacea

Rosacea is a chronic inflammatory skin condition that causes redness, pimples, and, in advanced stages, thickened skin on the face and around the eyes. The disease is characterized by frequent flushing of the center of the face and tends to flare in cyclic phases. Some researchers believe that rosacea is a disorder where blood vessels dilate too easily, producing the signature facial flushing and redness. The cause of rosacea is unknown, but it is believed that the condition is often hereditary.

Although there is no cure for rosacea, physicians can treat and control the disease by improving the health and appearance of the patient's skin. Topical antibiotics such as metronidazole and clindamycin, are often applied directly to the affected skin. In more severe cases, physicians may prescribe oral antibiotics, which tend to provide relief more quickly. Some of the most common oral antibiotics used to treat rosacea include tetracycline, minocycline, doxycycline, and erythromycin. Finally, electrosurgery and laser surgery reduce the visibility of blood vessels in the face and improve facial appearance.

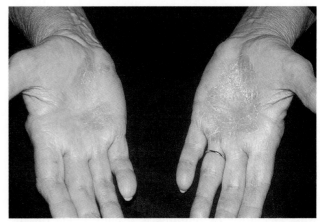

FIGURE 9.3. Psoriasis. This disorder appears as red, raised patches that have silvery scales called plaques. Reprinted with permission from Goodheart HP, MD. *Goodheart's Photoguide of Common Skin Disorders*, 2nd Edition. Philadelphia: Lippincott Williams & Wilkins, 2003.

Psoriasis

Psoriasis is a chronic, recurring disease characterized by red, raised patches that have silvery scales called **plaques**, as illustrated in Figure 9.3. The patches appear on the skin of the scalp, elbows, knees, back, or buttocks. These patches occur because of an abnormally high rate of growth of skin cells. The reason for the rapid cell growth is not known but is believed to be associated with an immune-system problem.

There is no cure for psoriasis but many patients go for long periods without flares, and there are a number of drugs and treatments that can relieve and control the disease. The primary goal of treatment is to suppress the growth of skin cells. Calcipotriene (Dovonex) is a prescription ointment that controls the overproduction of skin cells for mild to moderate psoriasis. As with treatment for eczema, phototherapy, or PUVA therapy, is extremely effective for moderate to severe plaque psoriasis. Finally, exposure to natural sunlight has been helpful in clearing up the skin.

Skin Infections

Skin is the primary barrier between the internal structures of the body and the outside world and functions to keep bacteria, viruses, fungi, and parasites away from body fluids, where they would otherwise multiply and attack the body. However, viruses, fungi, and other parasites can break down the skin as well; when this occurs, a skin infection develops. There are many types of skin infections that require diagnosis and treatment by a physician, three of the most common being bacterial infections, fungal infections, and viral infections.

Bacterial Infections

The skin is the body's first barrier against bacteria that cause infections. Humans are natural hosts for many bacterial species that live on skin and colonize it as normal flora. However, when a break in the skin occurs, bacteria can enter the body, grow, and reproduce,

---

QUICK CHECK 9.2 ✓

Indicate whether the following sentences are true (T) or false (F).

1. A hollowed-out or linear-crusted area caused by scratching, rubbing, or picking at the skin is called a telangiectasia.   T   F

2. Phototherapy uses UV light to kill certain cells that can cause skin disease.   T   F

3. Atrophic skin is typically paper thin and wrinkled.   T   F

4. Another word for itching is erythema.   T   F

5. Rosacea is a contagious condition.   T   F

causing a wide variety of skin infections. Some are limited to one small location; others can cover a large area.

Cellulitis

Cellulitis is an acute bacterial infection of the skin and underlying tissues. It can be caused by many different bacteria, but the most common are those in the *Streptococcus* species. This form of bacteria invades the skin to the deep dermis and spreads quickly, resulting in skin redness, swelling, and tenderness. As the skin is tense, it resembles the peel of an orange; physicians refer to **peau d'orange** when describing this characteristic. Diagnosis of cellulitis is usually made on the basis of the appearance of the skin, but blood cultures and skin biopsies may be ordered to confirm the diagnosis and determine the type of bacteria that is causing the infection.

Failure to treat cellulitis can result in multiple and sometimes life-threatening complications in other parts of the body. Strep cells released into the bloodstream can result in cardiac impairment as they infect the tissue in the heart muscle, a condition known as **bacterial endocarditis**. Infections of the lymph nodes may need to be drained. Most seriously **gangrene,** or tissue death, and flesh-eating bacteria can develop, necessitating amputation of the affected limb. As with other streptococcal infections, antibiotic treatment (such as penicillin) and cool, wet dressings on the infection site are used to control the spread of the infection. Treatment may require hospitalization if the infection is sufficiently severe to warrant intravenous antibiotics and close observation.

Impetigo

Impetigo is a contagious skin infection that leads to the formation of gradually expanding itchy, crusted, fluid-filled **bullae**, or scabs on the body. Impetigo commonly affects children and is spread by the fluid that oozes from the blisters. A child is more likely to develop impetigo if the skin has already been irritated or injured by other skin problems such as insect bites, poison ivy, or a skin allergy. Impetigo is caused primarily by staphylococci, which are spherical, parasitic bacteria that usually occur in grapelike clusters. It can also be caused by streptococci, which are oval-shaped bacteria that occur in pairs or chains. Impetigo results in groups of thin-roofed, pus-filled bullae that appear a few days after contact with the bacteria. The blisters are small at first but then slowly get bigger.

Impetigo is diagnosed by the appearance of the skin. A swab from a crusted area of skin may be sent to the laboratory to determine which germ is causing the outbreak and which antibiotic is most likely to be effective. With small areas of skin, treatment can include antibiotic ointment such as mupirocin (Bactroban)

applied directly to the rash. With larger areas of infection, a physician may prescribe an oral antibiotic such as dicloxacillin, erythromycin, or cephalexin to be taken to clear the lesions.

Folliculitis

Folliculitis is a bacterial infection of the hair follicles of the skin that develops when bacteria, the most common being *Staphylococcus aureus*, invade the skin. It results from a disruption of the function of the sebaceous glands that coat each hair shaft with sebum and is often caused by shaving or by wearing tight clothing. The infection appears as small, white-headed pustules that may dry out and crust over. Hair can grow through or alongside the pustules, which sometimes ooze and become uncomfortable. Left untreated, folliculitis can cause a **boil**, a warm, painful, pus-filled pocket of infection below the skin's surface; or **carbuncles**, clusters of abscesses that are connected to each other under the skin. The bacteria from a boil or carbuncle can then enter the bloodstream and travel to other parts of the body, affecting lymph nodes and other organ systems.

Nonprescription topical antibiotic creams such as bacitracin or neomycin applied to the affected area can clear up a small number of folliculitis pustules. More serious cases, or those in which the infection has spread to other body systems, require a course of oral antibiotics such as erythromycin, cephalexin, or dicloxacillin, all of which kill staphylococci.

Fungal Skin Infections

Fungal infections of the skin are a common occurrence. They are caused by microscopic organisms called **dermatophytes** that live on keratin, the protein that makes up skin, hair, and nails. Under appropriate conditions of warmth, moisture, or irritation to the skin, dermatophytes start to grow invasively, causing a skin infection. Some fungal infections simply multiply on the top layer of skin and cause irritation; others penetrate the deeper layers and cause itching, swelling, blistering, and scaling.

A fungal infection of the skin is also known as a **mycosis**. A person who studies, identifies, and classifies fungi according to their microscopic appearance and in culture is called a **mycologist**. Although most fungal skin infections are not serious, some can cause other health problems and require clinical care by a physician. The following are common types of fungal infections.

Tinea (Ringworm)

Tinea, also known as ringworm (because of the circular appearance of the fungal rash, not because it is caused by an actual worm), is a fungal infection of the skin. It manifests in a characteristic red, ring-shaped rash that spreads outward as it grows and is prevalent in warm, moist areas of the body, such as between the toes and in the groin area. The common types of a tinea infection include:

- **Tinea capitis**, involving the scalp or neck.
- **Tinea barbae**, involving the beard area.
- **Tinea corporis**, involving the arms, shoulders, and face.
- **Tinea cruris**, involving the groin (also called jock itch).
- **Tinea pedis**, involving the feet (also called athlete's foot).

The ring-like appearance of tinea lesions are unique and usually allow for a diagnosis simply based on the physical examination of the infected skin. In addition, a physician may order a culture or examination of a sample of the skin to confirm the diagnosis. Treatment for ringworm includes the use of a special shampoo to eliminate the fungus on the scalp. A physician may also add an oral antifungal medication or steroids to help destroy the fungus and reduce swelling of the skin. Because fungi can live indefinitely on the skin, treatment may be prolonged or repeated.

Candidiasis

Candidiasis, commonly called a fungal infection, yeast infection, or thrush, is an infection caused by the *Candida* species of fungi. *Candida* are thin-walled, small yeasts that reproduce by budding. Even though there are more that 150 species of *Candida*, no more than 10 cause disease in humans with any frequency. *Candida albicans* (transcribed as *C. albicans*) is probably the most common. Other species of *Candida* responsible for human disease include *C. tropicalis, C. glabrata, C. krusei,* and *C. lusitaniae.*

Yeast organisms are common in low concentrations on the skin and inside the digestive, respiratory, and reproductive organs. *Candida* are a member of normal flora found in the skin, mouth, vagina, and stool. They are usually prevented from uncontrolled growth by the body's immune system. However, when an imbalance occurs between these organisms and healthy flora in the body, either from a damaged or weakened immune system or some medication regimens, *Candida* increase in number and can invade the body's skin and mucosa, causing symptoms.

Cutaneous candidiasis is the term that describes infection of the skin with *Candida* and is the most common form of candidiasis. The infection involves the very outermost layers of the skin and, although not life-threatening, can be very irritating to the patient. Diaper rash and **intertrigo** (a rash erupting in the folds of the skin) are common manifestations of a cutaneous candidiasis.

Candidiasis can be treated with antifungal drugs, such as nystatin or clotrimazole creams, that are applied directed to the affected area. In addition, a physician may prescribe an antifungal drug, such as fluconazole, to be taken orally.

Viral Skin Infections

Viral infections are caused by a virus entering the skin and causing a variety of skin conditions that require treatment by a physician.

Warts

Warts, also called **verrucae**, are small, noncancerous skin growths caused by the *Papillomavirus.* Warts occur in the outer layers of the skin and are found most often on the hands, feet, and face. They can be mildly contagious and can spread to other parts of the body as well as to other people.

Plantar warts occur on the soles of the feet, where they become hard and flat from the pressure of walking. **Filiform warts** are narrow, small growths that appear on the eyelids, face, neck, or lips. Genital warts, also called **condyloma acuminata**, appear on or around the genitals. They are irregular, bumpy growths with the texture of a small cauliflower. Warts on the hands, arms, and legs are called common warts, or **verrucae vulgaris**, and typically have a rough surface.

Warts are usually harmless and often go away untreated after an extended period. Over-the-counter corrosive agents, applied daily over a period of several weeks, can treat unsightly warts. Warts can also be surgically removed with **cryotherapy** (freezing using liquid nitrogen), **electrocautery** (burning with an electrical current), or laser surgery.

Shingles (Herpes Zoster)

Shingles, or **herpes zoster**, is a viral infection of the nerves caused by a reactivation of the varicella-zoster virus that causes chickenpox. The rash appears as a group of small, painful blisters and can occur anywhere on the body. Chickenpox is the initial manifestation of the virus, and shingles is the re-emergence of the virus after it has lain dormant in the body's spinal or cranial nerves for several years. The virus may never reactivate; but if it does, it typically travels along nerve fibers, causing pain. When the virus reaches the skin, it erupts, creating a painful rash of small, red spots that turn into fluid-filled blisters resembling chickenpox.

During the acute phase of the illness when the rash is highly inflamed and tender, topical creams such as calamine lotion or sulfadiazine (Silvadene) can be used to relieve pain and discomfort. Meanwhile, physicians may prescribe oral antivirals to attack the virus in the body. Acyclovir (Zovirax) is used to reduce inflammation

TRANSCRIPTION TIP:

Physicians typically dictate a patient's physical examination to document physical findings. Although they often begin that section of the report by saying, "On physical exam …," do not type that directive as a heading ("ON PHYSICAL EXAM:") Instead, use standard heading text ("PHYSICAL EXAMINATION:") and proceed to transcribe the dictated findings; or you may type, "PHYSICAL EXAMINATION: On physical exam …"

and pain during an acute attack and can also reduce the likelihood of lingering pain after an attack, especially in older patients. Famciclovir (Famvir) is also helpful in reducing pain and hastening recovery from an attack. It is believed this drug works by preventing the virus from multiplying and damaging affected nerves. Finally valacyclovir (Valtrex) is another option in treating an acute attack of shingles.

Even after the shingles rash has abated, some people may continue to experience chronic pain in the area of the outbreak. This pain, called **postherpetic neuralgia** (PNH), may be present for weeks or months thereafter.

Skin Damage from Heat and Cold

The skin works to keep the body at a constant temperature—about 98.6°F—to ensure that its systems can function efficiently. Skin that has reddened from overexposure to sun or rosy cheeks caused by cold weather may be more serious than they appear to be. The skin is highly sensitive to heat and cold, which can cause damage to skin cells or even, in the extreme, vital organ systems.

Burns

A **burn** is an injury caused by heat, electricity, chemicals, or radiation, which damages and destroys layers of skin. Depending on the severity and extent of the burn, victims may require long-term medical care, rehabilitation, multiple surgeries, and psychological treatment.

Skin burns are classified according to the depth of the burn and extent of damage to the skin tissues:

- First degree: Also called **superficial burns**, first degree burns usually affect the epidermis and tend to be moist, red, and sensitive to touch. Usually there are no blisters, and these burns often heal quickly. Sunburns are a type of first degree burn.
- Second degree: Sometimes referred to as **partial-thickness burns**, second degree burns affect both the epidermal and dermal layers of skin, causing redness, pain, swelling, and blisters. These burns heal but leave a change in skin pigmentation.
- Third degree: Also called **full-thickness burns**, third degree burns destroy all the epidermal and dermal skin layers. The tissue damage extends below the hair follicles and sweat glands to the deep subcutaneous tissue. The skin becomes charred and leathery and often appears depressed compared to surrounding tissue.
- Fourth degree: Fourth degree burns are deep enough to involve muscle, bone, tendons and/or ligaments and are life-threatening.

Second, third, and fourth degree burns are serious because the destruction of skin over a large area inhibits the body's ability to control the rate at which water is lost to the outside environment or to regulate the temperature of the body to control infection. Someone who has lost over half the skin to second, third, or fourth degree burns is unlikely to survive.

Proper burn treatment involves appropriate and consistent wound management to minimize damage

QUICK CHECK 9.3 ✓

Match the definitions on the left with the terms on the right.

1. _____ Microscopic organisms that live on keratin.   A. cellulitis

2. _____ A rash erupting in the folds of the skin.   B. dermatophytes

3. _____ An acute bacterial infection of the skin and underlying tissues.   C. verrucae

4. _____ Another name for shingles.   D. herpes zoster

5. _____ Small, noncancerous skin growths caused by the Papillomavirus.   E. intertrigo

and complications and to promote healing and recovery. Some burns can be treated on an outpatient basis, whereas others may require advanced treatment at special burn centers. For minor skin burns, a topical antibiotic cream, such as silver sulfadiazine, and sterile bandages may be sufficient treatment. Deep or severe burns require additional treatments to promote healing and prevent infection. **Debridement** is a process by which dead tissue and debris are removed from the wound to expose and cleanse the area. The wound is then dressed and checked regularly to monitor the healing process. **Dressing** refers to the materials used to cover and protect a wound from the environment. Dressings can include the antimicrobial ointment applied to the wound along with cotton gauze or a synthetic bandage to cover the wound. **Dressing changes** refer to the process of removing old bandages and protective materials from the wound and replacing them with new, clean ones.

A **skin graft** is a layer of healthy skin taken from another area on the body and transferred to an area with a skin defect, such as burned tissues. A skin graft is constructed from the patient's own skin (called an **autograft**) or from the skin of a cadaver (called an **allograft**). In an autograft procedure, skin is taken from the patient's back or thigh, secured to the wound with staples or stitches, and then covered with a tight dressing. The graft heals by taking up a blood supply from the base of the wound, thereby allowing the grafted skin to survive. A **split-thickness skin graft** is a graft that includes the epidermal layer and part of the dermal skin layers. A **full-thickness skin graft** consists of both the epidermal and complete dermal skin layers. Skin flaps are used when the area requiring reconstruction lacks the blood supply needed to support a skin graft. A skin flap contains skin along with the underlying fat, blood vessels, and sometimes muscle, which is moved from a healthy part of the body to the injured site. The blood vessels in the flap are surgically reattached to the new site.

Infection, or in the case of cadaver skin, rejection is a primary concern in skin graft patients. Although cadaver skin can provide protection from infection and loss of fluids during a burn victim's healing period, a subsequent graft of the patient's own skin is often required. However, for patients with extensive, severe burns, skin grafts alone are not enough to help them heal completely: the body cannot act fast enough to manufacture the necessary replacement cells, or their burns may extend deep below the top layer of skin. Skin substitutes, or **artificial skin grafts**, help close wounds and coax the lower layer of the skin to regenerate. These artificial skin substitutes, created in the laboratory, are synthetic products mixed with certain components of donated skin tissue that, when applied, interact with clotting factors in the wound. That interaction causes the dressing to adhere better, forming a more durable protective layer over the wound. It takes about two weeks for the body to fill the artificial skin with blood vessels that bring infection-fighting immune cells to the wounds and create a new epidermal skin layer, although the scar tissue that heals over the wound lacks sweat glands and hair follicles.

Most of the biological component of artificial skin comes from donated neonatal foreskins removed during circumcision. Amazingly, one foreskin can yield enough cells to make *four acres* of grafting material! A common type of tissue cell called a **fibroblast** is extracted from the donated tissue. Fibroblasts are rich in collagen and other molecules that enable them to migrate and grow readily in tissue cultures. After they are tested for viruses or other infectious pathogens, such as HIV, hepatitis, or mycoplasma, the fibroblasts are mixed with other substances, where they grow on a mesh-type scaffolding structure in the laboratory. When the growth cycle is completed, the new tissue is rinsed with a nutrient-rich media, labeled, and stored in sterile containers until needed.

An artificial skin graft is more useful than grafts derived from the patient and cadavers. Because it is artificial, it eliminates the need for tissue typing for a suitable patient match. Since the artificial product does not contain immunogenic cells, it is not rejected by the body. It can be made in large quantities and frozen for storage and shipping, making it available in large quantities when needed. Finally, rehabilitation time is significantly reduced for the patient.

Frostbite

Frostbite is an injury to the skin and underlying tissues resulting from exposure to very cold temperatures. Frostbite occurs when the body is so cold that ice crystals begin to form in the tissues. These ice crystals cause the skin to rupture, killing the cells. Although frostbite can occur anywhere on the body, the most likely affected areas include the hands, feet, cheeks, nose, and ears.

Like burns, frostbite is identified by the appearance of the skin after exposure to cold, and the damage is measured in degrees of severity:

- First degree: First degree frostbite is characterized by numbed skin that turns white in color. The skin may feel stiff to the touch, but the tissue under is still warm and soft. Usually there is no blistering and the skin heals without any residual damage.
- Second degree: In second degree frostbite, the skin will turn white or blue and will feel hard and frozen on the surface, yet the underlying tissue is not damaged. Blistering is likely, but the skin will heal with proper treatment.
- Third degree: Third degree frostbite, also called *deep frostbite*, is extremely dangerous. As in second degree frostbite, the skin turns white or blue and

will blister, but the tissue underneath is hard and cold to the touch because the tissue cells are damaged or dead. In severe cases, amputation may be the final option available to avoid a skin infection.

Treatment for frostbite involves the warming of the affected area as quickly as possible. The area is then washed, dried, and wrapped in a sterile bandage to prevent infection and promote healing. Physicians will usually prescribe anti-inflammatory drugs such as ibuprofen to reduce inflammation, along with drugs to improve circulation to the affected area, such as heparin or dextrans. If infection develops, the patient is treated with antibiotics.

Skin Cancers

Skin cancer is the most common form of cancer in the United States. According to the National Institutes of Health (NIH), UV radiation, a component of sunlight, is the main cause of skin cancer, especially when the overexposure to sunlight results in sunburn or blistering. People who live in areas that receive high levels of UV radiation from the sun are more likely to develop skin cancer. Although most skin cancers appear after age 50, skin cancer is related to a lifetime of exposure to UV radiation. Therefore, protection should start in early childhood to prevent skin cancer later in life.

Skin cancer develops when DNA found in skin tissues becomes damaged and the body cannot repair the damage. These damaged cells begin to multiply and divide uncontrollably, forming a lesion, or tumor, on the skin. Because skin cancer develops in the deeper tissues of the skin and erupts on the surface, the tumor is easily visible, which makes most skin cancers detectable and treatable in their early stages.

Three types of cancer account for nearly all of the diagnosed cases of skin cancer. Each is named for the type of cell in which it originates. The most common types of skin cancer include basal cell carcinoma and squamous cell carcinoma, both of which have a high rate of cure if detected early. Melanoma, although less common than basal cell or squamous cell carcinoma, is potentially more serious.

Basal Cell Carcinoma

Basal cell carcinoma is the most common form of skin cancer and accounts for more than 90% of all skin cancers in the United States. It commonly occurs from sun exposure and typically occurs in the middle-aged or elderly. Although basal cell carcinoma almost never spreads to other parts of the body, it can cause damage to tissue by spreading to the skin surrounding it.

Basal cell carcinoma begins in the lowest layer of the epidermis, the stratum germinativum. It is usually identified by the appearance of the lesion on the skin. Some lesions are raised bumps or nodules, waxy or pearly in appearance, that break open and form scabs in the center, while others appear as flat patches that have a scarlike appearance. A definitive diagnosis is made by removing all or part of the growth and studying its features under a microscope to check for cancer cells.

Squamous Cell Carcinoma

Squamous cell carcinoma is a cancer that begins in the squamous cells located in the upper levels of the epidermis, usually on places that have been exposed to the sun. Squamous cell carcinoma occurs about one-fourth as often as basal cell carcinoma. Although it carries the risk factors common to basal cell carcinoma, some uncommon factors may predispose an individual to squamous cell carcinoma: exposure to arsenic, hydrocarbons, heat, or x-rays; or suppression of the immune system by infection or drugs. In addition, unlike basal cell carcinoma, squamous cell carcinoma can spread to other body systems. Squamous cell carcinoma is usually identified by the thick, scaly, irregular appearance of the skin. It usually begins as a red area with a scaly, crusted surface that does not heal. As it grows, the tumor may become somewhat raised and firm, similar to a wart. Eventually, the cancer grows down into underlying skin tissue.

Melanoma

Melanoma is usually a malignant skin cancer that arises from the melanocytes, the cells in the epidermis that produce melanin and give the skin its color. Melanoma is the most harmful of all skin cancers because it can **metastasize**, or spread, to other parts of the body and internal organs, where it continues to destroy tissue. Although the cure rate for melanoma is 95% if detected early, once it spreads, the prognosis is poor.

Melanomas are identified by the appearance of a dark pigmented lesion in the skin with an irregular shape, irregular borders, and multiple colors, as shown in Figure 9.4. Because melanocytes continue to produce melanin, the cancer produces mixed shades of tan, brown, or black in the lesion. Melanoma may appear suddenly, or may begin in or near a mole, appearing as an irregular dark patch or dark lump. Once it sets in, malignant melanoma progresses quickly and metastasizes all over the body.

Any new mole or changes to an existing one—such as enlargement, darkening, inflammation, bleeding, itching or pain—are warning signs of a possible melanoma. Physicians often evaluate lesions using the ABCD method, a useful tool to help in early diagnosis

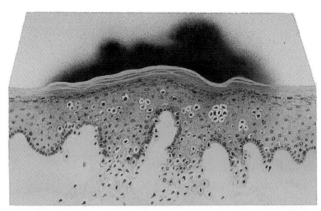

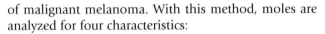

FIGURE 9.4. **Malignant Melanoma**. Melanoma occurs when melano-cytes beneath the skin's surface become malignant and subsequently appear as an abnormal-appearing mole or tumor on the surface of the skin. Asset provided by Anatomical Chart Co.

TRANSCRIPTION TIP:

Although the ABCD method of diag-nosing skin cancer has been used for decades, researchers at New York University have recom-mended expanding the acronym to ABCDE, adding an E to the classic teaching for *evolving* or *evolutionary change*, a characteristic that many dermatologists believe is the biggest indicator of a melanoma. Therefore, some dicta-tors may assess a skin lesion with factors that include **a**symmetry, **b**order irregularity, **c**olor variation, **d**iameter of more than 6 mm, and **e**volutionary change of the lesion.

of malignant melanoma. With this method, moles are analyzed for four characteristics:

A: Asymmetry. Most skin cancers are not symmetri-cal, meaning that instead of being evenly round they have an uneven or irregular shape.

B: Border irregularity. Physicians look to see if the borders of the mole are smooth or whether they are jagged or notched.

C: Color variation. Most moles are one shade, usu-ally brown. Various colors or shades of black, brown, or other colors may indicate skin cancer.

D: Diameter of 6 mm or more. Cancerous skin lesions tend to grow larger than regular moles.

Nearly all basal cell and squamous cell carcinomas can be successfully treated. There is a very high success rate for these cancers if caught in their early stages. Depend-ing on the location and size of the cancer, as well as on the patient's age and general health, physicians employ a variety of methods for removing skin cancer, including the following:

- Curettage and desiccation. **Curettage** is the proce-dure of removing the cancerous lesion by scooping it out of the skin using a spoonlike instrument called a curette. **Desiccation** is the additional application of an electric current to the area to con-trol bleeding and kill the remaining cancer cells. The skin heals without stitching.
- Surgical excision. In this method, the cancer is cut out of the skin, or **excised**. The resulting wound is then stitched closed.
- Radiation therapy. Doctors use radiation on cancers that are difficult to treat with surgery. In this treat-ment, high-energy x-rays are used to kill or shrink cancer cells. This form of radiation, called **external beam radiation**, involves directing a beam from a high-energy x-ray machine directly on the tumor. This type of radiation therapy can accurately target

the tumor with high doses of radiation, while min-imizing damage to surrounding tissue.
- Cryosurgery. Liquid nitrogen is applied to the car-cinoma to freeze and kill the abnormal cells.
- **Mohs micrographic surgery**. This technique in-volves removing a small piece of the tumor and examining it under a microscope during surgery. Because skin cancer cells often spread beyond the edges of the visible tumor, doctors use the Mohs technique to make sure they remove all of the can-cer, even that which is not visible to the naked eye. The surgeon first removes the visible tumor and then begins cutting away the edges of the wound bit by bit, examining each piece removed under the microscope for signs of cancer cells. This sequence of cutting and microscopic examination is repeated so that the lesion can be mapped and taken out without having to estimate or guess at the depth of the lesion. The surgery ends when there is no evi-dence of cancer cells on microscopic examination. This process has the dual advantage of eliminating all cancerous cells and leaving behind as much healthy tissue as possible.

The treatment for melanoma is similar to that for basal cell and squamous cell carcinoma, including surgical excision, radiation, and Mohs surgery. In ad-dition, amputation of a digit may be necessary.

TRANSCRIPTION TIP:

Mohs microscopic surgery was named after its inventor, Dr. Frederick Mohs. Transcriptionists frequently add an apostrophe to the name (*Mohs*) when typing reports that refer to Mohs surgery; this is incorrect.

Chemotherapy, the use of oral or intravenous drugs to kill cancer cells, is also used to treat melanoma.

Immunotherapy agents are also used to treat melanoma. These medications work with the body's immune system to stop or slow the growth of cancer cells. Immunotherapy may be used alone or in combination with chemotherapy to treat the cancer. Each medication is administered in carefully defined doses over a period of time that may extend to several months or more, depending on the response to therapy. Some of these medications include interleukin-2 (many times dictated as IL-2), interferon alpha, dacarbazine (Dicarbosil), and temozolomide (Temodar).

Many other types of medical treatment are also being investigated by researchers to treat melanoma. These include the use of **monoclonal antibodies**, which are specially formed antibodies that attach to cancer cells. A melanoma vaccine and a gene therapy are also being researched in an effort to identify new treatments for this potentially deadly skin cancer.

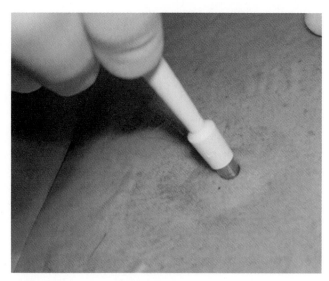

FIGURE 9.5. **Punch Biopsy.** A punch biopsy is obtained using a disposable punch tool. Reprinted with permission from Goodheart HP, MD. *Goodheart's Photoguide of Common Skin Disorders,* 2nd Edition. Philadelphia: Lippincott Williams & Wilkins, 2003.

DIAGNOSTIC STUDIES AND PROCEDURES

Diagnostic studies may be performed to diagnose bacterial or fungal skin infections as well as skin cancers. They are also performed to differentiate between malignant lesions and benign growths. Laboratory tests include special microscopic examinations of the skin.

Skin Biopsy

A **skin biopsy** is the removal of a sample of tissue under local anesthesia for laboratory analysis. A portion of a skin lesion is removed and then examined under a microscope to identify and diagnose various skin disorders. Skin biopsies are performed to diagnose bacterial or skin infections as well as skin cancer.

There are several techniques for performing a skin biopsy, depending on the location, size, and type of lesion to be examined. A **shave biopsy** uses a scalpel to slice a superficial specimen from the site and does not require closure with stitches. A **punch biopsy** is most often used for deeper skin lesions. Figure 9.5 illustrates how a small oval core of skin (usually the size of a pencil eraser) is removed from the dermis or subcutaneous tissue with a sharp, hollow instrument. The wound may require stitches if a large sample is taken. An **excisional biopsy** is the removal of the entire lesion, along with a small border of normal skin, for analysis. After removal, the wound is closed with stitches.

KOH Test

A **KOH test** is a microscopic examination of a sample of skin, hair, or nails for the presence of a fungus that infects these structures. The KOH test can be used to diagnose infections produced by dermatophytes that characterize skin disorders such as eczema and psoriasis. The test is named after the chemical formula for potassium hydroxide (KOH), which is used to dissolve skin cells, protein, and cell debris, making fungi easier to identify in the sample.

A sample of skin is taken by a light scraping of the affected area. The sample is placed on a microscopic slide with potassium hydroxide solution. The solution slowly dissolves the skin cells but not the fungus cells. The fungus cells are then visible under the microscope.

Tzanck Test

The **Tzanck test**, also called the "herpes skin test" or "chickenpox skin test," is a method of testing sores for the herpes simplex virus, which causes cold sores, fever blisters, and genital sores. It is also used to test sores for the presence of the varicella zoster virus, which causes chickenpox and shingles. In this test, a scraping of a sore is obtained and placed onto a microscope slide and examined. Positive findings of herpes-infected cells confirm an infection with one of two viruses tested.

CHAPTER SUMMARY

Our skin has many more functions than just to enhance our appearance. Familiarizing yourself with the function and design of the integumentary system as well as its conditions and diseases will give you a better understanding of this complex and dynamic system so vitally important to human health.

·I·N·S·I·G·H·T·

Hyperbaric Therapy Helps Skin Wounds

Most skin wounds heal on their own. Sometimes, however, destructive processes outpace healing time and a skin wound can become chronic, leaving the body vulnerable to infection. Researchers have found that hyperbaric oxygen therapy (HBOT) not only helps wounds heal, it helps the body fight infection and can shorten the healing time of open skin wounds.

Hyperbaric oxygen therapy is a method of delivering high doses of oxygen to the body. In this process, the patient is placed in a pressurized air chamber where 100% oxygen is breathed by means of a mask or hood. HBOT has been used for many years to help deep-sea divers recover from decompression sickness, or *the bends*. But recently, this therapy has been found to promote healing of ulcerous skin lesions due to diabetes, gangrenous lesions, compromised skin grafts, and even the side effects of skin damage from radiation therapy. Topical hyperbaric oxygen therapy is a process where high pressure oxygen is applied by means of a thin, transparent, disposable membrane bag that covers the legs and 75% of the torso. The bag is secured with tape to the patient below the breastbone and inflated with oxygen to the optimal pressure. This pressure must be maintained within rigid bounds or the treatment will not be effective or, worse, the skin lesion can be further damaged. The bag allows healthcare professionals to supersaturate or soak the body with high-pressure oxygen in a very controlled, closely monitored environment. This high-pressure dose of oxygen facilitates the growth of new blood vessels to injured tissue, which in turn reduces infection and helps heal damaged tissues. After treatment, lesions have healed without the formation of scar tissue and have better appearance and resistance to further breakdown than the surrounding untreated skin. Lesions extending to the bone have been successfully treated.

Although HBOT cannot improve the healing process in all open wounds, patients who have decreased oxygen in wound tissues gain significant improvement with this form of therapy when it is used in conjunction with other factors that promote good wound healing, such as regular wound care with debridement and topical dressings, appropriate antibiotics, adequate nutrition, and optimal control of blood sugar in patients with diabetes.

Common Soundalike Words

Word	Word Pronunciation	Soundalike	Soundalike Pronunciation
wheal: a smoothly, slightly elevated area on the body surface that is redder or paler than the surrounding skin; as in *wheal-and-flare* reaction.	wēl	**wheel:** the invention that revolutionized the world.	wēl
melanotic: the presence of melanin.	mel-ă-not′ik	**melenic:** marked by melena. Referring to gastrointestinal reports, this is the correct word, as in *melenic stools*, although commonly dictated in error as *melanotic stools*.	me-lē′nik
mottling: blotchy, as in skin.	mot′ling	**modeling:** a continuous process by which a bone is altered in size and shape during its growth by resorption and formation of bone at different sites and rates.	mod′ĕl-ing
bullous: relating to a bulla, a fluid-filled blister or bubblelike structure.	bul′ŭs	**bolus:** a single, relatively large quantity of a substance, usually one intended for therapeutic use, such as in a dose of a drug.	bō′lŭs
flare: a redness of the skin.	′flār	**flair:** a natural talent.	′flār
carbuncle: a cluster of connecting infected hair follicles (boils).	kar′bŭng-kel	**caruncle:** a small, fleshy protuberance, or similarly shaped structure.	kar′ŭng-kel
lipoma: a benign lump of fatty tissue.	li-pō′mă	**lymphoma:** a neoplasm consisting of lymphoid tissue.	lim-fō′mă
pruritic: pertaining to pruritus, or itching (such as a rash).	prū-rit′ik	**paretic:** relating to or suffering from paresis (paralysis).	pă-ret′ik
macula: a small, discolored patch or spot on the skin, neither elevated above nor depressed below the the skin's surface.	mak′yūla	**macula:** in ophthalmology, the center area of the retina responsible for central vision, seeing color, and distinguishing fine detail.	mak′yūla
papule: a small, circumscribed, solid elevation on the skin.	pap′yul	**papilla:** a small nipple.	pă-pil′ă

Combining Forms

Combining Form	Meaning	Combining Form	Meaning
adip-, adip/o	fat, fatty	lun/o	moon
albin/o, leuk/o	white	melan/o	black
caus/o	burning	necr/o	death
cellul/o	cell	onych/o	fingernail, toenail
coll/a	fibers that hold together	papill/o	elevations of dermis
cutane/o, cut/i	skin	papul/o	papule
derm-, derm/a, derm/o,	skin	phyt/o	plants
dermat/o, integument/o		pigment/o	pigment
diaphor/o	profuse sweating	pil/o	hair
elast/o	flexing, stretching	prurit/o, psor/o	itching
epiderm/o	outer layer of skin	sarc/o	connective tissue
erythem/o, erythemat/o	redness	seb/i, seb/o	sebum, sebaceous, tallow
esthes/o	sensation, feeling	squam/o	scalelike
excori/o	to take out skin	sud/o, sudor/o	sweat
exud/o	oozing fluid	topic/o	a specific area
follicul/o	follicle (small sac)	trich/o	hair, hairlike structure
fung/o, myc/o	fungus	ungu/o	relating to a nail
hidr/o	sweat, sweat glands	xanth/o	yellow
ichthy/o	scaly, dry (fishlike)	xen/o	foreign
kerat/o	hard, firm protein	xer/o	dry
lip/o, steat/o	fat		

Add Your Own Combining Forms Here:

_____

_____

_____

_____

_____

_____

ABBREVIATIONS

Abbreviation	Meaning	Abbreviation	Meaning
C	*Candida*	PUVA	psoralen and subsequent exposure to long-wavelength ultraviolet light
HBOT	hyperbaric oxygen therapy		
KOH	chemical abbreviation for potassium hydroxide	TCOM	transcutaneous oxygen monitoring
NIH	National Institutes of Health	TIMs	topical immunomodulators
PNH	postherpetic neuralgia	UV	ultraviolet

Add Your Own Abbreviations Here:

_____

_____

_____

_____

_____

TERMINOLOGY

Term	Meaning
allograft	A skin graft constructed from cadaver skin.
arrector pili muscles	Smooth muscle cells that surround hair follicles.
artificial skin graft	A skin substitute derived from synthetic materials created in the laboratory used to help close wounds and aid in regeneration of a patient's native skin.
atopic dermatitis	Another term for *eczema*.
autograft	A skin graft constructed from the patient's own skin.
bacterial endocarditis	An infection of the tissue of the heart.
basal cell carcinoma	A common form of skin cancer beginning in the basal cells of the epidermis.
basal cells	Living rounded cells in the basal layer of the skin.
boil	A warm, painful, pus-filled pocket of infection below the skin's surface.
bulb	The onion-shaped structure at the end of the root of hair.
bullae	Fluid-filled, honey colored blisters.
burn	An injury to the skin caused by heat, electricity, chemicals, or radiation.
Candida	Thin-walled, small yeasts that cause candidiasis.
candidiasis	An infection caused by the *Candida* species of fungi.

Term	*Meaning*
carbuncle	Clusters of abscesses that are connected to each other under the skin.
cellulitis	An acute bacterial infection of the skin and underlying tissues.
chemotherapy	The use of drugs to kill cancer cells.
cold sweat	Perspiration from the sweat glands activated by emotions, such as fear.
collagen	Along with fibrillin, a protein that gives skin elasticity, tone, and strength.
condyloma acuminata, syn. genital warts	Warts that appear on or around the genitals.
cryotherapy	Removal of a lesion by freezing with liquid nitrogen.
curettage	The procedure or removal of a new growth or irregular tissue with a curette.
cutaneous	The term that describes something relating to the skin.
cutaneous candidiasis	An infection of the skin with *Candida*.
debridement	The process of removing dead tissue to expose and cleanse the area.
dermatitis	Inflammation of the upper layers of the skin that results in a rash.
dermatophytes	Microscopic organisms that live on keratin and cause a fungal infection in the skin.
dermis	The inner layer of skin.
desquamation	The process of shedding dead skin cells from the epidermis and replenishing them from the deeper layers of the dermis.
desiccation	The application of an electrical current to an incision to control bleeding and kill remaining cancer cells.
dressing	Materials that cover and protect a wound from the environment.
dressing changes	The process of removing old bandages from a wound and replacing them with new, clean ones.
duct	A tubular structure giving exit to the secretion of a gland.
eczema	A skin disease characterized by a chronic, itchy rash, and dry, thickened skin.
edema	Another term for *swelling*.
electrocautery	Removal of a lesion by burning with an electrical current.
endocrine gland	A gland which releases its secretions directly into the bloodstream.
epidermis	The outermost, or superficial, layer of skin.
erythema	Another term for *redness*.
excise	To "cut out."
excisional biopsy	The removal of an entire lesion for laboratory analysis.
exocrine gland	A gland which drains its secretions through ducts, or tubes, to the surface of the body or other sites.
external beam radiation	A type of radiation that focuses on radiation from outside the body on a skin tumor.
fibrillin	Along with collagen, a protein that gives skin elasticity, tone, and strength.
fibroblasts	A common cell type, found in connective tissue, that is used in artificial skin grafts.
filiform warts	Narrow, small growths appearing on the eyelids, face, neck, or lips.
follicle	A pit in the skin containing the root of a shaft of hair.
folliculitis	A bacterial infection of the hair follicles of the skin.
frostbite	Injury to the skin and underlying tissues when the body is exposed to very cold temperatures.
full-thickness burn	Another term for *third-degree burn*.

Term	Meaning
full-thickness skin graft	A graft that includes both epidermal and complete dermal skin layers.
gangrene	Tissue death due to obstruction, loss, or diminution of blood supply to the area.
glands	A type of tissue that is made up of cells specialized for fluid secretions.
hair	A fine, threadlike structure composed of dead epithelial cells composed of keratin, arranged in columns around a central core.
herpes zoster, syn. shingles	A viral infection of the nerves caused by the reactivation of the varicella zoster virus that causes chickenpox.
immunotherapy agents	Medications that work with the body's immune system to stop or slow the growth of cancer cells.
impetigo	A contagious skin infection that leads to the formation of bullae on the body.
integument	The collective word for skin referred to by physicians.
integumentary system	The skin, including its corresponding layers, derivatives, and all of its components.
intertrigo	A rash erupting in the folds of the skin.
keratin	A tough, fibrous protein found in the epidermis, also found in the fingernails and hair.
keratinocyte	The principal cell of the epidermis.
KOH test	A microscopic examination of the skin, hair, or nails for the presence of a fungus that infects these structures.
lunula	The white half-moon shaped part located at the nail base.
maculopapular	A term that describes a lesion that contains both macules and papules.
mammary glands	A modified type of sweat gland that produces breast milk for the nourishment of offspring.
melanin	The pigment responsible for absorbing ultraviolet light and giving skin its dark appearance.
melanocytes	Pigment producing cells found in the basal layer of the skin.
melanoma	A dangerous skin cancer that arises from the melanocytes in the epidermis.
metastasize (metastasis)	The spreading of a tumor to the lymph and other organ systems.
mitosis	The basic process of cell division in which two identical cells are reproduced from a parent cell.
Mohs micrographic surgery	A technique of removing and examining a piece of tumor until the entire lesion is removed.
monoclonal antibodies	Specially formed antibodies that attach to cancer cells.
mycologist	A person who studies, identifies, and classifies fungi according to their microscopic appearance and in culture.
mycosis	A fungal infection of the skin.
nodule	An elevated, solid lesion on the skin.
onychomycosis	A fungal infection in the nail.
papillary layer	A thin layer of the dermis that connects to the epidermis.
Papillomavirus	The virus that causes verrucae, or warts, in humans.
paronychia	A bacterial infection caused by a tear in the skin at the side or base of a fingernail.
partial-thickness burn	Another term for second degree burn.
peau d'orange	A symptom of cellulitis that makes skin resemble the tight peel of an orange.
phototherapy	Exposure to ultraviolet light to decrease symptoms of some skin diseases.

Term	Meaning
plantar warts	Warts occurring on the soles of the feet.
plaques	Raised patches of silvery scales common in psoriasis.
postherpetic neuralgia (PNH)	Chronic pain that lingers in the area of a shingles outbreak.
pruritus	Another term for *itching*.
psoralen	A drug taken orally before exposure to ultraviolet light that lessens the effects of UV light on the skin.
psoriasis	A chronic, recurring disease characterized by silvery scales called plaques on the skin.
punch biopsy	The removal of a sample of skin for laboratory analysis with a sharp, hollow instrument.
PUVA therapy	The combination of using psoralen and UV light as a treatment of certain skin diseases.
rash	An inflammation in the skin affecting its appearance or texture.
receptors	Nerve endings in the skin that sense pain, touch, temperature, and pressure.
rosacea	A chronic inflammatory skin disease primarily affecting the face and around the eyes.
rubor	Another term for *rash*.
sebaceous cyst	A blockage in a sebaceous gland causing a backup of fatty material.
sebaceous glands	Glands that open into hair follicles and secrete sebum.
seborrheic dermatitis	An inflammation of the sebum-rich areas of the skin of the scalp and face and occasionally the trunk of the body.
sebum	An oily substance secreted by the sebaceous glands that softens and lubricates the skin.
shave biopsy	The removal of only superficial layers of skin for laboratory analysis.
skin	The soft outer covering of the body and the site of the sense of touch.
skin biopsy	The removal of a sample of skin for laboratory analysis.
skin graft	A layer of skin taken from a healthy area on the body and transferred to an area with a skin defect or burned tissues.
split-thickness skin graft	A graft that includes the epidermal and part of the dermal skin layers.
squamous cell carcinoma	A cancer that begins in the squamous cells in the upper levels of the epidermis.
squamous skin cells	Flattened cells that make the skin waterproof and provide the main barrier to skin infection.
stratum corneum	The uppermost epidural layer, also called the *horny layer*.
stratum germinativum	The bottom sublayer of the epidermis, or *basal layer*.
stratum granulosum	A grainy layer of skin above the spiny layer.
stratum lucidum	A thick, clear layer of skin that is particularly thick in the hands and soles of the feet.
stratum spinosum	A spiny layer of skin above the basal layer
subcutaneous	A word meaning "beneath the skin."
subcutaneous layer	The fat layer below the dermis.
subcuticular	Underneath the dermis.
superficial burn	Another term for *first degree burn*.
sweat	A salty, watery fluid secreted by the sweat glands in response to heat.
sweat glands	Glands that produce sweat.

Term	*Meaning*
tinea	Also known as *ringworm*, a fungal infection of the skin resulting in a characteristic red, ring-shaped rash as it grows.
tinea barbae	A fungal infection involving the beard area on the face.
tinea capitis	A fungal infection involving the scalp or neck.
tinea corporis	A fungal infection involving the nonhair parts of the body.
tinea cruris	Also called *jock itch*, a fungal infection involving the groin.
tinea pedis	Also called *athlete's foot*, a fungal infection involving the feet.
topical immunomodulators (TIMs)	A class of drugs that inhibit inflammatory skin reactions when treating for symptoms of some skin diseases.
tumor	A large nodule.
Tzanck test	A method of testing skin sores for the herpes simplex virus or varicella zoster virus.
urticaria	Another term for *hives*.
verrucae	Also called *warts*, small, noncancerous skin growths caused by the papillomavirus.
verrucae vulgaris	Also called *common warts*, they are found on the hands, arms, and legs.
warts	A common term for *verrucae*.

Add Your Own Terms and Definitions Here:

_____

_____

_____

_____

_____

_____

_____

_____

REVIEW QUESTIONS

1. List three different types of skin biopsies and describe the procedure used for each.
2. What skin infection occurs in as much as 85% of people with AIDS?
3. List the skin's specialized structures.
4. What is another name for a fungal infection of the skin?
5. Which type of skin cancer is considered to be the most dangerous and why?
6. What are the three layers of tissue that make up the skin?
7. What is another name for eczema?
8. What does the acronym PUVA stand for and what is PUVA therapy?
9. What is a sebaceous cyst?
10. Which virus causes shingles?

CHAPTER ACTIVITIES

Soundalike Word Choice

Circle the correct word in the following sentences.

1. (Melanoma, Melanin) is the most dangerous of all skin cancers.
2. The patient developed (pneuritis, pruritus) after taking that particular antibiotic.
3. (Cytotherapy, Cryotherapy) is the process of removing a skin lesion by freezing it.
4. Some patients develop postherpetic (neuroma, neuralgia) after shingles.
5. Ms. Lupita's malignant tumor was removed using (electrocautery, electrocutlery).
6. An infection caused by the species *Candida* is called (candidiasis, candiolysis).
7. The patient's skin sample was examined using a (KOH/KLH) test.
8. Living, rounded cells in the skin are called (basal/basil) cells.
9. Her skin was lacking (fibrinogen, fibrillin), giving it less elasticity.
10. (PUVA, PIVA) therapy uses psoralen and UV light to treat certain skin diseases.

Creating Medical Words

Search for and combine the following prefixes, suffixes, and combining forms in the following list to create a medical word that best fits the following definitions. Add missing consonants or vowels if needed to complete the word. Verify the spelling of the words you create with a medical dictionary. The first answer is provided for you.

erythr/o	-logy	xer/o	melan/o
-phyt/o	-osis	epi-	onych/o
-ar	-ia	squam/o	-sis
-ema	-itis	-derm	derm/a
seb/o	myc/o	urtic/o	-us
dermat/o	bio-	-esthesia	-opsy
-ic	-is	-ous	-cyte

Definitions

1. A mature red blood cell. ___erythrocyte___
2. An eruption of <u>itchy</u> wheals. _____
3. Describing a dark or black pigment to skin. _____
4. Any disease caused by a fungus. _____
5. Relating to the secretion of sebum. _____
6. A fungal infection in the nail. _____

7. The study of the diagnosis and treatment of cutaneous diseases and related systemic diseases.
_____

8. Relating to or covered with scales. _____

9. The process of removing tissue from patients for diagnostic examination. _____

10. The uppermost layer of skin. _____

Medical Word Equivalents

Write the correct medical term next to each English phrase or characteristic given.

1. eczema _____
2. boil _____
3. cradle cap _____
4. silvery scales _____
5. peau d'orange _____
6. flushing of the face _____
7. warts _____
8. athlete's foot _____
9. ringworm _____
10. "honey-colored" blisters _____
11. dandruff _____
12. carbuncle _____

Skin Disorder Differentiation

Indicate whether the following skin infections are bacterial (B), fungal (F), or viral (V).

1. impetigo _____
2. verruca vulgaris _____
3. folliculitis _____
4. tinea barbae _____
5. shingles _____
6. cellulitis _____
7. condyloma _____
8. onychomycosis _____
9. candidiasis _____
10. tinea corporis _____

Proofreading Exercise

Circle the errors in the following clinic report. Then retype the corrected report using the same format on a blank document screen. When finished, print one copy and save the corrected report as CHAPTER-9-NOTE.

SUBJECTIVE: The patent is here for complaint of ring worm, the patients father states the child has aras of hair loss and multiple spots on his scalp. He has had ringworm in the past; overall he is healthy and doing well. He is up-to-date with his immunizations.

OBJECT: Temperature 98.2, blood pressure 90-60, weight 41/2 pounds, height 43 inches, pulse 86, respiratory rate 24. On his scalp, he has multiple areas of patches and hair loss consistent with tinea capitus. There are no other lessons on his body or face. Head, ears, eyes, nose, and throat: PERLA. Tympanic membranes clear. Oropharynx: Clear. No lymphadenopathy. Cardiovascular: Regular rate and rhythm. Chest-clear. Extremities: No edima.

ASSESSMENT: Well child. Tinea capitus. Griseofulvin 20 mgs per kgm per day for a month. Return to clinic for followup as patient may need 4–6 weeks of therapy for this to clear up.

TRANSCRIPTION PRACTICE

Open your word-processing software. Insert the student CD-ROM and locate the dictation for this chapter. For each of the words in the "listen for these terms" list for each report, use a medical dictionary or other resource to identify and write down a brief definition of the terms on a separate sheet of paper to attach with your work. Then listen to the dictation and transcribe each report. Use the current date for each report where a date is indicated. Insert a heading into the document if the text requires a second page.

At the end of each report, indicate the name of the dictating physician under the signature line and insert reference initials. For date dictated and transcribed and date of admission, use the current date. Proofread your work, print one copy for your instructor along with your term definitions, and save the completed report to your student disk.

Report #T9.1: Operative Report
Patient Name: Monsanto Kato
Medical Record No.: 555-3990
Surgeon: Sabrina Scott, MD

Listen for these terms:
melanoma
sentinel node
sartorius muscle
saphenous vein
saphenofemoral junction
Prolene
hemostasis
JP drain

Report #T9.2: Discharge Summary
Patient Name: Sergio Garcia
Medical Record No.: 90XT-6721
Date of Admission: 02/15/xxxx
Date of Discharge: 02/17/xxxx
Attending Physician: Lilia Montero, MD
Dictating Physician: Michael Josephs, MD

Listen for these terms:
chemotherapy
lymph nodes
temporal lobe
Velban
gamma knife

Report #T9.3: Consultation Report
Patient Name: Earl Sines
Medical Record No.: 808-98881
Date of Service: (Current Date)
Attending Physician: Donny Dukes, MD
Consulting Physician: Lena Kushner, MD

Listen for these terms:
rosacea
iridectomy
blepharoplasty
tinnitus
CABG
Auricular

10

OPHTHALMOLOGY

OBJECTIVES

After completing this chapter, you will be able to:

- Describe and locate general anatomic structures of the eye.
- Understand and explain the visual process that enables people to see.
- Describe common visual impairments that affect eye function.
- Describe common structure disorders that affect vision.
- Discuss the diagnostic studies used to help identify disorders of the ocular system.

INTRODUCTION

Ophthalmology, one of the oldest branches of medicine, deals with the study of the eye, including diseases of the eye and their respective treatments. An **optometrist** is a professional who performs eye examinations to diagnose vision problems and eye diseases; an **optician** is a person who manufactures, verifies, and delivers lenses, frames, and other specially fabricated optical devices. An **ophthalmologist**, however, is a medical doctor who performs eye surgery as well as diagnoses and treats eye diseases and injuries.

Even though the eye itself is very small—about one inch in diameter on average—it is a delicate, complex structure that is often called the most complex organ in the body. The function of the eyes enables the brain to produce images that allow us to visualize not only objects but also shapes, colors, and dimensions of objects in order to interpret our surroundings.

Sight guides the human body. The eyes are constantly at work, adjusting the amount of light that enters them, focusing on objects, and producing continuous images that are transmitted to the brain as the gaze is shifted from distant objects to near objects. This chapter provides an introduction to the anatomy of the human eye and the process of vision; it also describes the procedures used to examine the eye as well as typical methods of diagnosis and treatment of common diseases of the eye.

ANATOMY OF THE EYE

The eye is essentially an opaque structure filled with a waterlike fluid. Its anatomic components are illustrated in Figure 10.1 and detailed below.

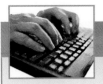

Outer Structures

The human eye is a spheroid structure that rests in a bony, cavernlike cavity called the **orbit**, or eye socket, located on the frontal surface of the skull. The eye sockets are actually formed by the convergence of several bones in the cheeks, the forehead, the temple, and the sides of the nose. The eyeball itself is cushioned within the orbit by pads of fatty tissue that protect the eye and enable it to move freely. The orbit also contains muscles, blood vessels, and a tear duct, or **lacrimal gland**, which produces tears that help provide lubrication for the eye and protection against infection. Tears help carry nutrients to and waste products away from the eye, provide a smooth refracting surface for visual acuity, and flush away foreign debris. The tears form a film over the eye and flow down to the inner corner of the eye to be collected by two tiny canals near the inner end of each eyelid. They then flow through the **nasolacrimal ducts**, which are small tubes that open into the nose. At times when the eye is dry, the eyelids will blink to help generate lacrimal fluid across the eye's surface. This protective mechanism keeps the eye moist and rids it of foreign debris. Tears represent an overflow of the lacrimal system.

The **eyelids** are folds of skin that act like shutters to protect the front of the eyeball. The eyelids are made up of connective tissue called **tarsus**, which is covered by skin on the outside. Numerous glands called **meibomian glands** located on the inside of the eyelids secrete oils that help lubricate the eye's surface. **Eyelashes** are hairs attached to the edge of the eyelids. Eyelashes are sensitive to touch and send warnings that an object such as an insect or debris is near, triggering the eyelid to close. The eyelids and eyelashes protect the eye from foreign matter, such as dust, dirt, and other debris, and from bright light that could damage the eye.

Inner Structures

The **cornea**, sometimes referred to as the "window of the eye," is a clear, paper-thin coating of cells located

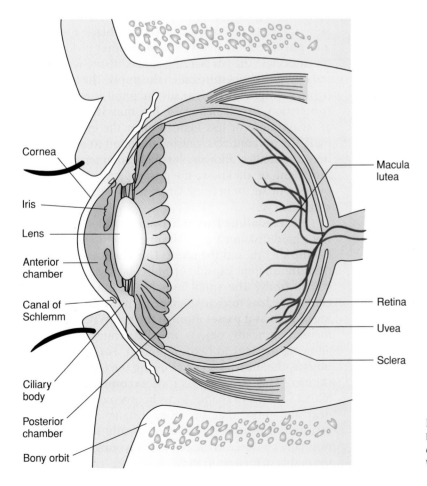

FIGURE 10.1. Gross Anatomy of the Human Eye.
Reprinted with permission from Pillitteri, A. *Maternal and Child Nursing*, 4th Ed. Philadelphia: Lippincott Williams & Wilkins, 2003.

at the front and center of the eye. The cornea covers the entire front of the eye and serves to protect it as well as to help focus light as it enters the eye. Like a camera lens, the cornea must have a perfect curvature because it is the front element of the optic system of the eye. The cornea bends the light coming in and works together with the lens to create an image on the retina. It is also very sensitive to temperature and to pain. Touching the cornea will cause the eyelid to instinctively close, and pain is registered when even a tiny speck of dust gets into the eye.

The **sclera**, often called the "white of the eye," is a tough layer of tissue that gives the eye its spherical shape. The purpose of the sclera is to provide strength, structure, and protection to the eye. Although only the front part of the sclera is visible and protected by the cornea, this layer extends all around the eye.

The sclera is attached to three pairs of muscles (a total of six muscles) in the orbit that help the eye pivot in different directions. Two pairs run straight to the bony orbit of the skull at right angles to each other: the superior rectus and the inferior rectus, and the lateral rectus and the medial rectus muscles. Another pair of muscles, the superior oblique and inferior oblique muscles, is placed at a bit of an incline. Together these six muscles, collectively called **extraocular muscles**, move the eye up and down, left and right, and diagonally in order to help centralize the focus of objects in the eye, as shown in Figure 10.2. The extraocular muscles and the muscles that move the eyelid are controlled by nerve impulses from cranial nerves III through VI that originate in the brain.

Nystagmus is an eye movement disorder characterized by involuntary rhythmic shaking or movement of

TRANSCRIPTION TIP:

Remember to distinguish between the singular or plural form of the terms *sclera* and *conjunctiva* when transcribing dictation about these anatomical structures. When referring to both eyes, the plural forms of these terms are *sclerae* and *conjunctivae*.

the eyes. The term is derived from the Greek word *nustagmos*, which was used to describe the wobbly head movements of a sleepy or inebriated individual. In police work, the **horizontal gaze nystagmus** test (where a person's pupil is observed as it follows a moving object) is used as a field test for sobriety.

Near the front of the eye, the sclera and inside of the eyelids are covered by a thin, clear layer of skin called the **conjunctiva**. The conjunctiva keeps bacteria and foreign material from getting behind the eye. Infections of this layer are often referred to as **conjunctivitis** or "pink eye."

The **iris**, or the colored part of the eye, is a circular mesh of interlocking fibers that control the amount of light entering the eye. The color of the iris is due to variable amounts of **eumelanin** (brown-black melanins) and **pheomelanin** (red-yellow melanins) produced by melanocytes. The iris is a ring-shaped tissue with a central opening or aperture called the **pupil**. The amount of light entering the eye through the pupil is regulated by contraction or expansion of the muscles of the iris, allowing more or less light to enter the eye. In bright light, the iris contracts, causing the pupil to constrict, or become smaller, allowing less light to enter the eye. In dim light or darkness, the iris expands, causing the pupil to dilate, or become larger, allowing more light to enter the eye.

The **crystalline lens**, often simply called the **lens**, is not a hard disk but a clear, flexible structure located just behind the iris and the pupil. The lens is enclosed in a thin, transparent capsule of muscular tissue called the **ciliary body**. The small muscles of the ciliary body enable the lens to change shape to allow for fine focusing of light as it passes through the eye. When the eye is focused on nearby objects, the ciliary muscles contract, allowing the lens to become thicker. For more distant objects, the muscles relax, allowing the lens to become thinner. This process is called **accommodation** and allows the lens to change focus between objects that are near and those that are more distant. As the pupils accommodate to keep an object clearly in focus, they normally converge as they constrict (young children like to try this maneuver to make their eyes "cross").

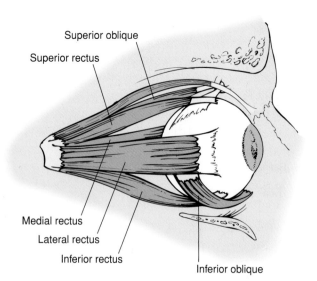

Superior oblique

Superior rectus

Medial rectus

Lateral rectus

Inferior rectus

Inferior oblique

FIGURE 10.2. Extraocular Muscles. Six sets of extraocular muscles provide movement of the eye in different directions. Reprinted with permission from Weber, J and Kelley, J. *Health Assessment in Nursing*, 2nd Ed. Philadelphia: Lippincott Williams & Wilkins, 2003.

The **retina** is a thin, light-sensitive layer of tissue that lines the inside of the back part of the eye. It receives light rays and converts the image cast on it to nerve signals that will eventually be carried to the brain. The center area of the retina is called the **macula**, which is responsible for central vision, seeing color, and distinguishing fine detail, whereas the outer portion of the retina allows for night vision and peripheral vision. The very center of the macula is called the **fovea centralis** (or "fovea") and is the part of the macula on which light rays coming into the eye focus precisely. If a portion of the fovea or macula is damaged, vision is reduced, resulting in central-vision blindness.

The inside of the eyeball is divided by the iris into two fluid-filled sections that nourish the internal structures of the eye and help to maintain its shape and pressure. The larger section at the back of the eye, extending to the retina, is called the **posterior chamber**. The smaller section in the front, extending from the inside of the cornea to the iris, is called the **anterior chamber**. The posterior chamber is filled with a clear, watery fluid called **vitreous humor**. The fluid that fills the anterior chamber is called the **aqueous humor**. Both the vitreous humor and aqueous humor maintain the shape of the eyeball and carry nutrients and oxygen to the cornea and lens. A circular canal called the **canal of Schlemm** provides a drainage system for the aqueous humor from the eye into the bloodstream. Blockages in the canal of Schlemm can cause the fluid to back up and result in increased pressure in the eye. When the pressure becomes higher than the optic nerve can tolerate, the optic nerve becomes damaged and an eventual loss of vision can occur.

The **optic nerve**, which is a bundle of more than one million nerve fibers, is located in the back of the eye and responsible for transmitting nerve signals from the retina to the brain, where the information is interpreted as a visual image. The region of the eye where the optic nerve meets the retina is called the **optic disc**. The optic disc is often referred to as the "blind spot" of the eye because it contains only nerve fibers and no light receptor cells.

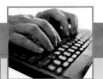

TRANSCRIPTION TIP:

The abbreviations *OD, OS,* and *OU,* which are often heard in the dictation of ophthalmology reports, stand for *oculus dexter* (right eye), *oculus sinister* (left eye), and *oculus uterque* (both eyes). Although these abbreviations are typically expanded in general text, it is appropriate, and even preferred, to use the abbreviated forms when the text is associated with visual testing and measured values, unless instructed otherwise by your employer.

VISUAL PROCESS

Vision is a complicated process that requires numerous components of the human eye and brain to work together to produce an image. Light rays bounce off all objects. One's ability to see begins when light is reflected from an object on which the eyes have focused. That light enters the eye and is then bent, or retracted, by the cornea. The perfect curvature of the cornea accounts for about 80% of the eye's ability to focus as it visualizes an object.

After the light passes through the cornea, it passes through the pupil and is then bent once more, this time by the lens, to a more finely adjusted focus. The lens changes its shape (accommodates) using the ciliary muscles to focus the light on the retina. The process of bending light to produce a focused image on the retina is called **refraction**. The closer an object is to the eye, the more focusing the lens must do to make the image clear.

The lens then projects the image onto the outermost layer of the retina called the **photoreceptor layer**. This layer is composed of over 125 million (in each eye) of light-sensitive cells called cones and rods. **Cones** function in bright levels of light, distinguish color and detail, and are responsible for central vision. Cones produce a sharp color image that is superimposed on the black-and-white image created by the rods. **Rods** see no color detail but function at reduced levels of light and are responsible for peripheral vision. When light is focused on the retina, a chemical change in the rods and cones causes them to convert the light to millions of nerve impulses that are transmitted along the optic nerve to the brain. For clear vision, light rays must focus directly onto the retina. When light focuses in front of or behind the retina, blurred vision results.

Because of the way in which the light rays have been bent as they enter each eye, the image of the object is actually upside down and facing in the opposite direction when it touches the retina. Each eye transmits signals of a slightly different inverted image to the brain, with the right eye signalling the left side of the brain and the left eye transmitting the image to the right side of the brain. Once they reach the brain, the brain analyzes the images and corrects them by turning them right-side-up again. The brain then combines the images to create the one that matches the object originally seen. The brain actually interprets most of our vision out of a lifetime of images stored in the visual cortex located in the back of the brain, the processor and storehouse for vision.

Common Visual Disorders and Treatments

Clear vision depends on how well the cornea and lens refract rays of light to fall onto the retina. If the cornea

QUICK CHECK 10.1 ✓

Match the definitions on the left with the terms on the right.

1. _____ The very center of the macula.

2. _____ The colored part of the eye.

3. _____ The "white of the eye."

4. _____ Secrete oils that lubricate the eyelids.

5. _____ A transparent capsule of muscular tissue.

A. meibomian glands

B. ciliary body

C. fovea

D. iris

E. sclera

or eye shape is abnormal, vision can become distorted because light does not fall exactly where it should on the retina. Disorders that cause improper focusing of the eye and subsequent blurring of vision are called **refractive errors**.

Myopia is another name for **nearsightedness**. When the shape of eye is too elongated or the light rays are refracted excessively by the cornea and lens, light will be focused at a point in front of the retina and be out of focus by the time it actually hits the retina. Consequently, objects that are far away will be difficult to see, even though objects at close range are seen clearly, as shown in Figure 10.3. Eyeglasses, contact lenses, or corneal sculpting with the use of lasers can correct nearsightedness.

Hyperopia is the medical term for **farsightedness**. The depth of the eye is too short, or the light rays are not refracted sufficiently by the cornea and lens, and light does not have a chance to achieve focus by the time it hits the retina and focuses at a point behind the retina. A person with farsightedness has difficulty visualizing objects at close range but often clearly sees those at a distance (see Figure 10.3). Hyperopia, like myopia, is corrected with prescription eyeglasses, contact lenses, or corneal sculpting with the use of lasers to correct the refractive error.

Astigmatism is the name given to a condition of impaired eyesight that often results from irregular con-

formation of the cornea. If the cornea is not perfectly spherical or has a slightly uneven surface curvature, light is focused irregularly in different parts of the eye, making the image out of focus and causing astigmatism. This abnormality can be corrected with eyeglasses, contact lenses, or corneal sculpting with the use of lasers.

Presbyopia, also called **aging eyes**, occurs when the lens loses the ability to focus due to the natural aging process. As a person becomes older, the lens gradually becomes more rigid and cannot change its shape as easily when it needs to focus, making activities such as reading difficult. Like other refractive errors, this condition can be corrected with eyeglasses, contact lenses, or laser eye surgery.

Diplopia, or **double vision**, results when light from an object is split into two images by a defect in the eye's optical system; or both eyes fail to point at the object being viewed and the images seen by the two eyes are fused into a single picture by the brain. Diplopia is treated with a series of eye exercises and/or realignment of the misaligned eye where possible and restimulation of the part of the pathway to the brain that is malfunctioning. Sometimes surgical straightening of the eye is required.

Amblyopia, or *lazy eye*, is a condition in which the brain does not fully "acknowledge" the images seen by one eye during a critical period of a child's development (birth to 6 years). If the image is not clear in one eye, or if the image is not the same in both eyes, the vision pathways will not develop properly and the good eye and the brain will compensate by suppressing use of the poorly focusing eye. This condition can be successfully treated in its early stages surgically in children over several weeks or by patching the good eye in order to cause the child to use the weaker eye and strengthen it. Sometimes drops or special eyeglasses are used to blur the vision in the good eye to make use of the weaker eye and make it stronger. If not detected and treated early, this condition can result in a permanent decrease in the vision in the nonfocusing eye that cannot be corrected with glasses, contacts, or laser surgery.

TRANSCRIPTION TIP:

PERRLA, (often dictated to sound like *PURR-la*), a common abbreviation used in an ocular examination, means that the **p**upils are **e**qual, **r**ound, and **r**eactive to **l**ight and **a**ccommodation. The examination abbreviation EOMI, meaning **e**xtra**o**cular **m**ovements (or muscles) are **i**ntact, means that the patient's eye successfully moves in all positions of gaze.

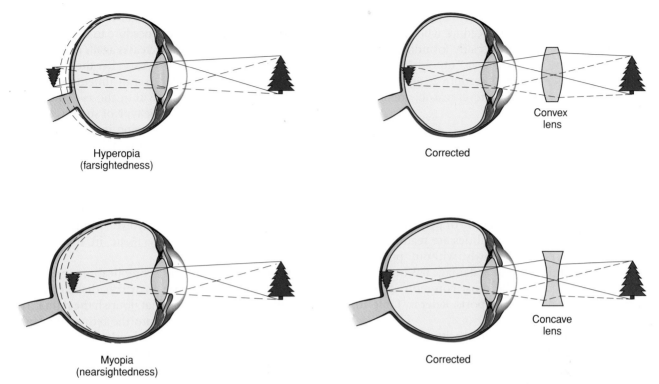

FIGURE 10.3. Refractive Errors. Improper focusing of the eye cause myopia and hyperopia. Reprinted with permission from Cohen BJ, Wood DL. *Member's the Human Body in Health and Disease*, 9th Ed. Philadelphia: Lippincott Williams & Wilkins, 2000.

Typically, vision errors are corrected by means of corrective lenses, a process that changes the manner in which light enters the eye. Many people, however, desire to reduce or eliminate their dependence on eyeglasses or contact lenses. There are several types of definitive corrective surgical procedures for refractive and visual disorders, such as myopia or presbyopia, some of which include:

- **Laser in situ keratomileusis (LASIK)** surgery. This procedure corrects the shape of the cornea and, hence, corrects nearsightedness by use of a computer-controlled laser and **microkeratome**, a surgical instrument that cuts the cornea and removes tissue. The reshaping of the cornea results in its flattening and consequent reduction of the myopia.
- **Photorefractive keratectomy (PRK)**. Like LASIK, PRK is a procedure in which the surface of the cornea is reshaped using a laser device, but the pro-

cedure does not involve cutting into the cornea with a microkeratome, and, thus, less time is required to achieve optimal vision. This procedure may be used to treat myopia, hyperopia, or astigmatism.
- **Radial keratotomy (RK)**. RK involves placing radial incisions in the peripheral cornea, which results in relaxation and flattening of the central cornea to correct myopia. However, the greater the nearsightedness, the more incisions are required to produce clear vision.
- **Astigmatic keratotomy (AK)**. This procedure is similar to RK but used to correct astigmatism. Instead of using a radial pattern of incisions in the peripheral cornea, the surgeon makes a curved pattern of incisions to optimally treat the astigmatism.
- **Laser thermokeratoplasty (LTK)**. This procedure treats hyperopia and involves the use of the **YAG laser**. YAG is an acronym for a rather complicated chemical compound that is used as the lasing medium for certain solid-state lasers. The laser beam causes shrinkage of collagen in the peripheral cornea, which results in reducing farsightedness by inducing a relative nearsightedness.
- **Conductive keratoplasty (CK)**. CK uses heat from low-level radiofrequency waves, rather than a laser or scalpel, to shrink the collagen in the peripheral cornea and change its shape. The radio waves are applied to the outer cornea, creating a constrictive band that increases the curve of the cornea and improves vision.

TRANSCRIPTION TIP:

In ophthalmology reports, physicians may refer to *forced duction*, which is a manual maneuver of conducting passive movement of the eyeball in a particular direction. Be careful to avoid the mistranscription of *forced adduction*.

- **Implantable collamer lens** (ICL) **procedure**. This is a lens replacement procedure whereby an ophthalmologist injects a specially formulated pliable lens into the eye, where it "unfolds" to correct nearsightedness. This procedure is an alternative for patients who, for whatever reason, are not candidates for LASIK surgery.

Common Structural Diseases and Treatments

Diseases and disorders that affect the eye prevent a person from leading a normal life or performing other tasks. Some of these abnormalities are readily visible, whereas others progress slowly without producing warning signs until irreparable damage has been done. The following describe the most common structural disorders found in dictated reports. Refer to Table 10.1 for a more comprehensive list.

A **cataract** is a clouding or opacity of the lens that causes light to be diffused as it enters the eye, impacting visual clarity and causing progressive, painless loss of vision, as illustrated in Figure 10.4. Cataracts are treated with a simple outpatient operative treatment, where the cloudy lens is removed from the eye in a process called **phacoemulsification**. The lens debris is flushed with fluid and the pieces of lens are removed from the eye by a suction device called an **irrigation-aspiration device**. Then the lens is replaced with a permanent, plastic lens called an **intraocular lens (IOL)** implant.

Glaucoma is a serious disease of the eye that causes damage to the optic nerve. Untreated, it can lead to total blindness. The precise cause of glaucoma is not known but is related to increased pressure in the eyeball due to obstruction of the outflow of aqueous humor through the canal of Schlemm. This pressure can lead to bleeding in the anterior chamber of the eye, a condition known as **hyphema**. Over time, this obstruction leads to a gradual, progressive, irreversible loss of vision.

Although currently vision loss due to glaucoma cannot be reversed, research into the cause of this disease and its treatment to prevent its progression is ongoing. There are a number of studies underway examining the genetics and heritability of glaucoma as well as new approaches to glaucoma therapy, including the use of anecortave acetate, a drug that is injected around the wall of the eye, which appears to decrease production of myocilin, a protein that clogs the pore system inside the eye where fluid drains. In the meantime, physicians have a variety of ways to treat glaucoma and help prevent further vision loss. Medicated eyedrops such as Timoptic, Betoptic, Trusopt, Azopt, Alphagan, and Xalatan, can be used to slow the progression of glaucoma. Physicians may also employ an argon laser procedure called **trabeculoplasty**, where the laser is focused into the eye in such a way as to let aqueous fluid leave the eye more efficiently. However, although nearly 80% of patients respond well enough to the procedure to delay or avoid further surgery, the pressure increases again in more than half of all patients within two years after the procedure.

If medication and initial laser treatments are unsuccessful in reducing pressure within the eye, incisional surgery may be performed. One type of surgery, called a **trabeculectomy**, creates an opening in the wall of the eye so that aqueous humor can drain. If the trabeculectomy fails, another type of surgery places a drainage tube into the eye between the cornea and iris. The tube drains to a plate that is sewn on the surface of the eye to help drain fluid from the eye. A third type of surgery, although infrequently used, involves using a laser or freezing treatment to destroy tissue in the eye that makes aqueous humor.

Diabetic retinopathy is a complication of diabetes. It is a degenerative disease in which diabetes causes damage to the blood vessels that nourish the retina. The damaged blood vessels leak into the retina, abnormal new blood vessels may grow, or blood vessels may break and cause bleeding, all of which leads to progressive vision loss in the central part of the retina, causing cloudy vision, blind spots (**scotomas**), or floaters, and, eventually, total loss of vision.

Vision loss and potential blindness can be prevented if diabetic retinopathy is detected and treated early. Laser surgery is used to treat retinopathy. Laser surgery is very effective at maintaining vision, but it cannot always restore vision that has already been lost. The laser destroys leaking blood vessels that lead to vision loss. In cases where the vitreous humor is filled with blood, a **vitrectomy** is performed to remove the liquid and replace it with a salt solution.

Age-related macular degeneration is a disease that is caused by the malfunction of the photosensitive cells in the macula, causing distortion of images in the center of the visual field, a darkened area in the center of an image, and diminished color perception. The macula slowly deteriorates, resulting in gradual, permanent loss of vision.

There are two forms of macular degeneration: **dry macular degeneration** and **wet macular degeneration**. The dry form, in which the cells of the macula slowly begin to break down, is diagnosed in approximately 90% of macular degeneration cases. **Drusen**, which are yellow waste deposits that accumulate under the retina, are common early signs of dry AMD. The risk of developing advanced dry AMD or wet AMD increases as the number or size of the drusen increases.

The wet form is diagnosed in approximately 10% of cases; however, it results in 90% of the visual impairment and is considered advanced AMD. Wet AMD is always preceded by the dry form of the disease. As the dry form worsens, some people begin to have abnormal blood vessels growing behind the macula. These vessels are very fragile and will leak fluid and blood (hence the term *wet* macular degeneration), causing rapid damage to the macula.

TABLE 10.1   Other Common Ocular Structural Disorders

Name of Disease or Disorder	Anatomic Site Affected	Definition of Disorder	Resulting Visual Problem or Defect	Treatment
Chalazion	Eyelids	Blockage of meibomian gland with oil secretion.	An enlargement of the oil gland, causing a meibomian or tarsal cyst on the eyelid.	A chalazion usually disappears in one to three months without treatment, or sooner with the application of hot compresses. In severe cases, a physician can drain the chalazion or apply a corticosteroid to the area.
Blepharitis	Eyelids	The chronic inflammation of the lid margins.	Redness of the lid margin with scaling of the skin, or in more severe cases, destruction or distortion of the follicles of the eyelashes.	Warm compresses and frequent washings to the area. A physician may also prescribe an antibiotic ointment such as bacitracin to treat or prevent infection.
Entropion	Eyelids	Abnormal inward curling of the eyelid into the eye.	Pain and redness of the cornea from rubbing of the eyelid and eyelashes on the globe.	Eyedrops and ointments are used to keep the eye moist and soothe irritation; or surgery may be indicated to preserve sight or for cosmetic reasons.
Ectropion	Eyelids	Abnormal outward curling of the eyelid away from the eye.	Tears overflow the eyelid, causing constant tearing and irritation of the skin.	Eyedrops and ointments are used to keep the eye moist and soothe irritation; or surgery may be indicated to preserve sight or for cosmetic reasons.
Conjunctivitis	Conjunctiva	An inflammation of the conjunctiva caused by viruses, bacteria, or fungi.	Conjunctiva becomes pink and irritated with a watery discharge. Vision may be blurred if cornea becomes infected.	The area is kept clean, and cool compresses can be applied to soothe irritation. Antibiotic eye ointments or drops, such as sulfacetamide or trimethoprim-polymyxin, are prescribed in cases of bacterial conjunctivitis. Other types of conjunctivitis may require oral antibiotics such as erythromycin, azithromycin, or doxycycline.
Stye (also called a hordeolum)	Eyelid	A small abscess of the hair follicle glands in the eyelid caused by a bacterial infection.	Swelling of the eye, redness, and pain. Eventually the stye bursts and the symptoms subside.	The treatment for a stye is to bathe it repeatedly with warm water. A physician may also prescribe an antibiotic ointment or drop to the area.
Scleritis	Sclera	A painful inflammation and purple discoloration of the sclera.	Eye tenderness increased tearing, and sensitivity to light. In severe cases, inflammation may cause perforation of the eyeball and loss of the eye.	Nonsteroidal antiinflammatory drugs (NSAIDs) or a corticosteroid such as prednisone is used to treat scleritis, as eye drops and ointments rarely affect this condition.
Superficial punctate keratitis	Cornea	An inflammation and death of cells on the surface of the cornea due to infection.	Eyes become bloodshot, painful, and sensitive to light. Vision may be blurred until normal vision is recovered from the application of antibiotics.	When the cause is a virus, usually no treatment is given and the disorder subsides on its own. If the cause is bacterial, antibiotics are used.

(continued)

TABLE 10.1   Other Common Ocular Structural Disorders (continued)

Name of Disease or Disorder	Anatomic Site Affected	Definition of Disorder	Resulting Visual Problem or Defect	Treatment
Keratoconus	Cornea	A gradual change in the shape of the cornea that causes it to become cone shaped.	Major changes in vision that require frequent changes in prescription for eyeglasses or contact lenses. In severe cases, a corneal transplantation may be needed to restore vision.	Contact lenses or glasses often correct the visual problem associated with this disorder. However, if the change in corneal shape is severe, corrective lenses will not be effective and corneal transplantation may be needed.
Trichiasis	Eyelashes/ Cornea	The eyelashes grow inward (due to entropion) and rub the cornea of the eye.	The eye becomes irritated and watery, with a feeling of a foreign body in it.	Trichiasis is treated by removing the ingrown eyelashes, or by surgery to correct the entropion, as above.
Xanthelasma	Eyelid	A yellow, fatty spot or bump on the inner corner of the upper eyelid, the lower eyelid, or both eyelids.	They cause no pain but are easy to see as a cosmetic defect.	Some xanthelasmas disappear on their own, whereas others require removal by a physician by freezing the growths with liquid nitrogen, which kills the fatty tissue.
Pterygium	Cornea	A wedge-shaped fleshy growth of tissue usually found in the inner corner of the clear front covering of the eye.	A pterygium may grow large enough to interfere with vision.	Eye drops or ointments can be spread in the eye, which may be used to soothe inflammation. If the pterygium is large, threatens sight, or is unsightly, it can be removed surgically.
Strabismus	Extraocular muscles	Also described as cross eyes or wandering eyes, strabismus is a vision condition in which a person cannot focus on the same target with both eyes simultaneously under normal conditions. One or both of the eyes may turn in, out, up, or down. Strabismus occurs when the extraocular muscles do not work properly to control eye movement.	When the eye muscles do not work correctly, the eyes may become misaligned, and the brain may not be able to merge the two images, causing double vision. Left untreated, amblyopia can develop.	Glasses, patching, and surgery are the most common. Glasses can sometimes correct strabismus when the eyes are only slightly misaligned. Patching may improve amblyopia by helping the eyes to align because they would be used equally. Surgery is used to correct severe strabismus. During surgery, the doctor changes the length or position of the extraocular muscles of the eye to help it align better.

TABLE 10.1   Other Common Ocular Structural Disorders (continued)

Name of Disease or Disorder	Anatomic Site Affected	Definition of Disorder	Resulting Visual Problem or Defect	Treatment
Amaurosis fugax	Blood vessels of the eye	Amaurosis fugax is a short-lived episode of blindness in one eye caused by a blockage within the main blood vessel supplying the eye. Blockages are usually a result of a small piece of plaque breaking off a larger artery and traveling upward to the eye, becoming lodged in the main artery supplying the eye, resulting in low or no blood flow to the brain and eye.	Temporary blindness in one eye, but in rare cases, it may be prolonged or permanent.	Treatment focuses on identifying and treating the source of the obstruction or low blood flow to the eye.

Although there is no known cure or treatment for AMD, laser therapy is often used as a treatment to remove scar tissue on the macula to save remaining vision. New treatment strategies are also being explored, including retinal cell transplants that will prevent or slow down the progress of the disease, radiation therapy, gene therapies, a computer chip implanted in the retina to help stimulate vision, and ways to prevent the growth of new blood vessels under the macula.

Diagnostic Studies and Procedures

Prompt diagnosis and management is essential to help prevent the progression of many visual and structural disorders. Ophthalmologists and optometrists use a series of diagnostic tools and methods to examine the eye to determine visual acuity and to detect abnormalities.

Assessing Visual Acuity

Visual acuity is the ability to perceive detail (acuity), color and contrast, and objects. A test of visual acuity is the most common clinical measurement of visual function. The word *acuity* comes from the Latin word *acuitas*, which means "sharpness." Visual acuity is determined by modalities that are based on the full cooperation and responses of the patient and are

---

QUICK CHECK 10.2 ✓

Circle the correct word in the following sentences.

1. (Entropion/ectropion) causes the skin around the eye to become irritated.

2. (Keraclonus/keratoconus) can cause the cornea to become cone-shaped.

3. The procedure used to correct astigmatism is called (AK/RK).

4. Elderly people often experience (presbytopia/presbyopia) and have difficulty reading.

5. Another word for farsightedness is (hypertropia/myopia).

Normal focus of light rays on the retina

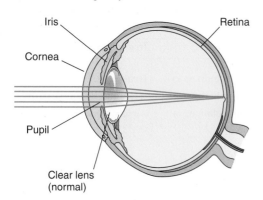

Light rays diffused by a cataract

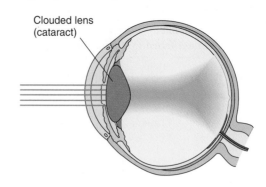

Normal daytime vision

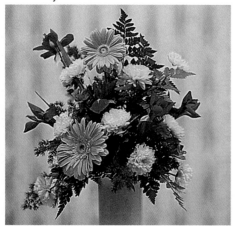

Simulation of daytime cataract vision

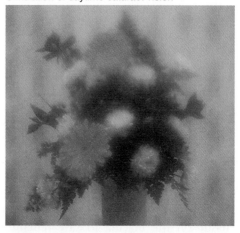

Normal nighttime vision

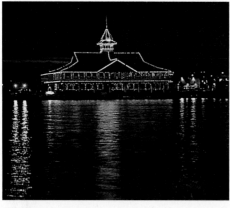

Simulation of nighttime cataract vision

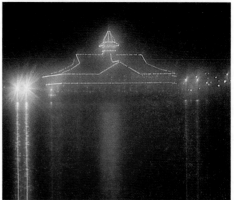

FIGURE 10.4. **The Visual Effect of Cataracts.** Reprinted with permission from Willis, MC. *Medical Terminology: A Programmed Learning Approach to the Language of Health Care.* Baltimore: Lippincott Williams & Wilkins, 2002.

entirely subjective as compared to other diagnostic studies and procedures.

Snellen Chart

Visual acuity is measured with a standard chart called the **Snellen chart**. This test requires the subject to identify a series of lines of letters from the alphabet from a distance of 20 feet (see Figure 10.5). The chart

was developed in 1862 by Dutch ophthalmologist Hermann Snellen. Snellen improved on an elementary idea of testing visual acuity in which, at the time, rather elaborate-looking characters and symbols were arranged on a chart to determine visual acuity. However, the characters were too difficult to create and reproduce to allow most clinicians to use the standard chart. Snellen's chart contained simple characters arranged in certain calibrations, printed in eleven lines

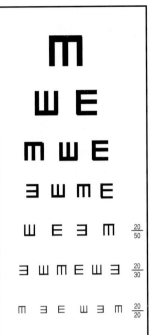

FIGURE 10.5. **Snellen Chart and the E Chart.** The Snellen chart consists of lines of different letters stacked one on top of the other. The E chart is configured just like the Snellen chart, but the characters on it are only E's, which face in all directions. Reprinted with permission from Weber J and Kelley J. *Health Assessment in Nursing*, 2nd Ed. Philadelphia: Lippincott Williams & Wilkins, 2003.

of blocked letters. The first line consists of one very large letter, *E.* Subsequent rows have increasing numbers of letters that decrease in size. The smallest row that can be read accurately indicates a patient's visual acuity in that eye. Only the nine letters C, D, E, F, L, O, P, T, and Z are used in the traditional Snellen chart. The chart could be easily reproduced by others and was quickly adopted worldwide.

For patients who cannot read or communicate verbally, an adapted version of the Snellen chart called the **E chart** is used. This chart is configured like the Snellen chart, but the characters on it consist of only the letter *E,* placed in different directions on the chart. The patient points to the direction in which the open *E* faces to assess visual acuity. Figure 10.5 shows both vision charts.

In a visual acuity test, a Snellen chart is placed 20 feet from the patient. At this distance, a patient with 20/20

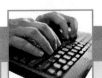

TRANSCRIPTION TIP:

The term **papilledema** refers to edema of the optic disc, often caused by increased intracranial pressure. Do not transcribe this term as *papal edema,* as it may sound in dictation.

vision is able to read the line composed of the smallest text. Therefore, at a 20-foot distance, (the top number in the fraction, or testing distance), a person with normal vision should be able to read the small 20/20 line on the Snellen eye chart. If a person can only read lines larger than the 20/20 lines, the visual acuity may be 20/30, 20/60, etc.—the more the second number (or denominator) of the fraction increases, the poorer the vision. For example, a person with 20/200 vision would have to come up to 20 feet to see a letter that a person with normal vision could see at 200 feet. Similarly, if the visual acuity is 20/15, it means that the patient's vision is better than normal.

Refraction

Refraction is a term that not only describes the process of bending light to produce a focused image on the retina, but also a procedure to determine refractive errors in the eye in order to provide a prescription for eyeglasses or contacts. This is done by the use of a **phoropter**, which is a device containing a complete range of corrective lenses to measure near-field and far-field vision. A clinician, with the use of a phoropter in conjunction with the Snellen chart, can determine the best strength of lens for correction of visual abnormalities such as myopia or hyperopia. Lenses of varying strengths are placed into the device; the patient looks through each lens and compares different levels of correction while viewing the Snellen chart. Based on the patient's responses as to how clearly he or she can view the Snellen chart with a particular combination of lenses, the clinician can prescribe the most appropriate corrective lenses or contacts.

Dilated Examination

A dilated examination of the eyes is a procedure using a specialized instrument to conduct a more extensive evaluation of the internal structure of the eye. The eye is dilated, a process called **mydriasis**, to permit enlargement of the pupil's diameter to allow the physician to observe the components of the internal eye more completely. In a darkened room, medicated eyedrops are used to dilate the pupil and make the interior structures easier to study. A physician then uses an **ophthalmoscope**, a handheld illuminated instrument containing an angled mirror and various lenses, to examine the internal structures of the eye. The physician will inspect each eye with the ophthalmoscope, which projects a beam of light and employs a magnifying lens that permits a good view of the central retina and vitreous humor. The ability to clearly examine these internal structures allows an ophthalmologist to detect signs and physiological effects of various circulatory, metabolic, and neurologic disorders such as high blood pressure and diabetes, as well as some tumors.

TRANSCRIPTION TIP:

The notation of visual acuity is transcribed as a fraction, with normal vision written as 20/20 (dictated as *twenty twenty* or *twenty over twenty*). The first number will always be 20, indicating the 20 feet between the chart and the patient. A dictated value that sounds like *twenty two hundred* would be transcribed as 20/200, not 2200 or 22/100.

Slit-Lamp Examination

A **slit lamp** is a device that consists of a table-mounted binocular microscope that shines a light into the eye to allow the doctor to examine the eye under high magnification. The slit lamp has better optics than the ophthalmoscope, providing magnification and a three-dimensional view, which allows measurement of depth. With the patient seated and the head stabilized by an adjustable chin rest and forehead strap, the physician can inspect the anterior structures of the eye such as the lens, iris, and cornea. Special lenses can be added to the slit lamp device to examine the back of the eye.

Visual Field Testing

The total area in which objects can be seen, without moving the head or eye, is known as the **visual field**. Analysis of the visual field is important in the detection of ocular disorders, particularly those of the optic nerve and brain. For example, optic nerve damage caused by glaucoma creates a very specific visual field defect. Other vision problems associated with blind spots developing within the visual field include optic nerve damage from disease or toxic exposure or dam-

age to the retina. **Visual field testing** is a series of diagnostic tests used to determine areas of impaired or absent vision due to retinal disease or some other ocular or neurologic abnormality.

Confrontation

A visual field confrontation test is a basic evaluation of the visual field performed by an examiner who sits directly facing the patient. As the patient looks into the examiner's eyes, a spot of light is moved from outside the visual field toward the center of the patient's vision. The patient is asked to indicate when he or she sees the spot of light. The test is often repeated using different sized spots of light.

Amsler Grid

The **Amsler grid** is a visual field test used to detect central visual field problems that occur in macular diseases such as macular degeneration. It consists of evenly spaced black horizontal and vertical lines printed on white paper, forming a grid. The patient is asked to look at the center of the grid where a dot is present, and to take notice of any distortion or disappearance of lines on the grid. A macular problem may exist if the lines of the grid do not appear straight and parallel areas appear to be missing.

Automated Perimetry

This test uses a computerized device called a **visual field analyzer**, which systematically plots the field of vision by determining retinal sensitivity in any given location in the visual field. In this procedure, the patient is seated with head held still in a chin rest in front of a concave dome. The patient stares at a central target within the dome. A computer-driven program flashes tiny spots of light at different locations within the dome's surface, and the patient presses a buzzer

QUICK CHECK 10.3 ✓

Indicate whether the following sentences are true (T) or false (F).

1. You cannot have better vision than 20/20.   T   F

2. Rods are responsible for vision in dim light.   T   F

3. The Snellen chart measures visual acuity.   T   F

4. The lens is mostly responsible for focusing light onto the retina.   T   F

5. The dictated figure *twenty forty* would be transcribed as *20–40*.   T   F

QUICK CHECK 10.4 ✓

Fill in the correct word in the following sentences.

1. The word *applanation* means _____.

2. The test that examines a patient's peripheral vision is called a _____ test.

3. _____ is used to evaluate the angle between the cornea and the iris.

4. The test that analyzes cornea curvature is called _____.

5. _____, a vegetable dye, is used to illuminate the retinal vasculature in the back of the eye.

---

when he or she sees the light appear in his or her peripheral vision. The lights are flashed in various levels of brightness to evaluate how sensitive the visual field is. In another version of the test, parts of the visual field are made to "shimmer," with the patient indicating which areas shimmer. At the conclusion of the test, the responses are compared to age-matched controls by the computer and the results printed out on a grid, with abnormal areas marked as black squares which represent visual-defect areas.

Applanation Tonometry

Applanation tonometry is a procedure that measures the **tension**, or balance of pressure, between the production and the drainage of the aqueous humor inside the anterior chamber of the eye, to evaluate for glaucoma. Applanation means *contact*, and in this type of tonometry the measuring device actually touches the eye. Usually drops are used to numb the eye. Then the doctor or technician will use a **tonometer**, often dictated as its brand name, **Tono-Pen**, to calculate the pressure from the change in the light reflected off the corneas and obtain a pressure reading. In noncontact tonometry, the device does not touch the eye; rather, it blows a puff of pressurized air into the eye and records the amount of pressure.

Gonioscopy

Gonioscopy is a diagnostic procedure used to evaluate the angle between the cornea and the iris. Using a slit lamp, an additional lens called a **gonio lens** is placed on the surface of the cornea under topical anesthesia (or it can be held in front of the eye) to allow examination of the angle to see if the angle where the iris meets the cornea is open or closed, showing if either open-angle or closed-angle glaucoma is present.

Fluorescein Angiography

Fluorescein angiography, also called **retinal photography**, is an eye test that uses an orange-colored fluorescent dye called **fluorescein** and a special camera to capture rapid-sequence photographs of the retinal vasculature in the back of the eye to determine if there is proper blood circulation in the retinal blood vessels. Fluorescein angiography is used for evaluation of patients with diabetic retinopathy, diseases that cause blockages to retinal veins and arteries, and some types of macular degeneration.

Fluorescein fluoresces, or glows, even in visible light. After eyedrops are administered to dilate the eyes, the dye is injected into a vein in the arm and travels to the blood vessels inside the eye. A digital camera equipped with special filters that highlight the dye then takes a series of rapid photographs of the back of the eye as the dye circulates through the blood vessels. The physician then analyzes the photographs, looking for any swelling or other abnormalities detected by the dye patterns in order to diagnose and treat the patient's condition.

Corneal Topography

Corneal topography is a test that uses a computer to analyze the curvature of the cornea. A device called a **corneal topographer** projects a series of illuminated rings onto the corneal surface; these rings are then reflected back into the instrument. The reflected rings of light are analyzed by the computer and a topographical map of the cornea is generated. The topographical map and computerized analysis reveals the corneal curvature and any distortions of the cornea, such as keratoconus or corneal scarring. This diagnostic procedure is used for patients considering laser procedures to correct refractive errors or as a followup procedure for patients who have undergone such surgical procedures.

CHAPTER SUMMARY

Although it is small, the eye is responsible for what is arguably the most important of the five senses—vision. This complex structure consists of an abundance of working parts relative to its size; the ability to see depends upon all of these parts working together properly. Remarkable advances in technology using laser light, new materials, and other high-tech tools to diagnose and treat ocular disorders have enabled physicians to achieve visual outcomes that not long ago were difficult to envision. Success in transcribing ophthalmologic reports requires familiarity with the specialized terminology used to describe the anatomy and physiology of the eye as well as a working knowledge of the diseases that affect the eyes, along with their respective treatments. A basic understanding of the visual process and common disorders that might impair vision will enable you to maximize your productivity when working in this very specialized field of human anatomy.

·I·N·S·I·G·H·T·

Stem Cells May Help Restore Eyesight

In a recent medical breakthrough, researchers discovered that stem cells may restore eyesight to people with otherwise irreversible damage to the cornea. More than a million Americans suffer corneal damage, and more than 40,000 people each year undergo cornea transplants for such injuries as chemical burns and side effects from inflammatory diseases such as lupus or shingles. According to the National Institutes of Health (NIH), corneal injuries and diseases are the leading cause of visits to eye care providers. The new study suggests that people who suffer corneal damage from chemical burn injuries or other damage may have their sight successfully restore from a corneal transplant using their own stem cells.

In the study, researchers took a small number of stem cells from the patient's undamaged limbus (the rim around the cornea) and grew the cells in the lab into viable tissue. The damaged corneal tissue was removed from the patient's eye, and the new tissue was grafted in its place. The experiment was carried out on 112 patients with corneas that were damaged by chemical burns, many of whom had been blind for years and had had unsuccessful operations to restore their vision. Sight was restored in several weeks to months, and ten years after the procedure, it was found that 78 percent of the test patients had retained their restored sight.

The breakthrough is exciting to ophthalmologists. The procedure is similar to organ transplants where the donor's body tissue must match the recipient's to avoid rejection. In this case, since the stem cells are from the patient's own body, tissue rejection would not be an issue and the patient would not need to take anti-rejection drugs. In addition, the technique is less invasive than taking a large tissue sample from the eye, lowering the chance of an eye injury.

While it is too early to be certain, the research suggests that one day this procedure may be used to save the eyesight of many patients as well as to treat other critical diseases of the eyes involving the retina or optic nerve.

Common Soundalike Words

Word	Word Pronunciation	Soundalike	Soundalike Pronunciation
cystitome: in ophthalmology, an instrument used to open the capsule of the lens of the eye. The cystitome spelled with the letter "i" pertains to the eye.	sis'ti-tōm	**cystotome**: in urology, an instrument used for incising the bladder.	sis'tō-tōm
recession: in ophthalmology, the moving of the head of an eye muscle and reimplanting it in a slightly different position for correction of strabismus.	rē-sesh'ŭn	**resection**: excision of a portion of an organ or of a structure.	rē-sek'shŭn
duction: in ophthalmology, a maneuver ("forced duction") to determine whether a mechanical obstruction is present in the eye.	dŭk'shŭn	**adduction**: movement of a body part toward the midline of the body.	ă-dŭk'shŭn
corneal: relating to the cornea of the eye.	kōr'nē-ăl	**cornual**: relating to the horns of the uterus where the fallopian tubes join the uterine cavity.	kōr'nyū-ăl
LASIK: acronym for laser-assisted in situ keratomileusis, a vision correction procedure.	lā'-sik	**Lasix**: a drug used to treat excessive fluid accumulation and swelling of the body.	lā'-siks
macula: the central part of the retina.	mak'yū-lă	**macule**: a small, discolored patch or spot on the skin, neither elevated above nor depressed below the skin's surface.	mak'yūl
esotropia: inward turning of the eye.	es-ō-trō'pē-ă	**exotropia**: outward turning of the eye.	ek-sō-trō'pē-ă
buckle: in ophthalmology, a technique for repair of retinal detachment ("scleral buckle").	bŭk'ăl	**buccal**: the cheek area of the mouth.	bŭk'ăl
intraocular: within the eye.	in'-tră-ok'yū-lăr	**intraauricular**: within the ear.	in'-tră-aw-rik'yu-lăr
scotoma: an isolated area of depressed vision (a blind spot).	skō-tō'mă	**scatoma**: a tumor in the rectum.	skă-to'ma

Combining Forms

Combining Form	Meaning	Combining Form	Meaning
ambly/o	dullness, dimness	ocul/o, ophthalm/o	eye
blephar/o	eyelids	opt/o, optic/o	vision
bulb/a	globe, eyeball	palpebr/a	eyelid
cili/o	eyelashes	phac/o, phak/o	lens
conjunctiv/o	conjunctiva	phot/o	light
core/o, pupill/o	pupil	presby/o	old
corne/o, kerat/o	cornea	retin/o	retina
dacry/o	tears, lacrimal duct or sac	scler/o	sclera
dipl/o	double	tars/o	tarsal plate
icter/o	jaundice	trich/o	hair (eyelashes)
ir/o, irid/o	iris	xer/o	dry
lacrim/o	tear		

Add Your Own Combining Forms Here:

_____

_____

_____

_____

_____

_____

ABBREVIATIONS

Abbreviation	Meaning	Abbreviation	Meaning
AK	astigmatic keratotomy	PERRLA	pupils equal, round, and reactive to light and accommodation
AMD	age-related macular degeneration	PRK	photorefractive keratectomy
CK	conductive keratoplasty	RK	radial keratotomy
CTK	laser thermokeratoplasty	YAG	An acronym for a rather complicated chemical compound used as the lasing medium in certain solid-state lasers used in vision correction surgery.
EOMI	extraocular muscles (or movements) intact		
ICL	implantable Collamer lens		
IOL	intraocular lens		
LASIK	laser in situ keratomileusis		

Add Your Own Abbreviations Here:

_____

_____

_____

_____

_____

_____

TERMINOLOGY

Term	Meaning
accommodation	The process of the lens becoming thicker or thinner in order to change focus between objects that are near and more distant.
age-related macular degeneration (AMD)	A disease that is caused by the malfunction of the photosensitive cells in the macula, causing distortion of images in the center of the visual field, darkened area in the center of an image, and diminished color a perception.
aging eyes	Another term for *presbyopia*.
amblyopia	A condition where the brain does not fully acknowledge the images seen by one eye, resulting in the abnormal development of vision pathways to the brain.
Amsler grid	A grid of evenly spaced black horizontal and vertical lines on a sheet of white paper with a dot in the center, used to evaluate for macular problems.
anterior chamber	The smaller, front section of the eye filled with fluid that nourishes the internal structures of the eye and helps maintain its shape and pressure.

Term	Meaning
applanation tonometry	A procedure that measures the pressure in the eye when evaluating for glaucoma.
aqueous humor	The waterlike fluid that fills the anterior chamber of the eye.
astigmatic keratotomy (AK)	A procedure to improve vision similar to RK, but using a curved pattern of incisions into the cornea rather than a radial pattern.
astigmatism	A condition of impaired eyesight resulting from the irregular conformation of the cornea, causing light to be focused irregularly in different parts of the eye, resulting in blurred vision.
canal of Schlemm	A circular canal that provides a drainage system for the aqueous humor from the eye into the bloodstream.
cataract	A clouding or opacity of the lens, causing loss of vision.
ciliary body	A thin, transparent capsule of muscular tissue containing the lens.
conductive keratoplasty (CK)	A procedure to improve vision that shrinks the collagen in the cornea by using heat from low-level radiofrequency waves.
cones	Cells in the photoreceptor layer that are responsible for fine color vision.
conjunctiva	A thin, clear layer of skin covering the sclera and eyelid.
conjunctivitis	An infection of the conjunctival layer of the eye.
cornea	The clear layer located at the front and center of the eye.
corneal topographer	A device that projects a series of illuminated rings onto the corneal surface of the eye in order to analyze and map the corneal curvature of the eye.
corneal topography	A test that uses a computer to analyze the curvature of the cornea.
crystalline lens	A clear, flexible structure that allows for fine focusing of light as it passes through the eye.
diabetic retinopathy	A degenerative eye disease in which diabetes causes damage to the blood vessels that nourish the retina.
diplopia	The result of light being split into two images by a defect in the eye's optical system.
double vision	Another term for *diplopia*.
drusen	Yellow waste deposits that accumulate under the retina.
dry macular degeneration	A form of macular degeneration in which the cells of the macula slowly begin to break down.
E chart	A chart configured like the Snellen chart but with different directions of the letter *E* placed on it for those patients who cannot read or have difficulty communicating verbally.
eumelanin	Brown-black melanins produced by melanocytes, which contribute to iris color.
extraocular muscles	Three pairs of muscles attached to the sclera that help move the eye in different directions.
eyelashes	Hairs attached to the edge of the eyelids.
eyelids	Folds of skin that protect the front of the eyeball.
farsightedness	Another term for *hyperopia*.
fluorescein	An orange-colored dye used in fluorescein angiography to help identify and photograph the retinal blood vessels.
fluorescein angiography, syn. retinal photography	An eye test that evaluates the retinal vasculature in the back of the eye.

Term	Meaning
fovea centralis ("fovea")	The center of the macula. The fovea is the point of the sharpest and most acute visual acuity.
glaucoma	A disease of the eye that causes damage to the optic nerve.
gonio lens	A special lens used in gonioscopic examination that indicates blockage or damage in the area where fluid drains from the eye.
gonioscopy	A diagnostic procedure used to evaluate the angle between the cornea and the iris when testing for glaucoma.
horizontal gaze nystagmus	An involuntary jerking or movement of the eyes that occurs as a person follows an object with the eyes to the side.
hyperopia	An ocular condition in which light rays are improperly focused behind the retina resulting in blurred vision.
hyphema	The presence of blood in the anterior chamber of the eye.
implantable Collamer lens (ICL) procedure	A surgical procedure whereby an ophthalmologist injects a specially formulated pliable lens into the eye that "unfolds" in the eye to correct nearsightedness.
intraocular lens	A permanent plastic lens that is implanted into the eye during cataract surgery.
irrigation-aspiration device	A device used in cataract surgery that flushes lens debris with fluid and then uses suction to remove pieces of lens from the eye.
iris	The colored part of the eye that controls the amount of light that enters the eye.
lacrimal gland	The gland that secretes tears.
laser in situ keratomileusis (LASIK)	A procedure that involves correcting the shape of the cornea, and, hence, nearsightedness.
laser thermokeratoplasty (LTK)	A procedure that treats hyperopia by shrinking the collagen in the cornea by means of a YAG laser.
lazy eye	Another term for *amblyopia*.
lens	A clear, flexible structure located just behind the iris and pupil that allows for fine focusing of light as it passes through the eye.
macula	The center area of the retina responsible for central vision, seeing color, and distinguishing fine detail.
meibomian glands	Glands in the eyelids that secrete oils that lubricate the eyelids.
microkeratome	A surgical instrument used to cut into the cornea and remove tissue.
mydriasis	Dilation of the pupils.
myopia	An optic condition in which light rays are improperly focused in front of the retina, resulting in blurred vision.
nasolacrimal ducts	Two tiny canals at the end of each eyelid that drain tears into the nose.
nearsightedness	Another term for *myopia*.
nystagmus	An involuntary rhythmic shaking or movement of the eyes.
ophthalmologist	A medical doctor who performs eye surgery as well as diagnoses and treats eye diseases and injuries.
ophthalmology	The study of the eye.
ophthalmoscope	A handheld illuminated instrument containing an angled mirror and various lenses to examine the internal structures of the eye.
optic disc	The region at the back of the eye where the optic nerve meets the retina, often called the "blind spot" of the eye.

Term	Meaning
optic nerve	The structure in the back of the eye responsible for transmitting nerve signals from the retina to the brain.
optician	An individual who manufactures, verifies, and delivers lenses, frames, and other specially fabricated optical devices.
optometrist	A professional who examines people's eyes to diagnose vision problems and eye diseases.
orbit	The bony eye socket located on the frontal surface of the skull.
papilledema	Edema of the optic disc caused by intracranial pressure.
phacoemulsification	A process whereby the cloudy lens is removed from the eye during cataract surgery.
pheomelanin	Red-yellow melanins produced by melanocytes that contribute to iris color.
phoropter	A device that contains a range of corrective lenses for measurement of near-field and far-field visual acuity.
photoreceptor layer	The outermost layer of the retina where light is focused and converted into nerve impulses.
photorefractive keratectomy (PRK)	A procedure to improve vision in which the surface of the cornea is reshaped using a laser device but without cutting into the cornea itself.
posterior chamber	The larger, back section of the eye filled with fluid that nourishes the internal structures of the eye and helps maintain its shape and pressure.
presbyopia	A condition that occurs when the lens loses the ability to focus due to the natural aging process.
pupil	The black opening or aperture in the iris where light enters the eye.
radial keratotomy (RK)	A procedure to improve vision that involves placing radial incisions in the peripheral cornea to correct myopia.
refraction	A process in which light is bent by the lens in order to produce a focused image on the retina. In optometry, an optical test which uses a device incorporating lenses of various strengths to measure near-field and far-field vision and to determine the corrective lens required for correction of such vision abnormalities as myopia or hyperopia.
refractive errors	Disorders that cause improper focusing of the eye and subsequent blurring of vision.
retina	A light-sensitive layer of thin tissue that lines the inside of the back part of the eye.
rods	Cells in the photoreceptor layer that are responsible for vision in dim light.
sclera	The tough outer white layer that gives the eye its spherical shape.
scotoma	An isolated area of varying size and shape, within the visual field, in which vision is absent or depressed; a *blind spot*.
slit lamp	A device that consists of a moveable light source and a binocular microscope that is used to examine the eye under high magnification.
Snellen chart	The standardized visual chart for measuring eyesight.
tarsus	Connective tissue making up the eyelids.
tension	A name given to the balance of pressure in the eye.
tonometer (Tono-Pen)	A device used to calculate the pressure in the eye from the change in the light reflected off the corneas.
trabeculectomy	A procedure to treat glaucoma where an opening is surgically created in the wall of the eye so that aqueous humor can drain.

Term	Meaning
trabeculoplasty	A procedure to treat glaucoma where the laser is focused into the eye in such a way as to let aqueous fluid leave the eye more efficiently.
visual acuity	The ability to perceive detail (acuity), color and contrast, and to distinguish objects.
visual field	The total area in which objects can be seen, without moving the head or eye.
visual field analyzer	A computerized device that analyzes the patient's response to the visual field test by charting the limits of the patient's peripheral vision.
visual field testing	Diagnostic tests that are used to determine areas of impaired or absent vision due to an ocular or neurologic abnormality.
vitrectomy	A procedure performed to remove the vitreous and replace it with a salt solution.
vitreous humor	The waterlike fluid that fills the posterior chamber of the eye.
wet macular degeneration	The form of macular degeneration that results after the dry form of the disease, when blood vessels grow abnormally behind the macula and begin to leak fluid and blood.
YAG laser	A type of solid-state laser used in vision correction surgery.

Add Your Own Terms and Definitions Here:

_____

_____

_____

_____

_____

_____

_____

REVIEW QUESTIONS

1. What is the primary (most powerful) focusing structure of the eye?
2. Which type of photoreceptor is most sensitive to bright light and color?
3. In which eye disorder does too much intraocular pressure damage optic nerve fibers?
4. What is the purpose of a visual field test?
5. As an increasing amount of light enters the eye, what does the pupil do?
6. What ocular disorder can develop if strabismus is not corrected?
7. What is the purpose of applanation tonometry?
8. What is the difference between an optometrist and an ophthalmologist?
9. What ocular disorder is the result of a complication of high levels of glucose?
10. What is fluorescein used for?

CHAPTER ACTIVITIES

Soundalike Word Choice

Circle the correct word in the following sentences.

1. (Florisil, Fluorescein) is a special dye used to photograph the retinal vasculature in the back of the eye.
2. Sarah's grandfather underwent a test for glaucoma using (approbation, applanation) tonometry.
3. On examination, the patient's pupils react briskly without (apparent, afferent) pupillary defect.
4. I discussed surgical correction of the patient's (nystagmus, nystatin) in depth with her.
5. Mr. Borello underwent a scleral (buckle, buccal) procedure to repair his retinal detachment last year.
6. The pain in the patient's left eye was caused by a (corneal, cornual) tear.
7. The pupils go through a process called (accumulation, accommodation) in order allow the lens to change focus between objects that are near and those that are more distant.
8. The irregular (refraction, reflection) of light by the cornea and lens established Mariah's myopia diagnosis.
9. After her (LASIX, LASIK) procedure, Janet found she no longer needed her glasses.
10. (Hyphema, Hyperemia), or bleeding in the anterior chamber of the eye, was eventually found to be the cause of the patient's loss of vision in the right eye.

Fill in the Blanks

Fill in the blanks with the correct term.

The human eye rests in a bony cavity called the _____, located on the frontal surface of the skull. The visible parts of the eye are composed of the clear layer in front of the eye called the _____, the white area called the _____, and the _____, which gives the eye its color. The sclera is attached to muscles in the eye called the _____. When light enters the eye, it travels through the _____ and is finely adjusted into focus by the _____, which then focuses the light onto the _____. Rods and cones are called _____, which convert the image into nerve impulses along the _____ to the brain.

Matching

Match the combining forms on the left with the definitions on the right.

Combining Form   **Definition**

_____ 1. xer/o   A. lens
_____ 2. scler/o   B. old
_____ 3. bulb/a   C. dry
_____ 4. irid/o   D. double
_____ 5. phot/o   E. vision
_____ 6. blephar/o   F. light
_____ 7. phac/o   G. (hair) eyelashes
_____ 8. dipl/o   H. pupil
_____ 9. trich/o   I. iris
_____ 10. optic/o   J. retina
_____ 11. presby/o   K. sclera
_____ 12. ambly/o   L. dullness, dimness
_____ 13. kerat/o   M. eyelids
_____ 14. retin/o   N. globe, eyeball
_____ 15. core/o   O. cornea

Medical Word Building

Build words by combining the correct root with the suffix appearing next to it. Write a definition for each term in the space at the right. Verify the spelling and definitions with a medical dictionary.

Root/Combining Form	Suffix	Word	Meaning
1. blephar/o	-plasty	_____	_____
	-itis	_____	_____
2. ophthalm/o	-logy	_____	_____
	-ic	_____	_____
3. retin/o	-ectomy	_____	_____
	-oid	_____	_____
4. kerat/o	-ectasia	_____	_____
	-graphy	_____	_____
5. scler/o	-ostomy	_____	_____
	-plasty	_____	_____
6. ocul/o	-dynia	_____	_____
	-ar	_____	_____
7. irid/o	-esis	_____	_____
	-ology	_____	_____
8. ambly/o	-scope	_____	_____
	-pia	_____	_____
9. tars/o	-itis	_____	_____
	-rrhaphy	_____	_____
10. core/o	-plasty	_____	_____
	-praxy	_____	_____

Multiple Choice

Circle the letter corresponding to the best answer to each of the following questions.

1. Visual acuity is tested by using a
    A. Snellen chart.
    B. Amsler grid.
    C. gonioscopy mirror.
    D. corneal topographer.

2. Another name for the tear duct is the
    A. corneal gland.
    B. tarsal gland.
    C. lacrimal gland.
    D. orbital gland.

3. The process of bending light to produce a focused image on the retina is called
    A. reflection.
    B. reorganization.
    C. refraction.
    D. remission.

4. PERRLA is an acronym that stands for
    A. pupils emergent, round, and reactive to light and accommodation.
    B. pupils equal, round, and reactive to light.
    C. pupils equal, raised, and reactive.
    D. pupils equal, round, and reactive to light and accommodation.

5. The correct name for *pink eye* is
    A. scleritis.
    B. conjunctivitis.
    C. blepharitis.
    D. retinal detachment.

6. The condition that causes irregularities in the central field of vision is called
    A. keratitis.
    B. macular degeneration.
    C. chalazion.
    D. myopia.

7. The part of the eye that is often called the "white of the eye" is called the
    A. pupil.
    B. cornea.
    C. iris.
    D. sclera.

8. The lens is enclosed in a capsule of muscular tissue called the
    A. ciliary body.
    B. retina.
    C. cilious tissue.
    D. cicatricial body.

9. Hyperopia refers to
    A. farsightedness.
    B. nearsightedness.
    C. double vision.
    D. crossed eyes.

10. During cataract surgery, the clouded lens is removed and replaced with a plastic lens called a (an)
    A. irrigation device.
    B. intravisual lens.
    C. intraocular lens.
    D. laser lens.

Understanding Medical Documents

Read the following excerpt from a procedure note and, using resource materials or the Internet to locate terms you do not know, answer the questions that follow.

S: This 15-year-old Hispanic male presents with mother for irritated eyes. He is having some drainage in the morning with some crusted lids. His brother had a similar episode in the past for a few weeks. He was put on Polytrim ophthalmic drops by a nurse practitioner and it improved, though did not completely resolve, and this patient also tried that with similar results. He is having nasal congestion and has a concern for allergies.

O: No acute distress. Blood pressure 120/83, heart rate 72, afebrile. OP within normal limits. Eyes are irritated and with some injected sclerae. Moderate nasal congestion. Lungs: Clear to auscultation. Heart: Regular rate and rhythm.

A: Probable seasonal allergies with allergic rhinitis and conjunctivitis.

P: Hold on the Polytrim drops. Start an over-the-counter allergy drop with pheniramine such as Naphcon-A. Erythromycin ophthalmic ointment for use at night. Continue loratadine and return to clinic if symptoms persist or worsen. Others in the family have a similar issue. If the Polytrim was not effective, likely this is allergies since it has lasted for several weeks.

Questions

1. What prescription medicine was tried without resolution of the symptoms?

   _____

2. What type of medical provider is mentioned in the report besides the physician?

   _____

3. What is the generic name for Polytrim?

   _____

4. What is the brand name for loratadine and what does it do?

   _____

5. What findings in the physical exam would lead the physician to believe this might be an allergic process and not an infectious process?

   _____

6. What do you think the "A" in Naphcon-A stands for?

   _____

7. What does OP stand for?

   _____

8. What is conjunctivitis?

   _____

9. What does the term *afebrile* mean?

   _____

10. Why did the physician conclude that the patient's presentation might be due to an allergic, as opposed to an infectious, process?

    _____

TRANSCRIPTION PRACTICE

Open your word-processing software. Insert the student CD-ROM and locate the dictation for this chapter. For each of the words in the "listen for these terms" list for each report, use a medical dictionary or other resource to identify and write down a brief definition of the terms on a separate sheet of paper to attach with your work. Then listen to the dictation and transcribe each report. Use the current date for each report where a date is indicated. Insert a heading into the document if the text falls on a second page.

At the end of each report, indicate the name of the dictating physician under the signature line and insert reference initials. For date dictated and transcribed and date of admission, use the current date. Proofread your work, print one copy for your instructor along with your term definitions, and save the completed report to your student disk.

Report #T10.1: Letter
Patient Name: Margaret Haldeman
Medical Record No.: 94527311
Consulting Physician: Sabrina Scott, MD
Attending Physician: James Davis, MD

Listen for this term:
dermatochalasis

Report #T10.2: SOAP Note
Patient Name: Michael Haldeman
Medical Record No.: 94527311
Attending Surgeon: Andrea Biggs, MD

Listen for these terms:
conjunctivitis
chalazion
ophthalmologist

Report #T10.3: Operative Report
Patient Name: Rayella Sadiqqi
Medical Record No.: 80345557
Attending Surgeon: Andrea Biggs, MD

Listen for these terms:
phacoemulsification
intraocular lens
diopters
ptosis
Cyclogyl
Ocuflox
Ocular
Super blade
retrobulbar
paracentesis
keratome
cystitome
capsulorrhexis
hydrodissection
Provisc
Kuglen hook

11

OTORHINOLARYNGOLOGY

OBJECTIVES

After completing this chapter, you will be able to:

- Describe and locate the general anatomic structures of the ear, nose, and throat.
- Understand and explain the process of hearing.
- Describe common diseases and disorders that affect the ears, nose, and throat and the medical treatments most commonly used to address them.
- Explain common diagnostic procedures used to investigate diseases and disorders of the ears, nose, and throat.

INTRODUCTION

The ears, nose, and throat all play important roles in the efficient functioning of the human body: The ears enable us to hear and also provide a sense of balance and equilibrium; the nose is responsible for our sense of smell and also helps us to breathe; the throat is involved in breathing, as well as in helping us to take in nourishment and to communicate with others. This chapter explores the anatomic features of the ears, nose, and throat (ENT) and also provides a basic understand-ing of the symptoms, mechanisms, and treatments of common ENT disorders.

WHAT IS OTORHINOLARYNGOLOGY?

Otorhinolaryngology—the study of the ear, nose, and throat—is the oldest medical specialty in the United States. The term derives from three Greek root words: *oto*, meaning *ear*; *rhino*, meaning *nose*; and *laryn*, meaning *throat*. The more commonly used term, otolaryngology, is actually the abbreviated form of otorhinolaryngology. Otolaryngologists, commonly referred to as ENT physi-cians, differ from general practice physicians in that they are trained in both medicine and surgery. In the last sev-eral years, the study of otorhinolaryngology has evolved from the ear, nose, and throat to a regional specialty of the head and neck. Otolaryngologists subspecialize in more than a dozen areas including otology (the study of the ear), neuro-otology (the branch of medicine con-cerned with the nervous system related to the auditory and vestibular systems of the ear), plastic surgery of the face and neck, nasal and sinus disorders, voice and swal-lowing problems, audiology (the diagnosis of disease through the evaluation of hearing loss), and upper air-way obstruction. In addition to providing medical care in the office, otolaryngologists also perform head and neck surgery, including treatments for the ear, nose, skull base, sinuses, pharynx, larynx, oral cavity, neck, thyroid, salivary glands, bronchial tubes, and esophagus, as well as cosmetic surgery of the face and neck. In addition, some otolaryngologists specialize in restoring hearing through microsurgical procedures that can correct deafness. Surgical techniques used by these specialists can also cure disease and infection and repair deformities present in the ear since birth. Finally, with their extensive knowledge of the head and neck, many otolaryngologists are also proficient in plastic reconstruction surgery of the nose, ears, jaw, and facial area to restore function and appearance.

ANATOMY OF THE EARS, NOSE, AND THROAT

The structures of the ears, nose, and throat are so closely connected to each other that an infection or disorder affecting one structure often passes to another. The anatomy and physiology of each structure, and how these structures relate to each other, is explained below.

Ear

The ears, positioned in the hollow spaces in the temporal bone on either side of the skull, are divided into three regions, each of which has its own function: the outer ear, the middle ear, and the inner ear. The **ear** is the organ responsible for hearing and balance and is the primary organ for two sensory systems: the **auditory system**, involved in the detection of sound, and the **vestibular system**, the part of the ear involved with maintaining the body's equilibrium (see Figure 11.1).

Sound waves traveling through the air are received by the ear and are changed first into mechanical vibrations and then into electrical nerve impulses, which are sent to the brain and interpreted as sounds. The ear also senses the body's position relative to gravity, sending information to the brain that allows the body to maintain its balance.

Outer Ear

The **outer ear** consists of the external, visible part of the ear, called the **pinna** or **auricle**, and the tubular passage leading inward to the eardrum, called the **external auditory canal**. The pinna is the outer, shell-like structure on

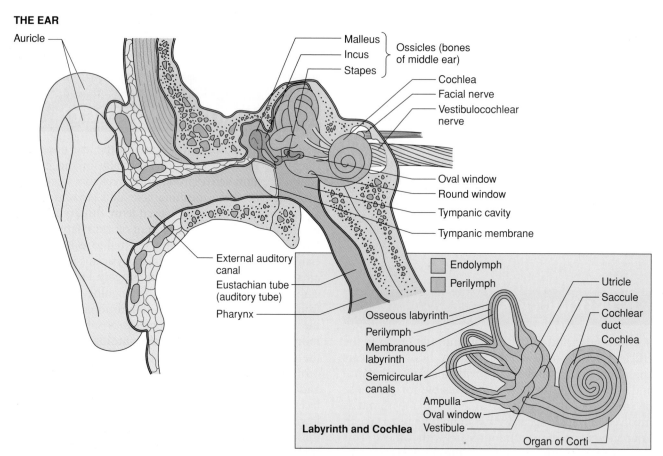

THE EAR

Auricle

Malleus
Incus
Stapes
} Ossicles (bones of middle ear)

Cochlea
Facial nerve
Vestibulocochlear nerve

Oval window
Round window
Tympanic cavity
Tympanic membrane

External auditory canal
Eustachian tube (auditory tube)
Pharynx

Osseous labyrinth
Perilymph
Membranous labyrinth
Semicircular canals

Endolymph
Perilymph

Utricle
Saccule
Cochlear duct
Cochlea

Ampulla
Oval window
Vestibule

Labyrinth and Cochlea

Organ of Corti

FIGURE 11.1. **Gross Anatomy of the Human Ear.** Reprinted with permission from Willis MC. *Medical Terminology: A Programmed Learning Approach to the Language of Health Care.* Baltimore: Lippincott Williams & Wilkins, 2002.

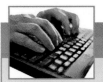

TRANSCRIPTION TIP:

Like ophthalmologists, ENT physicians often dictate abbreviations to indicate the left ear, right ear, and both ears. The abbreviations *AD, AS,* and *AU,* stand for *aurus dextra* (right ear), *aurus sinistra* (left ear), and *aures uterque* (both ears). However, the Institute for Safe Medication Practices (ISMP) has included these abbreviations among those that are frequently misinterpreted and involved in harmful medication errors. These abbreviations should be expanded when used in general reference; however, they should be abbreviated when associated with diagnostic testing and measured values. Check with your employer as to whether these abbreviations are acceptable when transcribing.

the side of the head. The pinna is a cartilaginous appendage that collects sound waves and funnels them into the external auditory canal to the **tympanic membrane**, commonly called the *eardrum*, a semitransparent membrane that separates the outer ear from the middle ear. The external auditory canal contains fine hairs and sweat glands that secrete **cerumen**, or ear wax, which protects the eardrum from damage by trapping dust and dirt. Cerumen usually dries up and falls out of the external auditory canal, but when it builds up, it can cause pain and hearing problems. The tympanic membrane lies at the end of the external auditory canal and divides the outer ear and the middle ear. Pearly gray in color, it reflects some of a physician's examining light shined on it, called a **light reflex**.

Middle Ear

The **middle ear** lies inside the skull with only a very thin layer of bone separating it from the brain. Located behind the eardrum, it consists of a small, air-filled chamber carved out of bone. It contains the **ossicular chain**, a chain of three movable tiny bones called **ossicles** that connect the eardrum to the middle ear. The three bones, the names of which are derived from the Latin terms for their shapes, are called the **malleus** (hammer), which is attached to the eardrum; the **incus** (anvil), the second bone in the chain; and the **stapes** (stirrup). If any one of these bones becomes damaged, the patient will experience a loss of hearing. Sound waves received by the tympanic membrane are converted by the ossicles into mechanical vibrations, which are then transmitted along the ossicular chain through the middle ear to the thin membrane that covers the opening to the inner ear called the **oval window**.

A short, narrow passage called the **eustachian tube** connects the middle ear to the back of the nose and throat. The eustachian tube functions to equalize air pressure on both sides of the eardrum, allowing air to enter the middle ear. This tube opens when a person swallows to allow air in or out for about one-tenth to one-thirteenth of a second, which helps to maintain equal pressure and prevents fluid, such as those from infections, from accumulating in the middle ear. Equal air pressure ensures that the eardrum vibrates maximally when struck by sound waves. If air pressure is not equal, the eardrum may bulge or retract, causing pain and distortion of sound. The act of swallowing or "popping the ears" relieves the buildup of pressure on the eardrum. The **Valsalva maneuver** is a maneuver that increases pressure in the nasopharynx, forcing air into the eustachian tube as all other outlets are blocked, which causes the "popping" of the ears.

Inner Ear

The **inner ear**, also called the **labyrinth**, lies deep in the temporal bones of the skull. By definition, a labyrinth is a complex system of paths and tunnels. In human anatomy, the term *labyrinth* refers to anatomic structures with numerous intercommunicating cells or canals. The inner ear consists of a maze of fluid-filled tubes running through the temporal bone, responsible for both hearing and balance. The inner ear functions to turn the mechanical vibrations received from the ossicles of the middle ear to nerve impulses. As it is not possible to view the inner ear during a clinical examination, this part of the ear is examined by testing of hearing and balance.

The inner ear consists of two major parts: the **cochlea**, a snail-shaped structure that is the organ of hearing, and the vestibular system, which regulates balance. The cochlea is filled with fluid and contains nerve fibers and specialized hair cells that detect different sound levels and frequencies. These cells vibrate when sound is transmitted from the middle ear to the inner ear, and the vibrations are picked up by the **organ of Corti**, the hearing mechanism housed in the cochlea. The organ of Corti contains specialized nerve endings that convert the vibrations into nerve impulses and

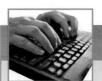

TRANSCRIPTION TIP:

When taking a patient's history, the physician may refer to the patient complaining of a sensation of *aural fullness* in the ear. Do not confuse the soundalike term *aural,* which relates to the ear, with *oral,* which relates to the mouth. A patient complaining of hearing difficulties would not complain of *oral fullness.*

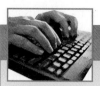

TRANSCRIPTION TIP:

The term *meatus* means a channel or *external opening* and is frequently heard in dictation regarding canals of the ears, nose, and throat. Keep in mind the plural of *meatus* is *meatus*, not *meati*, as often dictated; the term *meatus* is both singular and plural.

transmit them via the internal auditory canal to the auditory center of the brain, which interprets the impulses as sound.

Loud noise can damage and destroy the hair cells in the cochlea. Once these cells are damaged, they cannot grow back. Continued exposure to loud noise eventually causes progressive damage and hearing abnormalities such as ringing in the ears, called **tinnitus**.

The vestibular system consists of saclike structures called the **utricle** and **saccule**, and three **semicircular canals**. Collectively known as the **vestibular organs**, they sense the body's relationship to gravity, which keeps the body erect and maintains balance. The semicircular canals lie perpendicular to each other in order to sense movement. Depending on the direction of the movement of the head, fluid flows through the canals, initiating nerve impulses that travel to the brain and carry information about the position of the body. If the semicircular canals malfunction, a person's sense of balance may be impaired. For example, excessive stimulation of the semicircular canals results in motion sickness.

Nose

The **nose** is the organ of smell, or **olfactory** sense. It is also responsible for warming and saturating inspired air, filtering bacteria and debris, and conserving heat and moisture from expired air (Figure 11.2).

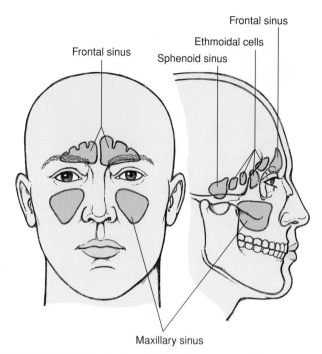

FIGURE 11.3. The Paranasal Sinuses. Locations of the paranasal sinuses that connect to the nose. Reprinted with permission from *Stedman's Medical Dictionary*, 27th ed. Baltimore: Lippincott Williams & Wilkins 2000.

The nose consists of the external nose and the nasal cavity, both of which are divided into right and left halves. The framework of the external nose is made up of a nasal bone, which forms the upper part, or **nasal dorsum**, of the nose, and the upper jaw bone, or **maxilla**. The **nasal septum** is a vertical wall made of bone and cartilage, which separates the nostrils into right and left sides. The flared cartilage on each side of the nostril is called the nasal **ala**.

By definition, a **sinus** is a hollow cavity or space in bone or other tissue. In the nose, a **nasal sinus** is an air-filled, mucus-lined cavity within the cranial or facial bone. The nasal cavities surrounding the nose are called **paranasal sinuses**, which connect to the nose through a small opening in each called the **ostium**. As shown in Figure 11.3, there are four groups of paranasal sinuses, each named after the facial bone in which it is located:

- **Maxillary sinuses**, one sinus on each side, located behind the skin of each cheek.
- **Ethmoid sinuses**, approximately 6 to 12 small sinuses per side, located around the bridge of the nose.
- **Frontal sinuses**, one sinus per side, located in the forehead
- **Sphenoid sinuses**, one sinus per side, located deep in the face behind the nose, near the center of the skull.

The nose itself is divided by the nasal septum into two nasal cavities, called the nostrils or **nares**. In nasal

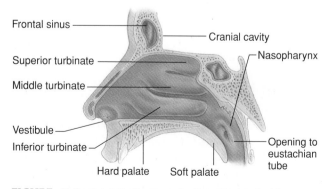

FIGURE 11.2. Nasal Cavity Cross-Section. Reprinted with permission from Bickley LS, Szilagyi, P. *Bates' Guide to Physical Examination and History Taking*, 8th ed. Philadelphia: Lippincott Williams & Wilkins 2003.

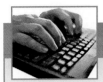

anatomy, a **nasal turbinate** or **concha,** is a long, narrow, and curled bone shelflike structure (shaped like an elongated seashell), which protrudes into the breathing passage of the nose. The side wall of the nose contains three nasal turbinates—the superior, middle, and inferior turbinates—the function of which is to trap particles entering the nasal passages. Each turbinate is a rounded projection that extends the length of the nasal cavity. The passage that is created by the overhanging edge of each of these turbinates is called a **meatus.** The nasal turbinates, or conchae, slow down inhaled air so that it can pick up warmth and moisture before entering the lungs. The middle turbinate (and sometimes other turbinates) that becomes filled with air cells is called **concha bullosa.** The term *bullosa* refers to a bubblelike structure, and this ballooning of the concha with air can cause nasal obstruction and facial pain and pressure from blockage of the sinus outflow tracts.

The nasal cavity is lined with **nasal mucosa,** a mucous membrane that produces **mucus,** a thick, slippery substance that lubricates and protects the delicate lining of the areas of body where mucous membranes are present—in this case, the lining of the inside of the nose.

Throat

The **pharynx,** also known as the *throat,* is the passageway that lies behind the mouth and nasal cavities just above the esophagus. The pharynx has openings to all three of these regions and functions as the passage for air as well as solid and liquid nourishment. It includes structures used in the processes of breathing, speaking, and swallowing. The pharynx also serves both the respiratory and digestive systems by receiving air from the nose and air and nourishment from the mouth. The pharynx is divided into three sections according to location: the nasopharynx, the oropharynx, and the hypopharynx.

Nasopharynx

The **nasopharynx** lies immediately behind the nose and extends to the **uvula,** which is the pendant, fleshy mass seen hanging from the soft palate, which is the muscular part of the back of the roof of the mouth. The uvula helps prevent food and fluids from entering the nasal cavity during swallowing. Air from the nose passes through the nasopharynx on its way down to the lungs. The eustachian tubes, which connect the middle ear to the throat, are found on the side walls of the nasopharynx.

Oropharynx

The **oropharynx** lies at the back of the mouth and includes the soft palate, the tonsils, the posterior third of the tongue, and the posterior wall of the throat.

Hypopharynx

The **hypopharynx,** also called the *laryngopharynx,* is the most distal—or most inferior—portion of the pharynx and is the part of the throat that connects to the esophagus. The hypopharynx lies below the aperture of the larynx and behind the larynx and extends from the vestibule of the larynx to the esophagus at the level of the inferior border of the cricoid cartilage.

The **tonsils** and **adenoids** are masses of lymphoid tissue in the pharynx. They are part of the defense system that the body uses to fight off infection. The tonsils are located on each side of the entrance to the oropharynx. The adenoids are situated in the nasopharynx. The eustachian tubes open in the pharynx very close to the adenoids. If the adenoids become inflamed, they can block the opening of the eustachian tubes. When this happens, infection can develop in the middle ear.

Larynx

The **larynx** is a tube-shaped structure leading from the pharynx to the **trachea** (commonly called the *windpipe*) and is part of the passageway for air between the pharynx above and the lungs below. It comprises a complex system of muscles, cartilages, and connective tissue and protects the trachea from the inhalation of food and liquids. The larynx also houses the vocal folds and the muscles that control the position and tension of these elements. This part of the larynx is also referred to as the voice box. Because of its location, the larynx plays a vital role in breathing, swallowing, and speaking. Part of the anatomy of the larynx includes a single U-shaped bone called the **hyoid.** The hyoid bone is isolated from all other bones. It is connected by ligaments to the styloid processes of the temporal bones. Muscles from the tongue, neck, pharynx, and larynx that attach to the hyoid bone contribute to the movements involved in swallowing and speech.

The superior or uppermost cartilage of the larynx is the **epiglottis,** a lidlike flap of cartilage that lies above and in front of the larynx. The epiglottis opens and closes to help direct food and liquid into the esophagus and to protect the vocal cords and airway during swallowing. The largest cartilage of the larynx, called the **thyroid cartilage,** can be felt at the front of the throat as what is commonly called the "Adam's apple." Other cartilages of the larynx include the **cricoid**, which lies below the thyroid cartilage and encircles the airway; the **arytenoids**, which are paired cartilages lying on top of the cricoid; and the **corniculate** and **cuneiform cartilages**, a pair of cartilages that strengthen the entrance of the larynx.

The larynx contains the two **vocal cords**, also referred to as *vocal folds*, which are two elastic folds of mucous membrane stretched horizontally across the larynx, and which are involved in voice production. The terms *vocal folds* and *vocal cords* are often used interchangeably in dictation. These vocal folds are often referred to in dictation as **true vocal folds** because immediately above them there is a second set of folds called **false vocal folds**, or **false vocal cords**. They are called *false* because in the early days of medicine, physicians examining a patient's throat often mistook these *false* folds for the *true* folds. The false vocal folds sit just above the true vocal folds. Although the false vocal folds do offer some protection to the true vocal folds, their role in vocalization is minimal (Figure 11.4).

The **glottis** is the gap between the vocal folds. During breathing the vocal cords are relaxed and the glottis widens. To produce sound, the gap narrows and the

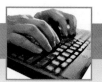

cords are tensed. When the air is forced through the vocal cords, they vibrate, generating sounds that can be modified by the tongue to produce speech. The vocal cords **abduct**, or open, during breathing and **adduct**, or close, during speaking, coughing, and swallowing.

THE PROCESS OF HEARING

Hearing occurs when sound waves travel through the ear by two pathways:

- **Air conduction**, which occurs when sound waves travel through the air, then through the external and middle ear to the inner ear.

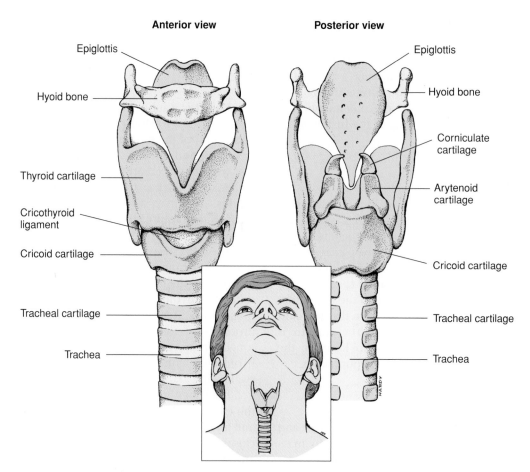

FIGURE 11.4. The Larynx. Reprinted with permission from *Stedman's Medical Dictionary,* 27th ed. Baltimore: Lippincott Williams & Wilkins 2000.

● **Bone conduction,** which occurs when sound waves travel through bone to the inner ear.

For sound to be heard, it must travel to the inner ear through air conduction, bone conduction, or both. In air conduction, sounds from the air are captured by the pinna, which directs the sounds through the external auditory canal to the tympanic membrane. From here the sound waves are relayed by vibration of the ossicles in the middle ear to the cochlea in the inner ear and the organ of Corti, located in the cochlea. There they disturb the cochlear fluid, which activates thousands of tiny hair cells in the organ of Corti. These sounds transform into electrical impulses that are relayed by nerve pathways to the brain. Different hair cells relay high-pitched and low-pitched sounds, with those in the deepest part of the cochlea receiving the lowest pitches. The brain not only extracts and processes the pitch and loudness of the sound impulses, but also processes other components such as timing and modulation—this in addition to combining sounds separately from each ear to form a single perception. These features can be compared to other acoustic patterns and stored in the brain, perhaps for the recognition of the voice of a family member or friend, or they can be processed as a new experience with a new sound or a new voice.

Bone conduction of sound works by conducting, or carrying, sound by means of the bones in the skull. The vibrations of the sound are transmitted directly from the vibrating part of the bone, through the skull, and to the cochlea, bypassing the outer and middle ears. When you wear earplugs, you will notice that your own voice still sounds fairly loud. This is because you hear it through bone conduction as opposed to air conduction.

COMMON OTOLARYNGOLOGIC DISEASES AND TREATMENTS

Although ear, nose, and throat disorders are rarely fatal, they still can be quite debilitating. Even a minor stuffed nose can make breathing and talking difficult. Ear disorders can disturb our equilibrium or compromise our hearing, impairing our ability to get along in life. Throat ailments can make it hard to eat, breathe, and talk.

Disorders of the Ear

Disorders of the ear include blockages, structural disorders, and infection that can affect hearing and balance.

Otitis Media

Otitis media, or a middle ear infection, is characterized by pain, redness of the eardrum, and possible fever. This infection occurs when the eustachian tube becomes inflamed from a cold, a sinus or throat infection, or an allergic reaction. If bacteria or viruses take hold, the resulting infection causes pain, an inflamed eardrum, and a buildup of fluids, pus, and mucus, typically behind the eardrum.

Treatment of ear infections consists of a course of antibiotics such as ampicillin, amoxicillin, or the combination drug trimethoprim/sulfamethoxazole (Bactrim). Acetic acid (Domeboro's Solution) also treats ear canal infections and prevents **otitis externa,** or "swimmer's ear," an infection of the external auditory canal.

In certain cases, a physician may perform ear-tube surgery. A **myringotomy,** or ear-tube surgery, may be performed on a child with persistent hearing loss or speech delay due to chronic ear infections and accumulation of pus or fluid in the middle ear. In this procedure, an opening is made through each eardrum to allow fluid to drain from the middle ear and help equalize the pressure in the ear. A tiny tube called a **tympanostomy tube** (also called a *pressure-equalization tube*) is inserted into the opening in each eardrum to help drain the fluid and allow air to enter the middle ear.

Vertigo

Vertigo is defined as sudden, brief feelings of dizziness and confusion with the change in the position of the

---

QUICK CHECK 11.1 ✔

Match the definitions on the left with the terms on the right.

1. _____ Connects to the nose.

2. _____ Located behind the mouth.

3. _____ Ear wax.

4. _____ Voice box.

5. _____ Labyrinth.

A. cerumen

B. inner ear

C. oropharynx

D. ostium

E. larynx

TRANSCRIPTION TIP:

When examining the ear, the physician will look for particular patterns produced by the ossicles on the tympanic membrane similar to the position of a prominent or well-known object in a particular landscape. These patterns are called **landmarks**. When the middle ear becomes infected, the tympanic membrane may appear opaque, obscuring these landmarks, which is what the dictator is referring to when using the phrases "landmarks are visible" or "landmarks are not visible."

head. **Benign paroxysmal positional vertigo** (BPPV) is the most common form of vertigo. The disorder, often called a "hallucination of movement," is characterized by the sensation of dizziness or "room-spinning" that occurs as a result of a disturbance in balance. It can occur when lying down from an upright position, turning over in bed, or even looking up. The feeling of vertigo is usually caused by a disorder in the nerves and structures of the inner ear that sense movement and changes in the position of the head, such as a blockage of fluid in the semicircular canals that detect body movement and regulate balance.

Treatment for vertigo, or dizziness, depends on identifying and eliminating the underlying cause. Ear infections causing the symptom of vertigo may be treated using the same antibiotics used to treat otitis media. Medications used to remedy dizziness include meclizine (Antivert) and diazepam (Valium). Vertigo caused by strokes, tumors, or diseases such as multiple sclerosis may require treatment with medication, radiation, or surgery.

Ménière Disease

Ménière disease, first described by French physician Prosper Ménière in 1861, is a balance disorder of the inner ear. It is also known as Ménière syndrome or endolymphatic hydrops. There are four main fluctuating symptoms of the disorder:

- Periodic episodes of vertigo
- Hearing loss in one or both ears, often in the lower frequency ranges
- Tinnitus
- A sensation of fullness or pressure in one or both ears

Although the cause of the disease is not known, some researchers suggest that it may result from an imbalance of fluids in the inner ear, a blood vessel pressing on a nerve in the inner ear, or an autoimmune

condition. The disease is diagnosed by several testing methods, including hearing and balance tests and MRI imaging of the head. There is no cure for Ménière disease, but the symptoms are often controlled successfully by reducing the body's retention of fluids with dietary changes (such as limitations on salt, caffeine, or alcohol) or by the use of medications to treat dizziness similar to those used to treat vertigo.

Cholesteatoma

A **cholesteatoma** is a sac or a cyst with an accumulation of dead cells and other debris, such as excessive cerumen, that accumulate in the middle ear, often the result of repeated ear infections. The cholesteatoma typically continues to fill with debris over time and, if not caught in time, can destroy the bones of the middle ear. Left untreated, a cholesteatoma can erode and destroy important structures within the temporal bone of the skull as well as cause central nervous system complications such as a brain abscess or meningitis. Cholesteatoma symptoms include a feeling of pressure, a foul-smelling discharge, earache, and hearing loss.

An examination by an otolaryngologist, including evaluation of balance and hearing, can confirm the presence of a cholesteatoma. Imaging studies such as x-rays and CT scans of the skull can confirm the size of the cholesteatoma and evaluate the extent of damage caused by the cholesteatoma. Initial treatment aims to stop the drainage in the ear by controlling the infection with the use of antibiotics and a careful cleaning of the ear. Large cholesteatomas require surgical removal.

Hearing Loss

Any loss of sensitivity produced by an abnormality anywhere in the auditory system results in the condition known as **hearing loss**. Hearing loss is defined as a deterioration in hearing; deafness is defined as profound hearing loss. Hearing loss may be partial or total and may develop gradually or suddenly. Patients have difficulty in hearing conversations. In addition, hissing, tinnitus, and vertigo may develop as hearing deteriorates.

Hearing loss can be categorized by determining the location or specific part of the auditory system that is damaged. **Conductive hearing loss** occurs as a result of disease or abnormality involving the outer or middle ear. Some causes of conductive hearing loss include cerumen buildup in the ear, otitis media, fluid in the middle ear space, perforation of the tympanic membrane, or hardening of the tympanic membrane, called **otosclerosis**. Once the cause is found and removed or treated, hearing usually is restored.

Sensorineural hearing loss, on the other hand, develops from disease or an abnormality that prevents nerve impulses of sound in the inner ear from being transmitted to the brain. The source may be located in the inner ear, in the nerve from the inner ear to the brain, or in the brain itself. Tumors in the inner ear can lead to sensorineural hearing losses, as can viral infections, Ménière disease, meningitis, and cochlear otosclerosis. Sensorineural hearing loss can also be the result of repeated, continuous exposure to loud noise, certain toxic medications, or an inherited condition. Generally, sensorineural hearing loss is irreversible; it is a permanent loss. Sudden sensorineural hearing loss can be catastrophic for the patient, and most physicians consider it a medical emergency.

Sometimes a conductive hearing loss occurs in combination with a sensorineural hearing loss. In other words, there may be damage in the outer or middle ear and in the nerves or structures of the inner ear. When this occurs, the hearing loss is referred to as a **mixed hearing loss**.

Diagnosis of hearing loss can be made by tests that measure the degree of hearing loss and the particular sound frequencies impaired. The treatment for hearing loss is relative to the cause. Infection or fluid buildup in the middle ear can be treated with antibiotics or the insertion of pressure-equalization tubes in the ears, as stated previously. However, in cases where there is no cure for the hearing loss, treatment involves maximizing the hearing that remains and compensating for the loss as much as possible. Hearing aids are devices that amplify sound to improve a person's ability to hear and communicate. In cases of severe hearing loss, a cochlear implant, which involves placing electrodes into the cochlea, may prove beneficial. An external microphone picks up sounds and, with the help of the implanted electrode, converts them into electrical impulses that stimulate the nerve pathways to the brain.

Disorders of the Nose

Because the nose projects from the center of the face, any structural abnormality on its surface is immediately noticeable. Some abnormalities are merely unsightly; others contribute to breathing problems.

Deviated Septum

A **deviated septum** is an abnormal configuration of the cartilage that divides the two sides of the nose, which may cause problems with breathing or nasal discharge. Although it is estimated that 80% of all nasal septums are off center, with one nostril narrower than the other, a deviated septum is one severely shifted away from the midline, resulting in difficulty breathing and repeated sinus infections due to inflammation of the sinuses and abnormal drainage from the nasal cavity.

A deviated septum can be corrected with a reconstructive procedure called a **septoplasty**, in which malformed portions of the septum may be removed entirely,

---

QUICK CHECK 11.2

Circle the letter corresponding to the best answer to the following questions.

1. By definition, any disruption in the flow of sound waves through the ear to the brain results in
   A. a cholesteatoma.
   B. hearing loss.
   C. tinnitus.
   D. vertigo.

2. One of the symptoms of Ménière disease is
   A. tinnitus.
   B. hoarseness.
   C. a deviated septum.
   D. cerumen.

3. The type of hearing loss that involves a disorder in the ear's nerve impulses is
   A. sensorineural hearing loss.
   B. regular hearing loss.
   C. conductive hearing loss.
   D. cerumen impaction.

4. The disorder often called a "hallucination of movement" is
   A. cholesteatoma.
   B. ossiculitis.
   C. otitis media.
   D. vertigo.

5. A sac or cyst containing dead cells in the middle ear is called a
   A. tympanic membrane.
   B. tympanostomy tube.
   C. cerumen blockage.
   D. cholesteatoma.

or they may be readjusted to straighten the deviation and facilitate better breathing through the nose.

Chronic Sinusitis

Sinus disorders are one of the most common of all medical problems and have a noticeable effect on a person's ability to breathe, sleep, and function in general. **Chronic sinusitis** is a condition in which sinuses become inflamed, causing improper drainage. As a result, bacteria grow continuously, causing nasal drainage, facial pressure, ear pain, teeth pain, and **postnasal drip** (PND), a condition in which mucus from the back of the nasopharynx drips down the back of the throat. Physicians do not know the cause of chronic sinusitis, but it seems to follow a viral infection, a severe allergy, or exposure to an environmental pollutant. A family history seems to be a factor as well.

The treatment of chronic sinusitis usually focuses on improving sinus drainage and curing the infection. Antibiotics are often prescribed, and some physicians may add a course of nasal steroid sprays to help blood vessels constrict and reduce inflammation in the mucous membranes. In severe cases, surgery called **endoscopic sinus surgery** (ESS) is required. ESS involves the removal of blockages in the sinuses to improve air flow through the sinuses and allow proper drainage through the nose. A thin, lighted instrument called an **endoscope** is inserted into the nose, and the doctor looks inside through an eyepiece to inspect the sinuses and see what is causing the blockage. Surgical instruments can then be used along with the endoscope to remove the blockages and improve breathing. The endoscope allows physicians to view the sinuses without cutting the face, and makes it possible to see parts of the sinuses that were formerly difficult to reach.

Epistaxis

Epistaxis is the medical term for nosebleed, which occurs when the lining of the inner nose is irritated or broken down enough to cause bleeding. Some common causes of epistaxis include forceful blowing; probing or picking at the nose, which inflames the nasal membranes; the repeated use of cocaine; or high blood pressure. Nosebleeds are generally treated with pressure and packing to stop the bleeding. Sometimes **electrocautery** (also called *nasal cautery* when used in the nose), which is the process of destroying tissue by means of electric current or caustic chemicals, is used to seal off the bleeding vessels. A small amount of a chemical called **silver nitrate** is applied over the area using a small stick for about 30 seconds to stop the bleeding. Electrocautery is then applied to stop the bleeding in larger vessels. For more severe or recurrent epistaxis, surgical procedures, including reconstruction of the nasal septum to close the site of bleeding, may be indicated.

Nasal Polyps

Nasal polyps are teardrop-shaped, fleshy outgrowths of the mucous membrane of the nose. Although polyps in other areas of the body (such as the colon or bladder) are associated with tumors or an increased risk of cancer, nasal polyps are simply a result of inflammation in the nose. Many people are not aware that they have nasal polyps, although may have the symptoms of nasal obstruction, chronic infections, sinusitis, and loss of the sense of smell. Medical treatment usually includes corticosteroids in the form of nasal sprays or oral tablets to shrink or eliminate the polyps. If the polyps block the airway or cause frequent sinus infections, nasal surgery to remove the polyps may be considered.

Disorders of the Throat

The throat plays an essential role in a person's ability to breathe, to swallow, and to communicate. The overall health of the throat, however, can be threatened by infectious diseases, chronic conditions, and structural abnormalities.

Obstructive Sleep Apnea

Obstructive sleep apnea (OSA) is a condition of interrupted breathing during sleep. The Greek word **apnea** means *without breath*. People with this sleep disorder literally stop breathing, often for a minute or longer, during sleep, as many as hundreds of times during a single night. This disruption is due to obstruction of the upper airway at any of several possible sites: The airway can be obstructed by excess tissue, large tonsils, or by a large tongue. Typically, too, the individual's airway muscles relax and collapse while sleeping. The primary risk factor for OSA is excessive weight gain, but narrow nasal passages, enlarged tonsils, and anatomic abnormalities are also factors that may contribute to OSA. The condition may also be related to the use of alcohol, tobacco, or sedatives. A **hypopnea** is a decrease in the rate and depth of breathing that is not as severe as an apnea. Like apneas, hypopneas usually disrupt the level of sleep.

Physicians use several methods to treat OSA. Significant weight loss appears to improve, if not completely eliminate, OSA. In addition, oral appliances can be used to help keep the airway open during sleep. A **mandibular advance device** is a mouth guard commonly used in contact sports; for this purpose, the mold for the lower teeth is advanced further forward than the mold for the upper teeth, moving the jawbone forward and opening the airway. A **tongue-retaining device**, similar to a suction cup, may be placed between the upper and lower teeth. Placing the tongue in the cup at night pulls it forward, eliminating obstruction caused by the base of the tongue.

More severe cases of sleep apnea are treated with a **continuous positive airway pressure** (CPAP) machine.

A CPAP machine blows pressurized air into the nose via a nose mask, keeping the airway open and unobstructed. This therapy is usually administered at bedtime by means of a nasal or facial mask held in place by Velcro straps around the patient's head, connected to an air compressor about the size of a shoe box. The air blown by the CPAP machine keeps the upper airway open and keeps it from collapsing. A bilevel positive airway pressure (BiPAP) machine is a variant of the CPAP machine, except that it blows air at two different pressures so that when a person inhales, the pressure is higher, and in exhaling the pressure is lower.

Sometimes surgery is used to correct OSA. **Uvulopalatopharyngoplasty** (UPPP) and a similar technique using the laser, called **laser-assisted uvulopalatoplasty** (LAU), are surgical procedures by which tissues in the back of the throat are removed, such as the uvula, the tonsils, and parts of the soft palate. Theoretically, these procedures increase the width of the airway at the throat opening and enhance palate movement and closure. Unfortunately, studies found these procedures did not prevent apnea episodes as often as hoped, and so these surgical procedures are used less frequently than they once were. **Somnoplasty** is a newer technique that uses microwave energy and has been found to be less painful and invasive. After a local anesthetic is administered, small needles are inserted into the tissue that needs shrinking. A very precise and controlled dose of radiofrequency waves is delivered to the target tissue only at the needle tips. The area around the needle tips is coagulated and absorbed, leaving only a tiny internal scar. This treatment results in an overall reduction in tissue volume.

Laryngopharyngeal Reflux Disease

Laryngopharyngeal reflux disease (LRD) is a condition in which the flow of digestive acids from the stomach backs up into the esophagus and into the tissues of the throat. Singers and professional speakers are at increased risk for LRD due to the use of their abdominal muscles to speak or sing, forcing stomach contents up into the larynx. There are various symptoms of LRD, including throat pain; a burning sensation in the throat; hoarseness; a chronic cough; or in some cases, difficulty breathing, which occurs when the vocal cords close to prevent aspiration of acid into the trachea (called **laryngospasm**). An otolaryngologist diagnoses LRD by performing an extensive head and neck exam, which frequently involves a visual examination of the lower throat and larynx. Indicators of LRD include abnormal thickening of the posterior portion of the larynx, called **pachydermia** or **cobblestoning**; redness and swelling of the vocal cords; and small ulcers in the posterior part of the vocal cords.

LRD is treated with a combination approach involving dietary and behavior modification and med-

ications to reduce the amount of acid in the stomach, which may irritate the esophagus and throat. Acid reflux drugs such as Aciphex, Nexium, Prevacid, and Zantac, may be prescribed. In some cases surgery to prevent reflux may be performed.

Vocal Cord Paralysis

Vocal cord paralysis is the inability to move the muscles that control the vocal cords. Although the exact cause is not known, the condition may be caused by head trauma, a neurologic insult such as a stroke, a neck injury, lung or thyroid cancer, a tumor pressing on a nerve, or a viral infection. Patients with vocal cord paralysis experience abnormal voice changes, changes in voice quality, and discomfort from vocal straining. For example, if only one vocal cord is damaged, the voice is usually hoarse or breathy. Changes in voice quality, such as loss of volume or pitch, may also be noticeable. Damage to both vocal cords usually causes difficulty in breathing as the air passage to the trachea is blocked. Treatment to improve vocal function includes voice therapy for the paralysis. After voice therapy, an operation that repositions or reshapes the vocal folds to improve vocal function, called **phonosurgery**, may also be indicated.

DIAGNOSTIC STUDIES AND PROCEDURES

Although a complete medical history and examination by a physician can confirm most ear, nose, and throat problems, further diagnostic testing and more extensive evaluation of the ears, nose, and throat may be necessary to establish a particular diagnosis.

Acoustic Studies

Acoustic studies evaluate overall hearing function. Various testing methods are used to diagnose hearing function disorders and their etiologies. Acoustic studies are the first-line screening method to decide if more in-depth tests, such as an MRI, are needed. They are also used in conjunction with other testing to diagnose specific disorders, such as Ménière disease.

QUICK CHECK 11.3

Fill in the blank with the correct term.

1. Light reflected on the tympanic membrane is called the _____.

2. Reconstruction of the septum can be achieved with a procedure known as _____.

3. Abnormal thickening of the posterior portion of the larynx is called _____.

4. _____ is the surgery that involves removing blockages in the sinuses.

5. A _____ occurs when the vocal cords close to prevent aspiration of acid into the trachea.

Otologic Examination

A visual inspection of the external auditory canal and tympanic membrane is called **otoscopy**. The physician performs the examination using an **otoscope**, which is a handheld instrument that directs light into the ear through a conical speculum attached to it. The tympanic membrane can be seen and assessed for infection or other problems in the middle ear. The physician can also get an idea of whether the eustachian tube is blocked when the patient performs the **Valsalva maneuver**, which is an attempt to forcibly exhale while keeping the mouth and nose closed, as mentioned previously. Normally the eardrum moves slightly during the maneuver. When the eustachian tube is blocked, the eardrum remains still.

Audiometry

Audiometry testing is used to identify and diagnose hearing loss. It involves a series of tests to evaluate the range of sounds that an individual can hear. The intensity of sound is measured in **decibels** (dB), and the frequency of sound is measured in **hertz** (Hz), or cycles per second. Testing is usually performed in a sound-proof testing room by an **audiologist**, who is a specialist in detecting hearing loss.

Pure Tone Audiometry

This procedure uses an **audiometer**, which is an instrument that emits sounds or tones at varying frequencies and pitches in order to determine the thresholds, or lowest intensity level, at which a patient can hear a set of test tones. The patient wears a set of headphones and listens for tones delivered to one ear at a time. At the sound of the tone, the patient responds, usually by raising a hand or finger, to indicate that the sound is detected. The audiologist lowers the volume and repeats the sound until the patient can no longer detect it. This test is repeated using different tones and frequencies to determine the exact nature of the patient's hearing deficit. The results are recorded on a grid or graph called an **audiogram**, which charts the frequencies and volume of tones used.

Tympanometry

Tympanometry evaluates the mobility of the tympanic membrane in response to air pressure change and thereby provides important information about the function of the middle ear, including the tympanic membrane, ossicles, and eustachian tube. In this test, a soft probe is placed into the ear canal and a small amount of pressure is applied. A microphone in the ear canal measures the intensity of the sound as it reflects off the eardrum. The results, recorded on a printout called a **tympanogram**, help determine how well the middle ear is functioning.

Air and Bone Conduction Tests

Air and bone conduction tests, also dictated as *tuning fork tests*, use vibrating tuning forks placed in contact with the head. A **tuning fork** is a metal instrument with a handle and two prongs or tines, similar to a table fork. The tuning fork, which is made of steel, aluminum, or magnesium-alloy, will vibrate at a set frequency to produce a musical tone when struck. The vibrations produced can be used to assess a person's ability to hear various sound frequencies. Two separate tests using a tuning fork help distinguish problems in the inner ear

TRANSCRIPTION TIP:

Some physicians abbreviate the term *decibels* in dictation as DBs, pronounced like *dee-bees*.

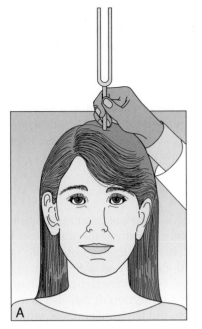

Bone conduction

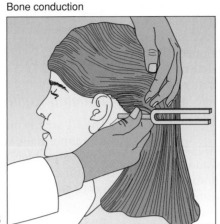

Air conduction

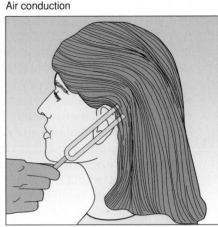

FIGURE 11.5. **Tuning Fork Testing. (A)** Weber test. **(B)** Rinne test. Reprinted with permission from Willis MC. *Medical Terminology: A Programmed Learning Approach to the Language of Health Care.* Baltimore: Lippincott Williams & Wilkins, 2002.

and central auditory pathways: the Rinne test and the Weber test, as shown in Figure 11.5.

The **Rinne test** compares bone conduction to air conduction in both ears. A vibrating tuning fork against the skull, usually on the **mastoid process** (the bone behind the ear), causes vibrations through the bones of the skull and inner ear. It is also held next to, but not touching, the ear to cause vibrations in the air next to the ear. The patient is asked to determine which sound is louder, the sound heard through the bone or through the air. Hearing loss is indicated if the patient hears a louder and longer tone when the tuning fork is held against the mastoid bone than when it is held next to the ear.

The **Weber test** evaluates bone conduction by placing the stem of a vibrating tuning fork at various points along the midline of the skull and face. The patient is then asked to identify which ear hears the sound created by the vibrations. The patient should perceive the sound equally in both ears. Varying volumes of sound vibrations conducted through the different parts of the skull and face can indicate which ear may have a hearing loss.

Otoacoustic Emissions Testing

Otoacoustic emissions (OAE) testing is used to assess the integrity and function of outer hair cells in the inner ear. A common test used to evaluate the hearing in newborns, OAE testing can also determine whether the cochlea is functioning. In this test, a sensitive microphone and speaker are inserted into the external auditory canal. Quiet tones are sent from the speaker, which travel through the middle ear and stimulate the hairs in the cochlea. The hairs respond by generating their own

sounds, which are detected by the microphone, indicating that the cochlea is functioning properly; if there is hearing loss, the hairs in the cochlea do not generate these minute sounds.

Brainstem Auditory Evoked Response Test

Brainstem auditory evoked response (BAER) is another testing screen that analyzes the brain's response to sound. In this procedure, the patient listens to a series of clicking sounds through headsets. The test measures the brain's activity in response to the sounds and indicates the results by displaying distinct waveforms on a computer screen.

Vestibular Studies

Vestibular studies assess the function of the vestibular portion of the inner ear for patients who are experiencing

TRANSCRIPTION TIP:

In the *diagnostic studies* portion of notes, listen for the following terms when transcribing the audiometric findings portion of reports: *audiogram; discrimination scores; otoacoustic emissions; pure tone thresholds; sound field testing; air-bone gap; evoked potentials;* and *type A, B, or C tympanogram.*

symptoms of vertigo, unsteadiness, dizziness, and other balance disorders. Some common vestibular studies include:

- **Electronystagmography** (ENG) records involuntary eye movements to determine whether ear nerve damage is the cause of dizziness or vertigo. In this test, electrodes are placed in particular locations around each eye. The electrodes record eye movements that occur when the inner ear and nearby nerves are stimulated by delivering cold and warm water to the ear canal at different times.
- Ocular motor assessment checks eye movement reactions to visual spatial stimuli that are observed and evaluated by computer analysis.
- **Barany caloric test**, also called a nystagmus test, is performed by irrigating the external auditory canal with either hot or cold water. This normally causes stimulation of the vestibular apparatus, resulting in **nystagmus**, which is a rapid, involuntary, oscillatory motion of the eyeball.
- Positional testing. The **Dix-Hallpike maneuver** is a test that determines whether vertigo is triggered by certain head movements. In this test, the patient is reclined rapidly from a sitting to a supine position with the head turned 45 degrees to the right and the neck extending 20 degrees over the examining table. After 30 seconds, the patient sits up and the eyes are observed for nystagmus. The timing and appearance of these eye movements will identify the cause of vertigo as either the inner ear or the brain. The test is then repeated with the patient's head turned in the opposite direction.

Nasal Studies

During an examination of the nose, a physician may need to look deep into the nose to check for evidence of congestion or obstruction.

Nasal Endoscopy

Nasal endoscopy, also referred to as *rhinoscopy*, is used to evaluate chronic and recurrent acute sinusitis. An

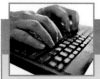

TRANSCRIPTION TIP:

When transcribing ENT notes, do not be confused with the soundalike abbreviated terms *EMG* and *ENG*. *EMG* is the abbreviation for *electromyelography*, which is a neurologic test to help isolate the cause of abnormal nerve function. In otolaryngology, *ENG* stands for *electronystagmography*, which is a test used by audiologists to evaluate balance and movement disorders.

endoscope is inserted into the nasal passages to the level of the larynx. The physician can then observe the internal structures of the nasal passageway and sinuses as the endoscope is introduced and withdrawn. The endoscope is equipped with a small light and a camera that enables the physician to view and record the terrain of the inner nose. Even the smallest nasal-related or sinus-related abnormalities can be identified through the endoscope. Bacterial cultures can also be taken from samples removed from the nasal cavity by the endoscope.

Imaging Studies

The CT scan is often used to view the paranasal sinuses for abnormalities. Usually isolating the cause of a chronic problem, it can be used to diagnose acute or chronic sinusitis and can also serve as a guide for surgeons during surgery. A CT scan may indicate inflammation and the extent of an infection. It can also detect problems that lie in deep, hidden air chambers, which might be missed on x-ray or nasal endoscopy. A CT scan can also indicate the presence of a fungal infection.

MRI is also used to evaluate the paranasal anatomy, but it is not as precise as a CT scan and, therefore, not typically used in cases of suspected sinusitis. However, it can help rule out fungal infections and may help identify inflammatory disease, malignant tumors, and complications within the skull.

Laryngeal Studies

A laryngeal examination typically includes diagnostic tests involving indirect laryngoscopy, or mirror examination; fiberoptic laryngoscopy; and videostroboscopy; and, to help diagnose OSA, polysomnography.

Mirror (Indirect) Laryngoscopy

Indirect laryngoscopy, also called a mirror exam of the throat, is used to view the patient's vocal folds and voice box structure by placing a mirror in the back of the patient's throat and reflecting a light down to the larynx, as shown in Figure 11.6. A small circular mirror on a long thin handle is inserted into the patient's mouth and turned so that the vocal cords are reflected on the surface. The otolaryngologist then shines a bright light on the mirror to examine the reflection of the vocal cords while the patient speaks. Although the examination is limited in scope, it can be done without special equipment.

Direct Laryngoscopy

Direct laryngoscopy permits a more detailed examination of the back of the throat, including the larynx and vocal cords. This examination uses a **fiberoptic laryngoscope**, a long, thin tube containing a fiberoptic

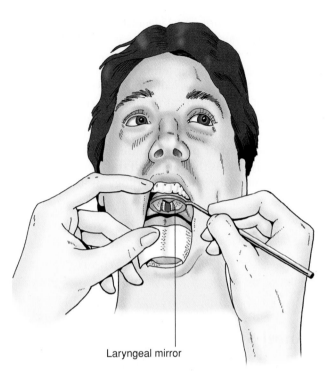

Laryngeal mirror

FIGURE 11.6. Mirror (Indirect) Laryngoscopy. A mirror and reflected light is used to visualize laryngeal structures. Reprinted with permission from Moore KL, Dalley AF. *Clinically Oriented Anatomy*, 4th ed. Baltimore: Lippincott Williams & Wilkins, 1999.

telescope, which allows a physician to get a more magnified view of the laryngeal structures than does a mirror examination.

A **rigid laryngoscopy** is an examination of the voice box in which a rigid telescopic tube is passed through the patient's mouth. The examiner then holds the patient's tongue while viewing the voice box. This examination provides the clearest magnified detail of the voice box, but the patient is unable to vocalize during the exam. A **flexible laryngoscopy**, on the other hand, allows the physician to view the voice box in action, or while the patient is producing sound. The otolaryngologist views laryngeal structures through a flexible viewing tube passed through the patient's nose to the back of the throat, thus allowing for visualization of the voice box while the patient speaks, sings, coughs, sniffs, etc.

Videostroboscopy

Videostroboscopy is an examination in which a strobe light is combined with rigid or flexible laryngoscopy to allow a slow-motion view of the vibrating vocal folds. The images are recorded on videotape and provide important information on the effects of a vocal fold abnormality on voice production. Videostroboscopy is used to document the state of laryngeal vibration for later comparison when following the course of a vocal disorder or evaluating the effect of treatment of a vocal disorder.

Polysomnography

Polysomnography, also known as a *sleep study*, is a diagnostic test during which a number of physiologic variables are measured and recorded during sleep. The test consists of a set of simultaneous measurements made over a period of hours while the patient is sleeping at night or napping during the day. Physiologic sensor leads are placed on various parts of the patient's body to record, among other things, brain electrical activity, eye movement, respiratory effort, and the levels of oxygen in the blood. These measurements are recorded and analyzed to reveal the pattern of changes or irregularities in stages of the patient's sleep, which can diagnose sleep disorders that lead to OSA. The **apnea-hypopnea index** (AHI) is an index of severity that combines apneas and hypopneas. Combining them both gives a measurement of the overall severity of sleep apnea, including sleep disruptions and oxygen **desaturations** (a low level of oxygen in the blood). The apnea-hypopnea index is calculated by dividing the number of apneas and hypopneas recorded by the number of hours of sleep. Another

---

QUICK CHECK 11.4 ✓

Indicate whether the following sentences are true (T) or false (F).

1. Bone conduction tests are also known as tuning fork tests.   T   F

2. In audiology, sound is measured in decibels and hertz.   T   F

3. A CT scan is not as useful as MRI in evaluating nose disorders.   T   F

4. Tympanometry evaluates middle ear function by measuring the movement of the eardrum in response to air pressure change.   T   F

5. An endoscope is a mirror used to evaluate the patient's nasal cavities.   T   F

index that is used to measure sleep apnea is the **respiratory disturbance index** (RDI). The respiratory disturbance index is similar to the apnea-hypopnea index; however, it also includes respiratory events that do not technically meet the definitions of apneas or hypopneas but do disrupt sleep.

CHAPTER SUMMARY

Earaches, runny noses, and sore throats certainly are among the most common conditions seen in primary care. In fact, it is not an exaggeration to state that primary care physicians see nearly as many acute and chronic ENT problems as ENT specialists; therefore, you will often encounter terms describing ENT disorders, diagnostic studies, and methods of treatment when transcribing medical reports. Learn to "develop an ear" for the variety of disorders and investigations typically used in this specialty. Rather than focusing on a single word or phrase, familiarize yourself with the specialty that is the subject of the dictation so that you can transcribe the terminology as used in this context.

· I · N · S · I · G · H · T ·

Why the Cochlea is Snail-Shaped

For years, scientists believed that the snail shape of the cochlea was merely a function of enabling many hearing structures to fit into a small space in the inner ear, and the shape had no effect on hearing function. However, researchers now realize that the unique shape of the cochlea effectively boosts the strength of vibrations caused by sound, especially for low pitches.

Starting with a simple model of a spiral, researchers calculated how the cochlea's curve affects movement of sound inside the inner ear. They found that as the sound waves progress, they accumulate increasingly near the outside edge of the spiral, rather than remaining evenly spread across it. Low frequencies travel the farthest into the spiral, so the effect is strongest for them.

Like the Whispering Gallery in St. Paul's Cathedral in London, where a whispered voice travels along the curved wall to be heard on the opposite side of the room, the researchers found that sound energy travels along the outer wall of the cochlea. The cochlea's gentle spiral adds a new twist: The increasingly tighter turns ensure that the waves of sound will focus steadily closer to the wall. The researchers calculated that the sensitivity increase in the center of the cochlea can be as much as 20 decibels, which corresponds to the difference between the hum of a quiet restaurant and the noise of a busy street. The ability to hear low-frequency sounds, which travel the farthest of all sounds, is especially important for communication and survival, and the entire shape of the cochlea itself contributes to amplifying these low frequencies.

Common Soundalike Words

Word	Word Pronunciation	Soundalike	Soundalike Pronunciation
aural: relating to the ear.	aw′răl	**oral**: relating to the mouth.	ōr′ăl
auricle: the outer structure of the ear.	aw′ri-kl	**oracle**: a wise person.	or′ri-kl
mastoiditis: an inflammation of any part of the mastoid process.	mas-toy-dī′tis	**mastitis**: an inflammation of the breast.	mas-tī′tis
nuchal: relating to the back of the neck.	nū′kăl	**knuckle**: a joint of the finger when the fist is closed.	nŭk′ĕl
otologic: pertaining to otology, or the study of the ear.	ō-tō-loj′ik	**audiologic**: pertaining to audiology, or the study of hearing disorders.	aw-dē-o-lōj′-ik
tympanic: relating to the tympanic membrane (eardrum).	tim-pan′ik	**tympanitic**: the quality of sound made when tapping the inflated intestines.	tim-pă-nit′ik
cerumen: ear wax.	sĕ-rū′men	**serum**: the fluid portion of blood obtained after removal of clots and blood cells.	sēr′ŭm
malleus: the largest of the three auditory ossicles in the internal ear.	mal′ē-ŭs	**malleolus**: the rounded bony prominence of the ankle joint.	ma-lē′ō-lŭs
tinnitus: the sensation of noises in the ear.	tin′i-tŭs	**tendonitis**: inflammation of a tendon.	ten-dŏ-nī′tis
shotty: having a feel to the touch like small, firm, discrete nodules; said of lymph nodes palpated through the skin.	shot′ē	**shoddy**: inferior quality, as in workmanship.	shod′ē

Combining Forms

Name	Definition	Name	Definition
acou/o	hearing	muc/o	mucus
aden/o	gland	myring/o, tympan/o	tympanic membrane (eardrum)
adenoid/o	adenoid		
audi/o, audit/o	sound, hearing	nas/o, rhin/o	nose
aur/i, aur/o, auricul/o, ot/o	ear	olfact/o	smell
cochle/o	cochlea (of the inner ear)	or/o	mouth
epiglott/o, epiglottid/o	epiglottis	osm/o	odor; smell
gloss/o	tongue	pharyng/o	pharynx
glott/o	glottis	sept/o	septum (dividing wall)
labyrinth/o	inner ear	sinus/o	sinus cavity
laryng/o	larynx (voice box)	sphen/o	wedge-shaped
lingu/o	tongue	tempor/o	temple (side of the head)
mandibul/o	mandible (lower jaw)	tonsill/o	tonsils
mast/o	mastoid process	trache/o	trachea
maxill/o	maxilla (upper jaw)	voc/o	voice

Add Your Own Combining Forms Here:

_____

_____

_____

_____

_____

_____

ABBREVIATIONS

Abbreviation	Definition	Abbreviation	Definition
AD	right ear	ENT	ear, nose, and throat
AHI	apnea-hypopnea index	ESS	endoscopic sinus surgery
AS	left ear	Hz	hertz
AU	both ears	LAUP	laser-assisted uvulopalatoplasty
BAER	brainstem auditory evoked response	LRD	laryngopharyngeal reflux disease
BiPAP	bilevel positive airway pressure	OAE	otoacoustic emissions
BPPV	benign paroxysmal positional vertigo	OSA	obstructive sleep apnea
CPAP	continuous positive airway pressure	PND	postnasal drip
dB	decibels	RDI	respiratory disturbance index
ENG	electronystagmography	UPPP	uvulopalatopharyngoplasty

Add Your Own Abbreviations Here:

_____

_____

_____

_____

_____

_____

TERMINOLOGY

Term	Meaning
abduct	To open or move away from.
adduct	To close or move toward.
adenoids	Two masses of lymphoid tissue located in the nasopharynx that fight off infection.
air and bone conduction tests, syn. tuning fork tests	A set of tests that use tuning forks to ascertain hearing loss.
air conduction	When sound waves travel through the air, then through the external and middle ear to the inner ear.
ala (plural *alae*)	The flared cartilage on each side of the nostril.
apnea	A term meaning *without breath*.
apnea-hypopnea index (AHI)	An index of severity that indicates the overall severity of sleep apnea.
arytenoids	Paired cartilages in the larynx that lie on top of the cricoid cartilage.

Term	Meaning
audiogram	A graph indicating the sound levels at which a person can hear different pitches.
audiologist	A specialist in detecting hearing loss.
audiology	The diagnosis of disease through the evaluation of hearing loss.
audiometer	An instrument that emits sounds or tones in order to test for hearing loss.
audiometry	Testing used to identify and diagnose hearing loss.
auditory system	The sensory system involved in the detection of sound.
benign paroxysmal positional vertigo (BPPV)	*Vertigo* for short, a sensation of dizziness as a result of a disorder or a blockage in the structures of the inner ear.
BiPAP	A machine that is a variant of the CPAP machine, except that it blows air at two different pressures into the nostrils so that when a person inhales, the pressure is higher, and with exhalation, the pressure is lower, in order to keep the airway open and unobstructed.
bone conduction	When sound waves travel through bone directly to the inner ear, bypassing the outer and middle ears.
brainstem auditory evoked response (BAER)	A hearing test that analyzes the brain's response to sounds.
Barany caloric test, syn. nystagmus test	A test that assess vestibular function of the ear.
cerumen	Ear wax.
cholesteatoma	A sac or cyst with an accumulation of debris located in the middle ear.
chronic sinusitis	A condition in which the nasal sinuses become inflamed, causing improper drainage.
cobblestone	A lumpy appearance of mucosa similar to a cobblestone pathway.
cochlea	A snail-shaped structure in the inner ear that is the organ of hearing.
concha (plural, *conchae*), syn. nasal turbinate	A long, narrow and curled bone shelflike structure (shaped like an elongated seashell), which protrudes into the breathing passage of the nose that helps traps particles entering the nasal particles.
concha bullosa	A condition in which a concha becomes filled with air, causing pain and nasal obstruction.
conductive hearing loss	Hearing loss caused by the prevention of sound waves from passing from the air to the ossicles of the middle ear.
continuous positive airway pressure (CPAP) machine	A machine that blows air under pressure into the nose via a nose mask, keeping the airway open and unobstructed.
corniculate cartilage	A small cartilage which, along with the cuneiform cartilage, helps strengthen the entrance of the larynx.
cricoid	The cartilage in the larynx that encircles the airway.
cuneiform cartilage	A small cartilage which, along with the corniculate cartilage, helps strengthen the entrance of the larynx.
decibel	The measure of loudness of sound.
desaturation	An indication of decreased oxygen in the blood.
deviated septum	An abnormal configuration of cartilage that divides the two sides of the nose.
direct laryngoscopy	An examination of the throat using a fiberoptic laryngoscope that is passed into the throat through the nose.
Dix-Hallpike maneuver	A test that determines whether vertigo is triggered by certain movements of the head.

Term	Meaning
ear	The organ responsible for hearing and balance.
electrocautery	The process of destroying tissue by means of electric current or caustic chemicals is used to seal off the bleeding vessels, such as those in the nose as a treatment for epistaxis.
electronystagmography (ENG)	A test that records involuntary eye movements to determine whether ear nerve damage is the cause of dizziness or vertigo.
endoscope	A thin, lighted instrument used to examine the nasal cavities and sinuses.
endoscopic sinus surgery (ESS)	A procedure that involves the removal of blockages in the sinuses to allow better air entry and proper drainage.
epiglottis	The part of the larynx that opens and closes in order to direct food and liquid into the esophagus and protect the airway during swallowing.
epistaxis	Profuse bleeding from the nose.
ethmoid sinuses	Approximately 6 to 12 sinuses on each side of the bridge of the nose.
eustachian tube	A short, narrow passage that equalizes air pressure on both sides of the eardrum.
external auditory canal	The tubular passage of the ear leading inward to the tympanic membrane (eardrum).
false vocal folds (false vocal cords)	A second set of folds above the true vocal folds that do not have a role in vocalization.
fiberoptic laryngoscope	A long, thin fiberoptic telescope used to examine the throat.
flexible laryngoscopy	A visual examination of the voice box while the patient is producing sound with the use of a flexible viewing tube passed through the patient's nose to the back of the throat.
frontal sinuses	One of a pair of sinuses located in the forehead.
glottis	The opening between the vocal cords.
hearing loss	A reduction in the ability to perceive sound.
hertz	A measure of the tone of sound.
hyoid	The single U-shaped bone that forms the larynx.
hypopharynx, syn. laryngopharynx	The part of the pharynx lying below the aperture of the larynx and behind the larynx. It extends from the vestibule of the larynx to the esophagus at the level of the inferior border of the cricoid cartilage.
hypopnea	An episode of decreased, but not absent, rate and depth of breathing.
incus	One of three ossicles of the middle ear, shaped like an anvil.
indirect laryngoscopy	Also called a *mirror exam*, an examination of the throat using a mirror and light reflected down into the larynx.
inner ear	The portion of the ear containing the organ of hearing and vestibular system for balance.
labyrinth, syn. inner ear	The internal ear, composed of the semicircular ducts, vestibule, and cochlea.
landmarks	In otorhinolaryngology, particular patterns produced by the ossicles on the tympanic membrane similar to the position of a prominent or well-known object in a particular landscape.
laryngopharyngeal reflux disease (LRD)	A condition in which the flow of digestive acids from the stomach flow backward into the esophagus and into the tissues of the throat.
laryngospasm	Closure of the vocal cords to prevent aspiration of acid into the trachea.
larynx, syn. voice box	A tube-shaped structure situated at the top of the trachea, it is the organ of voice production and also serves a protective function for the airway.

Term	Meaning
laser-assisted uvulopalatoplasty (LAUP)	A laser-assisted surgical procedure wherein certain excess tissue in the throat is removed to open the airway and help prevent apnea episodes during sleep.
light reflex	The light reflected off the tympanic membrane when light is shined upon it.
malleus	One of three ossicles of the middle ear, shaped like a hammer.
mandibular advance device	A type of mouth device that helps adjust the lower jaw to aid in preventing obstructive sleep apnea.
mastoid process	The bone located behind the ear.
maxilla, *syn.* jawbone	The upper jawbone in the face.
maxillary sinuses	One of a pair of sinuses located in each cheek on the face.
meatus	A passage or channel; in the nose, the passage created by the overhanging edge of each turbinate inside the nose.
Ménière disease, syn. Ménière syndrome or endolymphatic hydrops	A balance disorder of the inner ear.
middle ear	The portion of the ear between the eardrum and the inner ear.
mixed hearing loss	A combination of both conductive hearing loss and sensorineural hearing loss.
mucus	A thick, slippery substance that lubricates and protects the delicate lining of the areas of the body where mucous membranes are present (in this case, the nasal mucosa).
myringotomy	An opening made through the eardrum to allow fluid to drain from the middle ear and help equalize pressure in the ear.
nares, syn. nostrils	The two anterior openings located on either side of the nasal cavity.
nasal dorsum	The uppermost part of the nose.
nasal endoscopy, syn. rhinoscopy	A procedure using an endoscope to evaluate acute and chronic sinusitis.
nasal mucosa	The mucous membrane that lines the nasal passages.
nasal polyps	Fleshy outgrowths of the mucous membrane of the nose.
nasal septum	A thin partition of cartilage and bone that separates the nostrils in the midline.
nasal sinus	An air-filled, mucus-lined cavity within the cranial or facial bone.
nasopharynx	The part of the pharynx that lies behind the nose and extends to the soft palate of the mouth.
neuro-otology	The branch of medicine concerned with the nervous system related to the auditory and vestibular systems of the ear.
nose	The organ of smell, or olfactory sense.
nystagmus	A rapid, involuntary, oscillatory motion of the eyeball.
olfactory	Pertaining to the sense of smell.
organ of Corti	The actual hearing organ housed in the cochlea.
oropharynx	The part of the pharynx that lies at the back of the mouth.
obstructive sleep apnea (OSA)	A condition of interrupted breathing during sleep.
ossicles	Tiny bones that connect the eardrum to the middle ear.
ossicular chain	The term that collectively describes the three movable bones of the middle ear.
ostium	The openings from each paranasal sinus to the nose.
otitis externa	An infection of the external ear canal.
otitis media	An infection of the middle ear.
otoacoustic emissions (OAE)	A test performed on newborns to assess hearing function.

Term	Meaning
otolaryngologists	Physicians who specialize in the treatment of ear, nose, and throat disorders.
otolaryngology	The abbreviated form of the term *otorhinolaryngology*.
otology	The study of the ear.
otorhinolaryngology	The study of the ear, nose, and throat.
otosclerosis	Hardening of the tympanic membrane.
otoscope	A handheld lighted instrument that is used to inspect the external auditory canal and tympanic membrane.
otoscopy	A visual inspection of the structures of the outer ear.
outer ear	The external portion of the ear, including the pinna, external auditory canal, and tympanic membrane (eardrum).
oval window	The thin membrane that covers the opening to the inner ear.
pachydermia	Abnormal thickening of the posterior portion of the larynx.
paranasal sinuses	Air-filled, mucus-lined spaces that are connected by passages to the nose.
pharynx, syn. throat	A vertically elongated passageway that lies behind the mouth and nasal cavities just above the esophagus.
phonosurgery	An operation that repositions or reshapes the vocal folds to improve vocal function.
pinna, syn. auricle	The external part of the ear.
polysomnography, syn. sleep study	A diagnostic test during which a number of physiologic variables are measured and recorded during a patient's sleep to help diagnose sleep disorders.
postnasal drip (PND)	A condition in which mucus from the back of the nasopharynx drips down the back of the throat.
respiratory disturbance index (RDI)	An index of severity used to measure sleep apnea, which includes respiratory events that do not technically meet the definitions of apneas or hypopneas but do disrupt sleep.
rhinoscopy	Also called *nasal endoscopy*, a procedure using an endoscope to evaluate acute and chronic sinusitis.
rigid laryngoscopy	An examination of laryngeal structures with the use of a rigid tube that is passed through the patient's mouth.
Rinne test	A type of tuning fork test, performed to determine hearing loss.
saccule	One of three tiny organs of the vestibular system in the inner ear.
semicircular canals	One of three tiny organs of the vestibular system in the inner ear.
sensorineural hearing loss	Hearing loss caused by an abnormality or defect in the auditory nerve or hair cells of the inner ear, preventing nerve impulses from being transmitted to the brain.
septoplasty	A reconstructive procedure to correct a deviated septum.
silver nitrate	A special chemical used in cauterization for the treatment of epistaxis.
sinus	A hollow cavity or space in bone or other tissue.
somnoplasty	A procedure that uses microwave energy applied to tissues in the throat to reduce tissue volume and help prevent apnea episodes during sleep.
sphenoid sinuses	One of a pair of sinuses located behind the nose near the center of the skull.
stapes	One of three ossicles of the middle ear, shaped like a stirrup.
thyroid cartilage	The largest cartilage of the larynx.
tinnitus	Ringing in the ears.

Term	Meaning
tongue retaining device	A mouth device that moves the tongue out of the airway to assist in preventing obstructive sleep apnea.
tonsils	Two masses of lymphoid tissue located on each side of the entrance to the oropharynx that fight off infection.
trachea, *syn.* windpipe	The passageway for air between the pharynx above and the lungs below.
true vocal folds (true vocal cords)	The two elastic bands of tissue in the larynx responsible for speech.
tuning fork	A two-pronged metal instrument similar to a table fork used to perform hearing tests.
tympanic membrane, syn. eardrum.	A semitransparent membrane that separates the outer ear from the middle ear.
tympanogram	The printout of the results of a tympanometry study of the middle ear.
tympanometry	A hearing test that evaluates middle ear function.
tympanostomy tube, syn. pressure equalization tube	A tiny tube inserted into the opening of the eardrum to help drain fluid and allow air to enter the middle ear.
utricle	One of three tiny organs of the vestibular system in the inner ear.
uvula	The pendant, fleshy mass hanging from the soft palate above the root of the tongue.
uvulopalatopharyngoplasty (UPPP)	A surgical procedure wherein certain excess tissue in the throat is removed to open the airway and help prevent apnea episodes during sleep.
Valsalva maneuver	A maneuver that increases pressure in the nasopharynx, forcing air into the eustachian tube as all other outlets are blocked.
vertigo	A sensation of dizziness as a result of a disorder or blockage in the structures of the inner ear.
vestibular organs	The utricle, saccule, and semicircular canals located in the inner ear, which help maintain the body's sense of balance.
vestibular system	The sensory system involved in maintaining the body's equilibrium.
videostroboscopy	An examination in which a strobe light is used with rigid or flexible laryngoscopy to allow a slow-motion view of vibrating vocal folds in the throat.
vocal cord paralysis	The inability to move the muscles that control the vocal cords.
vocal cords, syn. vocal folds	Two elastic folds of mucous membrane that aid in vocalization.
Weber test	A type of tuning fork test to determine hearing loss.

Add Your Own Terms and Definitions Here:

_____

_____

_____

_____

_____

_____

REVIEW QUESTIONS

1. Name the three sections of the pharynx.
2. What are the two measurements of sound?
3. What part of the ear responds to gravity?
4. What is the purpose of the nasal turbinates?
5. What is the difference between an indirect laryngoscopy and a direct laryngoscopy?
6. Name the bones that make up the ossicular chain.
7. In what part of the pharynx are the adenoids located?
8. Name two symptoms of Ménière disease.
9. What are the four groups of sinuses connected to the nose?
10. What is a myringotomy?

CHAPTER ACTIVITIES

Soundalike Word Choice

Circle the correct word in the following sentences.

1. The patient's vestibular problems seemed to stem from the (labrum, labyrinth) portion of the ear.
2. Her vocal cords, situated in the (larynx, pharynx), appeared normal in size and shape.
3. Ms. Brown was diagnosed with nasal polyps after undergoing (rhinoscopy, pharyngoscopy).
4. The physician performed a lavage of the child's ears to clear them of (serum, cerumen), which improved his hearing.
5. The (tympanic, tympanitic) membranes appear intact bilaterally with no evidence of infection.
6. Her (aural, oral) cavity had no masses or lesions, and her tonsils appeared normal.
7. My mother was diagnosed with a deviated (septum, sepsis) last year.
8. The patient's hearing was evaluated using the (Weber, Wernicke) tuning fork test.
9. Mr. Hall was recommended to have a tracheostomy because his (glomus, glottis) was obstructing his airway.
10. The (tracheal, trabecular) rings in the throat were examined during inspiration and expiration and no clots were noted.

Understanding Medical Documents

Read the following excerpt from a procedure note and, using resource materials or the Internet to locate terms you do not know, answer the questions that follow.

After a topical anesthesia was applied and allowed to act, the fiberoptic laryngoscope was advanced into the right nasal cavity. His turbinates appeared to be normal in size with no masses. When the Mueller maneuver was performed, there was noted to be lateral collapse of the upper oropharynx and lower nasopharynx. The base of tongue did not retract at this point based on the Mueller maneuver. When the patient was then laid supine, there was also lateral collapse of the soft palate but minimal collapse of the base of the tongue. His true vocal folds were mobile bilaterally with no lesions. Next, the left nasal cavity was evaluated and there were no masses noted.

Questions

1. What is the Mueller maneuver?
2. What does the supine position look like?
3. In what part of the ENT system are the true vocal folds located?
4. What words in the first sentence tell you what kind of procedure this is?
5. What procedure is it?

Fill In The Blanks

Fill in the blanks of the following paragraph with the correct terms from the text. The same terms may be used more than once.

The ear includes both the _____ system, which detects sound, and the _____ system, which maintains the body's equilibrium. The ear is divided into three regions: the _____, _____, and _____. The tubular passage leading to the eardrum is called the _____. The _____ connects the _____ ear to the _____ ear. In the _____ ear, the _____ is the organ of hearing. The _____ ear also contains tiny organs that react to body movement called the_____, the _____, and the _____ canals. The _____ converts sound vibrations into nerve impulses and transmits them to the brain, which interprets the impulses as sound.

True or False

Read each statement and indicate whether it is true or false. If false, rewrite the sentence in the Correction column to make the statement true.

Statement	True (T) or False (F)	Correction, if False
1. The pharynx lies immediately behind the nose.	_____	_____
2. A cholesteatoma is a cyst that forms in the middle ear.	_____	_____
3. The nasal septum separates the nostrils at the midline.	_____	_____
4. Nasal polyp is a medical term for a nosebleed.	_____	_____
5. Phonosurgery involves removing blockages from the sinuses.	_____	_____
6. Ménière disease is a balance disorder of the middle ear.	_____	_____
7. Ear tube surgery is called indirect laryngoscopy.	_____	_____
8. The trachea can be found in the nasopharynx.	_____	_____
9. Videostroboscopy allows slow-motion viewing of the vocal folds.	_____	_____
10. Another name for ringing in the ears is vertigo.	_____	_____

ENT Terminology Word Search

Find the words in the grid. When you are done, the unused letters in the top half of the grid will spell out a hidden message. Pick them out from left to right, top line to bottom line. Words can go horizontally, vertically, and diagonally in all eight directions.

```
O  T  T  X  N  Y  R  A  H  P  O  P  Y  H  O  L  A  R  Y  N  G  O
L  U  O  G  I  G  N  I  N  O  T  S  E  L  B  B  O  C  S  T  S  A
R  R  S  E  S  P  E  C  O  S  S  I  C  U  L  A  R  C  H  A  I  N
Y  B  I  I  A  R  L  I  S  V  E  R  T  I  G  O  W  T  S  T  R  A
R  I  I  S  T  H  N  E  C  D  I  N  T  H  E  D  I  E  A  G  V  N
T  N  O  L  S  I  I  S  S  H  A  N  D  T  X  R  E  A  B  I  T  M
E  A  E  I  N  N  G  I  T  T  O  O  F  T  R  O  A  D  D  E  I  T
M  T  I  S  O  O  N  N  A  A  L  L  E  N  T  P  B  E  R  O  R  B
O  E  L  N  E  S  M  U  Y  S  P  E  L  X  A  O  E  M  X  D  H
I  S  Y  O  P  C  S  S  L  R  M  E  K  S  D  S  L  G  C  Y  V  L
D  Y  C  T  X  O  U  I  N  Q  A  E  S  Y  T  N  T  L  L  I  N  G
U  Y  T  M  W  P  C  T  Z  X  P  L  M  R  A  E  L  L  I  K  O  T
A  K  Q  F  N  Y  N  I  R  I  Q  O  O  S  M  V  A  W  M  X  N  V
R  I  N  N  E  D  I  S  S  L  T  B  O  N  R  H  K  T  L  H  A  X
B  Q  H  N  R  V  P  T  C  O  O  P  Q  N  N  T  Q  N  O  C  Z  M
N  V  P  N  Z  D  A  A  G  S  H  K  K  Y  T  W  E  K  L  M  N  L
N  H  H  T  Q  X  E  N  C  A  A  L  W  Z  N  M  R  G  G  N  A  N
J  Y  T  N  I  H  I  O  R  K  N  N  V  N  U  P  V  G  M  T  L  R
B  T  P  S  C  R  P  Y  K  G  N  K  M  R  X  D  H  F  N  R  T  V
T  D  X  A  Y  Y  N  T  T  V  I  M  E  N  T  F  X  Q  M  N  G  N
B  Q  R  M  R  X  P  F  G  M  P  C  K  B  J  K  L  H  X  G  N  H
R  T  D  I  O  C  I  R  C  T  S  O  P  V  H  Z  Q  V  W  M  L  P
```

www.WordSearchMaker.com

audiometry	myringotomy	tonsils
cerumen	nasopharynx	trachea
cholesteatoma	ossicular chain	turbinates
cobblestoning	pinna	vertigo
epistaxis	postcricoid	videostroboscopy
hypopharynx	rhinoscopy	voice box
incus	rinne	weber
laryngitis	sinusitis	
maxilla	stapes	

Hidden message: _____

Proofreading Practice

Proofread the following clinic note, which contains multiple errors in terminology, grammar, and context. Circle each error, then retype the document correctly. Print one copy and save your work to your student disk.

CHIEF COMPLAIN: Frequent ear infections.

HISTORY OF PRESENT ILLNESS: The patient is a 5 year old female brung in by mom and dad for evaluation of difficulties with frequent ear infections. Her initial ear infection reportedly occurred at approximately 6 weaks of age. Since that time, she has had several other episodes of otitis media requiring antibiotics. She has completed several courses of oral antibiotics in the past three years. The parents feel that her ear infections never completely resolve. She typically will tug pull or scratch at the ears and appears to have significantly discomfort in both ears. This results in difficulty sleeping at night and increased iritability. The patient has had fever on several occasionallys as well. there has been no drainage from ether ear. She does response at home appropriate to voice and environmental sounds.

MEDICATIONS: Amoxicallin 250 milligrams bid currently and Floxitine drops as prescribed by her pediatrician.

ALLERGIES: No one.

REVIEW OF SYSTEMS: Ear drainage nasal drainage skin rash, and difficulty breathing thru the nose.

PHYSICAL EXAMINATION: Vital signs? Temperature 98.9. The patient is a pleasant, happy appearing children who is in no acute distress. Ears: The left ear shows that the extreme auditory canal is clear. Tympanic membranes is mildly injected and otherwise unremarkable. Middle ear space shows evidence of effusion present. On the right, external auditing canal is clear. Tympanic memberane is injected and erythmatous. There is mucpurulent type infection present in the middle ear space. Nasal cavity. There is clear discharge anteriorly. Oral cavity: Clear. Plate intact. Tonsils are 2 plus and symemtric. Neck -Without lymphopathy or masses.

TESTS REVIEWED: Audiograph today demonstrates a mild hearing loss throughout all frequencies.

IMPRESSION:
  1. Acute right otitis medium.
  3. Mild conducive hearing loss secondary to number one.

RECOMMENDATIONS: Patient's exam findings were reviewed and discussed with mom and dad today. Treatment options include continued use of oral antibiotics as needed with a period of obervation to allow resolution of the acute otitis media and subsequent resolution of effusions. The second treatment option includes myringototomy and tube placement. The risks and benefits of both approaches were discussed. At this time they are advised to consider myringotomy dew to chronicity of the patient's symptoms and ottis as well as the componence of hearing loss which has been documented today. They are interest and will follow up for scheduling in 2 week's time.

TRANSCRIPTION PRACTICE

Open your word-processing software. Insert the student CD-ROM and locate the dictation for this chapter. For each of the words in the "listen for these terms" list for each report, use a medical dictionary or other resource to identify and write down a brief definition of the term on a separate sheet of paper to attach with your work. Then listen to the dictation and transcribe each report. Use the current date for each report where a date is indicated. Insert a heading into the document if the text falls to a second page.

At the end of each report, indicate the name of the dictating physician under the signature line and insert reference initials. For date dictated and transcribed and date of admission, use the current date. Proofread your work, print one copy for your instructor along with your term definitions, and save the completed report to your student disk.

Report #T11.1: Operative Report
Patient Name: Stevie Hutton
Medical Record No.: 773855
Surgeon: Kamraan George, MD
Assistant: Robert Maddox, MD

Listen for these terms:
adenotonsillar hypertrophy
red rubber catheter
myringotomy
Crowe-Davis retractor
Bovie cautery

Report #T11.2: Consultation Letter
Patient Name: Edward Staples
Medical Record No.: 77-21190
Consulting Physician: Michael Josephs, MD
Requesting Physician: Andrea Zaya, MD

Listen for these terms:
cholesteatoma
otalgia
tympanoplasty
mesotympanum
Hapex

Report #T11.3: Clinic Note
Patient Name: Toney Faro
Medical Record No.: FAR-2321
Attending Physician: Eugene Richards, MD

Listen for these terms:
polypoid
videostroboscopy
laryngoscopy
Hurricaine

12

PULMONOLOGY

OBJECTIVES

After completing this chapter, you will be able to:

- Identify the structures of the respiratory system and describe the function of each.
- Understand and explain the mechanism of breathing and exchange of gases in the respiratory process.
- Explain the process of mechanical ventilation.
- Describe common diseases and disorders that affect the respiratory system and the most commonly used medical treatments.
- Explain common diagnostic studies and procedures used to investigate pulmonary diseases and disorders.

INTRODUCTION

We seldom think about the act of breathing. Our lungs take in air approximately 12 to 20 times per minute, or nearly 25,000 times during a normal day. Once in the lungs, oxygen in the air must reach active tissues, which use it to keep all systems performing at optimal levels. When we breathe, the body consumes oxygen and produces carbon dioxide as a waste product, which must make its way back to the lungs in order to be ventilated from the body. This process, which takes place in the lungs, causes the body to exchange the carbon dioxide accumulated in the blood for oxygen in the airways that is inhaled with the air we breathe. The **respiratory system** is a collective term comprising the organs and tissues involved in the process of filtering incoming air, circulating oxygen to be used by the body through the blood, converting that oxygen to carbon dioxide, and eliminating carbon dioxide from the body. Because oxygen and carbon dioxide are both gases, the process of bringing one in and expelling the other is referred to as **gas exchange**.

In addition to its role in gas exchange as described, the respiratory system also performs other vital biological functions and is particularly important as a body defense. Although air is composed primarily of oxygen and nitrogen, it also contains elements that can hurt the lungs, such as bacteria, viruses, cigarette smoke, car exhaust, and other toxins. A healthy respiratory system prevents airborne particles and impurities from damaging the lungs or entering the bloodstream. Coughing is one way we attempt to clear the airway of noxious material and is a signal that our respiratory system is working to filter and clean the air that we breathe.

This chapter outlines the basic anatomy and physiology of the respiratory system, the process of respiration that takes place in the lungs, and the numerous physiological factors that affect optimal pulmonary function.

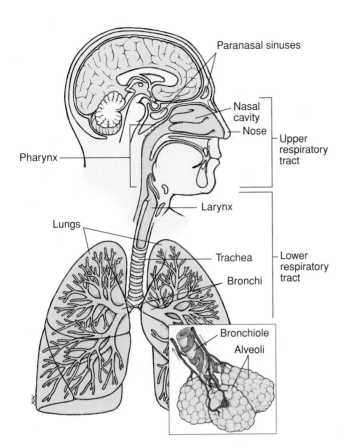

FIGURE 12.1. The Upper and Lower Respiratory System.
Reprinted with permission from *Stedman's Medical Dictionary,* 27th ed. Baltimore: Lippincott Williams & Wilkins, 2000.

ANATOMY OF THE RESPIRATORY SYSTEM

The anatomy of the respiratory system can be divided into two tracts: the upper respiratory tract and the lower respiratory tract, as shown in Figure 12.1.

Upper Respiratory Tract

The **upper respiratory tract** consists primarily of the nose, the nasal cavities, the sinuses, the mouth, and the pharynx. The nose, formed by bone and cartilage, is divided by the nasal septum into the right and left nasal cavities. Bony structures called **conchae** (singular, **concha**), also called **nasal turbinates**, divide the cavity into passageways that are lined with mucous membranes to help increase the surface area available to warm and filter incoming air. The two nostrils enable air to enter and leave the nasal cavity. Hair, mucus, and capillaries line the nasal cavity to filter, warm, and eliminate debris from the passing air on its way to the lungs. Particles trapped in the mucus are carried to the pharynx by fine hairs called **cilia,** which move the debris toward the esophagus, where it is swallowed and carried to the

stomach. The **pharynx**, located behind the mouth between the nasal cavities, receives the incoming air from the nasal cavities on its way to the larynx and, eventually, into the lower respiratory system. Besides warming and humidifying inhaled air, these structures enable taste, smell, and the chewing and swallowing of food.

Lower Respiratory Tract

The **lower respiratory tract** includes the larynx, the trachea (which conveys inhaled air into the lungs), the bronchi, and the lungs. The **larynx**, located below the pharynx, receives air from the oral cavity. A flap of cartilage called the **epiglottis** covers the upper region of the larynx during swallowing, which prevents food or other materials from entering the lungs.

The **trachea**, or windpipe, is a muscular tube that extends downward behind the esophagus and into the **thorax**, or chest cavity. The tracheal wall contains 20 C-shaped rings of cartilage, the open ends of which face posteriorly. The incomplete ends are filled with smooth muscle and connective tissue. These cartilage rings prevent the trachea from collapsing and blocking the airway, whereas the soft tissues that complete the rings in the back allow the esophagus next to the trachea to expand as food moves through it on the way to the stomach. A blocked trachea can cause a person to suffocate, or asphyxiate, in minutes. If a foreign object or swollen tissues obstruct a trachea, physicians can create a temporary opening in the tube in order for air to bypass the obstruction, a procedure called a **tracheostomy**.

In the chest cavity, the trachea splits, or branches off, at the **carina** (also called the **tracheal bifurcation**) into the two main air passages called the right and left **bronchi** (singular, **bronchus**). The word *carina* means any keel-shaped or ridged-shaped anatomic part (in fact, a section of the stomach is also called the carina). The word is derived from Latin, meaning *hull* or *keel of a ship.*

The bronchi lead to the lungs, with each bronchus entering the lung on its respective side. The branched bronchi further divide and branch into even smaller airways called **bronchioles**. The bronchi and bronchioles resemble an upside-down tree, which is why this part of the respiratory system is referred to as the bronchial

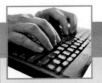

TRANSCRIPTION TIP:

Dictators will often interchange the words *tracheostomy* and *tracheotomy*, as these words are synonymous; therefore, the dictated abbreviated form *trach* could refer to either term and in this case, should not be expanded.

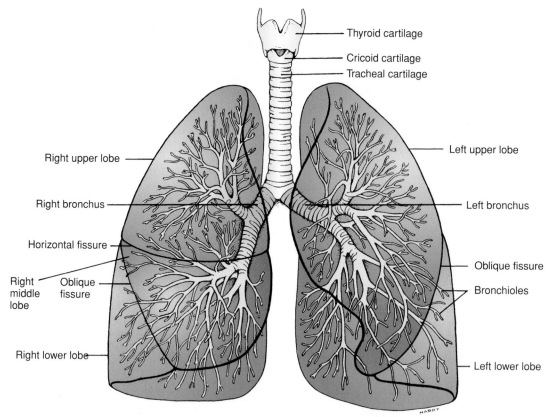

FIGURE 12.2. The Lobes and Bronchial Tree. The lungs consist of five lobes. The right lung has three lobes (upper, middle, and lower); the left has two (upper and lower). The lobes are further subdivided by fissures. The bronchial tree, another lung structure, inflates with air to fill the lobes. Reprinted with permission from Smelzter SC, Bare, BG. *Textbook of Medical-Surgical Nursing,* 9th ed. Philadelphia, Lippincott Williams & Wilkins, 2000.

tree. At the end of each bronchiole are thousands of **alveoli** (singular, alveolus), which are tiny, thin-walled sacs arranged in grapelike clusters that expand when the lungs fill with air. Together, the millions of alveoli provide a large surface area of thin layered cells through which the exchange of oxygen and carbon dioxide during the respiratory process can occur. Within the alveolar walls are tiny blood vessels called **capillaries**, which allow oxygen to move from the alveoli into the blood and for carbon dioxide to move from the blood in the capillaries into the alveoli where it is subsequently exhaled through the lungs.

The **lungs** are soft, spongy, cone-shaped organs located in the thoracic cavity. The lungs take in oxygen, which cells need to live and carry out their normal functions. The lungs also get rid of carbon dioxide, a waste product of the body's cells. They extend from the collarbone to the **diaphragm**, the dome-shaped muscle that separates the thoracic cavity from the abdominal cavity. One is located on the right side of the chest cage and one is on the left side; together they are the body's major respiratory organs. The left lung is slightly smaller than the right lung because it shares the space on the left side of the chest wall with the heart. Each lung is divided into sections called **lobes**: three in the right lung—the right upper lobe, middle lobe, and lower

lobe; and two in the left lung—the left upper lobe and lower lobe (Figure 12.2). The lobes are further subdivided by **fissures**, or crevasses, that separate the lobes. The lungs are surrounded by the ribs, the **sternum** (or breastbone), and the thoracic vertebrae of the spine. They are separated from each other by the **mediastinum**, which is a space in the thoracic cavity containing the heart, major blood vessels, esophagus, and many lymph nodes.

A clear, shiny coating called the **pleura** envelops the lungs. The inner layer of the pleura, called the **visceral layer**, attaches to the lungs, whereas the outer layer, called the **parietal layer**, attaches to the inside of the rib cage, or the chest wall. Pleural fluid holds these layers in place, similar to two glass microscope slides that are set and stuck together. The small amount of fluid in the pleura serves as a lubricant to provide a smooth surface for the lungs to inflate and deflate freely within the chest during respiration.

RESPIRATORY PROCESS

The function of the respiratory system is rather simple in concept: "to breathe," or bring in oxygen from the atmosphere and get rid of the carbon dioxide from the blood. The upper and lower respiratory tracts, as well as the diaphragm and **intercostal muscles**, which are the muscles located between the ribs, are all involved in breathing. There are two sites of exchange of oxygen and carbon dioxide: the lungs and the tissues of the body. The exchange of gases that takes place in the lungs is called **external respiration**. The exchange of gases between blood in the systemic capillaries and the cells of the body is called **internal respiration**. Respiration occurs through three processes:

- **Diffusion**, or gas movement through a semipermeable membrane from an area of greater concentration to one of lesser concentration (internal respiration occurs only through diffusion between capillaries and the cells of the body).
- **Pulmonary perfusion**, which is blood flow from the right side of the heart, through the pulmonary circulation, into the left side of the heart.
- **Ventilation**, which is gas distribution into and out of the lungs.

The respiratory process actually begins in the part of the central nervous system that controls breathing, called the **brainstem**. The brainstem is the respiratory drive center, responsible for sending motor impulses to tell the diaphragm and the muscles of the thorax to contract. It controls breathing and functions to move air in and out of the lungs whether we think about it or not.

However, if the brainstem is damaged in any way, the function of automatic breathing is impaired. When we breathe, air passes through the nose and into the nasal cavities where mucous membranes warm the air to body temperature and humidify it before it enters the lungs. The air then passes through the larynx and trachea into the right and left bronchi of the lungs. The intercostal muscles move the ribs upward and outward, and the diaphragm contracts and flattens. This draws air into the expanded lungs.

The inner surfaces of the larger airways are lined with special cell types that are designed to keep dust, debris, and bacteria from entering the lungs. Some of the cells produce mucus to trap inhaled debris and bacteria. Other cells produce a ciliary action in which the cilia, or tiny hairs, lining the passageway beat rhythmically toward the larynx, keeping dust, debris, and bacteria from entering the lungs and wafting it toward the throat where it may be swallowed or coughed up. Scavenger cells called **macrophages**, concentrated toward the alveoli, clean up debris and defend against invasion by bacteria.

When the inhaled air rushes into the alveoli they expand. When air is exhaled, the sacs relax and gas exchange takes place. The capillaries that surround each alveolus are filled with blood. When air is inhaled, oxygen from the air diffuses into the capillaries. These vessels take up oxygen and release carbon dioxide. The carbon

QUICK CHECK 12.2 ✓

Indicate whether the following sentences are true (T) or false (F).

1. The surfactants are tubes that deliver air to the alveoli.   T   F

2. When air is inhaled, oxygen from the air fills the capillaries.   T   F

3. The exchange of gases between blood in the systemic capillaries and the cells of the body is called internal respiration.   T   F

4. The heart plays no role in circulating oxygen-rich blood throughout the body.   T   F

5. The temporal lobe is the part of the brain that controls breathing.   T   F

---

dioxide is diffused from the blood capillaries, into the alveoli, and out of the lungs with each exhalation. The inner surfaces of the alveoli are also covered with a natural soapy film of fluid that contains a special chemical called **surfactant**. The surfactant keeps the lung air sacs open by helping to reduce the surface tension in the alveoli and keeping them from collapsing when air is exhaled.

The heart plays a role in circulating the oxygen-rich blood throughout the body. Oxygenated blood leaving the pulmonary capillaries enters the left ventricle of the heart. From the left ventricle, the blood is pumped, via the body's arterial circulation, to all the muscles, tissues, and organs. In this way the kidneys, brain, liver, heart, bones, and other tissues receive the vital oxygen they need to function. Deoxygenated blood then returns from these organs and tissues, via the venous system, to the right atrium of the heart. The blood that enters the right atrium has given up much of its oxygen to the tissues. After passing through the right atrium, this venous blood then goes to the right ventricle. From there it is pumped to the lungs, where it receives a fresh supply of oxygen, and the cycle then starts all over. Air is expelled through the lungs, the chest cavity returns to its normal size, and the diaphragm expands to its normal size, awaiting the next rush of inhaled air.

When lungs do not expand properly, there is a decrease in the total volume of air that the lungs are able to hold. Consequently, defects develop in the ability of the alveoli to diffuse oxygen into the blood and extract carbon dioxide from the blood, thereby hindering the gas exchange process. Some problems that interfere with proper lung expansion include **pleurisy**, which refers to an inflammation of the pleura. Any large volume of fluid, such as serum in some cases of viral infection or blood caused by a stab wound to the chest, must be removed from the lung. Expansion of the lung can also be hampered by the presence of air in the pleural cavity, known as **pneumothorax**. Pneumothorax

may occur spontaneously because of a rupture of an air space in the outer part of the lung or as a result of injury that leads to perforation of the chest wall.

A patient who has **dyspnea**, or difficulty breathing, may use the muscles of the neck and chest not normally associated with breathing, called **accessory muscles**, to aid in bringing air into the lungs. **Orthopnea** is discomfort in breathing except in an upright position. You may hear terms such as **two-pillow orthopnea** or **three-pillow orthopnea** when transcribing. This describes a patient's sleeping habits in which the patient requires two or three pillows, respectively, to breathe comfortably while sleeping. **Cheyne-Stokes respirations** refers to alternating periods of **apnea** (the absence of breathing) and deep, rapid breathing.

In addition, irregularities in the respiratory process are often identified by abnormal sounds heard on physical examination. Normal breath sounds are called **vesicular** breath sounds. Abnormal breath sounds are called **adventitious sounds**. Common abnormal lung sound terms heard when transcribing medical reports include the following:

- **Rhonchi,** which are loud, coarse, gurgling sounds occurring over the central airway during inspiration or expiration that sound like a whistle or a horn.
- **Wheezes,** which are high-pitched, whistling-type sounds heard over the large bronchi.
- **Rales,** which are sounds resembling a crackling sound like hairs being rubbed together, are usually heard during inspiration and indicate that the lung is partly filled with fluid. Rales are also referred to as **crackles**.
- **Rubs,** which are friction sounds like pieces of sandpaper being rubbed together, caused by inflammation of the pleura. A patient who breathes hard to inhale may display **flaring**, which is a widening of the nostrils to allow more air into the nose.

- **Grunting,** which refers to a grunting noise heard during expiration.
- **Stridor,** which is a crowing sound heard on inspiration that is caused by air whistling as it passed through swollen upper airways.

Reduction or absence of breath sounds over part of the chest wall can denote several abnormal conditions. Pneumothorax, as described above, is the name given to air in the pleural space. Collapse of lung tissue or incomplete expansion of a lung is called **atelectasis.** The presence of pus in the lungs is called **empyema;** the presence of blood, **hemothorax;** and the presence of fluid, **pleural effusion** or **hydrothorax.**

MECHANICAL VENTILATION

Mechanical ventilation is the use of a machine to mechanically assist patient's breathing when spontaneous breathing is absent or insufficient. The machine, called a **ventilator,** artificially induces alternating inflation and deflation of the lungs in order to regulate the exchange of gases in the blood. The most common type of ventilator delivers oxygen directly into the person's airway through a tube passed through the nose or mouth into the trachea, a process called **intubation.** If prolonged ventilation is required, a tracheostomy is performed and the tube is inserted into the patient's trachea.

The ventilator works by pushing air into the lungs, with a built-in computer mixing different levels of oxygen and pressures of air to sustain the patient. It can be adjusted to different modes depending on the patient's needs. For example, in the **assist/control, or A/C mode,** the patient sets his or her own breathing rate, but if the rate falls below a certain rate, the ventilator takes over. In the **intermittent mandatory ventilation (IMV)** mode, the ventilator delivers a set number of breaths each minute but allows the patient to breathe in between. Both modes have a preset **tidal volume,** which determines the volume of air that is inspired or expired in a single breath during regular breathing, in order to determine the size of the breath; and a preset **fraction of inspired oxygen (FiO$_2$),** which determines the amount of oxygen in each inspiration. In the A/C mode, the same tidal volume is delivered each time, but in the IMV mode, if the patient triggers a breath, it is at his or her own tidal volume. **Positive end-expiratory pressure, or PEEP,** is sometimes added to maintain extra pressure at the end of expiration to help prevent the alveoli from collapsing.

When the patient is ready to be **extubated,** or taken off the ventilator, the process of weaning begins. During weaning, the PEEP and FiO$_2$ are gradually decreased and the patient may be switched from the A/C mode to the IMV mode until he or she can breathe without assistance.

COMMON PULMONARY DISEASES AND TREATMENTS

Respiratory disorders are associated with abnormalities in any of the structures involved in the process of breathing and bringing oxygen into the lungs and blood. These disorders have a variety of distinct causes and account for a large number of illnesses and deaths each year. Each is named according to the sites affected. For example, bronchitis is a bacterial infection of the large airways and may follow viral infections of the upper respiratory tract. **Bronchiolitis** refers to infection of the finer airways. **Bronchiectasis** is the dilation of the large airways with the accumulation of secretions and chronic infection.

Pneumonia

Pneumonia is a serious lung disease in which inflammation of the alveoli, caused by bacteria, viruses, or both, results in the accumulation of fluid and cellular debris, thereby preventing gas exchange. An infection of the smaller bronchial tubes in the lungs is called **bronchopneumonia,** whereas infection caused by fluid and pus filling an entire lobe of the lung is called **lobar pneumonia** (Figure 12.3). The bacterium *Streptococcus pneumoniae* is the most common bacterium that causes **bacterial pneumonia.** This type of pneumonia usually occurs when an individual's resistance is lowered in some way due to conditions such as age, disease, alcohol consumption, or even malnutrition. Bacteria work their way in to invade part, or all, of the lobes of the lungs. The infected lobes then fill with fluid and pus, which in turn interfere with the lung's normal oxygen exchange. Other microorganisms responsible for pneumonia include *Staphylococcus aureus, Klebsiella pneumoniae,* and *Haemophilus influenzae.*

Viral pneumonia is usually acquired by inhaling airborne infected virus droplets from someone's sneezing or coughing. Viruses are responsible for half of all pneumonias. Some of these viruses include the influenza virus (types A, B, and C are the most common in adults), **respiratory syncytial virus** (RSV), parainfluenza virus, adenovirus, **cytomegalovirus** (CMV), and **Epstein-Barr virus** (EBV).

Mycoplasma pneumoniae is the bacterial species that causes the disease entity known as mycoplasma pneumonia, or **walking pneumonia.** The term *walking pneumonia* is used to describe pneumonia that is not severe enough to cause a person to be hospitalized. **Mycoplasmas** are the smallest free-living agents of disease in humankind. They share characteristics with both viruses and bacteria but are not classified as either. These mycoplasmas account for approximately 70% of all pneumonias in children ages 9 to 15.

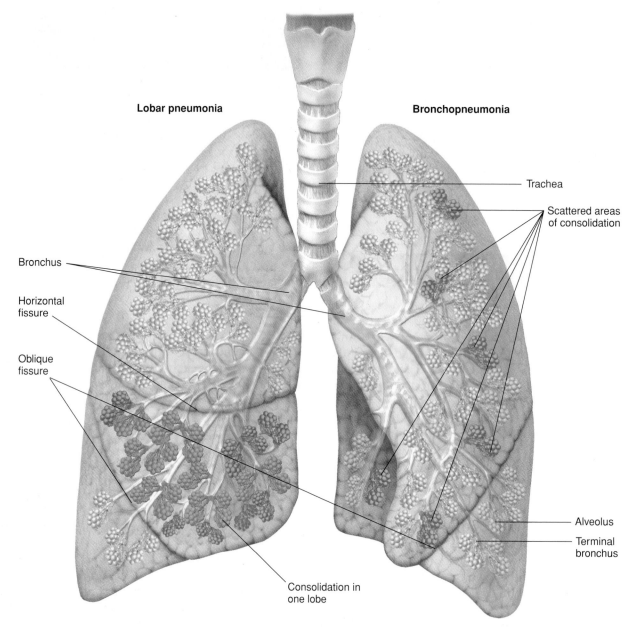

FIGURE 12.3. **Types of Pneumonia**. Lobar pneumonia (left) and bronchopneumonia (right). In bronchopneumonia, patchy areas of consolidation (infection) occur. In lobar pneumonia, an entire lobe is affected. Reprinted with permission from Anatomical Chart Co.

Some forms of pneumonia are caused by certain bacteria and viruses that typically invade the lungs, and are called **opportunistic infections.** These infections are illnesses caused by various organisms that usually do not cause disease in persons with normal immune systems. Opportunistic infections are often seen in patients with **acquired immunodeficiency syndrome** (AIDS), an illness that is most commonly spread by sexual contact or by sharing unsterilized intravenous needles. **Human immunodeficiency virus** (HIV), the virus that causes AIDS, invades and destroys a specific type of white blood cell, the CD4+ T cell, which is a chief component of the body's immune system. (Note: A more thorough discussion of HIV/AIDS is covered in

Chapters 16 and 19, *Obstetrics and Gynecology* and *Immunology*, respectively.)

Many viruses and bacteria usually do not cause healthy people to become ill, but because the immune system in patients with AIDS is so compromised, they are more susceptible to becoming ill from exposure to these infectious agents. Because the respiratory system is "open" to the environment, taking in air and any infectious material in the air, the lungs are the most susceptible to attack.

Pneumocystis carinii pneumonia (PCP), as the condition is commonly termed (although the causative organism has been renamed *Pneumocystis jiroveci*, pronounced *yee-row-vet-zee*), is an infection of the lungs that has an adverse effect on individuals with weakened immune systems because of HIV/AIDS. *Pneumocystis* is a genus of unicellular fungi found in the respiratory tracts of many mammals and humans. The organism was first described in 1909 and named in honor of Italian physician Antonio Carini. In 1976, Dr. Otto Jirovec isolated the organism from humans, and the organism responsible for PCP was renamed after him. PCP was rarely seen prior to the AIDS epidemic. Before the use of preventive antibiotics for PCP, up to 70% of individuals in the United States with advanced AIDS would develop PCP. Common drugs used to treat and prevent PCP include sulfamethoxazole and trimethoprim (Bactrim), pentamidine (NebuPent), dapsone (Aczone), clindamycin (Cleocin), atovaquone (Mepron), and tobramycin (Tobrex).

Treatment of pneumonia involves prescribing the appropriate antibiotic for the microorganism causing the illness. Bacterial pneumonia usually responds to penicillin, ampicillin plus clavulanic acid (Augmentin), and erythromycin. Other treatments for bacterial-type pneumonias include antibiotics such as cefuroxime (Ceftin), ofloxacin (Floxin), sulfamethoxazole and trimethoprim (Bactrim), clarithromycin (Biaxin), tetracycline (Sumycin), and azithromycin (Zithromax). Viral pneumonias do not respond to antibiotic treatment and usually resolve over time.

Asthma

Asthma is a common lung disease characterized by recurrent attacks of wheezing due to obstruction of the airways from excessive amounts of secretions. The airway obstruction arises when the airways of the lungs are inflamed and hyperreact to certain triggers such as viruses, smoke, dust, mold, animal hair, and pollen. Persons with asthma have acute episodes when the air passages in their lungs get narrower, and breathing becomes more difficult. This causes tightness in the chest, wheezing, shortness of breath, or a cough that never goes away and/or gets worse over time.

Several different medications are used in treating acute asthma attacks and for the long-term prevention of asthma. **Bronchodilators** help open the bronchial airways of the lungs, allowing more air to flow through them. They can be administered as pills, liquids, inhalers, or via an injection. For most people, inhaled bronchodilators are used first because they go right into the lungs and immediately relieve the symptoms of asthma. Some common bronchodilators include albuterol, Proventil, Levophed, Proventil, Serevent, and salmeterol.

Anti-inflammatory medicines reduce the swelling inside airways and decrease the amount of mucus in the lungs. They are administered using a metered-dose inhaler (MDI), swallowed as a liquid or a tablet, or taken as an injection. Although there are many different types of anti-inflammatory medicines, the ones that are used most often in people with asthma are corticos-

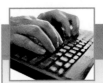

teroids, including Advair, Azmacort, betamethasone, prednisone, Flovent, and Solu-Medrol.

Leukotriene receptor antagonists are a class of drugs that block leukotrienes, byproducts of the metabolic process in the lungs that cause narrowing and swelling of the airways. Blocking leukotrienes can improve asthma symptoms and can help prevent asthma attacks. Because they come in tablet form, leukotriene antagonists can be a helpful preventive therapy for people who would rather not use an inhaled medicine or who have difficulty using their inhaler properly. A leukotriene receptor antagonist can be used instead of inhaled steroids to help prevent asthma attacks. Some common leukotriene receptor antagonist medications include montelukast (Singulair) and zafirlukast (Accolate).

Chronic Obstructive Pulmonary Disease

Chronic obstructive pulmonary disease (COPD) is a general term for a group of diseases that describes abnormalities in the lungs that lead to gradual loss of lung function. Generally, COPD refers to two diseases that are closely related: chronic bronchitis and emphysema. These diseases cause excessive inflammation that eventually leads to abnormalities in lung structure that permanently obstruct airflow and make it difficult to expel oxygen-depleted air normally (hence the term *chronic obstructive*).

Bronchitis

Bronchitis is an inflammation of the bronchi, or breathing tubes, which causes increased production of mucus and other changes. Although there are several different types of bronchitis, the two most common are acute and chronic.

When the cells of the bronchial-lining tissue are irritated beyond a certain point, the tiny cilia, which normally trap and eliminate pollutants, stop functioning. Consequently, the air passages become clogged by debris and irritation increases. In response, a heavy secretion of mucus develops, which causes the cough characteristic of bronchitis. Acute bronchitis is usually caused by an infection from bacteria or viruses and commonly evolves from a severe cold. It may also be

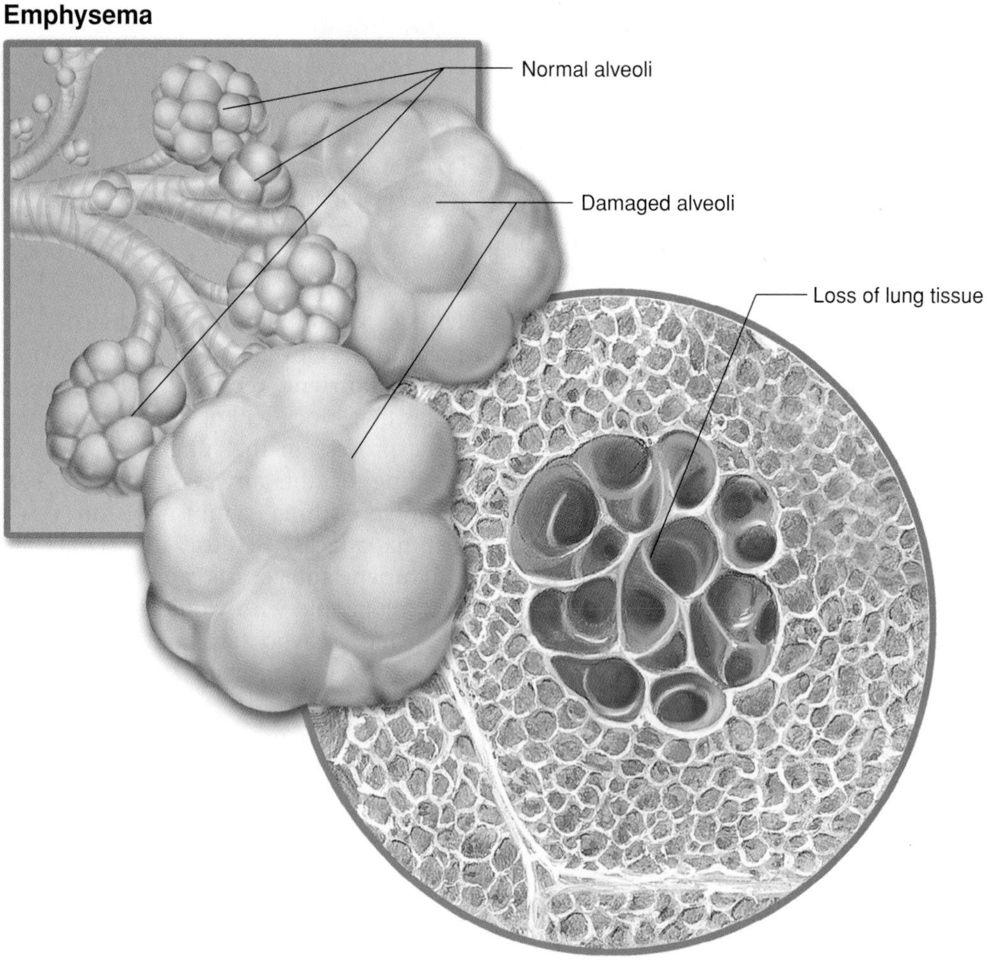

Emphysema

FIGURE 12.4. **Chronic Obstructive Pulmonary Disease: Emphysema.** Damage to the alveoli is irreversible and results in permanent holes in the tissues of the lower lungs. Reprinted with permission from Anatomical Chart Co.

caused by other agents such as dust, allergens, fumes from chemical cleaning compounds, or cigarette smoke. Acute bronchitis is usually a mild, self-limiting condition with complete healing and return to function.

Chronic bronchitis is the term given to bronchitis symptoms, such as excessive mucus secretion in the bronchi or a mucus-producing cough, that last three or more months and recur for two successive years. Sometimes the large and small airways of the lungs become narrowed, and the lining of the passageways may become scarred. This makes it hard to move air in and out of the lungs, resulting in shortness of breath.

Emphysema

Emphysema is a lung condition that often accompanies chronic bronchitis. Whereas chronic bronchitis mainly involves the larger airways, emphysema is a disease involving the very fine airways and alveoli. This breakdown of the walls of the alveoli causes a decrease in respiratory function and, often, breathlessness.

Emphysema begins with the destruction of the alveoli in the lungs, where oxygen from the air is exchanged

for carbon dioxide in the blood. The walls of the air sacs are thin and fragile. Damage to the air sacs is irreversible and results in permanent "holes" in the tissues of the lower lungs, as shown in Figure 12.4. As the alveoli become fractured or burst, the remaining alveoli become enlarged to make up for the loss. This results in fewer numbers of alveoli, or alveoli that do not work properly, to function in gas exchange. The lungs are able to transfer less and less oxygen to the bloodstream, causing shortness of breath. The lungs lose their elasticity and exhalation becomes difficult, causing air to remain in the alveoli. Consequently, the next breath is started with air in the lungs that should have been exhaled. The trapped "old" air takes up space, so the alveoli are unable to fill with enough fresh air to supply the body with needed oxygen when the person inhales. This results in the feeling of shortness of breath during exertion and, as the disease progresses, even while at rest.

Cigarette smoking is the major cause of emphysema, accounting for more than 80% of all cases. Emphysema usually occurs in people older than age 40 who have smoked for many years. Long-term exposure to second-hand smoke, as well as air pollution, environmental or occupational hazards, and genetic factors, may also play a role in emphysema.

In technical terms, COPD is a slowly progressive disease that is characterized by a decrease in the ability of the lungs to maintain the body's oxygen supply and remove carbon dioxide. The term **barrel chest** refers to a chest expanded in the shape of a barrel, a condition often seen in COPD patients because of chronic hyper-inflation of the lungs.

Cystic Fibrosis

Cystic fibrosis (CF) is an inherited (genetic) condition affecting the cells that produce mucus, sweat, saliva, and digestive juices.

The basis of CF lies in an abnormal gene. The result of this genetic defect is an atypical electrolyte transportation system within the cells of the body. This causes the cells in the respiratory system, especially the lungs, to absorb too much sodium and water. Normally, these secretions are thin and slippery, but in CF, the defective gene causes the secretions to become thick and sticky. Instead of acting as a lubricant, the secretions plug up tubes, ducts, and passageways (especially in the pancreas and lungs), becoming very thick and hard to remove. These thick secretions put a patient with CF at risk for constant infection and respiratory failure. The high risk of infection leads to damage in the lungs, lungs that do not work properly, and, eventually, death of the cells in the lungs.

CF is a chronic, progressive, and usually fatal disease. In general, individuals with CF live only into their 30s.

Tuberculosis

Tuberculosis, also known as TB, is an infectious, inflammatory disease caused by bacteria belonging to the genus *Mycobacterium*. The bacteria can attack any part of the body but usually attack the lungs. TB was once the leading cause of death in the United States.

The bacteria that cause TB are spread from person to person in infected droplets from the coughs of people who have untreated TB. These droplets are extremely tiny and can remain suspended in the air for several hours, and people nearby may inhale these bacteria and become infected. When a person breathes in TB bacteria, the bacteria can settle in the lungs and begin to grow. From there, they can move through the blood to other parts of the body, such as the kidney, spine, and brain.

Although we may think of TB as a disease of the past, it remains among the leading killers of adults. In the 1940s, scientists discovered the first of several drugs now used to treat TB. As a result, TB slowly began to disappear in the United States. However, once the country became complacent about TB and funding of TB pro-

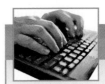

grams was decreased, the disease made a comeback. Recent increases in funding and attention to the TB problem are once again causing an all-time low in new cases of TB in as late as 2006, but TB is still a problem with more than 14,000 new cases reported annually in the United States.

Like any infectious disease, TB threatens the health of people everywhere. TB spreads easily among coworkers, friends, and family through casual contact (such as coughing, sneezing, or laughing) in a matter of hours. Tuberculosis is treated with a combination of antibiotics appropriate for the disease process. A combination is used because the TB bacteria are likely to develop drug resistance if only a single drug is used. The treatment usually takes six to nine months and sometimes longer in order to avoid recurrence. The oral drugs used to treat tuberculosis include isoniazid (INH), rifampin, ethambutol, and pyrazinamide.

Acute Respiratory Distress Syndrome

Acute respiratory distress syndrome (ARDS) is a life-threatening condition in which inflammation of the lungs and accumulation of fluid in the alveoli lead to low blood oxygen levels. When the alveoli are damaged, some collapse and lose their ability to receive oxygen. With some alveoli collapsed and others filled with fluid, the lungs become heavy and stiff; it becomes difficult for them to absorb oxygen and expel carbon dioxide. Within one or two days, progressive interference with gas exchange can bring about respiratory failure requiring mechanical ventilation.

The cause of ARDS remains unknown. It can appear after direct physical or toxic injury to the lungs, for example, by inhalation of smoke or other toxic fumes, or "bruising" of the lungs that usually occurs after a severe blow to the chest. Another mechanism, more common but less understood, is an indirect bloodborne injury to the lungs. When a person is very sick or the body is injured, the lungs react by becoming inflamed, causing lung failure. Examples of this type of indirect lung injury include the presence of severe infection or trauma.

ARDS patients are usually treated in the intensive or critical care unit of a hospital. Treatment consists of mechanical ventilation along with fluid maintenance and balance and breathing support as the patient's lungs heal. Treatment of the precipitating illness is conducted simultaneously. No specific pharmacological therapies currently exist for patients with ARDS, although many experimental therapies show promise, including the replacement of surfactant and the use of anti-inflammatory agents. The lungs can reorganize and recover but it may take as long as 6 to 12 months and sometimes longer, depending on the precipitating condition and the injury.

Lung Cancer

Lung cancer, like all cancer, is an uncontrolled proliferation of abnormal cells, in this case occurring in one or both lungs. It is actually a cancer of the bronchi of the airway, properly called **bronchogenic carcinoma**. Normal lung tissue cells reproduce to form healthy lung tissue, but cancerous cells reproduce too rapidly, forming a mass of tissue or tumor. Gradually the tumor invades and destroys healthy lung tissue, making it difficult for the lung(s) to function properly. See Figure 12.5. If untreated, the cancer cells may spread through the

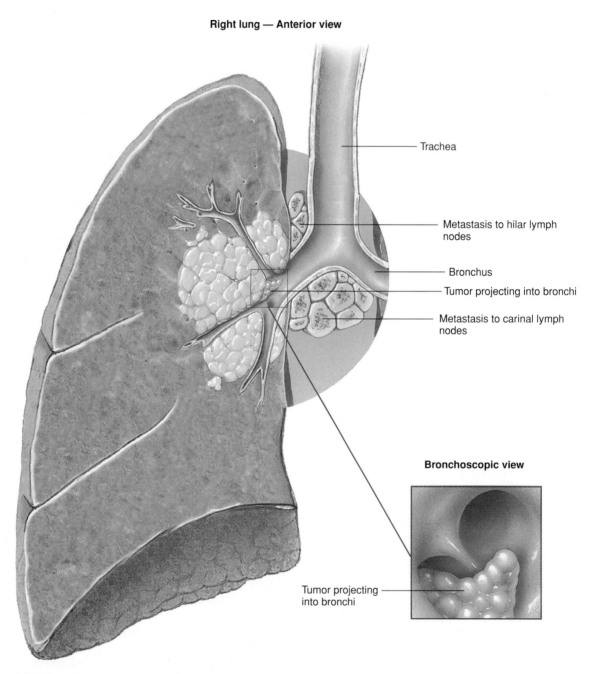

Right lung — Anterior view

Trachea

Metastasis to hilar lymph nodes

Bronchus

Tumor projecting into bronchi

Metastasis to carinal lymph nodes

Bronchoscopic view

Tumor projecting into bronchi

FIGURE 12.5. **Tumor Infiltration in Lung Cancer**. Reprinted with permission from Anatomical Chart Co.

blood and lymphatic system to other parts of the body, where they form new tumors.

Any of the tissues in the lung can become cancerous, but most commonly lung cancer forms from the lining of the bronchi. Lung cancer is not really thought of as a single disease but rather a collection of several diseases that are characterized by the type of cell from which the tumors form, the way in which these cells behave, and how they are treated. Cancers that begin in the lungs are divided into two major types: **small-cell lung cancer** and **non-small cell lung cancer**. The terms *small-cell cancer* and *non-small cell lung cancer* refer to the appearance of the cells under a microscope. Small-cell lung cancer cells appear as small rounded cells with prominent nuclei whereas the non-small-cell types of lung cancer cells are generally larger. There are also differences in how the cells group together when viewed under a microscope, as well as molecular differences between the two types of cancer cells. Thus, the staging of and treatment approaches to these two types of lung cancer are different.

Lung cancer is usually more aggressive than other cancers, and it is more dangerous. Unlike skin or breast tumors, lung cancer shows no external, visible signs and is often well developed by the time it is suspected or diagnosed.

Smoking is by far the most common cause of lung cancer, as smoking causes constant irritation and precancerous changes in the inner layer of cells lining the airway. Before cigarettes became popular, lung cancer was a relatively rare disease. Today lung cancer accounts for 25% of all cancer deaths in the United States. However, not all smokers develop lung cancer. Genetic predisposition, previous lung disease, and exposure to cancer-causing substances are also factors in the development of lung cancer. Exposure to asbestos is a common cause for **mesothelioma**, a rare form of cancer. In this disease, malignant cells develop in the **mesothelium**, the protective lining that covers most of the body's internal organs. It can occur in the lining of the abdominal cavity (**peritoneum**) or the sac that surrounds the heart (**pericardium**), but its most common site is the pleura of the lungs.

Like other cancers, the options for treatment for lung cancer generally revolve around surgery, radiation, or chemotherapy, or a combination of all three. Surgery is used to remove the cancerous lesion along with surrounding tissue. If a lobe of the lung is removed, it is called a **lobectomy**. If part of a lobe is removed, it is called a **wedge resection**. If the entire lung is removed, it is called a **pneumonectomy**.

High-energy radiation therapy is used to kill very small deposits of cancer cells that cannot be seen and removed during surgery. It can also be used to **palliate**, or relieve, symptoms of lung cancer such as pain, bleeding, difficulty swallowing, cough, and problems with metastasis to the brain. **External beam radiation** is delivered from outside the body and focused on the cancerous tumor.

Brachytherapy uses a small pellet of radioactive material placed by a bronchoscope directly into the lesion or into the airway next to the lesion. **Chemotherapy** is a treatment that involves anticancer drugs administered either intravenously or orally to kill cancer cells. These drugs enter the bloodstream and travel throughout the body, making this treatment useful for cancer that has metastasized to organs beyond the lung. Chemotherapy can be given as a single therapy or as an addition to surgery, called **adjuvant chemotherapy**. Chemotherapy drugs such as cisplatin or carboplatin, when combined with another drug such as gemcitabine (Gemzar), paclitaxel (Taxol), docetaxel (Taxotere), or vinorelbine (Navelbine), are an effective treatment regimen to kill cancer cells.

In recent years, researchers have developed other cancer drugs that actually interfere with the growth of individual cancer cells. Taken orally, these drugs work against protein **epidermal growth factor receptors (EGFRs)**, which are proteins found in the cell membranes. When activated, these receptors initiate a signaling process that regulates cell growth. Many cancers have an abnormal increase in the activity of EGFRs; therefore, drugs have been developed to inhibit their functioning. These drugs include gefitinib (Iressa), erlotinib (Tarceva), and cetuximab (Erbitux). Other innovative approaches used to treat lung cancer include a vaccine called GVAX, which is made from a patient's own tumor cells. These cells are genetically modified to secrete a hormone that stimulates the immune system to attack the tumor. In gene therapy, tumor-suppressor genes that reduce lung cancer are injected into a patient's lung in an attempt to kill cancer cells or slow their growth.

Pulmonary Edema

Pulmonary edema is a buildup of fluid in the lungs, most often due to heart failure from a heart attack or other myocardial disease or injury. It can also be caused by fluid overload, such as that caused when an individual is given too much intravenous fluid in the hospital. In these situations, the heart muscle weakens and is less able to pump blood forward into the atrial system. Pressure rises in the pulmonary veins, resulting in leakage of fluid into the air spaces and the lungs.

Treatment of pulmonary edema requires immediate removal of fluid from the lungs with an intravenous medication. This medication helps the kidneys to excrete fluid buildup (a process called **diuresis**) and strengthens the pumping ability of the heart. At the same time, the patient is treated for any underlying condition that has brought on the heart failure, such as an infection or heart attack.

Pulmonary Embolism

Pulmonary embolism (PE) is an obstruction of the pulmonary circulation by solid or cellular material that

QUICK CHECK 12.3 ✓

Circle the correct word in the following sentences.

1. The patient stated she had "walking pneumonia," or (mycoplasma, micoflora, mycopleuritis) pneumonia, approximately 3 years ago.

2. (CPPD, COPP, COPD) refers to abnormalities in the lung that lead to gradual loss of lung function.

3. The cause of (ARDS, ADDS, ARRD) remains unknown.

4. The patient was prescribed an antibiotic to treat her (bronchiosis, bronchitis, bronchopsis).

5. Cystic (fibroma, fibroplasia, fibrosis) is an inherited condition resulting from an abnormal gene.

has traveled from the venous circulation through the right side of the heart and lodged in an artery of the lungs, blocking the blood supply. It is usually caused by a blood clot from a vein in the lower leg called a **deep vein (or venous) thrombosis (DVT)**. The clot cuts off the blood supply to the lungs and also disrupts the flow of blood through the left side of the heart and the rest of the body. If the blockage is large enough, the output from the heart is disabled and body tissues die.

Intravenous drugs are used to dissolve the clot. Further clotting is prevented with anticoagulant drugs, also known as "blood thinners," which are used to stop clots from getting bigger and to prevent additional blood clots from forming. These drugs can be taken in pill form, such as warfarin (Coumadin), or as an injection or intravenously, such as heparin or enoxaparin (Lovenox).

Alternatively, a **vena cava filter** can be used instead of medication or when anticoagulant medication proves to be ineffective. This tiny device is inserted inside a large vein called the **inferior vena cava**, which is the vein that carries blood from the body back to the heart. The filter serves to catch the clots as they try to move through the body to the lungs. Although this treatment can prevent a clot from traveling to the lungs, it cannot stop other clots from forming.

Compression stockings worn on the legs from the arch of the foot to just above or below the knee can also be used to provide support and reduce the swelling in the leg after a blood clot has occurred.

DIAGNOSTIC STUDIES AND PROCEDURES

Pulmonary Function Testing

Pulmonary function testing, also called **spirometry**, is one of the basic tools for evaluating a patient's respiratory status. **Pulmonary function tests** (PFTs) are a series of measurements that evaluate the lungs' capacity to hold air, move air in and out, and to exchange oxygen and carbon dioxide. PFTs provide valuable feedback about the function of the lungs that can help determine the type and severity of lung disorders. PFTs are often the first diagnostic test employed in the workup for patients with suspected pulmonary disease. PFTs are also used for preoperative evaluation, managing patients with known pulmonary disease, and quantifying pulmonary disability.

Simple spirometry has become more common in the daily practice of medicine. As environmental pollutants continue to worsen, the rate of obesity continues to escalate, and the dangers of smoking continue to make themselves known, clinics and health centers are using PFTs as a routine diagnostic tool to quickly assess a patient's general lung function.

The instrument used to perform PFTs is called a **spirometer**. It is a device that consists of a small plastic breathing tube hooked to a computerized console that records and prints the data it obtains. The results are printed on a graph called a **spirogram**. The values obtained are indicated on the graph and are compared to predicted values that factor in a patient's gender, age, height, and weight.

There are more than 15 spirometry parameters measured and reported by physicians to evaluate lung function. The most common of these include:

- Tidal volume. This value indicates the amount of air inhaled or exhaled during normal breathing.
- **Forced vital capacity (FVC)**. This value indicates the volume of air that can be exhaled forcibly and quickly after the patient has taken in the deepest breath possible. This value is expressed in liters.
- **Forced expiratory volume measured in one second of time (FEV1)**. This is the measurement taken when the patient takes the deepest breath possible and blows into the console's breathing tube, but only the first second of time of the forced exhalation is recorded. This value is also expressed in liters.

- **FEV1-FVC ratio. This** is a comparison of the FVC and FEV1, expressed as a percentage. It indicates the percentage of the total forced vital capacity that was exhaled in the first second of forced exhalation.
- **Total lung capacity (TLC).** This measures the total volume of the lungs when maximally inflated.
- **Forced expiratory flow (FEF).** This value measures the average rate of flow during the middle half of forced vital capacity.
- **Diffusing capacity for carbon monoxide (DLCO).** This value analyzes the amount of carbon monoxide exhaled compared to the amount inhaled.

The information gathered during pulmonary function testing is useful in diagnosing certain types of lung disorders, but is most useful when assessing for obstructive lung diseases, such as asthma and COPD.

Pulse Oximetry

Pulse oximetry (often dictated as *"pulse ox"*) is a simple, noninvasive method of measuring arterial blood oxygen using a clip or probe attached to a sensor site, such as the tip of the finger. The percentage of hemoglobin that is saturated with oxygen is called **oxygen saturation** and is expressed as a percent value. The **pulse oximeter** is a small machine with a sensor attached that clips to the patient's fingertip or ear lobe, which is linked to a monitoring console. The monitor displays the percentage of hemoglobin saturated with oxygen, anywhere from 0% to 100% (which physicians often dictate as "O_2 sat," being slang for "saturation"). When saturation falls below a certain level, usually 85%, the patient is given supplemental nasal oxygen to help restore saturation to optimal levels.

Arterial Blood Gas Test

An **arterial blood gas** test, or ABG, is performed on a patient to measure the amounts of oxygen and carbon dioxide dissolved in the blood by measuring the **partial pressure of oxygen (PO_2)** and **partial pressure of carbon dioxide (PCO_2)**. This test also ascertains the **potential of Hydrogen (pH)**, or the acid or alkaline status of the blood. ABG results can reflect the overall cardiopulmonary and renal functions of the patient. Oxygen and carbon dioxide levels are important indicators of lung function because they reflect the extent to which the lungs are getting oxygen into the blood and getting carbon dioxide out of it. This test uses blood drawn from an artery, where the oxygen and carbon dioxide levels can be measured before they enter body tissues and become changed.

The ABG test measures the following parameters:

- pH, which is a measure of the acidic or alkaline nature of blood. A pH of less than 7 is acidic, and a pH greater than 7 is called alkaline. The pH of blood is usually close to 7.4.
- PO_2, which represents the overall content of oxygen in the blood and how well oxygen is able to move from the blood into the air space of the lungs.
- PCO_2, which indicates how well carbon dioxide is able to move out of the blood into the airspace of the lungs and out with exhaled air.
- **Bicarbonate** (HCO_3), which is the most important buffer in the blood. Buffers are chemical substances that keep the pH of blood within a normal range.
- Oxygen saturation, which provides information about the amount of oxygen in the blood.

Arterial blood gas analysis can help diagnose many disorders. If the PCO_2 is elevated due to **hypoventilation**, a state in which there is a reduced amount of air entering the alveoli (such as in asthma or COPD), the patient is said to have **respiratory acidosis**, or excess carbon dioxide retention. If the PCO_2 is low due to **hyperventilation**, a state in which there is an increased amount of air entering the alveoli (such as in pneumonia or a pulmonary embolus), then the patient is said to have **respiratory alkalosis**, which occurs when too much carbon dioxide is excreted. **Metabolic acidosis** indicates a condition in which the blood is too acidic. It may be caused by severe illness or bacteria in the bloodstream, called sepsis. **Metabolic alkalosis** indicates excessive blood alkalinity caused by an overabundance of bicarbonate in the blood or a loss of acid from the blood.

Peak Flow Monitoring

Peak flow monitoring measures the rate of air flow, or how fast air is able to pass through the airways. Measuring peak flow helps a healthcare provider manage a patient's asthmatic condition effectively. It gives an accurate measure of the severity of the disease and permits detection of airway obstruction before wheezing can be heard or symptoms can be felt.

Peak flow monitoring is measured with a device called a peak flow meter, which looks like a lightweight plastic tube about the size of a household flashlight. The peak flow meter measures how fast air is expelled

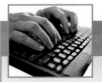

TRANSCRIPTION TIP:

In pulmonary function testing, the term tidal volume should not be transcribed as "title volume."

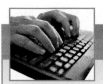

from the lungs. This rate, called the **peak expiratory flow (PEF)** is recorded in a chart or graph and provides an accurate picture of lung function in order for a clinician to make appropriate decisions regarding the effectiveness of the patient's medicine and treatment plan.

Bronchoscopy

A **bronchoscopy** is a medical procedure that allows a clinician to examine the larynx and airways through a flexible viewing tube in order to diagnose a lung problem such as a mass or infection, or to collect lung secretions or tissue specimens so they can be tested for cancer or other diseases. A thin, flexible lighted tube called a **bronchoscope** is inserted through the nose or mouth. The bronchoscope has a lighted viewing lens so that a physician can visually examine the larynx, bronchi, and bronchioles.

This procedure is used to examine the mucosal surface of the airways for abnormalities that might be associated with a variety of lung diseases and to investigate the source of bleeding. The bronchoscope can also be used to remove secretions, blood, pus, and foreign bodies as well as place drugs in specific areas of the lung. If a doctor suspects lung cancer, the airways can be examined using a bronchoscope to obtain small bits of tissue from any suspicious areas. It also can be used for **bron-**

choalveolar lavage (BAL), which is the process of washing the lining of the bronchi or bronchioles to obtain cells for culture to diagnose diseases.

Ventilation Perfusion Scan

A **ventilation-perfusion scan**, commonly referred to as a **V/Q scan** (the *q* stands for *quotient*) is used to assess distribution of blood flow and ventilation throughout both lungs. Effective gas exchange depends on a stable relationship between ventilation and perfusion, referred to as the **V/Q ratio**. Areas of poor blood flow and poor ventilation within the lungs show as increased uptake of radioactivity in the tissues.

A mismatch in ventilation and perfusion can affect all body systems. The following types of mismatch can occur:

- Need for more oxygen. Inadequate ventilation occurs when pulmonary circulation through the heart is adequate but not enough oxygen is available in the lungs. As a result, a portion of the blood flowing through the pulmonary capillaries does not receive oxygen. Perfusion without ventilation usually results from airway obstruction, such as that caused by pneumonia.
- Need for more blood. Inadequate perfusion occurs when ventilation is normal, but blood flow in the pulmonary capillaries is not adequate. Narrowed capillaries or blocked capillaries (such as from blood clots) commonly cause this occurrence.
- Need for more oxygen and blood. Inadequate ventilation and perfusion occurs when there is a lack of oxygen in the lungs (ventilation) and in the pulmonary circulation (perfusion). When this occurs, the body compensates by delivering blood flow to better ventilated lung areas. Chronic alveolar collapse from disease or blood clots can create this condition.

A V/Q scan is actually two tests that may be performed separately or together. During the ventilation

QUICK CHECK 12.4

Fill in the blanks with the appropriate answers.

1. A _____ is an instrument used to examine the larynx and airways.

2. _____ is the state in which there is a reduced amount of air entering the alveoli.

3. _____ helps a healthcare provider assess the patient's asthmatic condition.

4. The values indicated on a _____ are compared to predicted values when performing PFTs.

5. The process of measuring hemoglobin that is saturated with oxygen is called _____.

scan, a tracer gas is inhaled into the lungs. Pictures taken during this scan show areas of the lungs that are not receiving enough air or that retain too much air. The perfusion portion of the scan is performed by injecting radioactive albumin into a vein. It travels through the bloodstream and into the lungs. Pictures from this scan can show areas of the lungs that are not receiving enough blood.

If the lungs are working normally, blood flow on a perfusion scan matches air flow on a ventilation scan. A mismatch between the ventilation and perfusion scans may indicate a **pulmonary embolism**, which is blockage by foreign matter or by a blood clot.

CHAPTER SUMMARY

Lungs are for living. Breathing, controlled by the respiratory system, is a continuous process that brings us the oxygen we need to live. Without even thinking, we take a breath and exhale carbon dioxide every few seconds. In addition to providing air to the body, the pulmonary system also helps to protect the body from germs and pollutants. Although an individual can go for days without food and water and for hours without sleep, a failure in the function of the pulmonary system for even a few minutes is fatal.

·I·N·S·I·G·H·T·

Oxygen Use in Commercial Flight

Pulmonary researchers are now advocating that airlines increase the amount of oxygen used in the cabins during flight. Most commercial jets fly about 35,000 feet above sea level, where the air is too thin for anyone to survive. Thus, cabins are pressurized to the equivalent of about 6,000 to 8,000 feet above sea level. Even that pressure can cause a dangerous lack of oxygen for patients with weak or diseased lungs. A recent study of flyers of all ages on both long-term and short-term flights found that blood oxygen levels in more than half of the participants dropped by an average of 4% at cruising altitudes, to an average of 93% oxygen saturation. This drop in oxygen levels might not even be noticeable in healthy individuals, but this reduction of oxygen can lead to critically low levels, and hence life-threatening problems, for passengers with respiratory diseases.

Even those individuals who normally would not use oxygen during their daily activities may need supplemental oxygen during airplane flights. Therefore, senior citizens or those individuals with chronic lung conditions should consult with a physician about the possibility of obtaining supplemental oxygen before traveling by air.

Common Soundalike Words

Word	Word Pronunciation	Soundalike	Soundalike Pronunciation
pleural: relating to the delicate serous membrane that lines each half of the thorax.	plūr′ăl	**plural**: relating to more than one kind.	plūr′ăl
alveolar: referring to the alveoli of the lungs.	al-vē′ō-lăr	**areolar**: referring to the areola, or the human nipple.	ă-rē′ō-lăr
pleuritic: relating to pleurisy, an inflammation of the pleura of the chest.	plū-rit′ik	**pruritic**: pertaining to pruritus, or itching.	prū-rit′ik
perfusion: relating to the amount of blood reaching a tissue.	pĕr-fyū′zhŭn	**profusion**: relating to something that is present in abundance.	prō-fyū′zhŭn
atelectasis: reduction or absence of air in part or all of a lung, with resulting loss of lung volume.	at-ĕ-lek′tă-sis	**alkalosis**: a state characterized by a decrease in the hydrogen ion concentration of arterial blood below the normal level.	al-kă-lō′sis
hemoptysis: spitting of blood from the lungs.	hē-mop′ti-sis	**hemolysis**: alteration, dissolution, or destruction of red blood cells.	hē-mol′i-sis
bronchi: plural of *bronchus*, one of the two subdivisions of the trachea serving to convey air to and from the lungs.	brong′kī	**rhonchi**: an added sound with a musical pitch occurring during inspiration or expiration, heard while listening to the chest during a physical exam.	rong′-kī
coarse: rough or lacking refinement in tone (such as breath sounds).	koors′	**course**: a mode of action; a line or route along which something travels or moves.	koors′
effusion: the accumulation of fluid from the blood vessels or lymphatics into the tissues or a cavity.	e-fyu′zhŭn	**infusion**: the introduction of fluid other than blood, e.g., saline solution, into a vein.	in-fyū′zhŭn

Combining Forms

Combining Form	Meaning	Combining Form	Meaning
alveol/o	alveolus/air sacs in the lungs	muc/o	mucus
aspir/o	to breathe in or suck in	nas/o, rhin/o	nose
asthm/o	asthma	ox/o, ox/i	oxygen
bronch/i, bronch/o, bronchiol/o	bronchi/bronchiole	pector/o	chest
		pharyng/o	pharynx, throat
capn/o, capn/i	carbon dioxide	pleur/o	pleura
cost/o	ribs	pneum/o, pneumon/o, pneumat/o	lung, air
diaphragmat/o, phren/o	diaphragm		
effus/o	pouring out	pulmon/o	lung
embol/o	embolus	sinus/o	sinus
epiglott/o, epiglottid/o	epiglottis	spir/o	breathe
laryng/o	larynx (voice box)	thorac/o	thorax (chest)
lob/o	lobe	trache/o	trachea, windpipe
mediastin/o	mediastinum		

Add Your Own Combining Forms Here:

_____

_____

_____

_____

_____

_____

ABBREVIATIONS

Abbreviation	Meaning	Abbreviation	Meaning
A/C	assist control	FiO$_2$	fraction of inspired oxygen
ABG	arterial blood gas	FVC	forced vital capacity
AFB	acid-fast bacilli	HCO$_3$	bicarbonate ion
AIDS	acquired immunodeficiency syndrome	HIV	human immunodeficiency virus
ARDS	acute respiratory distress syndrome	IMV	intermittent mandatory ventilation
BAL	bronchoalveolar lavage	PCO$_2$	partial pressure of carbon dioxide
CF	cystic fibrosis	PCP	*Pneumocystis carinii* pneumonia
CMV	cytomegalovirus	PE	pulmonary embolism
CO$_2$	carbon dioxide	PEEP	positive end-expiratory pressure
COPD	chronic obstructive pulmonary disease	PEF	peak expiratory flow
CPR	cardiopulmonary resuscitation	PFTs	pulmonary function tests
DLCO	diffusing capacity for carbon monoxide	pH	potential of Hydrogen
DNR (or DNR/DNI)	do not resuscitate; do not intubate	PO$_2$	partial pressure of oxygen
		RSV	respiratory syncytial virus
DVT	deep vein (venous) thrombosis	TB	tuberculosis
EBV	Epstein-Barr virus	TLC	total lung capacity
EGFRs	epidermal growth factor receptors	V/Q	ventilation-perfusion (scan)
FEF	forced expiratory flow		
FEV$_1$	forced expiratory volume measured in one second		

Add Your Own Abbreviations Here:

_____

_____

_____

_____

_____

_____

TERMINOLOGY

Term	*Meaning*
accessory muscles	The muscles of the neck and chest not normally associated with breathing.
acid-fast bacilli	The pathogens that cause tuberculosis.
acquired immunodeficiency syndrome (AIDS)	An illness that is most commonly spread by sexual contact or by sharing unsterilized intravenous needles.
acute respiratory distress syndrome (ARDS)	A life-threatening condition in which inflammation of the lungs and accumulation of fluid in the alveoli leads to low blood oxygen levels.
adventitious sounds	Abnormal breath sounds heard on lung examination.
adjuvant chemotherapy	Chemotherapy given in addition to surgery.
alveoli (singular, alveolus)	Tiny sacs that hold air in the lungs.
apnea	Absence of breathing.
arterial blood gas (ABG)	A test performed to determine the amounts of oxygen and carbon dioxide dissolved in the blood, and to ascertain the acid base status of the blood.
assist control mode (A/C)	A setting in which the patient sets his or her own breathing rate, but if the rate falls below a certain rate, the ventilator takes over.
asthma	A disease in which the lung airways are inflamed and react with an oversensitivity of the lungs and airways to certain triggers.
atelectasis	Decreased or absent air in the entire or part of a lung resulting in lung collapse.
bacterial pneumonia	A pneumonia caused by bacteria.
barrel chest	A chest expanded in the shape of a barrel, a condition often seen in COPD patients due to chronic hyperinflation of the lungs.
bicarbonate (HCO_3)	A buffer in the blood that keeps the pH within a normal range.
brachytherapy	Small pellets of radioactive material placed by a bronchoscope directly into the lesion or into the airway next to the lesion.
brainstem	The part of the central nervous system that controls breathing.
bronchi (singular, bronchus)	The two main air passages that enter the right and left lung, respectively.
bronchiectasis	The dilation of the large airways with the accumulation of secretions and chronic infection.
bronchioles	The finer subdivisions of the branched bronchial tree.
bronchiolitis	An infection of the bronchioles, or finer airways of the lungs.
bronchitis	An inflammation of the bronchi, or breathing tubes, which causes increased production of mucus and other changes.
bronchoalveolar lavage (BAL)	The process of washing the lining of the bronchi or bronchioles to obtain cells for culture to diagnose diseases.
bronchodilators	A type of medication that helps open the bronchial airways of the lungs, allowing more air to flow through them.
bronchogenic carcinoma	A cancer of the bronchi of the airway, also called *lung cancer*.
bronchopneumonia	An infection of the smaller bronchial tubes of the lungs.
bronchoscope	A thin, flexible lighted tube used in bronchoscopy.
bronchoscopy	A medical procedure that allows a doctor to examine a person's airway in order to diagnose a lung problem.
bronchus (plural bronchi)	Either of the two main branches of the trachea.

Term	Meaning
capillaries	Tiny blood vessels around the alveoli.
carina, syn. tracheal bifurcation	The point at which the trachea divides into and is continuous with the two main or principal bronchi.
chemotherapy	A treatment that involves anticancer drugs administered either intravenously or orally to kill cancer cells.
Cheyne-Stokes respirations	A respiratory pattern that describes alternating periods of apnea and deep, rapid breathing.
chronic obstructive pulmonary disease (COPD)	A collective term for a group of respiratory tract diseases that are characterized by airflow limitation.
cilia	Tiny hairs within the cells of the bronchial-lining tissue.
conchae (singular, concha), syn. nasal turbinates	The bony structures that form the posterior walls of the nasal passages.
cystic fibrosis (CF)	An inherited (genetic) condition affecting the cells that produce mucus, sweat, saliva and digestive juices.
cytomegalovirus (CMV)	A virus that occurs in healthy individuals without causing symptoms, but in immunocompromised individuals, can cause pneumonia and other serious illnesses.
deep vein (or venous) thrombosis (DVT)	A blood clot in a vein in the lower leg.
diaphragm	The muscle that separates the thoracic cavity from the abdominal cavity that contracts and relaxes during breathing.
diffusing capacity for carbon monoxide (DLCO)	The amount of carbon monoxide exhaled compared to the amount inhaled.
diffusion	Gas movement through a semipermeable membrane from an area of greater concentration to one of lesser concentration (as in internal respiration).
diuresis	Removal of fluid from the lungs.
dyspnea	Difficulty breathing.
epidermal growth factor receptors (EGFRs)	A protein in cells that initiates a signaling process that triggers abnormal cell growth.
emphysema	A degenerative disease in which lung tissue loses its elasticity and the affected person must expend energy to exhale.
empyema	A collection of pus in the lung.
epiglottis	A flap of cartilage that covers the upper region of the larynx during swallowing, which prevents food or other materials from entering the lungs.
Epstein-Barr virus (EBV)	A type of virus that causes pneumonia.
external beam radiation	High-energy radiation that is delivered from outside the body and focused on the cancerous tumor.
external respiration	The exchange of gases that involves air from the external environment.
extubation	The process of being removed from the ventilator.
FEV_1-FVC ratio	A comparison of the FVC and FEV1, expressed as a percentage.
fissures	Crevasses that separate the lobes of the lungs.
flaring	A widening of an area, such as the nostrils. In pulmonary medicine, often dictated as "nasal flaring."
forced expiratory flow (FEF)	A measure of the average rate of flow during the middle half of forced vital capacity.

Term	Meaning
forced expiratory volume measured in one second (FEV1)	The measurement taken when the patient takes the deepest breath possible and blows into the console's breathing tube, but only the first second of the forced exhalation is recorded.
forced vital capacity (FVC)	The volume of air that can be expired forcibly and quickly after the patient has taken in the deepest breath possible.
fraction of inspired oxygen (FiO$_2$)	The amount of oxygen in each inspiration.
gas exchange	The process involving circulation of oxygen through the blood for use by the body, and the conversion of that oxygen to carbon dioxide for elimination by the body.
grunting	A grunting noise heard during expiration during a lung examination.
Haemophilus influenzae	A microorganism responsible for pneumonia.
hemothorax	The presence of blood in the lung.
human immunodeficiency virus (HIV)	The virus that causes AIDS.
hydrothorax	The presence of water or fluid in the lung.
hyperventilation	A state in which there is an excessive amount of air entering the alveoli.
hypoventilation	A state in which there is a reduced amount of air entering the alveoli.
inferior vena cava	The vein that carries blood from the body back to the heart.
intercostal muscles	The muscles located between the ribs.
intermittent mandatory ventilation (IMV)	A ventilator setting in which the ventilator delivers a set number of breaths each minute but allows the patient to breathe in between.
internal respiration	The exchange of gases between the blood in the capillaries and the cells of the body.
intubation	The insertion of a tube into the patient's trachea to assist in the breathing process.
Klebsiella pneumoniae	A microorganism responsible for pneumonia.
larynx	The cartilaginous structure at the top of the trachea that contains the vocal cords.
leukotriene receptor antagonists	A class of drugs that block leukotrienes, certain products of metabolism that cause narrowing and swelling of the airways in the lungs.
lobar pneumonia	An infection of the alveoli caused by fluid and pus filling an entire lobe of the lung.
lobectomy	Removal of a lobe of the lung.
lobes	Sections of the lung.
lower respiratory tract	The part of the respiratory system that includes the larynx, trachea, lungs, bronchial tubes, and alveoli.
lung cancer	An uncontrolled proliferation of abnormal cells occurring in one or both lungs; also called *bronchogenic carcinoma*.
lungs	Either of two respiratory organs in the chest that serves to remove carbon dioxide and provide oxygen to the blood.
macrophages	Scavenger cells that clean up debris and defend against invasion by bacteria.
mechanical ventilation	The use of a machine to mechanically assist patients breathing when spontaneous breathing is absent or insufficient.
mediastinum	The area of the body that contains the heart, the trachea, the esophagus, the thymus, and the lymph nodes.

Term	*Meaning*
mesothelioma	A rare form of cancer in which malignant cells develop in the mesothelium, the protective lining that covers most of the body's internal organs and commonly occurs in the pleura of the lungs.
mesothelium	The protective lining that covers most of the body's internal organs.
metabolic acidosis	A condition in which the blood is too acidic.
metabolic alkalosis	Excessive blood alkalinity caused by an overabundance of bicarbonate in the blood or a loss of acid from the blood.
Mycoplasma pneumoniae	The bacterial species that causes the disease entity known as mycoplasma pneumonia, also known as *walking pneumonia*.
mycoplasmas	The smallest free-living agents of disease in humankind that contain characteristics of both a virus and a bacterium but are not classified as either.
non-small-cell lung cancer	A disease in which malignant (cancer) cells form in the tissues of the lung.
opportunistic infections	Life-threatening diseases that are caused by microbes such as viruses or bacteria that usually do not make healthy people sick.
orthopnea	Discomfort in breathing except in the upright position.
oxygen saturation	The amount of oxygen in the blood.
palliate	"To relieve, but not to cure," such as when chemotherapy is used to relieve the symptoms of cancer.
parietal layer	Outer layer of the pleura.
partial pressure of carbon dioxide (PCO_2)	The value of how well carbon dioxide is able to move out of the blood into the airspace of the lungs and out with exhaled air.
partial pressure of oxygen (PO_2)	The overall content of oxygen in the blood and how well oxygen is able to move from the blood into the airspace of the lungs.
peak expiratory flow (PEF)	The rate of how fast air is expelled from the lungs.
peak flow monitoring	A test that measures the rate of air flow, or how fast air is able to pass through the airways.
pericardium	The membrane that surrounds the heart.
peritoneum	The membrane that lines the abdominal cavity.
pH	A measure of the acidity or alkalinity of a solution.
pharynx	The cavity at the back of the mouth.
pleura	A clear, shiny coating enveloping the lungs.
pleural effusion	A collection of fluid or blood in the pleural space around the lung.
Pleur-evac	A water-seal suction device for pulmonary procedures.
pleurisy	An inflammation of the pleura.
Pneumocystis carinii	The microorganism that causes interstitial plasma cell pneumonia in immunodeficient people.
Pneumocystis carinii pneumonia (PCP), now called *Pneumocystis jiroveci* pneumonia	An infection of the lungs caused by the pathogen *Pneumocystis carinii* (now renamed *Pneumocystis jiroveci*).
pneumonectomy	The surgical removal of a lung (usually to treat lung cancer).
pneumonia	A serious lung disease in which inflammation, caused by bacteria and/or viruses, results in the accumulation of fluid and cellular debris in the air spaces of the lungs, preventing gas exchange.

Term	Meaning
pneumothorax	The abnormal presence of air in the pleural cavity resulting in the collapse of the lung.
positive end-expiratory pressure (PEEP)	A ventilator setting to which maintains extra pressure at the end of expiration to help prevent the alveoli from collapsing.
potential of Hydrogen (pH)	The measure of the acidity or alkalinity of a solution.
pulmonary edema	A buildup of fluid in the lungs.
pulmonary embolism (PE)	A blockage of the pulmonary artery by foreign matter or by a blood clot.
pulmonary function tests (PFTs)	A test with multiple values that measures the rate and volume of gas exchange in the respiratory system.
pulmonary perfusion	Blood flow from the right side of the heart, through the pulmonary circulation, into the left side of the heart.
pulse oximeter	A small machine that displays the percentage of hemoglobin saturated with oxygen, anywhere from 0% to 100%.
pulse oximetry	A noninvasive method of measuring oxygen saturation in the blood.
rales, syn. crackles	Wet, crackling lung noises heard on inspiration, which indicate fluid in the air sacs of the lungs.
respiratory acidosis	A name given to a state in which there is a decreased amount of air entering the alveoli from hypoventilation.
respiratory alkalosis	A name given to a state in which there is an increased amount of air entering the alveoli from hyperventilation.
respiratory syncytial virus (RSV)	A type of virus that causes pneumonia.
respiratory system	A collective term for the organs and tissues involved in filtering incoming air, circulating oxygen to be used by the body through the blood, converting that oxygen to carbon dioxide, and eliminating carbon dioxide from the body.
rhonchi	Abnormal dry, leathery sounds heard in the lungs, which indicate congestion and mucus in the bronchial tubes.
rubs	Friction sounds in the lungs caused by inflammation of the pleura.
small-cell lung cancer	A type of lung cancer in which the cells appear small and round when viewed under the microscope and tend to spread quickly through the body via the blood.
spirogram	A tracing that shows the values of expiratory volumes and flow rates.
spirometer	A device that consists of a small plastic breathing tube hooked to a computerized console that records and prints the data it obtains.
spirometry	A test that provides measurable feedback about the function of the lungs.
Staphylococcus aureus	A microorganism responsible for pneumonia.
sternum, syn. breast bone	A flat, dagger-shaped bone located in the middle part of the anterior wall of the thorax that, along with the ribs, forms the rib cage.
Streptococcus pneumoniae	The most common bacteria that cause bacterial pneumonia.
stridor	A whistling sound heard on inspiration that indicates obstruction of the trachea or larynx.
surfactant	A special chemical in the lining of the alveoli that helps to reduce the surface tension in the alveoli and keep them from collapsing when air is exhaled.
thorax	The chest cavity.
three-pillow orthopnea	A description of the patient's sleep habits in which the patient requires three pillows to breathe comfortably while sleeping.

Term	Meaning
tidal volume	Indicates the amount of air inhaled or exhaled during normal breathing.
total lung capacity (TLC)	The total volume of the lungs when maximally inflated.
trachea	The membranous tube that conveys inhaled air from the larynx to the bronchi.
tracheostomy	A temporary opening created in the trachea, allowing air to bypass an obstruction.
tuberculosis (TB)	An airborne infection caused by *Mycobacterium tuberculosis*, bacteria that attack the lungs.
two-pillow orthopnea	A description of the patient's sleep habits in which the patient requires two pillows to breathe comfortably while sleeping.
upper respiratory tract	The part of the respiratory system that includes the nose, nasal cavities, sinuses, mouth, and pharynx.
vena cava filter	A device inserted inside the inferior vena cava to catch clots as they try to move through the body to the lungs.
ventilation	The distribution of gas into and out of the lungs.
ventilator	A machine that mechanically assists the patient in the exchange of oxygen and carbon dioxide.
vesicular	A term that describes breath sounds that are normal.
visceral layer	Inner layer of the pleura.
V/Q ratio	The relationship between ventilation and perfusion.
V/Q scan, syn. ventilation-perfusion scan	A scan used to assess distribution of blood flow and ventilation throughout both lungs.
walking pneumonia	A type of pneumonia caused by the bacterium *Mycoplasma pneumoniae*, which is a pneumonia that is not severe enough for an infected person to become bedridden or hospitalized.
wedge resection	Removal of part of a lobe of the lung.
wheezes	Airy, whistling-type sounds made on exhalation.

Add Your Own Terms and Definitions Here:

_____

_____

_____

_____

_____

_____

_____

REVIEW QUESTIONS

1. What is another name for mycoplasma pneumonia?
2. What is the difference between the parietal pleura and the visceral pleura?
3. During the respiratory process, what system returns blood from organs and tissues to the right atrium of the heart?
4. What is a spirometer and what is it most often used for?
5. What is pneumothorax and what can cause it?
6. How does emphysema destroy lung tissue?
7. What is gas exchange?
8. What are FVC and FEV1?
9. What are the two diseases commonly associated with COPD?
10. What are cilia and what do they do?

CHAPTER ACTIVITIES

Soundalike Word Choice

Circle the correct word in the following sentences.

1. Three common values obtained during an arterial blood gas test include pH, PO_2, and (PGO_2, PCO_2).
2. The patient's chest x-ray showed an inflammation in the (plural, pleural) cavity.
3. The patient had a large (effusion, infusion) in the right lung base, which seems to be her principal problem at this time.
4. A (bronchoscopy, rhinoscopy) was performed, showing only a mild tracheitis and no masses.
5. He had pulmonary function tests that showed an (FBV1, FEV1) of 4.2 liters.
6. Even though her tuberculosis skin test was positive, Mom denies child was exposed to anyone with (TV, TB).
7. We started a course of (diuresis, enuresis) to help remove fluid from the patient's lungs.
8. The child exhibited nasal (flaring, flaming) due to her difficulty breathing.
9. The (diagram, diaphragm) is the muscle that separates the thoracic cavity from the abdominal cavity.
10. (Rales, rails) are sounds resembling crackles indicating that the lung is partly filled with fluid.

Multiple Choice

Circle the letter corresponding to the best answer to the following questions.

1. A term used to describe a sudden, uncontrollable attack of difficulty breathing at night, usually waking a person from sleep is known as
    A. paradoxical nocturnal dyspnea.
    B. paroxysmal nocturnal dyspnea.
    C. persistent nocturnal dyspnea.
    D. paroxysmal nontruncal dyspnea.

2. The term that describes coughing or spitting up blood from the respiratory system is
    A. hematemesis.
    B. hemeptosis.
    C. cardiomyopathy.
    D. hemoptysis.

3. FEV1 stands for
    A. forced expiratory volume measured in one second.
    B. fast expiratory volume.
    C. forced extreme volume.
    D. forced one-time volume.

4. Partial pressure of carbon dioxide is written as
    A. PCD.
    B. PO_2.
    C. CO_2.
    D. PCO_2.

5. An infection of the alveoli is known as
    A. pharyngitis.
    B. asthma.
    C. pneumonia.
    D. gas exchange.

6. A clear, shiny coating that envelopes the lung is called the
    A. pleura.
    B. plasma.
    C. plexus.
    D. paroxysm.

7. What are the two sites of exchange of oxygen and carbon dioxide?
    A. the larynx and tissues
    B. the lungs and tissues
    C. the lungs and rib cage
    D. the heart and diaphragm

8. The most common bacterium that causes bacterial pneumonia is
    A. *Steptophyllis pneumoniae.*
    B. *Streptococcus pneumonia.*
    C. *Staphylococcus pneumoniae.*
    D. *Streptococcus pneumoniae.*

9. Generally, COPD refers to
    A. pneumonia and emphysema.
    B. asbestosis and bronchitis.
    C. asthma and pneumonia.
    D. chronic bronchitis and emphysema.

10. ARDS stands for
    A. adult reactive distress syndrome.
    B. adult respiratory delay syndrome.
    C. acute respiratory distress syndrome.
    D. abnormal respiratory distress site syndrome.

11. Pulmonary function testing is also known as
    A. spirometry.
    B. spirography.
    C. oximetry.
    D. spiral cytometry.

12. A comparison of FEV1 and FVC is expressed
    A. as a fraction.
    B. in milliequivalents.
    C. as a dollar value.
    D. as a percentage.

13. A small machine with a sensor that is attached with a plastic clip to the patient's finger or ear lobe, which is linked to a monitoring console, is called a
    A. pulse odometer.
    B. pulse oximeter.
    C. spirometer.
    D. pulmonary oximeter.

14. The *q* in V/Q scan stands for
    A. quotient.
    B. quality.
    C. q.d.
    D. quasi.

15. The exchange of gases between blood in the systemic capillaries and the cells of the body is called
    A. internal respiration.
    B. external respiration.
    C. on-site respiration.
    D. mediastinal inspiration.

Converting Nouns to Adjectives

Convert each of the following nouns into its adjective form.

1. bronchus   _____

2. vein   _____

3. hemolysis   _____

4. pleura   _____

5. artery   _____

6. emphysema   _____

7. stenosis   _____

8. hemorrhage   _____

9. obstruction   _____

10. infection   _____

Misspelled Terms

Look at the following terms and determine if they are misspelled. For each misspelled term, write the correct term in the space provided. If the term is spelled correctly, write the word "correct" in the space provided.

1. ronchi   _____
2. ortopnea   _____
3. trachea   _____
4. hemoptisis   _____
5. empyema   _____
6. weezes   _____
7. Klebsiela   _____
8. dispnea   _____
9. parietal   _____
10. macrofages   _____
11. plurisy   _____
12. vena cava   _____
13. ascultation   _____
14. diuresis   _____
15. gama knife   _____
16. hemuthorax   _____
17. broncioles   _____
18. croup   _____
19. strider   _____
20. tachipnea   _____

Fill in the Blanks

Fill in the blanks with the correct terms.

The anatomy of the respiratory system is divided into two tracts: the _____ and the _____. The two _____ enable air to enter and leave the nasal cavity. The _____ receives air from the pharynx. In the chest cavity, the trachea splits into two smaller branches called the right and left _____. The lungs are divided into sections called _____. The two sites of gas exchange in the body are the _____ and the _____. Scavenger cells that clean up debris and defend against invasion are called _____. A person who has _____ has difficulty breathing _____ is the name given to air in the pleural space _____ is the most common bacterium that causes bacterial pneumonia.

TRANSCRIPTION PRACTICE

Open your word-processing software. Insert the student CD-ROM and locate the dictation for this chapter. For each of the words in the "listen for these terms" list for each report, use a medical dictionary or other resource to identify and write down a brief definition of the term on a separate sheet of paper to attach with your work. Then listen to the dictation and transcribe each report. Use the current date for each report where a date is indicated. Insert a heading into the document if the text falls to a second page.

At the end of each report, indicate the name of the dictating physician under the signature line and insert reference initials. For date dictated and transcribed and date of admission, use the current date. Proofread your work, print one copy for your instructor along with your term definitions, and save the completed report to your student disk.

Report #T12.1: Operative Report
Patient Name: Ahmed El-Jalal
Medical Record No.: 584300
Surgeon: Samuel Voorhees, MD
Assistant: Jeremy Simpson, MD

Listen for these terms:
washings
biopsies
Xylocaine
lidocaine
Cetacaine
fiberoptic bronchoscope
bronchial tree
bronchus intermedius
carina

Report #T12.2: Pulmonary Function Tests
Patient Name: Elsie Gray
Medical Record No.: 12-003
Attending Physician: Kerry Gutmann, MD
Dictating Physician: Lena Kushner, MD

Listen for these terms:
spirometry
bronchodilator
plethysmography

Report #T12.3: Discharge Summary
Patient Name: Maria Velez
Medical Record No.: 900-3002
Attending Physician: Robert Novale, MD
Dictating Physician: Michael Josephs, MD

Listen for these terms:
patent foramen ovale
thrombocytopenia
ventricular flutter
implantable cardioverter-defibrillator (ICD)
bubble study
ventilation perfusion scan
hypoxia
V/Q scan
Sildenafil

CARDIOLOGY AND THE CARDIOVASCULAR SYSTEM

OBJECTIVES

After completing this chapter, you will be able to:

- Describe the functions of the cardiovascular system.
- Name and describe the anatomic structures of the heart and associated blood vessels.
- Explain cardiac conduction and describe the cardiac cycle.
- Discuss blood pressure measurement and how blood pressure readings are obtained.
- Describe common diseases and disorders related to the heart and their treatments.
- Discuss common laboratory tests and diagnostic studies used to identify heart disease.

INTRODUCTION

Cardiology is a medical speciality dealing with the diagnosis and treatment of diseases and disorders of the heart. The term derives from the Latin word *cardium*, which is borrowed from the Greek word *kardia*. *Cardium* is used to describe the heart using the combining forms card/i and cardi/o, such as **cardiopulmonary** (relating to the heart and lungs) and **cardiovascular** (relating to the heart and blood vessels or circulation).

The heart is a complex organ that supplies the body with the blood and oxygen it needs to function properly. Relatively simple in function, the heart's primary purpose is to pump blood, 24 hours a day, 70 to 80 times a minute. With each beat, the heart pumps blood that delivers life-sustaining oxygen and nutrients to 300 trillion cells. The rhythmic beating of the heart is a continuous activity, beginning before birth and ceasing only at the end of life.

The heart pumps blood through a closed pathway of blood vessels that circulates throughout the body, delivers nutrients and other essential materials to cells, and removes waste products as it passes through the various areas of the body in a continuous loop. This pathway uses a transportation system in the body called the **circulatory system**. The circulatory system consists of two subsystems: the cardiovascular system and the lymphatic system (see Chapter 19, *Immunology*, for further discussion of the lymphatic system). The **cardiovascular system** is the pathway of blood vessels that the heart uses to pump blood containing oxygen and nutrients from the heart to every part of the body. The blood picks up waste products for disposal by the kidneys and other organs before proceeding back through the cardiovascular system to enter the heart again for another trip.

Although major advances have occurred in physicians' understanding of the heart and ways to treat cardiac disorders, the workings of the heart and the diseases that affect it still present the medical profession with diagnostic and therapeutic challenges. This chapter reviews the function of the cardiovascular system as well as the anatomy and function of the heart, common diseases and disorders affecting heart function, and the clinical tests and procedures used to diagnose and treat heart disease.

THE CARDIOVASCULAR SYSTEM

Blood vessels—a network of interconnecting arteries, arterioles, capillaries, venules, and veins—provide the pathway in which blood is transported between the heart and the body's cells.

The blood vessels of the body each have a different function:

- Arteries and arterioles—distribute
- Capillaries—exchange
- Veins and venules—collect

Arteries carry blood away from the heart to supply organs and tissues with oxygen and nutrients. All arteries, except the pulmonary artery (and the umbilical artery in the fetus) carry oxygenated blood. The largest artery in the body is the **aorta**, which carries blood from the heart to the rest of the body. It branches off from the heart and divides into many smaller arteries called **arterioles,** which adjust their diameter to increase or decrease blood flow to a particular body tissue. **Capillaries** are thin-walled vessels that are actually just the extension of the lining of arteries and veins. They allow oxygen and nutrients to pass from the blood in the arterioles into tissues and allow waste products to pass from tissues into the blood. Some tissues do not have capillaries, such as the epidermis, cartilage, and the lens and cornea of the eye. Most tissues, however, have extensive capillary networks. At the site of exchange, substances move from the blood to tissue fluid, and others move from tissue fluid to the blood. Gases move by **diffusion**, a process whereby oxygen passes from the blood to the tissue fluid, and carbon dioxide moves from the tissue fluid to the blood to be brought back to the lungs and exhaled. **Filtration** is a process whereby plasma and dissolved nutrients are forced out of the capillaries into tissue fluid. This is how nutrients such as glucose, vitamins, and other substances are brought to cells.

Blood then flows from the capillaries into very small veins called **venules**. Venules are small vessels that gather blood from the capillaries; these venules, in turn, drain into **veins**, the larger vessels that carry deoxygenated blood back to the heart. All veins, except the pulmonary vein (and the umbilical vein in the fetus) carry deoxygenated blood. See Figure 13.1 to better understand the structure of the artery, arteriole, capillary, venule, and venous network.

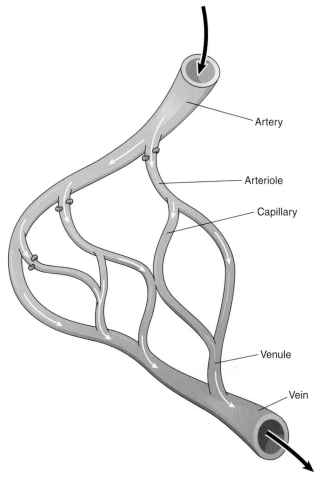

FIGURE 13.1. The Structures of the Vascular System. These structures conduct the 'major business' of the vascular system of providing the pathway in which blood is transported between the heart and body cells. Reprinted with permission from Cohen BJ, Taylor JJ. *Memmler's The Human Body in Health and Disease*, 10th Edition. Baltimore: Lippincott Williams & Wilkins, 2005.

ANATOMY OF THE HEART

The human heart is a four-chambered muscular organ that works to pump blood through the body. Although most of the hollow organs of the body do have muscular layers, the heart is composed almost entirely of muscle.

Although it is convenient to describe the flow of blood through the right side of the heart and then through the left side, it is important to realize that the heart is actually two different, but anatomically connected, pumps that contract at the same time. The right side of the heart receives blood from the body and pumps it into the lungs to gather oxygen, whereas the left side receives the oxygenated blood from the lungs and pumps it to the rest of the body, where oxygen and nutrients are delivered to tissues and waste products are transferred to the blood for removal by other organs, such as the kidneys.

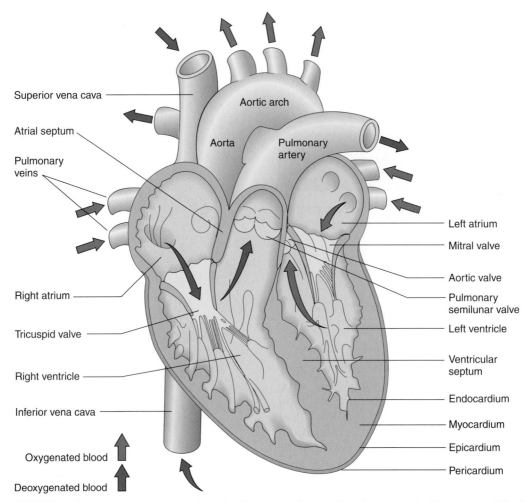

FIGURE 13.2. Anatomy of the Heart. The red and blue arrows show the flow of oxygenated and de-oxygenated blood through the heart muscle. Reprinted with permission from Willis MC. *Medical Terminology: A Programmed Learning Approach to the Language of Health Care.* Baltimore: Lippincott Williams & Wilkins, 2002.

The heart is located in the middle of the chest, behind and slightly to the left of the sternum, and is composed of membranous layers, chambers, valves, and a variety of blood vessels, as shown in Figure 13.2.

Layers

A double-layered membrane called the **pericardium** surrounds the heart like a transparent sac. The outer layer of the pericardium is attached by ligaments to the spinal column, diaphragm, and other parts of the body. The inner layer of the pericardium is attached to the heart itself. Three layers of tissue form the heart wall: the outer layer of the heart wall is the **epicardium**; the middle layer, or heart muscle itself, is the **myocardium**; and the inner layer that lines the heart's chambers and covers its valves is the **endocardium**.

Chambers

Chambers are compartments of the heart through which blood flows. The internal cavity of the heart is divided into four chambers, two on the left and two on the right. Each of the two upper chambers is called the left and right **atrium** (plural, **atria**). The atria serve as reservoirs for blood. Each atrium is connected by its own valve to a chamber below it. The two lower chambers are called the left and right **ventricles**, which are responsible for collecting blood from the right and left atria and pumping it out of the heart. The left atrium

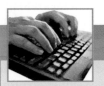

TRANSCRIPTION TIP:

To remember the location of the atria, visualize the architecture of a Roman house, from where the term *atrium* derives. The atrium was an entrance where a person was greeted before moving into other rooms. The atria are the first chambers in the heart to receive blood before it empties into the ventricles to be pumped throughout the body.

and ventricle are responsible for receiving oxygen-rich blood from the lungs and pumping it throughout the body. The right atrium and ventricle are responsible for receiving deoxygenated blood from veins returning from various areas of the body and pumping it to the lungs so that gas exchange can occur.

Valves

A valve is a device used to control the flow of liquids. Pumps require valves to keep fluid flowing in one direction, and the heart is no exception. The heart's **valves** are the structures that open and close with each heartbeat to ensure the proper sequence of bloodflow through the heart. The **tricuspid valve** is located between the right atrium and right ventricle. The **pulmonary valve** is located on the right side of the heart. It opens from the right ventricle to the pulmonary artery. The **mitral valve** is located between the left atrium and left ventricle. Finally, the **aortic valve** is between the left ventricle and the **aorta**, the major arterial blood vessel that begins in the left ventricle and delivers oxygenated blood to the rest of the body. The aortic valve controls blood flow out of the left ventricle. Each valve contains flaps, called **leaflets**, which open and close like spring-loaded doors that open in one direction only to regulate blood flow and prevent backflow of blood from ventricles to the atria during a heartbeat.

Coronary Arteries and Vessels

The heart's role is to pump oxygen-rich blood to every cell in the body. The **coronary arteries** comprise a network of blood vessels that supply oxygen- and nutrient-rich blood directly to the heart's muscle tissue (Figure 13.3). The **right coronary artery** (RCA) supplies the right side and bottom of the heart with blood. The **left coronary artery** (LCA) supplies the majority of blood to the heart and, like the RCA, branches from the aorta near the top of the heart. The main branch of the RCA is called the **posterior descending artery** (PDA). The initial segment of the left coronary artery branches into two slightly smaller arteries called the **left anterior descending artery** (LAD) and the **left circumflex artery** (LCA). The LAD is located on the surface of the front side of the heart and supplies the front wall and septum of the heart

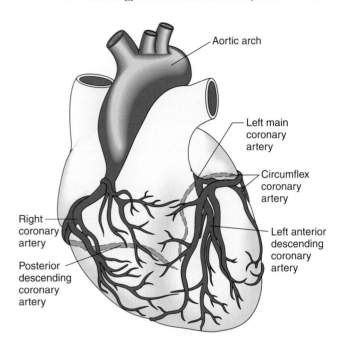

FIGURE 13.3. **The Coronary Arteries and Veins.** Coronary arteries (in red) arise from the aorta and encircle the heart. Coronary veins (above) are shown in blue. Reprinted with permission from Smeltzer SC, Bare BG. *Textbook of Medical-Surgical Nursing,* 9th ed. Philadelphia: Lippincott Williams & Wilkins, 2000.

with blood, whereas the LCA circles around the left side of the heart and is embedded in the surface of the back of the heart. The lesser coronary vessels include the two **diagonal branches** (D1 and D2) which arise from the LAD, and the two **obtuse marginal branches**, which arise from the LCA (OM1 and OM2).

The two main channels for pumping blood through the body are the aorta and the pulmonary artery. The aorta is the great arterial trunk that carries blood from the heart and distributes it through branched vessels throughout the body. The pulmonary artery carries deoxygenated blood from the heart to the lungs for gas exchange before being returned to the heart for circulation throughout the body via the aorta.

Unrestricted flow of blood through the heart's blood vessels is crucial for optimal heart function. When arteries narrow or are blocked to the point of obstructing the flow of blood through a coronary artery, the cardiac muscle tissue fed by the coronary artery beyond the point of the blockage is deprived of oxygen and nutrients, which prevents this area of tissue from functioning properly. This condition is called a **myocardial infarction** (MI), or a heart attack.

CARDIOVASCULAR CIRCULATION

There are two major pathways of the vascular circulation of blood in the body: pulmonary and systemic.

TRANSCRIPTION TIP:

The term *aorta* means *that which is hung.* Aristotle was the first to apply the name to this artery because the arching curve of the aorta as it exits the heart and descends into the body looks something like a modern-day clothes hanger.

Pulmonary circulation is the part of vascular circulation that begins at the right ventricle of the heart, and **systemic circulation** is the part that begins at the left ventricle. Pulmonary circulation begins when the right ventricle contracts and pumps blood into the main pulmonary artery. This major artery branches off into two pulmonary arteries (right and left), which deliver deoxygenated blood to the corresponding lung. In the lungs, each artery branches into smaller arteries and arterioles, and then into capillaries. Gas exchange of oxygen and carbon dioxide takes place between the pulmonary capillaries and the alveoli of the lungs. The capillaries unite to form venules, which merge into veins, and finally into two main pulmonary veins, one from each lung, that return oxygenated blood to the left atrium. This oxygenated blood then travels through the systemic circulation to the rest of the body and the pulmonary circulation begins again.

In systemic circulation, the left ventricle pumps blood into the aorta, which branches off into other arteries that take oxygenated blood into arterioles and capillary networks throughout the body. After exchange of oxygenated blood and waste products, the capillaries merge to form venules and veins to send deoxygenated blood back to the heart via two major veins: the superior vena cava and the inferior vena cava. The **superior vena cava** is the vein that carries blood from the upper body to the right atrium (it is called *superior* because it means *near the top*). The **inferior vena cava** carries blood from the lower body to the right atrium (*inferior*

means *situated below*). Blood in the right atrium empties in to the right ventricle, and the process starts again.

CARDIAC CYCLE

Like all pumps, the heart requires a source of energy in order to function. The heart's pumping energy comes from an electrical conduction system within the heart muscle. **Cardiac conduction** is the name given to the electrical conduction system that controls the heart rate. This system generates electrical impulses that cause the heart muscle to contract and relax, enabling it to pump blood throughout the body. This contracting and relaxing of the heart muscle is a two-part pumping action commonly called a **heartbeat**.

The **cardiac cycle** is the sequence of events in one heartbeat. Throughout the cardiac cycle, the right and left atria continuously accept blood returning to the heart from the body while the two ventricles push blood out of the heart to be circulated into the body. In its simplest form, the cardiac cycle is the simultaneous contraction of the two atria, followed a fraction of a second later by the simultaneous contraction of the two ventricles. The cardiac cycle has two basic components: The contraction phase, called **systole**, occurs when blood is ejected from the chambers of the heart. The relaxation phase, called **diastole**, occurs when the heart is at rest and the chambers fill with blood in preparation for the next contraction.

Figure 13.4 illustrates the process of the cardiac cycle. The electrical stimulus for the pumping of the heart begins with the **sinoatrial (SA) node**, a small mass of specialized tissue located near the rear wall of the right atrium that causes the heart to beat. The SA node is often called *the heart's natural pacemaker* because it sets the rate and rhythm of the heartbeat. The SA node generates an electrical impulse, which begins traveling down through the conduction pathways in the heart muscle, similar to the way electricity flows through power lines from a power plant. When this impulse fires, it spreads through the walls of the right and left atria, which are filled with blood. The impulse causes the atria to contract so that blood will flow from the atria into the ventricles.

The impulse then travels to another section of nodal tissue called the **atrioventricular (AV) node**, which lies on the right side of the partition that divides the atria. Located near the center of the heart, the AV node is like a bridge between the atria and ventricles and serves as a kind of gatekeeper, delaying the electrical impulse from the atria for about one tenth of a second before relaying it on to the ventricles. This pause is important because it permits the atria to complete their contraction and empty their blood into the ventricles. This allows the ventricles to fill before they contract, or open, releasing the blood to its destination—from the

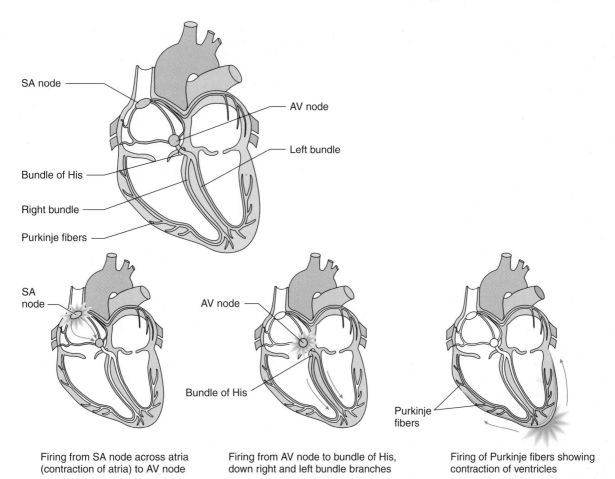

Firing from SA node across atria
(contraction of atria) to AV node

Firing from AV node to bundle of His,
down right and left bundle branches

Firing of Purkinje fibers showing
contraction of ventricles

FIGURE 13.4. **The Cardiac Cycle.** This SA node fires and follows the impulse to the AV node, the bundle of His, the bundle branches, and finally to the Purkinje fibers. Reprinted with permission from Willis MC. *Medical Terminology: A Programmed Learning Approach to the Language of Health Care.* Baltimore: Lippincott Williams & Wilkins, 2002.

right ventricle to the lungs, and from the left ventricle to the aorta for distribution to the body.

From here, the impulse travels on to the right and left ventricles by way of a system of specialized nerve fibers that carry the electrical signals throughout the ventricles. The impulse travels to the first of these fiber bundles called the **bundle of His** (pronounced like *hiss*). The impulse moves along the bundle of His as it divides into the right and left pathways called **bundle branches**. At the base of the heart, the right and left bundle branches further divide into microscopic muscle branches called the **Purkinje fibers.** When the impulses reach these fibers, they trigger the ventricles to contract and push blood out into the lungs and body.

As the blood moves from the ventricles into the pulmonary artery and aorta for circulation throughout the body, the atria relax and are filled once again with blood by the veins, and the cycle begins again. This cycle lasts, on the average, six sevenths of a second. This series of contractions is repeated over and over again, increasing in frequency during times of exertion or stress and decreasing in frequency during times of rest.

HEART SOUNDS

The sounds associated with the heartbeat, called **heart sounds**, are heard when listening to the heart through a stethoscope, called **auscultation**. Heart sounds are vibrations in the tissues and blood caused by closure of the valves and provide important information to the physician about the condition of the heart.

Heart sounds are usually divided into normal and abnormal heart sounds. A healthy heart makes a sound described as a **lub-dub**, which occurs with each heartbeat. This sound comes from the valves closing inside the heart during each heartbeat. The *lub* sound, called the first heart sound (S1 or S_1), is caused by the closure of the mitral and tricuspid valves as the blood enters the ventricles from the atria and is a loud, long sound with a deep pitch. These mitral and tricuspid valves close to prevent blood from flowing back into the atria. The *dub* sound, called the second heart sound (S2 or S_2), is a shorter sound caused by the closure of the aortic and pulmonary valves at the end of ventricular systole, or when blood is released from the ventricles. As the ventricles empty, the valves close. A brief period of silence between S1 and S2 represents diastole, or ventricular relaxation as the ventricles fill with blood coming from the atria.

The sounds of the heart should be sharp and crisp, with a brief moment of silence between each heartbeat. If the valves do not close properly and leak, the sound will not be clear but blurred and abnormal. Abnormal heart sounds may sound like *lub-shhh-dub* or *lub-dub-rumble* when heard through a stethoscope. These sounds do not necessarily indicate a disease or disorder, and not all heart disorders cause abnormal sounds.

A **murmur** is a heart sound caused when blood does not normally flow through a valve or other orifice. Murmurs can be described as *melodic, innocent, early peaking, high-frequency, crescendo/decrescendo, functional, holosystolic, diastolic, systolic ejection,* and *regurgitant.*

Murmurs are classified, or graded, based on the degree to which they are audible. This six-point grading system is indicated by numerals (grades 1 to 6), with grade 1 being barely detectable and grade 6 being so loud it can be heard with a stethoscope just above the chest wall. Express murmurs with a virgule (slash) between the murmur grade and the scale used. For example, a murmur may be dictated as "a 2 over 6 murmur," which would indicate the murmur is a grade 2 on a scale of 1 to 6. This value is transcribed as a *grade 2/6 murmur.* Roman numerals are not used to categorize cardiac murmurs. Some other examples:

Other abnormal heart sound terms that may be transcribed by a medical transcriptionist include the following:

- A **rub** is an abnormal sound that is caused by the friction between the beating heart and the pericardium. Also referred to as a *pericardial friction rub,* it resembles the sound of squeaky leather and often is described as grating, scratching, or rasping. It is used in the diagnosis of pericarditis, discussed below.
- A **gallop** is a tripling or quadrupling of heart sounds that includes three or four sounds that resemble the cantering of a horse. These sounds occur during the heart's relaxation phase, or when it fills with blood.

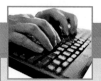

TRANSCRIPTION TIP:

When transcribing objective findings of the heart, listen for the terms S1 and S2. The letter *S* refers to sounds of the heart. S1 and S2 refer to the first and second heart sounds, which generally are always heard. When mention is made of an S3 or S4, the physician is referring to a murmur or some other type of abnormality of the heart.

TRANSCRIPTION TIP:

A **bruit** is an abnormal sound made by blood rushing past an obstruction in an artery. The plural form of this term is *bruits,* but because of the term's French origin, the *s* is not pronounced, although often heard in dictation. Therefore, both the singular and plural forms of the term are correctly pronounced as *broo-ee.* Sometimes dictators will mispronounce the term as *broot.* Do not transcribe the term as *brute.*

Dictated:	grade 2/6 diastolic murmur
Transcribed:	grade 2/6 diastolic murmur
Dictated:	grade 2 and a half over 6 murmur
Transcribed:	grade 2.5/6 murmur
Dictated:	grade 2 to 3 over 6 murmur
Transcribed:	grade 2/6 to 3/6 murmur
	Not grade 2-3/6 murmur
Dictated:	grade 3 over 6 crescendo decrescendo murmur
	Grade 3/6 crescendo-decrescendo murmur

- A **click,** or *systolic click,* is a short, high-pitched sound heard when a valve is not functioning properly and may be indicative of valvular disease. Clicks are characterized in the same manner as murmurs, as above.
- A **thrill** is a high-frequency vibration felt on the chest wall over the heart, which may be indicative of a structural defect of the heart.

HEART RATE AND RHYTHM

A healthy adult has a resting heart rate, or pulse, of about 60 to 80 beats per minute. A normal heart rate is called **sinus rhythm. Arrhythmia** means a lack of a normal heart rhythm (indicated by the prefix *a-*). A more accurate term to describe what are commonly referred to arrhythmias is dysrhythmia, which means an abnormal heart rhythm. Some common terms used to describe dysrhythmia are as follows:

- **Bradycardia,** a slow heartbeat, usually defined as less than 60 beats per minute.
- **Tachycardia,** a fast heart rate, defined as greater than 100 beats per minute.
- **Atrial flutter,** an arrhythmia in which the atrial rhythm is regular, but the rate is abnormally fast.
- **Fibrillation,** an uncoordinated, irregular contraction of the heart muscle that may originate in the atria (called **atrial fibrillation**) or the ventricles (called **ventricular fibrillation**).

- **Heart block**, an impaired conduction of the heart's electrical impulses, leading to a slow heartbeat.
- **Paroxysmal atrial tachycardia**, a rapid heart rate that starts and stops suddenly and unpredictably.
- **Premature atrial contraction**, an extra heartbeat that originates from the atria before it should.

Sometimes abnormal heart rhythms can lead to **cardiac arrest**, which occurs when the heart suddenly stops pumping effectively and begins to flutter wildly, failing to pump blood to the vital organs of the body. If the heart's normal rhythm is not reestablished immediately, death will follow within minutes.

One way physicians treat an abnormal heart rate is with a pacemaker. A **pacemaker** is a small device that is placed in the chest or abdomen to help control abnormal heart rhythms. This device uses electrical pulses to prompt the heart to beat at a normal rate. Pacemakers also can monitor and record the heart's electrical activity and heart rhythm. Newer pacemakers can monitor blood temperature, breathing rate, and other factors and adjust the heart rate to changes in a patient's activity. Pacemakers can be temporary or permanent. Temporary pacemakers are used to treat temporary heartbeat problems, such as a slow heartbeat that is caused by a heart attack, heart surgery, or an overdose of medication. Permanent pacemakers are used to control long-term heart rhythm problems.

Physicians treat abnormal rhythms with a device called an **implantable cardioverter defibrillator (ICD)**, or simply *defibrillator*. Like a pacemaker, this device is implanted in the chest or abdomen. The device uses electrical pulses or shocks to help control life-threatening or irregular heartbeats, especially those that could cause sudden cardiac arrest. An ICD has wires with electrodes on the ends that connect to your heart chambers. The ICD continually monitors the heart rhythm. If the device detects an irregular rhythm in the ventricles, it will use low-energy electrical pulses to restore a normal rhythm. If the low-energy pulses do not restore normal heart rhythm, the ICD will switch to high-energy electrical pulses for defibrillation.

BLOOD PRESSURE

The beats of the heart create a pulsating force that keeps blood moving to all parts of the body through the arteries. **Blood pressure** is the measurement of this force, or the pressure exerted by the circulating volume of blood on the walls of the arteries, the veins, and the chambers of the heart each time the heart pumps. Blood pressure is at its highest when the heart pumps blood, or the contraction of the left ventricle, and called the **systolic pressure** and is the top number given in a blood pressure measurement. When the heart is at rest, between beats, the pressure falls to its lowest point; this is called **diastolic pressure** and is

the bottom number given in a blood pressure measurement. Blood pressure varies constantly according to time of day, level of physical exertion, and with anxiety, stress, emotional changes, or other factors.

Nearly every encounter with a medical provider includes a blood pressure reading that is entered into the medical record. Blood pressure can be measured manually with an instrument called a **sphygmomanometer**, which measures the maximum pressure (systolic) and lowest pressure (diastolic) made by the beating of the heart. In this process, an inflatable cuff is wrapped around a patient's upper arm and is kept in place with Velcro. A tube leads out of the cuff to a rubber bulb. Another tube leads from the cuff to a gauge with an indicator on it that points at a number corresponding to the blood pressure reading. Air is then forced into the cuff, increasing the pressure and tightening the cuff around the patient's upper arm. The person taking the blood pressures places the stethoscope to the patient's arm and listens to the pulse while the air is slowly released from the cuff.

Blood pressure is measured in terms of **millimeters of mercury** (mmHg). A blood pressure reading is expressed as a fraction—for example, 120/80. The systolic blood pressure, or the top number, represents the maximum pressure in the arteries as the heart contracts and pumps blood into the arteries. It is measured when the pulse is first heard through the stethoscope. The diastolic pressure, which is the bottom number, reflects the minimum blood pressure as the heart relaxes following a contraction and is measured from the moment the sound of the pulse is no longer audible.

A blood pressure reading of 90/60 mmHg or lower is known as **hypotension**. Hypotension usually occurs from a loss of blood volume. **Orthostatic hypotension** is the sudden temporary decrease in systolic blood pressure that occurs when a person changes position, resulting in a feeling of lightheadedness. The term *orthostatic* pertains to the upright position of the body. A physician may check for orthostatic hypotension during a physical exam by taking individual blood pressure readings when the patient is lying down, sitting, and standing. The diagnosis of orthostatic hypotension is made when the systolic blood pressure declines 20 mmHg or the diastolic pressure declines 10 mmHg within five minutes of rising from a seated or lying position to standing. These values are transcribed by the medical transcriptionist in the physical exam portion of a report along with other vital signs.

COMMON CARDIAC DISEASES AND TREATMENTS

Heart disease affects the heart and the blood vessels that supply the heart muscle. Some disorders of the blood vessels can also affect the heart directly. Common terms

QUICK CHECK 13.1

Indicate whether the following sentences are true (T) or false (F).

1. The tricuspid valve is located in the right atrium.   T   F

2. Three layers of tissue form the heart wall.   T   F

3. Abnormal heart sounds are called systoles.   T   F

4. Veins carry oxygen-rich blood away from the heart.   T   F

5. The cardiac cycle is the sequence of events in one heartbeat.   T   F

---

that may be heard when transcribing symptoms of cardiac problems include **cyanosis**, a bluish discoloration of the skin and mucous membranes resulting from a lack of oxygen in the blood, or **pallor**, which means paleness or a decrease or absence of color in the skin. **Edema** refers to an accumulation of abnormal amounts of fluid in the intercellular tissues, pericardial sac, and other tissues of the body. **Diaphoresis** refers to profuse sweating associated with elevated body temperature, physical exertion, or stress. Finally, **angina**, also called **angina pectoris**, is severe chest pain that lasts for several minutes and results from an inadequate supply of oxygen and blood flow to the heart muscle.

Hypertension

Hypertension, or high blood pressure, describes a condition in which the pressure of the blood in the arteries is too high, raising the possibility of damage to the heart and to the walls of the blood vessels. This can occur when the heart pumps blood too forcefully around the body, or when arteries narrow, inhibiting blood flow. There are two types of hypertension: **primary hypertension**, in which there is no identifiable cause; and **secondary hypertension**, in which another disease or medication is the cause. Hypertension causes a number of health complications, including heart disease and stroke. In most cases, the cause of hypertension is unknown, but some researchers believe that a family history of hypertension, smoking, and a diet high in salt and fat, resulting in obesity, are contributing factors. Stress and excessive alcohol consumption are also thought to play a role.

Because of the role hypertension plays in stroke and heart attacks, the first line of treatment is to attempt to bring blood pressure under control with diet and lifestyle modification. Drug therapy is the next step. Depending on the circumstances, various types of drugs are available to treat hypertension:

- **Diuretics**. Diuretics decrease blood pressure by eliminating extra sodium and fluid from the body. The blood vessels do not have to hold so much fluid to circulate, and, thus, blood pressure is reduced. Diuretic medications may include triamterene/hydrochlorothiazide (Dyazide), furosemide (Lasix), or spironolactone (Aldactone).

- **Beta-blockers**. Beta-blockers decrease heart rate and the amount of blood the heart pumps out with each beat, and relax the blood vessels, which reduces blood pressure. Examples of these drugs include atenolol (Tenormin), metoprolol (Lopressor), or propranolol (Inderal).

- **Angiotensin-converting enzyme (ACE) inhibitors.** These drugs are used to inhibit the formation of a naturally occurring substance, angiotensin II, which is a very potent chemical that causes the muscles surrounding blood vessels to contract and thereby narrows the blood vessels. The narrowing of the vessels increases the pressure within them, causing blood pressure to rise. Angiotensin II is formed from angiotensin I in the blood by the angiotensin converting enzyme. ACE inhibitors prevent production of angiotensin II and as a result, blood vessels dilate and blood pressure drops. These drugs may include lisinopril (Prinivil), benazepril (Lotensin), enalapril (Vasotec), quinapril (Accupril) or ramipril (Altace).

- **Calcium channel blockers**. Calcium channel blockers inhibit the movement of calcium into the muscle cells of the heart and arteries. Calcium is needed for these muscles to contract. Calcium channel blockers work to decrease the force of the heart's pumping action (cardiac contraction) and to relax the muscle cells in the walls of the arteries, which helps them to open and reduce blood pressure. Commonly prescribed calcium-channel blockers include verapamil (Calan), diltiazem (Cardizem), and nifedipine (Procardia XL).

- **Angiotensin II receptor blockers (ARBs)**. Like ACE inhibitors, ARBs block the action of the enzyme that causes blood vessels to narrow. As a result, blood vessels may relax and open up. This makes it easier for blood to flow through the vessels, which reduces blood pressure. Additionally, these drugs increase the release of sodium and

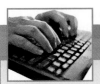

TRANSCRIPTION TIP:

Listen for the term **essential hypertension**, which refers to high blood pressure with no identifiable cause. Do not mistranscribe this as *central hypertension*, which is not a valid cardiac term.

water into the urine, which also lowers blood pressure. ARBs reduce blood pressure as effectively as ACE inhibitors but without some of the side effects (such as a cough) associated with ACE inhibitors. Medications commonly prescribed in this category include losartan (Cozaar), olmesartan (Benicar), telmisartan (Micardis), and valsartan (Diovan).

Coronary Artery Disease

Coronary artery disease (CAD) refers to the narrowing of the coronary arteries to the extent that the heart muscle no longer receives an adequate supply of blood. CAD is also called **cardiac ischemia**. The term ischemia comes from the combining form *isch/o*, to hold back, and *–emia*, meaning a blood condition. Cardiac ischemia is the name for lack of blood flow and oxygen to the heart muscle.

CAD is caused by the gradual buildup of fatty deposits called **plaques** in the coronary arteries. This buildup of plaques, called **atherosclerosis**, causes the arteries to become narrow and to harden, thereby reducing the flow of blood through them. The lay term for this disorder is *hardening of the arteries* (Figure 13.5).

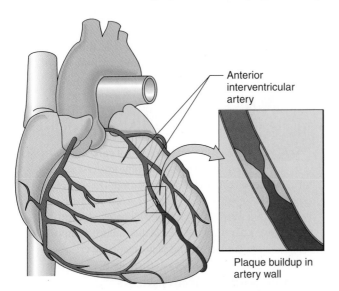

Anterior interventricular artery

Plaque buildup in artery wall

FIGURE 13.5. Coronary Artery Disease. Plaque buildup in the arteries narrows vessels, inhibiting blood flow through the heart. Reprinted with permission from Willis MC. *Medical Terminology: A Programmed Learning Approach to the Language of Health Care.* Baltimore: Lippincott Williams & Wilkins, 2002.

The medical term for the narrowing of any blood vessel, valve, or passage is **stenosis**. Eventually, the diminished blood flow due to the stenosed artery may cause conditions such as angina, **dyspnea** (shortness of breath), or myocardial infarction.

Over time, CAD can weaken the heart muscle and prevent it from pumping blood the way it should, a condition known as **heart failure**. **Congestive heart failure** (CHF) is a condition that occurs when the heart's weak-pumping action causes a buildup of fluid, called **congestion**, in the lungs and other body tissues. The lung congestion that results from heart failure may cause some people to experience breathing difficulties while lying down. This condition, called **orthopnea**, requires a person to keep his or her head elevated by sitting or standing in order to be able to breathe comfortably. **Paroxysmal nocturnal dyspnea** (PND) is a sudden onset of breathing difficulty occurring at night, usually an hour or two after the individual has fallen asleep. The term derives from the terms **paroxysmal**, relating to the sudden onset of a symptom; **nocturnal**, pertaining to the hours of darkness or night; and dyspnea, which, as mentioned before, means shortness of breath or difficulty breathing.

CAD is treated in a variety of ways. A number of medications can help reduce angina and minimize the chance of blood clots forming at the sites of blockages. **Nitrates**, such as nitroglycerin, relieve angina by dilating blood vessels, making it easier for the heart to pump a sufficient amount of blood through the body. Many of the antihypertensive medications described previously are also used to treat CAD.

In severe cases, surgical intervention may be required. **Angioplasty**, also called **percutaneous transluminal coronary angioplasty** (PTCA), is a procedure that opens narrowed arteries by using a **catheter**, which is a thin, flexible tube to which a tiny balloon is attached. First, the catheter is inserted into an artery in the leg and guided to the site of the **stenosis**, or narrowed portion, of the coronary artery. The catheter's position at the artery site is confirmed by **fluoroscopy**. Fluoroscopy is a process in which a continuous x-ray beam is passed through a body part being examined and then transmitted to a monitor so that the body part and its motion can be seen in detail. Physicians will often refer to the use of fluoroscopy in procedures by dictating the phrase, "under fluoroscopic guidance . . . " or "images obtained by fluoroscopy . . . "

Once the catheter's position is confirmed, the physician introduces a tiny balloon into the catheter. The balloon is directed through the narrowed portion of the artery and inflated, flattening the plaque against the artery wall and widening the channel through which blood can flow. The balloon and catheter are then removed from the body.

To keep the artery from re-stenosing, or narrowing again after an angioplasty procedure, an expandable

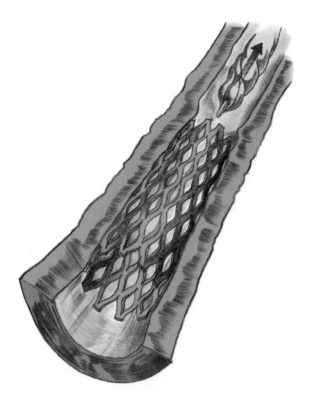

FIGURE 13.6. **Vascular Stent Used in Coronary Angioplasty.** When the stent expands, each rectangle stretches to a diamond shape. The expanded stent supports the artery and helps prevent restenosis. Reprinted with permission from *Nursing Procedures,* 4th ed. Ambler: Lippincott Williams & Wilkins, 2004.

stent is implanted at the site of the blockage to keep the artery from collapsing. A stent is a mesh-like stainless steel tube that has a rectangular design, as shown in Figure 13.6. In this procedure, a balloon is attached to the catheter, as in standard angioplasty, but in this procedure, the balloon is used to deploy and dilate the stent at the site of the narrowed artery in order to reduce the rate of arterial restenosis and acute reclosure following angioplasty.

The stent is crimped over a balloon and inserted into the area of a blockage after the artery has been expanded by angioplasty. When the stent is in position, the balloon is inflated, allowing the stent to be expanded until it hugs the arterial wall. The balloon is then deflated and removed from the body with the catheter while the stent stays in position. Like scaffolding on a building, the stent supports the artery walls to prevent them from narrowing again. Stents are being used with increasing frequency in association with angioplasty procedures.

When the blockage in an artery is calcified or so dense that a balloon cannot be placed to widen the artery wall, other devices are used. Plaque can be cut out, ablated with a laser, or bored out using a surgical drill bit (a procedure called **atherectomy**).

Coronary artery bypass graft surgery (CABG, pronounced like *cabbage*) is a more extensive surgical procedure that restores circulation when occluded, or blocked, coronary arteries prevent normal blood flow to the heart muscle. In this procedure, occluded arteries are replaced with segments (called **grafts**) from vessels in other parts of the body, which are used to bypass the blocked coronary artery and improve blood flow.

Conventional CABG surgery is done by opening the patient's chest with an incision over the **sternum** (breast bone) and dividing it to expose the heart. Bypasses may be performed using different blood vessels: Vessels in the chest wall called the **left internal mammary artery** (LIMA, pronounced "leema") or **right internal mammary artery** (RIMA) may be used as grafts; but more often, the **greater saphenous vein**, which is a large vein located in the leg and thigh, is removed (surgeons refer to this as *harvesting* the vein) to be used for the bypass procedure. This harvested vein is referred to as a **saphenous vein graft** (SVG).

During the CABG operation, the patient is connected to a **heart-lung machine**. This machine is used to provide circulation and oxygenate the blood while the heart is stopped by the surgical team in order to perform the bypass. Depending on the number and location of the blockages, the surgeon might perform between one and seven bypasses. The new healthy artery or vein graft then carries the oxygenated blood around the blockage in the coronary artery. When the bypass procedure is completed and the graft is in place, the heart is restarted. Once the heart beats normally, the patient is removed from the heart-lung machine, the sternum is closed with stainless steel wire sutures, and the chest and leg wounds are closed with sutures or clips.

Cardiomyopathy

Cardiomyopathy is a general term for the progressive impairment of the structure and function of the

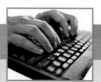

TRANSCRIPTION TIP:

The classification of cardiac failure widely used by physicians was developed by the New York Heart Association. This system ascribes the severity of a patient's cardiac failure using Roman numerals I through IV, with I being asymptomatic and IV denoting severe cardiac failure, symptomatic at rest. Transcribe this value using lowercase *class,* followed by a roman numeral (I through IV). Examples:

New York Heart Association class II.

NYHA class I.

IMPRESSION: Cardiac failure, class III.

myocardium, or muscle tissue of the heart. The term is derived from the components *cardi/o* (heart), *my/o* (muscle), and *-pathy* (disease). Damage prevents the heart from functioning normally, or the walls of the tissue thicken or harden, causing the heart to resist filling to capacity. Cardiomyopathy progresses in most cases, and it is one of the main diseases requiring heart transplantation.

Dilated cardiomyopathy refers to overall enlargement (**dilation**) of the heart chambers, especially the ventricles. Although this enlargement is a key part of dilated cardiomyopathy, it is not the initial problem but rather the heart's own response to a weakness of heart muscle and poor pumping ability, resulting in heart failure. **Hypertrophic cardiomyopathy** is an overgrowth of heart muscle that can impair blood flow both into and out of the heart. The walls of the ventricles thicken (a condition called **hypertrophy**) and become stiff, even though the workload of the heart is not increased. **Restrictive cardiomyopathy** is a disorder in which the ventricles become stiff, but not necessarily thickened, and do not fill normally with blood between heartbeats. Cardiomyopathy may be caused by chronic cardiac disease, excessive alcohol intake, infection due to viruses, or vitamin deficiency disorders. The most common cause, however, is scarring and dilation of the heart muscle as a result of a previous heart attack or other forms of atherosclerosis.

Cardiomyopathy cannot usually be reversed or cured. However, depending on the type of cardiomyopathy, drugs may be prescribed to decrease the heart's workload, regulate the heartbeat, and help prevent blood clot formation and fluid accumulation in the body. These drugs include ACE inhibitors, **anticoagulants** (commonly called *blood thinners*), and diuretics to remove excess fluid from the body.

Valvular Heart Disease

Heart valves regulate the flow of blood through the heart's four chambers. If these valves malfunction, the heart's ability to pump blood can be impeded. If heart valves do not close completely, blood can leak back through the valves. This leakage of blood back through the valve is called **regurgitation**. Valves may not open completely, which results in blood pumping through a blocked or narrowed opening, called stenosis. Regurgitation and stenosis can affect any of the heart valves and are named according to the site of the defect, such as mitral valve regurgitation, tricuspid regurgitation, and aortic regurgitation; or mitral valve stenosis, aortic stenosis, and tricuspid stenosis.

Mitral valve prolapse is a disorder in which the mitral valve does not regulate the flow of blood between the left atrium and left ventricle of the heart properly, causing regurgitation of blood back through the valve and into the atrium. Physicians diagnose mitral valve prolapse after hearing the characteristic clicking sound of the disorder through a stethoscope; hence, this disorder is also referred to as **click-murmur syndrome**. Although prolapse may involve any valve or combination of valves, the mitral valve is the most common site of prolapse.

In most cases, mitral valve prolapse is harmless, does not cause symptoms, and does not need to be treated. In a small number of cases where it causes severe mitral regurgitation, it may require treatment with surgery. Patients with mitral valve prolapse may be prescribed antibiotics before surgical, dental, or medical procedures to prevent the risk of **bacterial endocarditis**. Bacterial endocarditis is an invasion of bacteria from the bloodstream that can lead to deformity and destruction of the valve leaflets.

Pericarditis

Pericarditis is an inflammation of the pericardium that surrounds the heart. There is a small amount of fluid between the inner and outer layers of the pericardium. When the pericardium becomes inflamed, the amount of fluid between its two layers increases, compressing the heart and interfering with its ability to function properly.

Pericarditis may be acute or chronic. The sharp chest pain associated with acute pericarditis occurs when the pericardium rubs against the heart's outer layer. In some cases, the inflammation causes fluid to accumulate in the pericardial sac, a condition known as **pericardial effusion**. This collection of excess fluid in the pericardium can place pressure on the heart, squeezing it, and interfering with its ability to fill adequately and pump blood efficiently. This disorder, known as **cardiac tamponade**, results in less blood leaving the heart, causing a dramatic drop in blood pressure and literally smothering the life out of it. If left untreated, even for a few minutes, cardiac tamponade can be fatal.

Pericarditis may be caused by a bacterial or fungal infection, invasion by cancer cells, or by certain diseases such as AIDS, cancer, or tuberculosis. It may also be precipitated by a heart attack or serious chest injury. Pericarditis also can develop shortly after a major heart attack because of the irritation of the underlying damaged heart muscle. In addition, a delayed form of pericarditis may occur weeks after a heart attack or heart surgery because of antibody formation. This delayed pericarditis is known as **Dressler syndrome**. Many experts believe Dressler's is the result of an autoimmune response, a mistaken inflammatory response by the body to its own tissues—in this case, the heart and pericardium.

Treating pericarditis often involves consideration of the underlying cause as well as the severity of the pericardial inflammation. Mild cases of pericarditis may get better on their own without treatment. People with more severe cases may need to be hospitalized for treatment, which typically includes anti-inflammatory medications or corticosteroids to reduce inflammation, and analgesics or narcotics to ease pain. Fluid may be drained from the pericardium using a technique called **pericardiocentesis**, also referred to as a **pericardial window**. In this procedure, a surgeon uses a sterile needle or a catheter to remove and drain the excess fluid from the pericardial cavity. In cases of long-term inflammation and chronic recurrences that permanently thicken and scar the pericardium, a surgical procedure called a **pericardiectomy** is performed, in which the portion of the pericardium that has become rigid, compromising the functioning of the heart, is removed.

Congenital Heart Disorders

A congenital heart defect is a structural problem in the heart acquired at birth. A baby's heart begins to develop shortly after conception. During development, structural defects can occur. The abnormality can be the result of an inherited disorder or acquired while the fetus is growing in the uterus because of exposure to a substance that causes abnormal development. These defects can involve the walls of the heart, the valves of the heart, and the arteries and veins near the heart.

Atrial Septal Defect

An **atrial septal defect** (ASD), sometimes referred to as a "hole in the heart," is a hole in the atrial septum that separates the atria of the heart. The defect allows blood to flow from one atrium to the other, usually from the left side to the right side, causing extra blood flow in the right atrium, in the right ventricle, or to the lungs. Left untreated, ASD can lead to arrhythmias, stroke, and eventual damage to the arteries and the small blood vessels in the lungs. Most ASDs close on their own as the heart grows during childhood. Large holes that do not close on their own are usually corrected with surgery. Once the defect has been closed or repaired, most children need no additional treatment.

Ventricular Septal Defect

A **ventricular septal defect** (VSD) is a hole, or defect, in the wall that separates the ventricles of the heart. In the normal heart, the ventricular septum prevents blood from flowing directly from one ventricle to the other. In a heart with a VSD, blood can flow between the two ventricles. Children with large VSDs may develop congestive heart failure from extra blood flow from the left ventricle through the right ventricle to the lungs. Bacterial endocarditis, an infection of the lining of the heart, valves, or arteries, can develop as a result of VSD, as can ventricular arrhythmias. As with an ASD, most VSDs close on their own or are so small that they do not need

treatment. On occasion, children and adults may need surgery or other procedures to close the VSD, but no further treatment is required after the VSD is repaired.

Patent Ductus Arteriosus (PDA)

Patent ductus arteriosus (PDA) is a condition in which there is an abnormal circulation of blood between two of the major arteries leading from the heart, the aorta and pulmonary arteries. Before birth, these two arteries are connected by a blood vessel called the **ductus arteriosus**, which is an essential part of the fetal circulation. After birth, the vessel is supposed to close within a few days as part of the normal changes that occur in the baby's circulation. In some babies, however, the ductus arteriosus remains **patent**, or open. This opening allows blood to flow directly from the aorta into the pulmonary artery, which can put a strain on the heart and increase the blood pressure in the pulmonary artery. In most cases, the PDA will shrink and go away completely. If it does not close, corrective surgery can be performed.

Transposition of the Great Vessels

Transposition of the great vessels occurs when the location of the aorta and pulmonary artery, jointly referred to as "the great vessels," is anatomically switched. The aorta comes off the right ventricle instead of the left, and the pulmonary artery comes off the left ventricle instead of the right. Therefore, instead of the oxygen-rich and nutrient-rich blood that is meant to pass through the aorta, blood without oxygen is pumped to the body. Babies born with transposition are cyanotic, or have a bluish coloration to the skin, shortly after birth because of the low oxygen in their blood.

The most common surgical procedure for correction of this defect is called an arterial switch operation, in which the major arteries are switched, connecting the aorta to the left ventricle and the pulmonary artery to the right ventricle, thereby allowing oxygenated blood to flow to the body.

Tetralogy of Fallot

Tetralogy of Fallot (pronounced as *fa-LOW*) is a condition that causes lower-than-normal oxygen levels in the blood, which leads to cyanosis. This congenital defect actually consists of a combination of four different heart defects (hence the prefix, *tetra-*): a VSD; obstructed outflow of blood from the right ventricle to the lungs, called **pulmonary stenosis**; a displaced aorta, which causes blood to flow into the aorta from both the right and left ventricles; and an abnormal enlargement of the right ventricle, called **right ventricular hypertrophy**. The severity of the symptoms is related to the degree to which the flow of blood from the right ventricle is

QUICK CHECK 13.2 ✓

Circle the letter corresponding to the best answer to the following questions.

1. Coronary artery disease is also known as
   A. CABG.
   B. cardiac angiography.
   C. cardiac ischemia.
   D. hypertension.

2. A buildup of plaque in the coronary arteries is known as
   A. atherosclerosis.
   B. arteriomyosis.
   C. angina pectoris.
   D. MI.

3. Blood pressure is measured with an instrument called a(an)
   A. syringometer.
   B. stethoscope.
   C. EKG monitor.
   D. sphygmomanometer.

4. A heart defect or problem present at birth is known as a
   A. ventriculomegaly.
   B. atrial heart defect.
   C. myocardial heart defect.
   D. congenital heart defect.

5. Progressive impairment and function of the myocardium is known as
   A. cardiomyopathy.
   B. ventricular septal defect.
   C. patent ductus ateriosus.
   D. pericarditis.

obstructed. Surgery to repair heart defects is always done when the infant is very young. Sometimes more than one surgery is needed. The first surgery may be done to help increase blood flow to the lungs, and a surgery to correct the underlying problem is done at a later time.

DIAGNOSTIC STUDIES AND PROCEDURES

There is no single test for the wide variety of coronary diseases experienced by patients. The diagnostic test used depends on a number of factors, especially the severity of the symptoms and the type of disease those symptoms represent. A physician may perform some tests to rule out other etiologies for a patient's symptoms, or others to check the severity of symptoms before making a diagnosis.

Blood Tests

Blood tests that measure different components in the blood to determine the overall health of the blood and the heart include the following:

- C-reactive protein test (CRP). **C-reactive protein** is a substance found in the blood when inflammation occurs, such as fatty buildup in artery walls. CRP levels help predict cardiac risk.

- **Homocysteine**. Homocysteine is an amino acid that is normally found in small amounts in the blood. Higher levels of homocysteine are associated with increased risk of heart attack and other vascular diseases. The levels may be high due to a deficiency of folic acid or vitamin B12, resulting from heredity, old age, kidney disease, or certain medications.

- **Lipoprotein (a)** or Lp(a). Lipoprotein (a), dictated as *L P little A*, is a biochemical in the body; high concentrations of Lp(a) are associated with premature coronary disease.

- Cholesterol particle test. The cholesterol particle test measures the size of the **low-density lipoprotein** (LDL) cholesterol, called *bad cholesterol*, particles in the blood. "Pattern A" particles are larger and lighter, whereas "Pattern B" particles are smaller and more dense. People with Pattern B LDL cholesterol are more likely to have atherosclerosis and heart disease. This test is dictated as "*Pattern A*" (or "*Pattern B*") *particle size*, where the word *pattern* and the *A* or *B* are enclosed in quotation marks.

- Lipid profile. This test evaluates the risk of coronary heart disease in a patient. It measures total cholesterol; LDL; **high-density lipoprotein** (HDL), called *good cholesterol*; and triglycerides.

- Blood sugar (glucose). This test detects the presence of diabetes and glucose intolerance, both of which indicate a significant cardiac risk.

- **B-type natriuretic peptide** (BNP). This test measures the amount of the BNP hormone in the blood. BNP is made by the heart, and if the heart is working harder over an extended period (such as from heart failure), the heart releases more BNP and the value will be elevated.
- Cardiac enzyme studies. These blood values measure the levels of the cardiac enzymes **troponin, creatine kinase** (CK), **myocardial band enzymes of creatine kinase** (CK-MB), **creatine phosphokinase** (CPK), and **myocardial band enzymes of creatine phosphokinase** (CPK-MB) in the blood. Elevated levels of cardiac enzymes indicate heart muscle damage. These enzymes, normally found in high numbers inside the cells of the heart, are needed for those cells to function. When these cells are injured, such as during a heart attack or other cardiac trauma, these enzymes are released into the bloodstream. By measuring the levels of these enzymes, physicians can determine if cardiac tissue has been damaged, the size of an adverse heart event (such as a heart attack), and approximately when the event occurred.

Electrocardiogram

An **electrocardiogram** (EKG, also called ECG) is a diagnostic test that analyzes the electrical activity of the heart. An EKG is a recording made from electrodes attached to the surface of the body. The recording produced is a graphic representation or tracing of the electrical activity of the heart as it contracts and relaxes. The EKG can detect abnormal heartbeats, some areas of damage, inadequate blood flow, and heart enlargement.

During the test, electrodes used to measure electrical impulses, called **leads**, are placed on the patient's arms and legs and across the chest wall. The leads are then connected to the EKG machine. These leads, 12 in all, are transcribed as a combination of letters and numbers according to their location on the body as leads I, II, and III, aVR, aVL, and aVF, and, finally, leads V1 through V6. Each electrical impulse detected by the leads is recorded onto a strip of paper as a **waveform**. Any deviation from the shape of the waveform or the interval between waveforms on the strip is indicative of a possible heart disorder. Figure 13.7 illustrates a waveform tracing showing normal sinus rhythm compared to the waveform appearance of abnormal rhythms.

A. Normal Sinus Rhythm (NSR)

B. Bradycardia

C. Tachycardia (sinus)

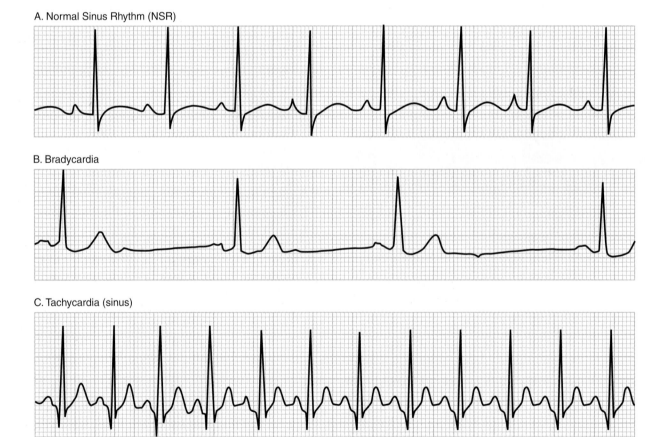

FIGURE 13.7. Electrocardiographic Wave Form. These electrocardiogram tracings show two types of arrhythmia compared to normal. **(A)** Normal sinus rhythm. **(B)** Bradycardia. **(C)** Tachycardia. Reprinted with permission from Willis MC. *Medical Terminology: A Programmed Learning Approach to the Language of Health Care.* Baltimore: Lippincott Williams & Wilkins, 2002.

Below are same common terms used to transcribe EKG terminology.

EKG leads (including augmented limb and precordial leads):

- lead I, lead II, lead III
- aVR, aVL, aVF
- V1, V2, V3, V4, V5, V6, V7, V8, V9
  or V_1, V_2, V_3, V_4, V_5, V_6, V_7, V_8, V_9
  or sometimes dictated as sequential leads: V1 through V9 (V_1 through V_9)
  not V1 through 5 or V_1 through $_5$ (even if dictated)
  not V1-5 or V_{1-5}

Tracing terms (in general, use all capital letters but larger and smaller letters may be used when denoting electrocardiographic deflections):

- Q wave, q wave
- R wave, r wave
- S wave, s wave
- T wave
- T-wave inversion
- QRS complex
- QT interval
- ST segment
- ST-T elevation

Echocardiogram

An **echocardiogram**, often dictated as *echo* for short, is a test in which ultrasound is used to examine the anatomy of the heart. This procedure can display a cross-sectional "slice" of the beating heart, including the chambers, valves, and the major blood vessels that exit from the left and right ventricles. The echocardiogram reveals important information about the anatomy of the heart, detects heart valve abnormalities, and evaluates congenital heart disease. A transducer is placed on the chest, and high-frequency sound waves are directed at the heart wall and valves. The sound waves bounce, or echo, off the cardiac structures, providing a two-dimensional image of the beating heart, which is viewed on a computer screen. By applying the transducer at particular areas of the chest, most of the important cardiac structures can be imaged by the echocardiogram.

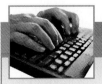

TRANSCRIPTION TIP:

For terms such as *T wave*, in which there is no hyphen, insert a hyphen when the term is used as an adjective, such as *T-wave abnormality*.

TRANSCRIPTION TIP:

Exercise capacity in a stress test is measured by the **Bruce protocol**, sometimes abbreviated as BPR, named after the developer of the standardized treadmill test for diagnosing and evaluating heart and lung diseases. The measurement of aerobic exercise capacity is expressed in **metabolic equivalents** (METS). For example: "The patient's exercise duration was 10 minutes using the Bruce protocol to a peak workload of 10.5 METS."

Cardiac Stress Test

A **cardiac stress test**, sometimes called a **treadmill stress test**, is an exercise test to evaluate the heart for problems that show up only when the heart is working hard. As the body works harder during the test, it requires more oxygen; thus, the heart must pump more blood. This test can show if the blood supply is reduced in the arteries that supply the heart.

In the basic stress test, EKG leads are placed on the patient's chest to provide electrocardiographic signals that are monitored during the test. The patient's heart rate and rhythm are observed while the test progresses from a slow walk on the treadmill to a faster pace and walking on an incline; certain changes in the rate and rhythm may suggest the heart itself is not receiving enough blood.

A **nuclear scan**, or *thallium stress test*, is sometimes used along with a treadmill or bicycle stress test. The scan can show areas of the heart that lack blood flow and are damaged, as well as revealing problems with the heart's pumping action. When the patient reaches his or her maximum level of exercise, a small amount of radioactive material called **thallium** is injected into a vein where it travels through the bloodstream. Then the patient lies down on a special table under a **gamma camera,** a special camera that can see the thallium and take pictures as the thallium mixes with the blood in the bloodstream and heart's arteries and enters heart muscle cells. A less-than-normal amount of thallium detected in the heart muscle cells is an indicator that this part of the heart muscle does not receive a normal blood supply and might be damaged.

Cardiac Catheterization and Coronary Angiography

Cardiac catheterization, along with a **coronary angiography**, is a procedure that allows the visualization of the heart and the coronary arteries that supply blood to the heart muscle. This procedure can evaluate blockages in coronary arteries, the function of the valves and other

QUICK CHECK 13.3 ✓

Fill in the blank with the correct meaning of the following abbreviations.

1. EKG _____

2. CABG _____

3. CK _____

4. HDL _____

5. BNP _____

heart structures, and coronary circulation and structural disorders. A thin catheter is inserted into an artery or vein and threaded through major blood vessels into the heart chambers. At the tip of the catheter, various instruments may be attached that measure the pressure of blood in each chamber, view the interior of blood vessels, or remove a tissue sample from inside the heart for examination later. During the coronary angiography portion of the examination, a radiopaque dye is inserted through the catheter into the openings of the heart (called ostia). The movement of the dye through the arteries provides clear images of the blood vessels as the heart pumps and the images are recorded on a video.

Multiple Gated Acquisition Scan

A **multiple gated acquisition (MUGA)** scan is a noninvasive test that uses a radioactive isotope called **technetium** to evaluate the functioning of the heart's ventricles. The MUGA scan is performed to determine if the heart's left and right ventricles are functioning properly and to diagnose abnormalities in the heart wall. During the MUGA scan, leads are placed on the patient's body so that an EKG can be conducted simultaneously. Then a small amount of technetium is injected into an arm vein, and a special camera is used to follow the movement of the technetium through the blood circulating in the heart. The camera displays multiple images of the heart in motion and records them on a computer for later analysis.

CHAPTER SUMMARY

The heart, which pumps blood through the circulatory system, is vital to survival. Body tissues need a continuous supply of oxygen and nutrients, and metabolic waste products have to be removed. Without these essential processes, cells soon undergo irreversible changes that lead to death. A critical understanding of the anatomy and function of the heart and familiarity with the ongoing diagnostic and therapeutic advances in managing heart disease are key factors in success at transcribing medical reports in the field of cardiology.

·I·N·S·I·G·H·T·

The Heart Brain

Western science has long believed that the brain's responses to external stimuli were the sole source of human emotion, whereas the hollow muscle of the heart possessed no emotion or intellect of its own. However, neurophysiologists have discovered that the heart is, in fact, a sensory organ with its own functional intrinsic "brain" that communicates with and influences the brain via the nervous system and other pathways.

Dr. J. Andrew Armour, associate professor of pharmacology, University of Montreal, pioneered the concept that the "heart brain" is a network of neurons, neurotransmitters and proteins that send messages to the body. Through his research, he found that, like the brain, the heart contains support cells and a complex electrical circuitry that enable it to act independently, learn, remember, and transmit information from one cell to another. According to these studies, the type of information sent from the heart to the brain can influence human perceptions, emotions, and thought processes. Some evidence to support this theory includes the documented testaments of heart-transplant patients who have taken on the habits, tastes, and memories of their dead donors. This led many researchers to conclude that the same type of memory-encoding neurons found in the brain is also found in the heart.

With new discoveries supporting the existence of a connection between the heart and the brain, neurocardiology is becoming increasingly relevant in the management of heart disease. Researchers hope that an understanding of how the neurons of the heart can exert dynamic control over emotions will help patients to focus on the power of the heart to facilitate beneficial changes in all parts of the body.

Common Soundalike Words

Word	Word Pronunciation	Soundalike	Soundalike Pronunciation
atherosclerosis: a form of arteriosclerosis in which plaques containing cholesterol and other material are formed within the arteries.	ath′er-ō-skler-ō′sis	**arteriosclerosis**: a clogging or hardening of the arteries. **arthrosclerosis**: a stiffening or hardening of the joints.	ar-tēr′ē-ō-skler-ō′sis ar′thrō-skler-ō′sis
median sternotomy: an incision through the midline of the sternum usually used to gain access to the heart, mediastinal structures, and great vessels.	mē′dē-an stĕr-not′ŏ-mē	**mediastinotomy**: incision into the mediastinum.	mē′dē-as-ti-not′ŏ-mē
BNP (B-type natriuretic peptide): a cardiac laboratory test as an indicator for myocardial infarction or congestive heart failure, which will always be a one-number value.	bee-en-pee	**BMP (basic metabolic panel)**: a panel of blood tests, containing several evaluations with several values.	bee em-pee
cor: another term for the heart.	kōr	**core**: the central part of anything.	kōr
ejection: the act of driving or throwing out by physical force from within (as in ejection fraction). In cardiology, the measurement of the blood pumped out of the ventricles.	ē-jek′shŭn	**injection**: the introduction of a medicinal substance or nutrient material into subcutaneous tissue, muscular tissue, or other places.	in-jek′shŭn
infarction: a blockage in an artery causing tissue death due to lack of oxygen-rich blood.	in-fark′shŭn	**infraction**: a violation or encroachment upon something (as the law).	in-frak′shŭn
arrhythmia: loss of rhythm; denoting especially an irregularity of the heartbeat.	ă-rith′mē-ă	**erythema**: redness of the skin due to capillary dilation.	er-i-thē′mă
stent: a device used to provide support for a bodily orifice or cavity.	stent′	**stint**: an unbroken period of time during which something is done.	stint′
pericardial: surrounding the heart.	per-i-kar′-dē-ăl	**precordial**: relating to the precordium or the front of the heart.	prē-kōr′dē-ăl
nitrate: a salt of nitric acid; found in cardiac medications.	nī′trāt	**nitrite**: a salt of nitrous acid; found on urinalysis.	nī′trīt

Combining Forms

Combining Form	Meaning	Combining Form	Meaning
ablat/o	take away	lipid/o	lipid (fat)
anastom/o	establish an opening	lumin/o	lumen (opening)
angi/o, vas/o, vascul/o	vessel	my/o	muscle
aort/o	aorta	ox/o	oxygen
arter/o, arteri/o	artery	palpit/o	to throb
ather/o	fatty plaque	pericardi/o	pericardium
atri/o	atrium	perone/o	fibular (lower leg bone)
cardi/o, coron/o	heart	phleb/o, ven/o	vein
cholesterol/o	cholesterol	regurgitat/o	flow backward
congest/o	accumulation of fluid	rhythm/o	rhythm
cyan/o	blue	sphygm/o	pulse
ectop/o	outside of a place	sten/o	narrowness; constriction
fibrillo/o	muscle fiber/nerve fiber	steth/o	chest
infarct/o	area of dead tissue	thromb/o	clot
isch/o	keep back, block	valv/o, valvul/o	valve
jugul/o	jugular (throat)	ventricul/o	ventricle

Add Your Own Combining Forms Here:

_____

_____

_____

_____

_____

_____

ABBREVIATIONS

Abbreviation	Meaning
ACE	angiotensin-converting enzyme
ARB	angiotensin II receptor blocker
ASD	atrial septal defect
BNP	B-type natriuretic peptide
CABG	coronary bypass artery graft
CAD	coronary artery disease
CHF	congestive heart failure
CK	creatine kinase
CPK	creatine phosphokinase
CRP	C-reactive protein
EKG (also called ECG)	electrocardiogram
HDL	high-density lipoprotein, or *good* cholesterol
ICD	implantable cardioverter defibrillator
LAD	left anterior descending artery
LCA	left coronary artery
LCA	left circumflex artery

Abbreviation	Meaning
LDL	low-density lipoprotein, or *bad* cholesterol
LP(a)	lipoprotein (a)
METS	metabolic equivalents
MI	myocardial infarction
mmHg	millimeters of mercury
MUGA	multiple gated acquisition scan
PDA	posterior descending artery OR patent ductus arteriosus
PND	paroxysmal nocturnal dyspnea
PTCA	percutaneous transluminal coronary angioplasty
RCA	right coronary artery
SA	sinoatrial (node)
TIMI	thrombolysis in myocardial infarction
VSD	ventricular septal defect

Add Your Own Abbreviations Here:

_____

_____

_____

_____

_____

_____

TERMINOLOGY

Term	Meaning
angina, *syn.* angina pectoris	Severe chest pain that lasts for several minutes and results from an inadequate supply of oxygen and blood flow to the heart muscle.
angioplasty, *syn.* percutaneous transluminal coronary angioplasty (PTCA)	A procedure that opens narrowed arteries by use of a catheter with a balloon on its tip.
angiotensin-converting enzyme (ACE) inhibitors	Drugs that prevent the formation of angiotensin II in the blood vessels, enabling blood vessels to dilate and decrease blood pressure.
anticoagulant	A substance that hinders the clotting of blood; commonly called *blood thinner*.
aorta	The main trunk of the arterial system that begins in the left ventricle.
aortic valve	The outgoing valve of the left ventricle.
angiotensin II receptor blockers (ARBs)	Drugs that block the action of the enzyme that causes blood vessels to narrow; similar to ACE inhibitors but without some of the side effects associated with ACE inhibitors.
arrhythmia	An irregular heartbeat.
arteries	Larger vessels that carry oxygen-rich blood away from the heart.
arterioles	Smaller branches of the arteries that distribute blood to body tissues.
atherectomy	A procedure in which a high-speed drill on the tip of a catheter is used to shave plaque from blocked arterial walls.
atherosclerosis	A buildup of plaques in the coronary arteries, causing the arteries to become hardened and narrowed.
atrium	The upper chamber of the heart (one on the left and one on the right).
atrial fibrillation	An uncoordinated, irregular contraction of the heart muscle that may originate in the atria.
atrial flutter	An arrhythmia in which the atrial rhythm is regular, but the rate is abnormally fast.
atrial septal defect (ASD)	A hole in the atrium septum that separates the atria of the heart.
atrioventricular (AV) node	The electrical connection between the atria and ventricles where electrical impulses are delayed for a fraction of a second to allow the ventricles to fill completely with blood.
auscultation	The process of listening to heart sounds through a stethoscope.
bacterial endocarditis	An infection leading to deformity and/or destruction of the inner layer of the heart.
beta-blockers	Drugs that slow the heart rate and reduce the force of the heartbeat.
blood pressure	The force of blood exerted on the inside walls of blood vessels.
blood vessels	A network of interconnecting arterial, arterioles, capillaries, venules, and veins that provide the pathway in which blood is transported between the heart and body cells.
bradycardia	A slow heartbeat, usually less than 60 beats per minute.
Bruce protocol	The standardized treadmill stress test used for diagnosing and evaluating heart and lung diseases.
bruit	An abnormal sound made by blood rushing past an obstruction in an artery.
B-type natriuretic peptide (BNP)	A hormone in the blood made by the heart.

Term	Meaning
bundle branches (right and left)	Pathways that branch off the bundle of His that help carry the electrical signals of cardiac conduction to the ventricles.
bundle of His	Specialized nerve fibers that help carry the electrical signals of cardiac conduction to the ventricles.
calcium channel blockers	Drugs that inhibit the movement of calcium into the muscle cells of the heart and arteries, resulting in a decrease in the force of the heart's pumping action and relaxing of muscle cells in the walls of the arteries, which helps them to open and reduce blood pressure.
capillaries	Thin-walled vessels that allow oxygen and nutrients to pass from blood to tissues.
cardiac arrest	A condition that occurs when the heart suddenly stops pumping effectively and begins to flutter wildly, failing to pump blood to the vital organs of the body.
cardiac catheterization	A procedure using a catheter threaded into the heart chambers that identifies possible problems with the heart or its arteries.
cardiac conduction	The name given to the electrical conduction system that controls the heart rate.
cardiac cycle	The sequence of events of one heartbeat.
cardiac ischemia	The name for lack of blood flow and oxygen to the heart muscle.
cardiac stress test, *syn.* treadmill stress test	An exercise test that evaluates the heart for problems which appear when the heart is working hard.
cardiac tamponade	Compression of the heart caused by blood or fluid accumulation in the space between the myocardium (the muscle of the heart) and the pericardium (the outer covering sac of the heart).
cardiology	The medical specialty dealing with the diagnosis and treatment of diseases and disorders of the heart.
cardiomyopathy	Progressive impairment of the structure and function of the myocardium.
cardiopulmonary	Relating to the heart and lungs.
cardiovascular	Relating to the heart and blood vessels or circulation.
cardiovascular system	The pathway of blood vessels that the heart uses to pump blood containing oxygen and nutrients from the heart to every part of the body.
catheter	A small, thin, flexible tube.
chambers	The compartments of the heart through which blood flows.
circulatory system	A transportation system of blood vessels that circulates blood and other fluids throughout the body, delivers nutrients and other essential materials to cells, and removes waste products from the body.
click, syn. *systolic click*	A short, high-pitched sound heard when a valve is not functioning properly
congestion	Buildup of fluid in an organ or tissue.
congestive heart failure	A condition that occurs when the heart's weak pumping action causes a buildup of fluid in the lungs and other body tissues.
coronary angiography	The part of the cardiac catheterization procedure in which a dye is inserted through the catheter to view images of the blood vessels as the heart pumps.
coronary arteries	The network of blood vessels that supply oxygen-rich and nutrient-rich blood directly to the heart's muscle tissue.
coronary artery bypass graft (CABG)	A surgical procedure in which a section of vein or artery from another part of the body is used to bypass a blockage in a coronary artery so that blood flow is not hindered.

Term	*Meaning*
coronary artery disease (CAD)	The narrowing of the coronary arteries sufficiently to prevent adequate blood supply to the heart muscle; also called *cardiac ischemia*.
C-reactive protein	A substance in the blood that is secreted when inflammation in the artery walls occurs.
creatine kinase (CK)	A cardiac enzyme.
creatine phosphokinase (CPK)	A cardiac enzyme.
cyanosis	A bluish coloration to the skin.
diagonal branches (D$_1$, D$_2$)	Lesser coronary vessels that branch off the left coronary artery.
diaphoresis	Profuse sweating associated with elevated body temperature, physical exertion, or stress.
diastole	The part of the cardiac cycle when blood fills the heart chambers.
diastolic pressure	The bottom number in a blood pressure reading that represents the minimum blood pressure as the heart relaxes following a contraction.
diffusion	A process whereby oxygen passes from the blood to the tissue fluid and carbon dioxide moves from the tissue fluid to the blood to be brought back to the lungs and exhaled.
dilation	Another word for *enlargement*.
dilated cardiomyopathy	Overall enlargement of the heart chambers, especially the ventricles.
diuretics	Drugs that act on the kidneys to promote the excretion of excess water in the body.
Dressler syndrome	A delayed form of pericarditis that may occur weeks after a heart attack or heart surgery because of antibody formation.
ductus arteriosus	A blood vessel that connects the aorta and pulmonary artery.
dyspnea	Shortness of breath.
echocardiogram	A test in which ultrasound is used to examine the heart anatomy.
edema	An accumulation of abnormal amounts of fluid in the intercellular tissues, pericardial, sac, and other tissues of the body.
electrocardiogram (EKG, also called ECG)	A graphic record of the electrical activity of the heart.
endocardium	The inner layer of the heart wall.
epicardium	The outer layer of the heart wall.
essential hypertension	High blood pressure that has no identifiable cause.
fibrillation	An uncoordinated, irregular contraction of the heart muscle.
filtration	A process whereby plasma and dissolved nutrients are forced out of the capillaries into tissue fluid.
fluoroscopy	A continuous x-ray beam that is passed through a body part being examined, then transmitted to a TV-like monitor so that the body part and its motion can be seen in detail.
gallop	A tripling or quadrupling of heart sounds that includes three or four sounds that resemble the cantering of a horse.
graft	A section of vein or artery from another part of the body transplanted to another part of the body.

Term	Meaning
gamma camera	A special scanning camera used during a stress test that takes pictures as thallium mixes with the blood in the bloodstream and heart's arteries and enters heart muscle cells.
greater saphenous vein	A large subcutaneous vein located in the leg and thigh.
heart block	An impaired conduction of the heart's electrical impulses, leading to a slow heartbeat.
heart failure	A condition in which the heart muscle does not pump the way it should.
heart sounds	The sounds associated with the heartbeat when listening to the heart through a stethoscope.
heartbeat	An electrical impulse from the heart muscle.
heart-lung machine	A machine that provides circulation and oxygenates the blood while the heart is stopped during a coronary bypass procedure.
high-density lipoprotein (HDL)	A type of cholesterol known as *good cholesterol.*
homocysteine	An amino acid used in cardiac risk factor testing.
hypertension	A condition in which the pressure of the blood in the arteries is too high; also called *high blood pressure.*
hypertrophic cardiomyopathy	Overgrowth of the heart muscle that can impair blow flood in and out of the heart.
hypertrophy	A term meaning increase in size or thickening.
hypotension	A blood pressure reading of 90/60 mmHg or lower.
implantable cardioverter defibrillator (ICD)	A small device implanted in the chest or abdomen that uses electrical shocks to help control life-threatening or irregular heartbeats.
inferior vena cava	The major vein that carries blood from the lower body to the right atrium.
leads	Electrodes on an EKG/ECG machine used to measure electrical impulses of the heart.
leaflets	Flaps in the valves that regulate blood flow from the heart.
left anterior descending artery (LAD)	A smaller artery that branches off the left main coronary artery.
left circumflex artery (LCA)	A smaller artery that branches off the left main coronary artery.
left coronary artery (LCA)	A major coronary artery in the heart.
left internal mammary artery (LIMA)	A vessel located on the left side of the chest wall.
left main coronary	The initial segment of the left coronary artery.
lipoprotein (a)	A biochemical in the body measured in cardiac risk factor testing.
low-density lipoprotein (LDL)	A type of cholesterol known as *bad cholesterol.*
lub-dub	The normal sound of a heartbeat.
metabolic equivalents (METS)	The measurement of aerobic exercise capacity.
millimeters of mercury (mmHg)	A unit used to measure blood pressure.
mitral valve	The incoming valve of the left ventricle.
mitral valve prolapse, syn. *click-murmur syndrome*	An abnormality of the mitral valves in which one or both mitral valve flaps close incompletely.
multiple gated acquisition scan (MUGA)	A test that uses technetium to evaluate the function of the heart's ventricles.

Term	Meaning
murmurs	Abnormal heart sounds.
myocardial band enzymes of creatine phosphokinase (CK-MB)	A cardiac enzyme found in the cells of the heart.
myocardial band enzymes of creatine phosphokinase (CPK-MB)	A cardiac enzyme found in the cells of the heart.
myocardial infarction (MI), *syn.* heart attack	The sudden insufficiency of arterial or venous blood supply to an area of the heart muscle, usually as a result of occlusion of a coronary artery.
myocardium	The middle layer of the heart wall.
nitrates	A type of medication that relieves chest pain by dilating blood vessels.
nocturnal	Pertaining to the hours of darkness or night.
nuclear scan	A scan that shows areas of the heart that may lack blood flow.
obtuse marginals (OM1, OM2)	Lesser coronary vessels that branch off the left coronary artery.
orthopnea	Breathing difficulty while lying down.
orthostatic hypotension	The sudden temporary decrease in systolic blood pressure that occurs when a person changes position, resulting in a feeling of lightheadedness.
pacemaker	A small device implanted in the chest or abdomen to help control abnormal heart rhythms.
pallor	A paleness or decrease or absence of color in the skin.
paroxysmal	Pertaining to the sudden onset of a symptom.
paroxysmal atrial tachycardia	A rapid heart rate that starts and stops suddenly and unpredictably.
paroxysmal nocturnal dyspnea (PND)	Difficulty breathing, experienced when lying down, which is caused by lung congestion that results from partial heart failure and occurring suddenly at night.
patent	Another word for *open*.
patent ductus arteriosus (PDA)	A condition in which there is abnormal circulation of blood between the aorta and pulmonary artery.
percutaneous transluminal coronary angioplasty (PTCA)	A procedure that opens narrowed arteries by using a catheter with a balloon on its tip.
pericardectomy	The surgical removal of the portion of pericardium that has become rigid, compromising the function of the heart.
pericardial effusion	A condition in which fluid accumulates in the pericardial sac.
pericardiocentesis, *syn.* pericardial window	The drainage of excess fluid from the pericardial cavity with a catheter.
pericarditis	An inflammation of the pericardium.
pericardium	A double-layered membrane that surrounds the heart like a sac.
plaques	Fatty deposits that build up in the coronary arteries, causing the arteries to become narrow and to harden.
posterior descending artery (PDA)	The main branch off the right coronary artery.
premature atrial contraction	An extra heartbeat that originates from the atria before it should.
primary hypertension	A form of hypertension in which there is no identifiable cause.
pulmonary circulation	The part of vascular circulation that begins at the right ventricle of the heart.

Term	Meaning
pulmonary stenosis	A condition of obstructed outflow of blood from the right ventricle to the lungs.
pulmonary artery	The main blood vessel that takes blood from the heart to the lungs.
pulmonary valve	The outgoing valve of the right ventricle.
pulmonary veins	The vessels responsible for carrying blood from the lungs to the heart.
Purkinje fibers	Specialized nerve fibers that help carry the electrical signals of cardiac conduction to the ventricles.
regurgitation	Leaking or backward flow.
restrictive cardiomyopathy	A disorder in which the ventricles become stiff but not necessarily thickened, and do not fill with blood normally between heartbeats.
right coronary artery (RCA)	A major coronary artery in the heart.
right internal mammary artery (RIMA)	A vessel located on the right side of the chest wall.
right ventricular hypertrophy	An abnormal enlargement of the right ventricle.
rub, syn. *pericardial friction rub*	An abnormal heart sound that is caused by the friction between the beating heart and the pericardium.
saphenous vein graft	The harvested vein used in a coronary artery bypass graft (CABG) procedure.
secondary hypertension	A form of hypertension in which another disease or medication is the cause.
sinoatrial (SA) node	A specialized cluster of cells in the heart that initiates the heartbeat.
sinus rhythm	A normal cardiac rhythm.
sphygmomanometer	An instrument that measures blood pressure.
stenosis	Narrowing of a blood vessel.
stent	A meshlike metal tube placed in an artery to keep it open.
sternum	The breast bone.
superior vena cava	The major vein that carries blood from the upper body to the right atrium.
systemic circulation	The part of vascular circulation that begins at the left ventricle.
systole	The part of the cardiac cycle in which the heart muscle contracts, forcing the blood into the main blood vessels.
systolic pressure	The top number in a blood pressure reading that represents the maximum pressure in the arteries as the heart contracts.
tachycardia	A resting heart rate of greater than 100 beats per minute.
technetium	A radioactive isotope used to reveal abnormalities in the heart wall.
tetralogy of Fallot	A condition that causes insufficient oxygen levels in the blood.
thallium	Radioactive material that is injected into a vein to show damaged areas of heart muscle.
thrombolysis in myocardial infarction (TIMI)	A grading system (grade 0 to 3) that evaluates reperfusion of blood flow. Achieved by thrombolytic therapy in a patient with myocardial infarction.
transposition of the great vessels	A condition in which the location of the aorta and pulmonary artery is switched.
tricuspid valve	The incoming valve of the right ventricle.
troponin	A cardiac enzyme found in the cells of the heart.
valve	In the heart, the structures that open and close with each heartbeat to ensure the proper sequence of blood flow through the heart.
veins	Larger vessels that carry oxygen-poor blood back to the heart.

Term	Meaning
ventricles	The lower chambers of the heart that collect blood from the right and left atria and pump it out of the heart.
ventricular fibrillation	An uncoordinated, irregular contraction of the heart muscle that may originate in the ventricles.
ventricular septal defect (VSD)	A hole in the wall that separates the ventricles of the heart.
venules	Small vessels that gather blood from the capillaries; these venules, in turn, drain into the larger veins that carry deoxygenated blood back to the heart.
waveform	The visual representation of each electrical impulse detected by leads during an EKG/ECG.

Add Your Own Terms and Definitions Here:

_____

_____

_____

_____

_____

_____

_____

REVIEW QUESTIONS

1. Describe the four chambers of the heart and the purpose of each.
2. Name the three layers of the heart wall.
3. Why is the heart considered to be double pump?
4. Explain the difference between diastole and systole.
5. What is the difference between primary hypertension and secondary hypertension?
6. What is a congenital heart disorder?
7. What is the role of a stent in an angioplasty procedure?
8. Name the three vessels that can be used as a graft in a coronary artery bypass procedure.
9. How are diuretics used to lower blood pressure?
10. Name the four valves of the heart and where they are located.

CHAPTER ACTIVITIES

Soundalike Word Choice

Circle the correct word in the following sentences.

1. Her laboratory data reflected a (BMP, BNP) of 47.5.
2. (Cor, Cord): Regular rate and rhythm with no murmurs.
3. His next exam revealed faint (brutes, bruits) on the right.
4. Nitroglycerin is a kind of (nitrate, nitrite) medication.
5. The patient was diagnosed a year ago with a non-Q-wave myocardial (infraction, infarction).
6. The echocardiogram was normal with an (ejection, infection) fraction of 70%.
7. Today the patient states he is doing quite well without any complaints of dyspnea on exertion (PND, PMD) or orthopnea.
8. Her lipid profile is satisfactory with normal total cholesterol, triglycerides, (HGL, HDL) and (LGL, LDL).
9. The cardiologist performed an angioplasty with placement of a (stent, stint) in the right coronary artery.
10. (Carbonate, Calcium) channel blockers decrease the heart's pumping strength to help lower blood pressure.

Creating Cardiology Words

Search for and combine the following prefixes, suffixes, and combining forms in the list below to create medical word that best fit the definition. Verify the spelling of the word you create with a medical dictionary. The first answer is provided for you.

tachy-	-gram	electr/o
scler/o	-osis	peri-
-ia	card/i, cardi/o	rhythm/o
angi/o	cyan/o	brady-
a-	-ic	-itis
-plasty	end/o	-logy
ather/o	nas/o	-ism

1. Inflammation of the endocardium.   _____

2. Abnormally rapid heart rate.   _____

3. A graphic trace of heart function.   _____

4. Inflammation of the pericardium.   _____

5. The study of the heart.   _____

6. Abnormally slow heart rate.   _____

7. Relating to turning blue.   _____

8. Hardening of the arteries.   _____

9. Abnormal heart rhythm.   _____

10. Surgical recanalization or dilation a blood vessel.   _____

Fill in the Blanks

Fill in the blanks with the correct terms.

1. What is the abbreviation for myocardial infarction?   _____

2. Name the medical specialty dealing with the heart.   _____

3. Which atrium receives blood from the body?   _____

4. What is the adjectival form of the word *ventricle*?   _____

5. What is the abbreviation for electrocardiogram?   _____

6. Which chamber contains the tricuspid valve?   _____

7. What is a normal heart rate called?   _____

8. Which test uses exercise to evaluate the heart?   _____

9. What is a leakage of blood back through a valve called?   _____

10. What condition is referred to as a *hole in the heart*?   _____

Combining Forms Practice

For each of the following terms, circle the correct combining form that corresponds to the meaning given.

1. vein	van/o	ven/o	vein/i
2. pulse	sphygm/o	angi/o	atri/o
3. blue	valv/o	ventricul/o	cyan/o
4. oxygen	ox/o	phleb/o	steth/o
5. chest	arteri/o	steth/o	vas/o
6. vessel	ven/o	vascul/o	thromb/o
7. aorta	rhythm/o	angi/o	aort/o
8. fatty plaque	ather/o	ven/o	pericardi/o
9. muscle	vas/o	my/o	coron/o
10. heart	cardi/o	aort/o	sphygm/o

Matching

Match the following abbreviations on the left with their corresponding meanings on the right.

_____   1. EKG

_____   2. PTCA

_____   3. ASD

_____   4. RCA

_____   5. CHF

_____   6. CABG

_____   7. MI

_____   8. HDL

_____   9. ACE

_____ 10. BNP

_____ 11. LIMA

_____ 12. SVG

_____ 13. LDL

_____ 14. CK

_____ 15. MUGA

A. A *hole in the heart.*

B. Heart attack.

C. Drug used to prevent formation of angiotensin-II.

D. Graph of the electrical activity of the heart.

E. A vessel in the chest wall used as a graft.

F. A cardiac enzyme.

G. *Good* cholesterol.

H. Buildup of fluid in lungs or body tissues.

I. Another name for an *angioplasty* procedure.

J. A graft from the vein in the thigh and leg.

K. A test that uses technetium to evaluate the ventricles.

L. *Bad* cholesterol.

M. A hormone made by the heart.

N. A major coronary artery.

O. Cardiac bypass surgery.

TRANSCRIPTION PRACTICE

Open your word-processing software. Insert the student CD-ROM and locate the dictation for this chapter. For each of the words in the "listen for these terms" list for each report, use a medical dictionary or other resource to identify and write down a brief definition of the term on a separate sheet of paper to attach with your work. Then listen to the dictation and transcribe each report. Use the current date for each report where a date is indicated. Insert a heading into the document if the text falls to a second page.

At the end of each report, indicate the name of the dictating physician under the signature line and insert reference initials. For date dictated and transcribed and date of admission, use the current date. Proofread your work, print one copy for your instructor along with your term definitions, and save the completed report to your student disk.

Report #T13.1: Clinic Note
Patient Name: Joseph Watson
Medical Record No.: WAT-34499
Attending Physician: Lena Kushner, MD

Listen for these terms:
percutaneous
luminal
dobutamine
orthostatic hypotension
jugular venous pressure
PMI
hydrochlorothiazide
isosorbide

Report #T13.2: Operative Report
Patient Name: Maria Figueroa
Medical Record No.: 80345112
Attending Surgeon: Andrea Biggs, MD
Assistant: Michael Hubbard, MD

Listen for these terms:
cardiopulmonary arrest
pacing wires
pressors
Cordis (stent)
Swan-Ganz catheter

Report #T11.3: Consultation Letter
Patient Name: Larry Jones
Medical Record No.: J-74901
Attending Physician: Andrea Biggs, MD
Requesting Physician: Priti Chawla, MD

Listen for these terms:
gout
cholecystectomy
sickle cell disease
scleral icterus
apical murmur

14

GASTROENTEROLOGY

OBJECTIVES

After completing this chapter, you will be able to:

- Identify the components of the digestive system and their functions.
- Describe the process of digestion of food through the gastrointestinal tract.
- Describe common disorders and diseases affecting different parts of the gastrointestinal system.
- Explain common laboratory tests, imaging studies, and other techniques used to diagnose and treat gastrointestinal disorders.

INTRODUCTION

Gastroenterology is the study of the group of organs in the body that is responsible for digesting food and extracting nutrients necessary to sustain life. *Gastr/o* is a Greek word meaning *stomach*; the combination form *enter/o* means *intestine*; and the suffix *–ology* means *study*. Thus, gastroenterology is primarily the study of the stomach and intestines. However, this medical specialty is actually quite broad and includes the anatomy and physiology of several organs and other structures

bordered by the abdominal wall in the anterior, the spinal column in the posterior, the diaphragm superiorly, and the pelvic organs inferiorly. A **gastroenterologist** is a medical specialist who cares for patients with a wide variety of diseases and disorders that affect this body system. A gastroenterologist may treat simple symptoms of abdominal discomfort as well as highly specialized and complex issues such as gastrointestinal organ resections. This chapter examines the anatomy and structure of this multiorgan system as well as the disorders and diseases that affect the digestive tract, and the common diagnostic and treatment protocols associated with each.

ANATOMY OF THE GASTROINTESTINAL SYSTEM

At its simplest, the gastrointestinal system (also known as the **alimentary canal**, the **gastrointestinal** (GI) **tract**, or simply the digestive tract) is a coiled tube that begins at the mouth and ends at the anus. It consists of a system of organs in the body that takes in food, digests it to extract energy and nutrients, and expels the remaining waste. The sole purpose of the GI tract is to break down ingested food so that nutrients can be extracted and transported by the circulatory system for dissemination around the body. The GI tract consists of the

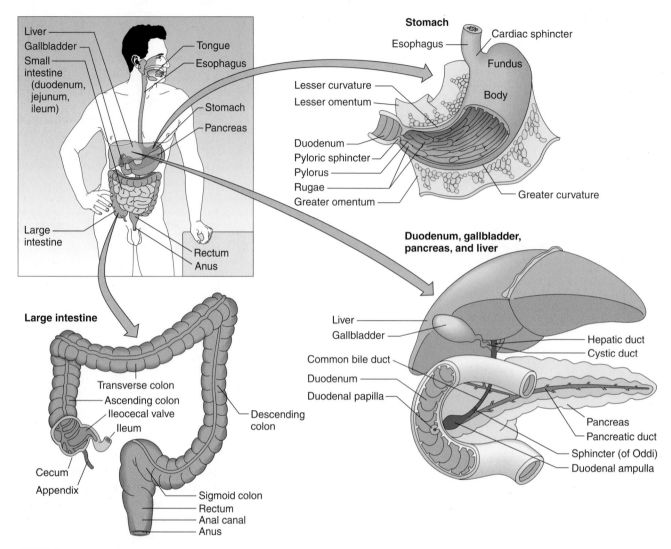

FIGURE 14.1. The Digestive System. Reprinted with permission from *Stedman's Medical Dictionary,* 27th ed. Baltimore: Lippincott Williams & Wilkins, 2000.

mouth, throat, esophagus, stomach, small intestine, large intestine, rectum, and anus. It also includes accessory organs that lie outside the digestive tract, such as the salivary glands, liver, gallbladder and biliary tract, and the pancreas (Figure 14.1).

The digestive system contains intestinal bacteria, also called gut flora, that perform a variety of functions:

- They help to create energy for the body by breaking down food products.
- They help train the immune system to identify and attack harmful organisms.
- They stimulate cell growth and protect the body from harmful bacteria, including *Staphylococcus aureus,* *Neisseria mengitidis,* and *Streptococcus pneumonia,* the bacteria that can cause toxic shock syndrome, pneumonia, and meningitis, respectively. The millions of colonies of gut flora prevent these harmful bacteria from growing to dangerous levels by dominating the resources in the digestive tract and creating a barrier effect that inhibits their growth.

Mouth and Throat

The digestive tract begins with the **oral cavity**, or the mouth. Chewing allows food to be mashed into a soft mass by the teeth. There are a total of 32 teeth in a complete adult set, which are used for biting and grinding. The roof of the mouth is called the **palate**. The anterior portion of the palate, called the **hard palate**, is formed by bone; and the posterior part, called the **soft palate**, is formed by soft tissue. The **tongue** is a mobile mass of muscular tissue covered with mucous membrane, occupying the cavity of the mouth and forming part of its floor. It is the organ of taste and assists in the chewing and swallowing of food as well as articulating speech. The **uvula** is a small piece of soft tissue hanging down from the soft palate over the back of the tongue, which is used primarily in speech production. With the aid of saliva, the structures in the mouth break down food and make it easier to swallow and pass to the throat.

The **oropharynx** lies at the back of the mouth and includes the soft palate, the tonsils, the posterior third of the tongue, and the posterior wall of the throat. The **pharynx**, or throat, lies behind the mouth. When food and fluids are swallowed, they pass through the oropharynx and into the throat. The **epiglottis**, a flap of cartilage that lies at the root of the tongue, opens and closes to prevent food and fluids from entering the airway.

Esophagus

The **esophagus** is a muscular channel that connects the throat to the stomach. It carries food and liquids that have been chewed and softened in the mouth from the throat to the stomach for further digestion. Food is forced downward to the stomach by powerful waves of muscle contractions passing through the walls of the esophagus. The esophagus has a ring of muscle at the bottom that contracts and closes after food passes from the esophagus into the stomach so that it does not flow back into the esophagus or throat.

Stomach

The **stomach** is a muscular, saclike organ that continues the process of digestion of food received from the esophagus. The stomach acts as a storage area for food and breaks it down so it can move into the intestines more easily. The **cardia** is the top portion of the stomach; it surrounds the opening of the esophagus to the stomach, which is called the **esophageal sphincter**. The **fundus** is the left upper portion of the stomach, whereas the **body** is the large central part of the stomach. The **antrum** is the lower portion of the stomach where food is ground down into small pieces. The outlet of the stomach into the small intestine is called the **pylorus**, and the ring of muscle that opens and closes to regulate the passage of food into the intestines is called the **pyloric sphincter**.

Small Intestine

The **small intestine**, also called the **small bowel**, is a long tube that connects the stomach to the large intestine. It is here that the actual digestion of food takes place. The small intestine is composed of three main parts: the **duodenum**, the first part of the small intestine, located at the top nearest to the stomach; the

jejunum, the middle portion; and the **ileum**, located at the end of the small intestine. Food enters the duodenum through the pyloric sphincter in amounts that can be digested by the small intestine. The jejunum and ileum work to absorb fat and other nutrients for use by the body and transport the remaining residues to the large intestine. An obstruction in the lower part of the small intestine is called an **ileus**.

Large Intestine

The **large intestine**, also called the **colon**, is a long tube-like organ that moves waste material from the small intestine to the rectum to be excreted by the body. It frames the coiled small intestine in the abdominal cavity, beginning at the lower right-hand side of the body and ending on the lower left-hand side. The main job of the large intestine is to absorb the remaining water from the food residue passing through the intestines and to form solid waste material called **stool** that can be excreted from the body. The first half of the colon absorbs fluids and recycles them into the bloodstream. The second half compacts the waste into feces and secretes mucus, which binds and lubricates the substances in order to ease their passage and protect the colon. The inability of the colon to pass stool is called **obstipation**.

The first portion of the large intestine is the **cecum**, which is a tubelike structure located at the beginning of the large intestine that receives undigested food material from the small intestine. The main job of the cecum is to absorb fluids and salts that remain after completion of intestinal digestion and to pass the remaining solid portion of waste into the main body of the colon. Attached to the cecum is a narrow fingerlike appendage called the **vermiform appendix** (commonly referred to simply as *the appendix*). Although the appendix has no obvious function, some scientists believe it helps support the immune system to prevent inflammation of the gastrointestinal tract.

The greater part of the large intestine is divided into a series of sections that succeed one another, forming a continuous arch, framing the abdominal cavity, and are referred to collectively as the colon. The colon absorbs water from waste and turns the waste into solid matter to be excreted by the body. The first section, located on the patient's right side, is called the **ascending colon** and extends from the cecum to the **hepatic flexure**, which is the name given to the turn of the colon next to the liver. The **transverse colon** is the top portion of the colon, which extends from the hepatic flexure to the **splenic flexure**, the name given to the turn of the colon next to the spleen. The left-sided segment, called the **descending colon**, extends from the splenic flexure to the beginning of the sigmoid colon. The **sigmoid colon** is the bottom part of the colon, located between the descending colon and the rectum. The **rectum** is a

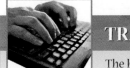

TRANSCRIPTION TIP:

The homonyms *ilium* and *ileum* are often confused. A helpful way to distinguish *ilium* from *ileum* is to think of the *e* in *ileum* being similar to the loops of the small and large intestines.

chamber that begins at the end of the large intestine, immediately following the sigmoid colon. Solid waste passes from the descending colon into the rectum, where it is stored temporarily and allowed to accumulate until **defecation**, or excretion of waste from the body, occurs. Finally, the **anus**, which is connected to the rectum, is the opening at the end of the digestive tract through which stool leaves the body. A muscular ring called the **anal sphincter** keeps the anus closed until defecation.

Accessory Organs

The salivary glands, liver, gallbladder, and pancreas are not part of the digestive tract, but they play a vital role in digestive activities, secreting fluids necessary for the processing of food into the digestive tract. For this reason, they are called **accessory organs**.

Salivary Glands

Ducts connect the mouth with three pairs of **salivary glands,** which help to moisten food during chewing, as follows:

- **Parotid**, located at the side of the face and in front of and below the external ear.
- **Submandibular**, located beneath the **mandible**, or lower jaw.
- **Sublingual**, located under the tongue.

These glands secrete saliva into the oral cavity, where it is mixed with food during the process of chewing. Saliva contains water, mucus, and **amylase**, a digestive enzyme that breaks down starches.

Liver

The **liver** is the largest organ in the body, occupying the entire upper right quadrant of the abdomen. A fold of tissue called the **falciform ligament** divides the liver into right and left sections, or **lobes**. Overall, the liver performs more than 500 vital functions in the body, among them is acting as a filter to remove toxins and waste products from the blood. These toxins include alcohol, drugs, and chemicals produced by microorganisms. The liver also stores nutrients, such as vitamins, minerals, and iron, and plays a role in managing levels of certain chemicals and proteins in the body, such as cholesterol, hormones, and sugars. The liver helps the body digest food by producing **bile**, a yellow-brown fluid that is released into the duodenum through a series of ducts, which allows blood and other substances to enter and leave the liver. In addition to water, bile contains cholesterol, **bile salts** (natural detergents that break up fat), and **bilirubin** (a chemical waste product formed from the breakdown of old red blood cells). Bile assists in the digestion and absorption of

fats, and transports toxins neutralized by the liver out into the intestines for excretion.

Gallbladder and Biliary Tract

The **gallbladder** is a sac-shaped accessory organ firmly attached to the lower surface of the liver. It receives bile from the liver through a series of ducts, collectively known as the **biliary tract**, and stores it for release at the appropriate time into the small intestine, where it aids in the digestive process. The ducts that comprise the biliary tract are named according to the structures to which they are connected. The **hepatic ducts (right and left)** begin in the liver and carry bile either to the gallbladder (by joining with the **cystic duct**), to the pancreas (by joining with the **pancreatic duct**), or to the duodenum. The **common bile duct**, therefore, is a convergence of the right and left hepatic ducts, which carries bile from the liver to the gallbladder, duodenum, and pancreas through appropriate separate ductal channels, as shown in Figure 14.2.

Pancreas

The **pancreas** is a large glandular structure that lies in front of the upper spine and behind the stomach. It secretes enzymes through the biliary ducts into the interior of the duodenum, aiding in the breakdown of proteins, fats, and carbohydrates. The pancreas is also part of the endocrine system, producing hormones and other chemicals that help regulate blood sugar.

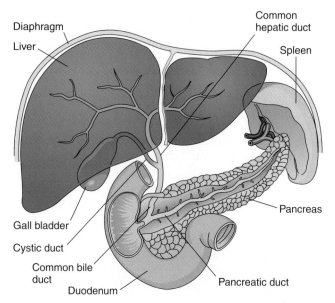

FIGURE 14.2. The Biliary Tract. The ducts in the biliary tract comprise a path by which bile is secreted by the liver and transported to the small intestine during digestion. Reprinted with permission from Cohen BJ, Wood DL. *Memmler's The Human Body in Health and Disease,* 9th Ed. Lippincott Williams & Wilkins, 2000.

QUICK CHECK 14.1

Match the anatomic structure in the left column with its function in the right column.

Anatomic Structure   *Function*

  A. liver   _____ Also part of the endocrine system.

  B. small intestine   _____ Manufactures bile.

  C. pancreas   _____ Where actual digestion takes place.

  D. rectum   _____ Receives food from the esophagus.

  E. stomach   _____ A "holding area" in the colon.

THE DIGESTIVE PROCESS

Digestion is the process whereby food and liquid are broken down into smaller parts and converted into forms of energy the body can use to maintain life and health. Digestion involves the mixing and physical breaking down of food; the movement of food through the digestive tract; and the chemical breakdown of molecules of food into components that are absorbed and used by the body. The digestive process also involves the creating of waste to be eliminated.

Digestion begins in the mouth, with both chemical and mechanical components. Foodstuffs are broken down mechanically, with saliva added as a lubricant. Crushing and grinding of food by the teeth, called **mastication** or chewing, allows food to be mashed into a soft mass, and the enzymes present in saliva break down food and make it easier to swallow and pass into the throat. The tongue and the mouth move to push the food to the back of the throat in preparation for it to be swallowed. The epiglottis closes off the trachea to make sure that swallowed food enters the esophagus and not the windpipe and lungs.

Upon entering the esophagus, the food is forced downward to the stomach by **peristalsis**, powerful wave-like movements of muscle that contract in syncopated pulses to move food through the digestive system. Before entering the stomach, the food passes through a one-way valve called the **esophageal sphincter**, which contracts to close after food enters the stomach in order to keep the contents from flowing back into the esophagus.

The food enters the stomach, which then performs three tasks: First, it stores swallowed food and liquid; this requires the muscles of the stomach to relax and accept large volumes of swallowed material. Second, it produces digestive acids that are mixed with the food and liquid by the muscle action of the lower part of the stomach. The resulting product is a mushy liquid called

chyme. At the same time, the cells of the stomach produce an acid that kills germs in the food that could harm the body. Finally, the stomach empties its contents slowly into the small intestine for further processing.

The small intestine receives the chyme from the stomach through the pyloric sphincter. Ducts that empty into the duodenum deliver digestive fluids from the pancreas that contain enzymes to help break down fats and protein. Bile is released from the gallbladder and travels through the bile ducts to reach the small intestine and mix with the fat in the food. The bile dissolves the fat into watery contents much like detergents that dissolve grease from a frying pan. Carbohydrates are broken down to simple sugars by enzymes that are released from the lining of the small intestine. All of these liquid elements are then absorbed through the cell walls of the small intestine, released into the bloodstream, and circulated throughout the body. What remains (waste) is passed through the ileum and into the large intestine to be eliminated.

Waste left over from the digestive process passes through the colon by means of peristalsis, first in a liquid state and ultimately in solid form as stool. As stool passes through the cecum and into the main body of the colon, any remaining water is absorbed, leaving only solid waste. Stool passes through the ascending and transverse colon until it reaches the descending colon, where it is stored until it is emptied into the rectum to

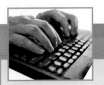

TRANSCRIPTION TIP:

The stool softener docusate is frequently mistranscribed because it is mispronounced. The correct pronunciation of the medication sounds like *DOCK-yoo-sate*, but dictators sometimes pronounce the word as *DUCK-a-sate*.

QUICK CHECK 14.2 ✓

Fill in the blanks with the correct answers.

1. The liver produces _____ that is stored in the gallbladder.

2. Food is forced into the stomach by a wavelike motion known as _____.

3. The one-way valve that contracts to allow food into the stomach is the _____.

4. The stomach mixes food into a mushy liquid called _____.

5. _____ is added as a lubricant in the mouth to help break down food.

---

begin the process of elimination. When stool enters the rectum, sensors send a message to the brain, giving a person the sensation of an impending bowel movement. At this point, the anal sphincter relaxes and the rectum contracts, expelling its contents through the anus.

COMMON GASTROINTESTINAL DISEASES AND TREATMENTS

Diseases and medical problems affecting the gastrointestinal system are called **digestive disorders**. Every section of the GI tract has its own unique disorders. Some cause only irritation and discomfort that may lead to a change in lifestyle; others can affect several parts of the digestive system, becoming debilitating and even fatal.

Peptic Disorders

Peptic disorders involve damage to the lining of the esophagus, stomach, or duodenum as a result of the presence of excess stomach acids, enzymes, or infection with bacteria, and may include the following:

Gastritis

Gastritis is a peptic disorder that refers to inflammation of the lining of the stomach, although the term is often used to encompass a variety of symptoms including burning or discomfort. Gastritis occurs when the normal mechanisms that protect the stomach lining are overwhelmed and irritation occurs. As a result, the lining of the stomach becomes irritated and inflamed, causing an attack of pain lasting a day or two. Over time, continual irritation can wear away the stomach lining. Gastritis can be caused by irritation from certain types of corrosive foods or substances, particular medications (such as anti-inflammatories), or a backflow of bile into the stomach. The most common cause of true gastritis is an infection with *Helicobacter pylori* bacteria, or *H pylori*, a microorganism whose outer layer is resist-

ant to the normal effects of stomach acid in breaking down bacteria.

Gastroesophageal Reflux Disease

Gastroesophageal reflux disease (GERD) is a condition whereby excess gastric and duodenal acids and other contents flow backward through the esophageal sphincter into the esophagus, as shown in Figure 14.3. This occurs when the esophageal sphincter does not function properly. This backflow of acid results in inflammation of the lining of the esophagus and causes symptoms such as a burning pain under the breastbone called heartburn, belching, nausea, vomiting, and difficulty swallowing. Other complications include narrowing of the esophagus, called esophageal stricture, which makes swallowing solid foods difficult. In addition, GERD can cause hoarseness, a sensation of a lump in the throat called **globus sensation**, and chronic sinusitis.

Recurrent untreated gastroesophageal reflux may lead to a precancerous condition of the lower esophagus called **Barrett esophagus**. Barrett esophagus is not just an irritation but is an actual *change* in the cells in the lining of the esophagus caused by chronic reflux of stomach and duodenal contents into the esophagus. In Barrett esophagus, the normal cells that line the esophagus, called squamous cells, change into columnar cells, a type of cell not usually found in the lining of the esophagus. Chronic damage to the lining of the esophagus causes these abnormal changes, increasing the risk of esophageal cancer. **Metaplasia** is the process in which normal adult cells in a tissue transform into a type of cell that is abnormal for that tissue, such as in the case of Barrett esophagus. Patients with Barrett esophagus usually undergo a diagnostic endoscopy, described below, every two to three years to ensure that the condition is not progressing to cancer.

Peptic Ulcer Disease

Peptic ulcer disease (PUD) is a condition whereby a **peptic ulcer**, a small open lesion, develops in the stomach

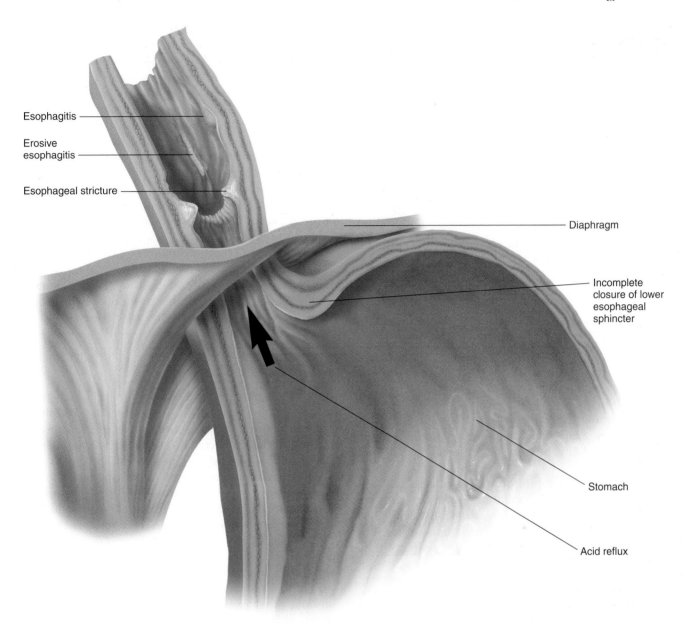

Esophagitis

Erosive esophagitis

Esophageal stricture

Diaphragm

Incomplete closure of lower esophageal sphincter

Stomach

Acid reflux

FIGURE 14.3. GERD. The reflux of stomach acid into the esophagus causes a variety of symptoms. Reprinted with permission from Anatomical Chart Co.

(called **gastric ulcer**) or duodenum (called **duodenal ulcer**) where the lining of the stomach or duodenum has been eaten away by stomach acids and digestive juices (Figure 14.4). Infection with the bacterium *H pylori* is the most common cause of duodenal and gastric ulcers. Other causes include the use of certain drugs that irritate the lining of the stomach, such as aspirin or nonsteroidal anti-inflammatory medications; smoking; and even psychological stress, which can increase acid production and play a role in peptic ulcer disease.

Left untreated, ulcers may bleed, causing a person to vomit blood (**hematemesis**) or pass black, tarry stools because of bleeding in the stomach (**melena**). If the ulcer perforates the stomach wall, stomach contents may spill into the abdominal cavity, causing **peritonitis**,

which is an infection caused by the inflammation of the clear membrane that covers all of the abdominal organs and the inside walls of the abdomen, known as the **peritoneum**. Peritonitis is caused by the introduction of bacteria into the peritoneum from a perforation of the wall of an organ. This rupture causes bacteria to spill into the bloodstream, resulting in infection.

The symptoms of peptic disorders can be relieved with drugs that neutralize or reduce the production of stomach acid, which promotes resolution of the disorder and its complications regardless of the cause. Drugs that produce this effect include the following:

- **Antacids,** which are used to neutralize acid already present in the stomach and relieve acute symptoms (but not cure the underlying disorder).

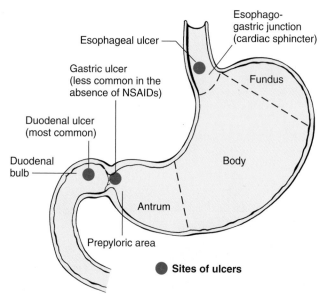

Esophago-gastric junction (cardiac sphincter)

Esophageal ulcer

Gastric ulcer (less common in the absence of NSAIDs)

Fundus

Duodenal ulcer (most common)

Duodenal bulb

Body

Antrum

Prepyloric area

● **Sites of ulcers**

FIGURE 14.4. Peptic Ulcer Disease. Sites of various types of ulcers in the digestive tract. Reprinted with permission from Nettina, Sandra M. *The Lippincott Manual of Nursing Practice,* 7th ed. Lippincott Williams & Wilkins, 2001.

- **Histamine-2 (H2) blockers,** a class of drugs that relieves symptoms and promotes healing of the stomach lining by reducing the secretion of acid in the stomach.
- **Proton pump inhibitors (PPIs),** a class of drugs that block the production of acid in the stomach. Often used concurrently with H2 blockers, PPIs reduce acid production in the stomach and promote healing of ulcers in a shorter period of time than do H2 blockers alone.
- **Antibiotics,** used when infection from bacteria, such as *H pylori,* is part of the problem.

When medical therapy fails, surgical intervention may be necessary. Anti-reflux procedures may help patients who have persistent symptoms despite medical treatment. The most common procedure is called a **Nissen fundoplication,** named after Dr. Rudolph Nissen who first performed the procedure in 1951. In this procedure, surgeons reconstruct the area of the lower esophageal sphincter, the muscle that separates the stomach and esophagus. The fundus (*fundo-*) of the stomach is wrapped (*-plication*) around the lower esophagus and positioned in such a way as to create a barrier, preventing the flow of acids from the stomach into the esophagus and strengthening the valve between the esophagus and stomach.

Other operations to repair damage resulting from chronic stomach acid problems are shown in Figure 14.5. **Vagotomy** is the surgical cutting of the vagus nerve adjacent to the esophagus to reduce acid secretion in the stomach. Deriving its name from the Latin word meaning *wanderer* because of its wide distribution, the **vagus**

nerve helps control function of the esophagus, larynx, stomach, intestines, lungs, and heart. Part of this nerve splits into branches that go to different parts of the stomach. Stimulation from these branches causes the stomach to produce acid, resulting in ulcers that may eventually bleed or perforate the stomach wall. Vagotomy is usually done in conjunction with an **antrectomy,** the surgical removal of the lower part of the stomach, which produces a hormone that stimulates the secretion of gastric juices.

Resective surgical procedures on the stomach include the **Billroth procedure,** named after the German surgeon Theodor Billroth who performed the first resection of the stomach in 1881. The **Billroth I** procedure, also called a **gastroduodenostomy,** involves performing an antrectomy, as above, and surgically attaching the remaining portion of the stomach to the duodenum. In the **Billroth II** procedure, also called a **gastrojejunostomy,** the remaining portion of the stomach is attached to the jejunum.

Gallbladder Disease

Gallbladder disease includes inflammation, infection, stones, and obstruction of the gallbladder. Although the exact cause of these disorders is unknown, several factors—including heredity, diet, hormones, obesity, and infection—are believed to play a role.

The most common disorder involving the gallbladder is the formation of **gallstones,** which are lumps of rocklike material that form inside the gallbladder, a condition called **cholelithiasis.** The term derives from the root words *chole-,* meaning bile, and *lith-,* meaning a stone or calculus. What causes gallstones to form is not clearly understood, but an abnormality in the function of the gallbladder causes it to remove an excessive amount of water from the bile, causing the substance that remains to form into hardened masses in the gallbladder. Consisting mainly of cholesterol, blood, bile, and calcium, the stones can range in size from a grain of sand to a golf ball.

TRANSCRIPTION TIP:

Remember that names of entities derived from the names of persons or places are called eponyms, and, as such, do not take the possessive form if the eponym is followed by a noun; for example, Barrett esophagus, *not* Barrett's esophagus. However, if the eponym is not followed by a noun or falls at the end of a sentence, the possessive form is used; for example: *The patient suffers from Barrett esophagus. The patient suffers from Barrett's.*

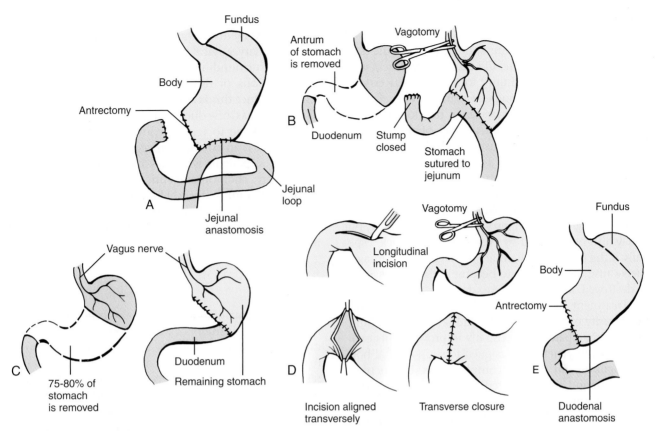

FIGURE 14.5. Surgical Procedures for a Peptic Ulcer. (A) Gastrojejunostomy (Billroth II); (B) antrectomy and vagotomy; (C) subtotal gastrectomy; (D) vagotomy; (E) gastroduodenostomy (Billroth I). Reprinted with permission from Nettina, Sandra M. *The Lippincott Manual of Nursing Practice*, 7th ed. Lippincott, Williams & Wilkins, 2001.

Gallstones can also be present in the common bile duct, a condition called **choledocholithiasis**, a term that derives from the root words *choledocho-*, meaning common bile duct, and *lith-* meaning a stone or calculus. **Cholecystitis** refers to a sudden inflammation of the gallbladder, causing severe abdominal pain. Gallstones are the main cause of cholecystitis, but severe illness, alcohol abuse and, rarely, tumors of the gallbladder may also cause an acute attack.

Most people with gallstones do not display any symptoms, but if gallstones cause disruptive, recurrent attacks of pain, physicians typically recommend surgical removal of the gallbladder, a procedure called **cholecystectomy**. The body can function well without a gallbladder, and removing it is a common treatment for gallstones that are causing symptoms.

Traditionally, cholecystectomy involved the removal of the gallbladder through a large surgical incision in the abdomen; this is called an **open cholecystectomy**. Today, however, nearly all cholecystectomies are performed by **laparoscopic cholecystectomy**, a minimally invasive procedure that uses a small fiberoptic tube called a **laparoscope, which** magnifies the body's internal structures and projects the images onto a video monitor in the operating room. In this procedure, very small incisions of up to half an inch are made in the patient's body at the operative site. The laparoscope and surgical instruments are then introduced through these incisions, allowing access to the patient's internal abdominal organs. The camera transmits an image of the organs onto a television monitor. The surgeon performs the procedure while viewing the organs on the monitor. Very thin surgical instruments locate the gallbladder, and the cystic duct and artery are cut and tied off. The gallbladder is removed through the incision sites and the incisions are closed. Because the incisions are so much smaller, this procedure results in less postoperative discomfort as well as much smaller scars. The patient has a quicker recovery time and earlier return to full activities.

Pancreatic Disorders

Pancreatitis is a disease in which the pancreas becomes inflamed and damaged. Damage to the pancreas occurs when its own digestive enzymes, which normally do not become active until they are released to the small intestine during the digestive process, become active prematurely in the pancreas and begin attacking the pancreas itself. In severe cases, there may be tissue damage, infection, and cysts. Enzymes and toxins may enter the bloodstream from a damaged pancreas and seriously injure other organs, such as the heart, lungs, and kidneys.

Acute pancreatitis occurs suddenly (hence the term *acute*) and may be a severe, life-threatening illness with many complications. If injury to the pancreas continues, such as when a person persists in drinking alcohol, a chronic form of the disease may develop, bringing severe pain and reduced functioning of the pancreas that affects digestion and causes weight loss.

Chronic pancreatitis is a slow, ongoing inflammation of the pancreas that occurs when digestive enzymes attack and destroy the pancreas and nearby tissues over time, causing scarring and pain. Chronic pancreatitis is usually brought on by many years of alcohol abuse, but it may also be triggered by even one acute attack, especially if the pancreatic ducts are damaged. The damaged ducts cause the pancreas to become inflamed, tissue to be destroyed, and scar tissue to develop.

Treatment of pancreatitis depends on the source and severity of the attack. If no kidney or lung complications occur, pancreatitis usually improves on its own. Treatment, in general, is designed to support vital bodily functions and prevent complications. If pancreatic cysts occur and are considered large enough to interfere with the healing process of the pancreas, the cyst may be drained or surgically removed. In the case of the pancreatic duct or bile duct being blocked by gallstones, causing an acute attack, removal of the gallbladder is usually required.

Pancreatic cancer is a disease in which cancerous cells are found in the tissues of the pancreas. Pancreatic cancer is a dangerous and difficult cancer to treat because it spreads rapidly and is seldom detected in its early stages, which is a major reason why it is a leading cause of cancer death. Signs and symptoms may not appear until the disease is quite advanced. By that time, the cancer is likely to have spread to other parts of the body and surgical removal is no longer possible. The most common type of pancreatic cancer is called an **exocrine tumor**, which is a tumor arising in the area of the pancreas that produces digestive juices, called the **exocrine pancreas**. These tumors are almost always malignant.

Treatment of pancreatic cancer is primarily based on the stage of the cancer, not its exact type. At one time, it was not possible to remove an exocrine tumor with surgery because of the blood vessels that passed through the tumor. Surgical advances, including the Whipple procedure, have found a way around that obstacle. The **Whipple procedure** is now the most common surgical treatment for cancer involving the head of the pancreas. Also called a **pancreaticoduodenectomy**, this procedure generally includes the removal of the head of the pancreas, the duodenum, a portion of the stomach, and other nearby tissues. This operation was first described by Dr. Alan O. Whipple of New York Memorial Hospital (now called Memorial Sloan-Kettering) in 1951.

Since that time, there have been many modifications and improvements of the procedure, but it continues to be the primary surgical treatment for tumors of the pancreas and surrounding structures. In the Whipple procedure, portions of the upper gastrointestinal tract are removed. Once this is complete, the remaining portions of the pancreas, bile duct, and stomach are sutured back to the intestine to restore continuity of the GI tract. Because this is an extensive procedure, the goal is to operate only on patients who may have removable tumors. Postsurgery, chemotherapeutic agents can be used to kill the remaining cancer. Fluorouracil or 5-flurouracil (5-FU), gemcitabine (Gemzar), and erlotinib (Tarceva) are the chemotherapeutic drug agents of choice in treating this type of cancer.

Hepatitis

Hepatitis is an inflammation of the cells of the liver, resulting in their injury or destruction. Hepatitis can be caused by a number of agents, including bacteria, drugs, toxins, a virus, or excess alcohol. Hepatitis can also result from an autoimmune condition in which cells in the body's immune system that normally serve to prevent infection attack the body's own liver cells as invaders, for no known reason. Hepatitis can begin suddenly and have a limited course, called **acute hepatitis**; or it can be slowly progressive and persist for prolonged periods, called **chronic hepatitis**.

Alcoholic hepatitis is an inflammation of the liver caused by alcohol. Alcohol is a poison if taken in more than modest amounts. Although it can adversely affect stomach lining, heart muscle, and brain tissue, the liver is a primary target because alcohol travels to the liver after leaving the intestines. **Nonalcoholic steatohepatitis** (NASH, dictated as an acronym, *nash*), also referred to in dictation as *fatty liver disease*, has features similar to that of alcohol-induced hepatitis but causes inflammation and liver injury related to the presence of fat. Severe obesity and diabetes are the major risk factors for NASH.

The most serious form of hepatitis occurs when any one of several hepatitis viruses infect the liver and begin replicating, a condition known as **viral hepatitis**. These viruses are delineated by type using the letters A through E, with the most common three listed below:

- Hepatitis A virus (HAV): Also referred to as **infectious hepatitis**, hepatitis A is the most common hepatitis virus. It is spread primarily by fecal-oral contamination, often by food handlers who prepare food with unwashed hands, and in crowded, unsanitary conditions. It may also be acquired from eating contaminated food—food or drinking water contaminated with fecal matter that contains the virus. A vaccine is available for those at high risk of contracting the virus.

- Hepatitis B virus (HBV): This disease is caused by the hepatitis B virus. It is spread by blood and other body fluids. It may be transmitted by sharing needles used for injection or by sexual contact. Most patients recover, but the disease may be serious and may even lead to liver cancer. There is an effective vaccine to prevent HBV infection, given in a series of three shots from birth to six months of age.

- Hepatitis C virus (HCV): HCV is a mild, slowly progressive virus that is spread by direct contact with infected blood or blood products, such as from blood transfusions (now rare), the sharing of IV drug needles or body piercing instruments, or even razors contaminated by microscopic amounts of blood. There is no vaccine for HCV because the genetic makeup of the virus mutates easily into new variations. These genes, called **genotypes,** vary in how they respond to treatment. Currently there are at least six distinct HCV genotypes with different subtypes, which are dictated as Arabic numbers from 1 to 6, with genotype subtypes classified alphabetically as *a, b, c,* etc. Example: *HCV, genotype 1a.*

Hepatitis is usually diagnosed through a series of blood tests that check the levels of many of the enzymes for which the liver is responsible. In addition, blood tests called **antigen tests** are conducted, which indicate the presence of the virus in the blood, as well as **antibody tests** to test for the body's reaction to the infection. These results are transcribed as being positive or negative. *Example: The patient's hepatitis B surface antigen is negative.*

Regardless of the cause or type of hepatitis diagnosed, however, treatment of the disease is required or liver failure may result. Drug treatments for hepatitis B and C are focused on reducing or preventing liver damage and boosting the immune system to promote attack on the viruses by the body.

All current treatment protocols for hepatitis C are based on the use of various preparations of the antiviral agent **interferon alpha,** which is administered by injection. **Interferon** is a protein naturally produced by the body to fight viruses by boosting the immune system. The medication interferon alpha is a synthetic reproduction of the naturally produced interferon, which is used in the treatment of chronic hepatitis C to try to arrest or stop the hepatitis C virus from damaging the liver. It can stop the inflammation in the liver in some patients and sometimes rids the patient of the hepatitis C virus entirely. However, it does not improve the scarring already present in the liver. A variety of names for preparations of this drug may be heard in dictation and include peginterferon alpha (pegylated interferon or Peg Intron) as well as Pegasys. Injections of interferon are usually combined with oral doses of ribavirin (Rebetol, Copegus), a broad-spectrum antiviral medication. Treatment usually takes from six months

TRANSCRIPTION TIP:

According to *The Book of Style for Medical Transcription,* 3rd Ed., when transcribing hepatitis terminology, the word hepatitis is not capitalized, but capital letters are used to designate type. Example: *The patient was diagnosed with hepatitis A.*

to one year and is successful in about 40% of people with HCV.

For people who develop life-threatening liver disease, a liver transplant may be necessary. Transplantation involves the surgical removal of the person's infected liver, which is then replaced with a donor liver. Although many times chronic hepatitis recurs after transplantation, the disease in this form is usually mild and not life-threatening.

Cirrhosis

Cirrhosis is a condition in which normal liver cells are damaged and replaced by scar tissue. This scarring causes distortion of the normal liver architecture, which interferes with blood flow through the liver and inhibits the ability of the liver to perform its biochemical functions.

The most common cause of cirrhosis is alcohol abuse, but chronic hepatitis can also lead to cirrhosis. Some terms describing complications of cirrhosis that may be dictated in the physical exam portion of medical reports include the following:

- **Spider angiomas,** tiny clusters of red veins close to the surface of the skin.
- **Ascites,** a condition that occurs when fluid accumulates in the abdomen due to abnormal liver function.
- **Jaundice** (also called **icterus**), a yellowish cast to the skin that occurs because the liver cannot process bilirubin.
- **Palmar erythema,** a condition in which the palms of the hands may be reddish and blotchy.
- **Xanthomas,** small fatty yellow lumps that develop on the eyelids, hands, and elbows.
- **Steatorrhea,** a condition in which the feces contain excessive fat, causing them to float and to be very foul smelling.
- **Hepatomegaly,** or an enlarged liver.

Cirrhosis is usually progressive, and there is no known cure for the disease. A person may stop drinking and prevent further destruction of liver tissue, but scar tissue, once formed, remains indefinitely. Treatment for cirrhosis includes the withdrawal of the toxic agents that damage the liver, along with proper nutrition and supplements. Liver transplantation is considered for patients with advanced cirrhosis, but a transplanted liver will also develop cirrhosis if the person continues to abuse alcohol; therefore, a patient must demonstrate that he or she is alcohol-free for a certain period before being considered as a candidate for transplantation.

Another complication of a diseased liver includes **esophageal varices**, which are abnormally enlarged veins within the wall of the lower part of the esophagus that develop when normal blood flow to the liver is blocked. Patients with cirrhosis develop portal hypertension, a condition of increased blood pressure within the portal vein of the liver. When portal hypertension occurs, blood flow through the liver is diminished. Thus, blood flow increases through the blood vessels within the esophageal wall. As this blood flow increases, the blood vessels begin to dilate. These stretched veins in the esophageal wall can rupture, resulting in a life-threatening event due to internal bleeding. Variants of esophageal varices are **gastric varices**. Gastric varices are abnormally dilated blood vessels that are found predominantly in the stomach. This, too, can be a life-threatening event if the vessels rupture and bleeding occurs.

The treatment for esophageal varices is directed immediately to control the bleeding endoscopically, followed by long-term medical therapy with beta-blockers for hypertension. These medications allow the pressure within the veins to decrease, thereby reducing the chance that bleeding will occur. Other treatments for upper GI bleeding associated with esophageal varices include vasopressin (Pitressin) and somatostatin (Stilamin). A common procedure option includes a **transjugular intrahepatic portosystemic shunt** (TIPS, pronounced like *tips* in dictation) procedure, which is a procedure to treat bleeding from varices in the esophagus or stomach as well as ascites in the abdomen caused by portal hypertension. In this procedure, a radiologist uses x-ray guidance to create a tunnel through the liver with a needle, connecting the portal vein to one of the **hepatic veins** (the veins connected to the liver). A metal stent is placed in this tunnel to keep the tunnel open. The tunnel reroutes blood flow in the liver and reduces pressure in all abnormal veins, not only in those of the stomach and esophagus, but also in the bowel and the liver.

This relieves the pressure of blood flowing through the diseased liver and can help stop bleeding and fluid backup.

Irritable Bowel Syndrome

Irritable bowel syndrome (IBS) is a chronic disorder of motility of the digestive tract characterized by abdominal pain, constipation, and diarrhea. The word **syndrome** means *a group of symptoms*. IBS is a syndrome rather than a disease because it manifests several symptoms without a particular cause or formal disease. It is a

functional disorder, which means the abnormality is caused by an alteration in which the body works, rather than by a structural or biochemical problem. Because it is a functional disorder, it cannot be diagnosed like other GI problems for which an anatomic cause can be determined, such as with blood work, scope procedures, or imaging studies. The diagnosis is usually made in the absence of other physical evidence of GI disease.

The causes and mechanisms of IBS are not clearly understood. Researchers believe it may be influenced, at least in part, by a malfunction of the **brain-gut axis** (see the Insight at the end of this chapter). A miscommunication between the brain and gut causes pain or spasms even when the GI tract is functioning normally. This explains the role of emotional factors in IBS, but diet, drugs, or hormones may also precipitate or aggravate heightened GI motility.

There is no cure for IBS, and treatment varies from person to person. Typical protocols include antispasmodics to slow bowel contractions, laxatives to treat constipation, and even antidepressants, which, when given in low doses, actually are helpful to IBS patients as they have acknowledged GI effects. In addition, stress management techniques (to aid in a patient's emotional health) and dietary changes (to avoid foods that trigger IBS attacks) are also effective in relieving IBS symptoms.

Inflammatory Bowel Disease

Inflammatory bowel disease (IBD) refers to a group of disorders that cause the intestines to become chronically inflamed and swollen. The two main types of IBD are ulcerative colitis and Crohn disease. **Ulcerative colitis** refers to an ulcerated inflammation of the top layer of the large intestine (colon), often starting at the rectum. Ulcerative colitis can affect the entire colon, a condition called **pancolitis**, or it may be limited to the rectum (**proctitis**). Symptoms of IBD include diarrhea (particularly bloody diarrhea) and abdominal pain. **Hematochezia** is the term that describes the passage of bloody stool.

Ulcerative colitis differs from Crohn disease in that it is limited to the structures of the colon and can be cured with surgery. Crohn's cannot be cured with surgery because of its tendency to recur either near the site of the prior surgery or at an entirely new place in the intestine. **Crohn disease** usually involves the proximal portion of the colon and, less commonly, the terminal ileum. Named after the American surgeon Burrill Crohn who first described it in 1932, this condition causes open sores affecting all layers lining the wall of the intestine, characterized by flare-ups and remissions.

When inflamed, the lining of the intestinal wall becomes red and swollen; it can become ulcerated and bleed, creating a characteristic cobblestone appearance. Absorption is impaired and small-bowel obstruction may result. Other complications of IBD include the formation of a **stricture**, a narrowing of part of the intestine; a **fistula**, which is an abnormal opening or passageway between two organs or from an internal organ to the surface of the body; or a **fissure**, which is a crack in the anal skin. Irritability and spasms associated with Crohn disease may lead to narrowing of the bowel.

The exact cause of IBD is unknown; as with IBS, a diagnosis is made after other possible causes of the inflammation, such as infection with parasites or bacteria, have been excluded. Stool samples and blood studies may be used to evaluate for bacteria or other foreign substances. A physician also may perform a biopsy, taking tissue samples from the lining of the rectum to examine microscopically for cancer or other tumors.

Although there is no cure for IBD, treatment is focused on controlling inflammation, correcting nutritional deficiencies, and reducing symptoms. Drug therapies to reduce inflammation include sulfasalazine (Azulfidine), corticosteroids such as prednisone, or immune system suppressers such as azathioprine (Imuran) and 6-mercaptopurine (often dictated simply as *6-MP*). Antibiotics such as metronidazole (Flagyl) are also prescribed to kill germs in the intestines, especially in the case of Crohn's. Avoidance of foods that cause a flare of the disease, as well as the addition of nutritional supplements and diet modification may also be considered.

In severe cases of ulcerative colitis and/or Crohn disease, surgery is required to relieve symptoms and correct complications such as blockage, perforation, or bleeding in the intestine. A limited surgical procedure called a **stricturoplasty** is used to widen narrowed areas of the intestines due to stricture from scarring. In this procedure, the surgeon cuts open the strictured segment lengthwise and then sews the tissue closed crosswise, relieving obstruction in the bowel and preserving bowel length. A common procedure for Crohn's is a **small-bowel resection**, in which a diseased portion of the small intestine is removed. The two healthy ends of bowel are then rejoined in a surgical procedure called **anastomosis**. If it is necessary to spare the intestine from its normal digestive work while it heals, an **ileostomy** may be performed, which involves bringing the end of the small intestine, the ileum, out through a surgical opening in the abdomen, called a **stoma**. The contents of the intestine and unformed waste are thereby diverted and expelled through this opening into a bag called an **ostomy bag**. A **colostomy** is a similar procedure in which the end of the colon is brought out through a stoma in the abdominal wall. Waste is expelled through an ostomy bag.

Crohn's or ulcerative colitis may also be treated with a **colectomy**, in which a part or all of the colon may be removed; or a **proctocolectomy**, in which the entire colon and rectum are removed. After the colectomy, a stoma in the abdomen is created, allowing for the drainage of stool from the large or small intestine, with a pouch worn over the opening to collect waste outside the body. However, recent surgical techniques eliminate the need for an outside pouch to collect waste. In an **ileal pouch anal anastomosis** (IPAA), the colon and rectum are removed, and an internal pouch is created from the very small end of the intestine (the ileum), called a **J pouch**. The pouch is then pulled down and attached to the anus. In this way, waste can leave the body through the anus, avoiding the need for a pouch to be worn outside the body.

Intussusception

Intussusception is a type of intestinal obstruction typically found in children between the ages of three months and six years. Intussusception occurs when a portion of the intestine folds like a telescope, with one segment slipping inside another segment. The walls of the "telescoped" sections of intestine press on each other, causing irritation and swelling and difficulty digesting food. Eventually, the blood supply to that area is cut off, and, if not treated, intussusception can cause serious damage to the intestines, leading to internal bleeding and a severe abdominal infection called peritonitis.

In some instances, intussusception will correct itself, or it can be repaired surgically. Under anesthesia, the surgeon will make an incision in the abdomen, locate the intussusception, and push the "telescoped" sections back into place. The intestine will be examined for damage, and, if any sections are not working correctly, they will be removed, and the two sections (or ends) of healthy intestine will be sewn back together. If a large segment of the intestine has been damaged, a colostomy may be done so that the digestive process can continue. With a colostomy, the two remaining healthy ends of intestine are brought through an opening in the abdomen. Stool will pass through the stoma and then into a collection bag. The colostomy may be temporary or permanent, depending on the amount of intestine that is removed.

Diverticular Disease

Diverticular disease is a disorder of the large intestine characterized by the presence of small, balloonlike pockets called **diverticula** (singular, diverticulum) that protrude through the muscular layer of the colon (Figure 14.6). The presence of these diverticula is called **diverticulosis**. If these diverticula become inflamed, the condition is known as **diverticulitis**. Diverticulitis causes symptoms of abdominal pain, fever, nausea, vomiting, diarrhea, and constipation. It is believed that chronic constipation as a result of a low-fiber diet is the main cause of diverticular disease. The condition is common only in developed or industrialized countries, where low-fiber diets are prevalent; it is rare in countries such as Africa and Asia, where people eat high-fiber vegetable diets. Blocked or infected diverticula can lead to

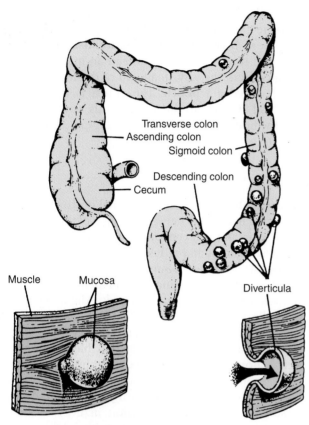

FIGURE 14.6. Diverticulosis. Diverticula are balloon-like pockets that protrude through the muscular layer of the colon. Reprinted with permission from Nettina, Sandra M. *The Lippincott Manual of Nursing Practice*, 7th ed. Lippincott Williams & Wilkins, 2001.

strangulation of the bowel tissue, preventing it from receiving nutrients and thus causing it to weaken and die. If not treated, the bowel wall could perforate, resulting in an abscess or life-threatening infection in the abdomen.

Treatment of diverticular disease, like the treatment for other bowel disorders, consists of changing the diet to one high in vegetables and fiber, as well as ingesting supplements with bulking agents. Antibiotics such as metronidazole (Flagyl), tetracycline (Sumycin), and amoxicillin (Amoxil) are commonly used when there is infection present. Surgery for obstruction or perforation caused by complicated diverticular disease is focused on resecting the diseased segment of bowel while, at the same time, actively managing any destruction of tissue by bacteria.

Colorectal Cancer

The most common sites for GI tract cancer are the colon and rectum, together referred to as **colorectal cancer**. Colorectal cancer ranks among the most frequent causes of cancer death in the United States in both men and women. Most of these cancers begin as a **polyp**, which

is a fleshy growth of tissue that starts in the lining and grows into the center of the colon or rectum. A polyp that could become cancerous is referred to as an **adenoma**. The removal of the polyp early may prevent it from becoming cancer. Cancers of the cells that line the inside of the colon and rectum are known as **adenocarcinomas** and are the most common type of colorectal cancer.

While the exact cause of colorectal cancer is not known, certain risk factors are known to increase a person's chances of getting the disease. The risk increases over age 50, with more than 9 out of 10 people found to have colorectal cancer being older than 50. Other factors include a prior history of colon polyps; a history of an inflammatory condition such as ulcerative colitis or Crohn disease; or a family history of colorectal cancer. Race and ethnic background seem to play a role, in that some studies have found that Jews of Eastern European descent (Ashkenazi Jews) and African Americans seem to have high numbers of colorectal cancer cases reported. Finally, lifestyle factors such as a diet high in fat and processed meats, lack of exercise, excess weight, and smoking all have been linked to an increased risk of colorectal cancer.

As with other cancers, treatment for cancer of colorectal cancer involves, primarily, removal of the cancerous tissue to stop the progression of the disease and tests to determine whether the cancer has spread to other organs. Surgery is the main treatment for colon cancer and usually involves removing the cancer along with a length of normal colon on either side of the cancer as well as nearby lymph nodes. However, if the cancer is caught early enough, it can be removed with a colonoscope. Such procedures, including a **polypectomy** (the removal of the polyp) or **local transanal resection** (removing only the tumorous tissue in the rectum) can be done with instruments placed into the anus, without having to cut through the skin.

In addition to surgery, treatments for cancer may include concurrent chemotherapy and radiation therapy as well as hormone-blocking drugs, or even a combination of these options (see Chapter 20, *Oncology*, for a more detailed discussion of chemotherapy and radiation treatments for cancer).

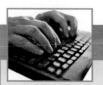

TRANSCRIPTION TIP:

A typical dictation error concerns the plural of the word *diverticulum*, which is *diverticula*, not *diverticulae*, *diverticulas*, or *diverticuli*. Be sure to transcribe the plural form of *diverticulum* correctly, even if the dictated form is incorrect.

DIAGNOSTIC STUDIES AND PROCEDURES

In addition to obtaining a thorough medical history, practitioners employ a variety of laboratory tests, imaging studies, and endoscopic procedures to treat a patient's digestive problems.

Laboratory Tests

Microscopic examinations of blood and stool can uncover unusual elevations or deficiencies in certain chemical compounds present in the body symptomatic of a digestive disorder. Analysis of blood can detect elevations in liver enzymes and proteins, which can indicate possible liver disease or injury, or a drop in red blood cell count, which could indicate bleeding in the GI tract. Electrolytes and minerals that are important for the body to function properly can be analyzed to help determine whether extra fluids might be needed to help restore hydration and mineral loss. Some common serum studies involving the digestive system include:

- Blood test to assess liver function. Certain enzymes are excreted by the liver during abnormal functioning due to metastases, obstruction, or other conditions, which include total protein, albumin, globulin, bilirubin alkaline phosphatase, aspartate aminotransferase (AST), and alanine aminotransferase (ALT).

- Blood tests to analyze pancreatic function. **Amylase** is a pancreatic enzyme that is active in the digestion of starches and sugars. The amylase level is often elevated with pancreatic damage. **Lipase** is an enzyme produced by the pancreas that aids in digestion. This test is ordered, often along with an amylase test, to help diagnose and monitor acute pancreatitis, chronic pancreatitis, and other disorders that involve the pancreas.

- Total cholesterol test, which measures the circulating levels of free cholesterol in the blood.

The **Model for End-Stage Liver Disease** (MELD) score is a system for allocating livers for transplantation in patients with liver disease. The score is based on a mathematical equation that calculates a patient's likelihood of dying within three months from liver disease in the absence of a transplant. In the past, the system of liver allocation was confusing and inaccurate. Patients were considered for available organs based on the length of time they had been on a waiting list and a physician's subjective criteria to determine placement on the waiting list. In addition, the public became disenchanted with the system after reading reports of celebrities and sports figures being placed at the top of the transplant list over thousands who were already waiting, many of whom were on the verge of death. This led to the development of the MELD system of evaluating a patient's need for liver transplantation based on a mathematical equation as opposed to subjective criteria, favoritism, or financial means.

Under this system, the sickest patient is given priority for a transplant. This disease severity score is determined by the values of three blood tests—the bilirubin and prothrombin time (PT), which are measured as the **International Normalized Ratio** (INR), and creatinine, which measures kidney function. The final score enables providers to evaluate a patient's need for transplant objectively and to allocate organs to appropriate transplant candidates based purely on medical urgency.

Stool studies are used to evaluate for digestive disorders as well. A **fecal fat test** is a measurement of the fat contained in a sample of stool. Elevated levels indicate a condition called **malabsorption**, in which the intestinal tract cannot digest fats as well as it should, enabling elevated amounts to pass into the stool. A **fecal occult blood** test checks for **occult**, or hidden, blood in the stool, indicating a possible bleed or perforation in the GI tract. A **stool culture** checks for the presence of abnormal bacteria in the digestive tract that may be causing diarrhea and other problems. A biopsy involves examining body tissue for a variety of factors, including cancerous or precancerous cells. An **ova and parasites** (O&P) test checks a stool sample for parasites or eggs (ova) that are associated with intestinal infections.

Imaging Studies

Imaging studies are used to view internal structures and locate abnormalities that would not otherwise be detected in blood work or laboratory analysis. Typical imaging studies involving the GI tract include the following:

TRANSCRIPTION TIP:

When dictating, physicians may refer to bilirubin values in various ways. Bilirubin may be express as *total bilirubin* or *direct bilirubin*, or both, and as brief forms such as *bili, direct bili, total bili,* or *T bili.* You should avoid the use of these brief forms and transcribe the term in full, for example, *bilirubin, direct bilirubin,* and *total bilirubin.*

Upper Gastrointestinal Series

An **upper gastrointestinal (GI) series**, also called a **barium swallow**, is an x-ray examination of the esophagus, stomach, and duodenum. In order for these structures to show up on radiographic images, the upper gastrointestinal tract must be coated with a contrast material called **barium sulfate**, which appears bright white in x-ray images. The patient drinks the barium, which coats the lining of the intestinal tract, making these organs visible on the x-ray. Depending on the degree to which the barium is absorbed by the various organs, the images can show a blockage, abnormal growth, ulcer, or other problem in the way of the degree to which an organ is working.

An **esophagram** (syn. esophagogram) is the portion of an upper GI series that examines the throat and esophagus. Sometimes dictated as a **cine-esophagram** (pronounced SIN-ee-esof-o-gram), this study focuses on the function and appearance of the esophagus and swallowing process. As the patient drinks a mixture of barium and water, rapid-sequence x-ray images are taken; the images are then viewed in sequence, essentially creating a motion picture of the swallowing mechanism.

Gastric Emptying Study

A **gastric emptying study** (GES) is a procedure to evaluate the speed at which food empties from the stomach and enters the small intestine. In this test, the patient eats some solid food (such as oatmeal or a hard-boiled egg) mixed with a small amount of radioactive material. A scanner is then placed over the patient's stomach to monitor the amount of radioactivity in the stomach for several hours after the test meal is eaten. As the food empties from the stomach, the amount of radioactivity in the stomach decreases, reflecting the rate of emptying.

Lower Gastrointestinal Series

A **lower gastrointestinal (GI) series** is an x-ray examination of the large intestine, including the rectum. It is also called a **barium enema** because of the contrast material, barium sulfate, which is administered to the patient by enema prior to the exam. This procedure shows problems like growths, ulcers, or other abnormal tissues in the colon. In this procedure, the entire large intestine is filled with barium liquid. The contrast dye coats the colon and rectum and makes these structures visible on radiographic images. In addition to determining the size and shape of the colon and rectum, this procedure can make any abnormalities visible.

Hepatobiliary Iminodiacetic Acid Scan

A **hepatobiliary iminodiacetic acid (HIDA) scan** is an imaging test used to examine the function of the liver, gallbladder, and bile ducts. This test, also referred to as **cholescintigraphy**, is named for the tracer medicine, hepatobiliary iminodiacetic acid, which is injected into the body for the scan. In this procedure, the patient is given a small dose of the radioactive tracer through an intravenous line. The tracer travels to the liver and into the bile ducts. A scanner is placed over the body to track the movement of the tracer through the biliary tract while making images of the liver, gallbladder, and bile ducts. The images are then examined by a radiologist for obstructions, gallbladder disease, or other abnormalities.

Abdominal Ultrasound

Many digestive tract abnormalities can be detected by abdominal ultrasound; it is most commonly performed to diagnose gallstones. A gel is applied to the patient's abdomen, as in a traditional ultrasound, and a transducer is run over the area. The soundwaves bounce off the gallbladder and are displayed as an image on a monitor. Gallstones appear on the screen as solid round objects. Ultrasound can detect gallstones as small as 2 mm in diameter with an extremely high rate of accuracy; ultrasound can also detect a thickening of the gallbladder wall, indicative of cholecystitis.

Endoscopic Procedures

An **endoscopy** is a nonsurgical procedure used to examine the digestive tract. A flexible tube with a light and camera attached to it, called an **endoscope**, is inserted into the body, and the images of internal structures transmitted by the camera are viewed on a television-type monitor. The endoscope varies in length depending on the procedure to be performed, and it contains different optical fibers along its channel to direct light on the area to be examined, to pump air or fluids in and out of the tube, or to pass surgical instruments through the tube to obtain a biopsy or perform reparative procedures. An **endoscopic ultrasound** (EUS) involves attaching an ultrasound wand to the end of the endoscope to examine and obtain images of various parts of the digestive tract.

Endoscopies are performed in many parts of the gastrointestinal system. Each procedure has its own name depending on the part of the body it is intended to investigate, as indicated below.

Esophagogastroduodenoscopy

An **esophagogastroduodenoscopy (EGD)**, also referred to as **upper endoscopy**, is a procedure in which a physician can examine the esophagus, stomach, and duodenum. During this procedure, the endoscope is guided into the mouth and throat, then into the esophagus, stomach, and duodenum. The endoscope allows the physician to visualize the internal surfaces of these organs as well as to insert instruments through the scope to obtain tissue for a biopsy, if necessary. The scope can also be used to examine individual structures in the upper GI tract such as the esophagus (**esophagoscopy**), the stomach (**gastroscopy**), and the duodenum (**gastroduodenoscopy**).

Colonoscopy

A **colonoscopy** is a procedure that allows the physician to view the entire length of the large intestine, and can often help identify abnormal growths or polyps, inflamed tissue, ulcers, and bleeding. A specialized endoscopic tool called a **colonoscope** is inserted into the rectum and up into the colon. This procedure allows the physician to see the lining of the colon, remove tissue for further examination, and possibly treat some problems that are discovered. A shorter colonoscopic procedure is called a **sigmoidoscopy**, which is used to investigate only the sigmoid colon, or lower part of the large bowel.

Endoscopic Retrograde Cholangiopancreatography

An **endoscopic retrograde cholangiopancreatography** (ERCP), also called **cholangiography**, is a procedure used along with x-ray imaging to evaluate and treat problems in the bile ducts, gallbladder, and pancreas, such as a blockage in the hepatobiliary ducts, jaundice, or abdominal pain. It involves the injection of contrast dye in a retrograde direction—that is, against the normal flow of bile and pancreatic fluids through the ducts—enabling x-rays to be taken of the bile duct system and pancreas. In this procedure, an endoscope is passed through the mouth and throat, then through the esophagus, stomach, and into the duodenum. Then a smaller catheter is inserted through the endoscope, directed into either the pancreatic or common bile duct. The catheter allows a radioactive tracer contrast material to be injected backwards—retrograde—through the ducts. A special camera documents the path of the contrast material as it passes from the liver to the gallbladder, and x-rays are taken to document any abnormalities (a process called **cholangiopancreatography**). With examination of the flow of the dye, widening, narrowing, or blockage of the biliary ducts can be pinpointed.

The examination of the biliary and pancreatic ducts with MRI is called **magnetic resonance cholangiopancreatography (MRCP)**. In MRCP, a contrast agent, usually gadolinium for this type of imaging, is injected through a catheter inserted through the endoscope. Images are then obtained using the MRI, which uses radiofrequency radiation in a high magnetic field to produce high-resolution images of the body.

QUICK CHECK 14.4 ✓

Indicate whether the following sentences are true (T) or false (F).

1. An endoscopy can be used in conjunction with ultrasound.   T   F

2. A fecal fat test measures the fat contained in a sample of stool.   T   F

3. A HIDA scan is also called a cholescintigraphy.   T   F

4. A laparoscopy is a procedure used to examine the throat and esophagus.   T   F

5. A gastric emptying study examines the large intestine, including the rectum.   T   F

CHAPTER SUMMARY

The gastrointestinal system is responsible for the digestion and assimilation of nutrients essential to survival. Digestive disorders are so common (some estimates suggest more than half the US population is affected) that medical reports concerning the illnesses related to digestion and the methods used to treat them are a major part of a medical transcriptionist's workload. Understanding the fundamental workings of this complex system as well as the health problems that affect the functions of the GI system is a tremendous aid in transcribing these documents effectively.

· I · N · S · I · G · H · T ·

The Brain-Gut Axis

Although the brain influences the digestive system, the opposite also is true. As stressful events can trigger digestive symptoms, so, too, can gastrointestinal disorders trigger stress, anxiety, and other psychological symptoms. Researchers refer to this reciprocal relationship as the brain-gut axis.

Researchers believe that the cause of functional GI disorders lies somewhere in the nervous system of the brain and the gut. Just as the brain has a network of nerve cells that enables it to communicate with the rest of the body, the GI tract has its own nervous system. This system of nerve cells performs several functions: coordinating the wavelike movements of the GI tract muscles as they digest food, determining when digestive chemicals are released into the stomach and intestines, and triggering the reflex that causes the urge to defecate.

Frequently it has been observed that some individuals with more severe digestive symptoms have coexisting psychological distress. Because the digestive system and the brain are so highly interactive, physicians find that a psychological evaluation often can be helpful in trying to understand the full impact of a gastrointestinal ailment when, in many cases, patients appear healthy and a physical examination does not reveal anything unusual. This is not to suggest that the problem is imagined or made up, but is an acknowledgement on the part of the medical profession that psychosocial stress may be a factor in the patient's digestive symptoms. All in all, for as many as 50% of people with digestive disorders, psychological factors play an important role.

Consideration of the broad scope of the brain-gut connection can help the doctor and the patient work together to address gastrointestinal symptoms and formulate an effective treatment plan.

Common Soundalike Words

Word	Word Pronunciation	Soundalike	Soundalike Pronunciation
aphagia: inability to eat.	ă-fā′jē-ă	**aphasia**: absent comprehension or production of speech due to a lesion of the dominant cerebral hemisphere of the brain.	ă-fā′zē-ă
dysphagia: difficulty in swallowing.	dis-fā′jē-ă	**dysphasia**: impairment in the production of speech and failure to arrange words in an understandable way, caused by an acquired lesion of the brain.	dis-fā′zē-ă
ileum: the third portion of the small intestine.	il′ē-ŭm	**ilium**: broad, flaring portion of the hip bone.	il′ē-ŭm
cirrhosis: a chronic disease interfering with the normal functioning of the liver.	sir-rō′sis	**serositis**: inflammation of the serous tissues of the body.	sēr-ō-sī′tis
fecal: relating to feces, or solid matter, discharged from the body.	fē′kăl	**thecal**: relating to a sheath, as a tendon sheath. **cecal**: relating to the cecum.	thē′kăl sē′kăl
pancreas: a bodily organ/gland, located in the left upper quadrant just beneath the stomach and spleen.	pan′krē-as	**Pancrease/pancrease**: an enzyme, capitalized as a brand name of medication; lowercased for the naturally occurring enzyme.	pan-krē-ās′
parental: relating to a parent.	pă-ren′tăl	**parenteral**: by some means other than through the gastrointestinal tract (as in nutrition).	pă-ren′tĕr-ăl
perianal: surrounding the anus.	per-i-ā′năl	**perinatal**: pertaining to the periods before, during, or after the time of birth.	per-i-nā′tăl
bile: the yellowbrown or greenish fluid secreted by the liver and discharged into the duodenum to aid in digestion.	bīl	**bowel**: the digestive tube passing from the stomach to the anus.	bow′el
succussion: an abnormal sound heard on examination of the abdomen.	sŭ-kŭsh′shŭn	**succession**: the action of following in order.	sŭk-se′-shŭn
		percussion: a diagnostic procedure designed to determine the density of a part by the sound produced by tapping the surface with the finger or a plessor.	pĕr-kŭsh′ŭn

Combining Forms

Combining Form	Meaning	Combining Form	Meaning
abdomin/o, lapar/o	abdomen	gloss/o	tongue
an/o	anus	hemorrhoid/o	hemorrhoid
append/o, appendic/o	appendix	hepat/o, hepatic/o	liver
bil/i	bile	herni/o	hernia
cec/o	cecum	ile/o	ileum
celi/o	abdomen, belly	inguin/o	groin
cheil/o	lip	jejun/o	jejunum
cholangi/o	bile duct	or/o, stomat/o	mouth
cholecyst/o	gallbladder	pancreat/o, pancreatic/o	pancreas
choledoch/o	common bile duct	phag/o	eating; swallowing
col/o, colon/o	colon	pharyng/o	pharynx
cyst/o	bladder or sac	peritone/o	peritoneum
diverticul/o	diverticulum	proct/o	rectum and anus
doch/o	duct	pylor/o	pylorus
duoden/o	duodenum	rect/o	rectum
emet/o	vomiting	saliv/o	saliva
enter/o	small intestine	sialaden/o	salivary glands
esophag/o	esophagus	sigmoid/o	sigmoid colon
fec/a, fec/o	feces, stool	splen/o	spleen
gastr/o	stomach		

Add Your Own Combining Forms Here:

_____

_____

_____

_____

_____

_____

ABBREVIATIONS

Abbreviation	Meaning
EGD	esophagogastroduodenoscopy
ERCP	endoscopic retrograde cholangiopancreatography
EUS	endoscopic ultrasound
GERD	gastroesophageal reflux disease
GES	gastric emptying study
GI	gastrointestinal
HAV	hepatitis A virus
HBV	hepatitis B virus
HCV	hepatitis C virus
HIDA	hepatobiliary iminodiacetic acid

Abbreviation	Meaning
IBD	irritable bowel disease
IBS	irritable bowel syndrome
INR	international normalized ratio
IPAA	ileal pouch anal anastomosis
MELD	Model for End-Stage Liver Disease
MRCP	magnetic resonance cholangiopancreatography
NASH	nonalcoholic steatohepatitis
O&P	ova and parasites
PUD	peptic ulcer disease

Add Your Own Abbreviations Here:

_____

_____

_____

_____

_____

_____

TERMINOLOGY

Term	Meaning
accessory organs	The structures in the abdomen that are not part of the digestive tract but have a role in digestive activities necessary for the processing of food—specifically, the salivary glands, liver, gallbladder, and pancreas.
acute hepatitis	Hepatitis that begins suddenly and has a limited course.
acute pancreatitis	The sudden inflammation of the pancreas.
adenocarcinoma	A cancer of the cells that line the inside of the colon and rectum.
adenoma	A polyp in the colon or rectum that could become cancerous.
alcoholic hepatitis	An inflammation of the cells of the liver from any cause.
amylase	An enzyme produced by the pancreas that aids in digestion by breaking down starches.

Term	Meaning
anal sphincter	The muscular ring around the anus that keeps it closed until defecation occurs.
anastomosis	The joining together of two healthy sections of tubular structures in the body after the diseased portion has been surgically removed.
antacid	A medication that neutralizes stomach acids.
antibiotic	A drug used to inhibit the growth of organisms that cause infection.
antibody test	A blood test to indicate the body's reaction to infection.
antigen test	A test to indicate the presence of a virus in the blood.
antrectomy	The surgical removal of the lower part of the stomach.
antrum	The lower portion of the stomach where grinding of food into smaller pieces takes place.
anus	The opening at the end of the digestive tract through which stool leaves the body.
ascending colon	The right-sided portion of the colon extending from the cecum to the hepatic flexure.
ascites	A condition that occurs when fluid accumulates in the abdomen.
barium sulfate	A contrast material used for radiographic study of the gastrointestinal tract.
Barrett esophagus	A precancerous condition of the lower esophagus as a result of chronic damage to the lining of the esophagus, increasing the risk of cancer.
bile	A yellow-brown fluid produced by the liver that assists in the digestion and absorption of fats and is responsible for the elimination of waste products from the body.
bile salts	Natural detergents that break up fat.
biliary tract	A series of ducts which, along with the gallbladder, convey and store bile.
bilirubin	A chemical formed from the degradation of hemoglobin in the blood, which is processed by the liver and then secreted into the bile.
Billroth procedure	A resective surgical procedure of the stomach.
Billroth I procedure, syn. gastroduodenostomy	A procedure that involves the surgical removal of the lower part of the stomach and attaching the remaining portion to the duodenum.
Billroth II procedure, syn. gastrojejunostomy	A procedure that involves surgically removing the lower part of the stomach and attaching the remaining portion to the jejunum.
body	The large central part of the stomach.
brain-gut axis	A communication of the nerve cells between the digestive system and the brain.
cardia	The top portion of the stomach.
cecum	The pouch at the beginning of the large intestine.
cholangiopancreatography	The portion of an ERCP procedure where x-rays are taken to document abnormalities in the bile ducts, gallbladder, or pancreas.
cholecystectomy	The surgical removal of the gallbladder.
cholecystitis	A sudden inflammation of the gallbladder.
choledocholithiasis	A condition in which gallstones form inside the common bile duct.
cholelithiasis	A condition in which gallstones form inside the gallbladder.
chronic hepatitis	Hepatitis that is slowly progressive and persists for long periods.

Term	Meaning
chronic pancreatitis	A slow, ongoing inflammation of the pancreas that occurs when digestive enzymes attack and destroy the pancreas and nearby tissues over time, causing scarring and pain.
chyme	A mushy liquid to which food is converted by the stomach.
cirrhosis	A condition in which normal cells of the liver are damaged and replaced by scar tissue.
colectomy	The surgical removal of all or part of the colon.
colonoscope	A flexible, elongated endoscope used to view the inside of the entire colon and rectum.
colonoscopy	A procedure in which the endoscope is used to evaluate the entire large intestine.
colorectal cancer	A term used to refer to cancer that originates in the colon or rectum.
colostomy	A procedure in which the end of the colon is brought out through a stoma in the abdominal wall and waste is expelled through an ostomy bag.
common bile duct	The duct that carries bile from the liver and gallbladder into the duodenum.
Crohn disease	A condition causing open sores affecting all layers lining the entire wall of the large and/or small intestine.
cystic duct	The duct that joins the common bile duct to the gallbladder.
defecation	The discharge of solid waste from the body.
descending colon	The left-sided portion of the colon extending from the splenic flexure to the beginning of the sigmoid colon.
digestion	The process by which food and liquid are broken down into smaller parts and converted into forms of energy the body can use to maintain life and health.
digestive disorders	Diseases and medical problems affecting the gastrointestinal system.
diverticula (singular, diverticulum)	Small, balloonlike pockets that protrude through the muscular layer of the colon.
diverticular disease	A disorder of the large intestine characterized by diverticula that protrude through the muscular layer of the colon.
diverticulitis	An inflammation of diverticula in the colon.
diverticulosis	The presence of diverticula in the colon.
duodenal ulcer	An ulcer that develops in the duodenum.
duodenum	The first portion of the small intestine nearest the stomach.
endoscope	A flexible tube with a light and camera attached that is used to examine the interior surfaces of an organ.
endoscopic retrograde cholangiopancreatography (ERCP), syn. cholangiography	A procedure in which the endoscope, along with x-ray imaging, is used to evaluate and treat problems in the bile ducts, gallbladder, and pancreas.
endoscopic ultrasound	An endoscopy used in conjunction with ultrasound imaging.
endoscopy	A nonsurgical procedure used to examine the digestive tract using a flexible tube with a light and camera attached to it.
epiglottis	A flap of cartilage at the root of the tongue that prevents food and fluids from entering the airway.
esophageal sphincter	A one-way valve located between the esophagus and stomach that regulates the entry of food into the stomach.
esophageal stricture	Narrowing of the esophagus that makes swallowing solid foods difficult.

Term	Meaning
esophageal varices	Abnormally enlarged veins in the lower part of the esophagus that develop when normal blood flow to the liver is blocked.
esophagogastroduodenoscopy (EGD), syn. upper endoscopy	A procedure in which the endoscope is used to evaluate the esophagus, stomach, and duodenum.
esophagoscopy	A procedure in which an endoscope is used to evaluate the esophagus.
esophagram, syn. esophagogram	The portion of an upper GI series that examines the esophagus.
esophagus	A muscular channel that connects the throat with the stomach.
exocrine pancreas	The area of the pancreas that produces digestive juices.
exocrine tumor	A tumor arising in the area of the pancreas that produces digestive juices (exocrine pancreas).
falciform ligament	The fold of tissue dividing the right and left lobes of the liver.
fecal fat test	A measurement of the fat contained in a sample of stool.
fecal occult blood	A test that checks for hidden blood in the stool.
fissure	A crack in the anal membrane.
fistula	An abnormal, infected tunnel connecting two organs, draining fluid into or out of the body.
functional disorder	An abnormality that is caused by an altered way in which the body works, rather than by a structural or biochemical problem.
fundus	The enlarged portion of the stomach to the left and above the cardia.
gallbladder	A sac-shaped accessory organ attached to the lower surface of the liver that absorbs bile and releases it to the small intestine when food is present.
gallstones	Lumps of rocklike material that form inside the gallbladder.
gastric emptying study (GES)	A procedure to evaluate the rate at which food empties from the stomach and enters the small intestine.
gastric ulcer	An ulcer that develops in the stomach.
gastric varices	Abnormally dilated submucosal veins in the stomach that develop when normal blood flow to the liver is blocked.
gastritis	A peptic disorder that involves inflammation of the lining of the stomach.
gastroduodenoscopy	A procedure in which the endoscope is used to evaluate the stomach and duodenum.
gastroenterologist	A medical specialist who cares for patients with diseases and disorders of the gastrointestinal system.
gastroenterology	The study of the series of organs in the body responsible for digesting food and extracting nutrients necessary to sustain life.
gastroesophageal reflux disease (GERD)	A condition whereby an excessive amount of stomach acids and enzymes flow backward from the stomach into the lower esophagus.
gastrointestinal (GI) system, syn. alimentary canal	The system of organs in the body contained in a long coiled tube extending from the mouth to the anus that takes in food, digests it to extract energy and nutrients, and expels the remaining waste.
gastroscopy	A procedure in which the endoscope is used to evaluate the stomach.
genotype	The genetic makeup of an organism or virus.
globus sensation	The sensation of a lump in the throat.
hard palate	The anterior portion of the palate, or roof of the mouth, formed by bone.

Term	Meaning
hematemesis	Vomiting of blood.
hematochezia	The passage of bloody stool.
hepatic ducts (right and left)	The ducts that merge to form the common bile duct that carries bile from the liver into the duodenum.
hepatic flexure	The name given to the turn of the colon next to the liver.
hepatic veins	The veins connected to the liver.
hepatitis	An inflammation of the cells of the liver.
hepatitis A virus, syn. infectious hepatitis	The most common hepatitis virus, spread primarily by fecal-oral contamination or from eating contaminated food.
hepatitis B virus	A form of hepatitis spread by blood and other body fluids.
hepatitis C virus	A mild, slowly progressive form of the hepatitis virus that is spread by direct contact with infected blood or blood products, such as from blood transfusions (now rare), the sharing of IV drug needles or body piercing instruments, or even razors contaminated by microscopic amounts of blood.
hepatobiliary iminodiacetic acid (HIDA) scan, syn. cholescintigraphy	An imaging test used to examine the function of the liver, gallbladder, and bile ducts.
hepatomegaly	Enlarged liver.
histamine-2 (H2) blockers	A class of drugs that reduce the production of acid in the stomach.
icterus	Another word for *jaundice*.
ileal pouch anal anastomosis (IPAA)	A surgical procedure in which the colon and rectum are removed and an internal pouch is created from the end of the small intestine, which is then attached to the anus.
ileostomy	A procedure that involves bringing the end of the small intestine out through a stoma in the abdomen.
ileum	The end portion of the small intestine.
ileus	An obstruction in the lower part of the small intestine.
inflammatory bowel disease (IBD)	A group of disorders that cause the intestines to become chronically inflamed and swollen.
interferon	A protein naturally produced by the body to fight viruses by boosting the immune system.
interferon alpha	A synthetically produced antiviral medication used to treat chronic hepatitis.
International Normalized Ratio (INR)	A measurement of bilirubin and prothrombin time (PT) in the blood.
intussusception	A type of intestinal obstruction that occurs when a portion of the intestine folds like a telescope, with one segment slipping inside another segment.
irritable bowel syndrome (IBS)	A chronic disorder of motility of the digestive tract.
J pouch	An internal pouch created from the very end of the small intestine that is attached to the anus during an ileal pouch anal anastomosis (IPAA) procedure.
jaundice	A yellowish cast to the skin and eyes.
jejunum	The middle portion of the small intestine.
laparoscope	A specialized endoscope used to evaluate the interior of the abdomen, pelvic cavity, and other parts of the body.

Term	Meaning
laparoscopic cholecystectomy	A minimally invasive procedure using the laparoscope and small incisions to remove the gallbladder.
large intestine, syn. colon	A long, tubelike organ that moves waste material from the small intestine to be excreted by the body.
lipase	An enzyme produced by the pancreas that aids in digestion.
liver	The largest organ in the body that plays a major role in the function of the body, including drug detoxification and the metabolism of sugars, fats, and proteins in the blood.
lobes	The two sections (right and left) of the liver.
local transanal resection	A noninvasive procedure whereby tumorous tissue is removed from the rectum.
lower gastrointestinal (GI) series, syn barium enema	An x-ray examination of the large intestine using contrast material.
magnetic resonance cholangiopancreatography (MRCP)	Similar to ERCP, except images are obtained using the MRI rather than x-ray.
malabsorption	A condition in which the intestinal tract cannot digest fats as well as it should.
mandible	The lower jaw.
mastication	The process of crushing and grinding of food by the teeth.
melena	Passage of black, tarry stools due to bleeding in the digestive system.
metaplasia	A process that occurs when the normal adult cells in a tissue transform into a type of cell that is abnormal for that tissue.
Model for End-Stage Liver Disease (MELD)	A scoring system for allocating livers for transplantation in patients with liver disease.
Nissen fundoplication	A surgical procedure in which the fundus of the stomach is wrapped around the lower part of the esophagus to prevent the backflow of acid into the esophagus.
nonalcoholic steatohepatitis (NASH)	An inflammation of the liver caused by the presence of fat.
obstipation	The inability for the colon to pass stool.
occult	Another name for *hidden*.
open cholecystectomy	The traditional procedure of removing the gallbladder that involves a large surgical incision in the abdomen.
oral cavity, syn. mouth	The beginning of the digestive tract, used to bite and chew food.
oropharynx	The first component of the digestive tract.
ostomy bag	A container attached to a stoma in the abdomen that collects the contents of the small intestine and unformed waste after an ileostomy procedure.
ova and parasites (O&P)	A test that checks a stool sample for parasites or eggs (ova) associated with intestinal infections.
palate	The roof of the mouth.
palmar erythema	A condition in which the palms of the hands may be reddish and blotchy.
pancolitis	Ulcerative colitis that affects the entire colon.
pancreas	A large gland that lies in front of the upper spine and behind the stomach, which allows digestive enzymes to flow into the duodenum.
pancreatic cancer	A disease in which cancerous cells are found in the tissues of the pancreas.
pancreatic duct	The duct that joins the pancreas to the small intestine.

Term	Meaning
pancreatitis	Inflammation of the pancreas.
parotid (glands)	A pair of salivary glands located at the side of the face and in front of and below the external ear.
peptic disorders	Gastrointestinal disorders that involve damage to the lining of the esophagus, stomach, or duodenum by stomach acids, enzymes, or infection with bacteria.
peptic ulcer	A nonmalignant sore that develops in the lining of the stomach or duodenum.
peptic ulcer disease (PUD)	A condition whereby a peptic ulcer develops in the stomach.
peristalsis	Powerful wavelike movements of muscle that contract in syncopated pulses.
peritoneum	The clear membrane that covers all the abdominal organs and the inside walls of the abdomen.
peritonitis	A dangerous inflammation and infection of the lining of the abdominal wall.
pharynx	Another name for the *throat*.
polyp	A fleshy growth of tissue that starts in the lining and grows into the center of the colon or rectum.
polypectomy	The removal of a polyp in the colon or rectum.
proctitis	A form of ulcerative colitis limited to the rectum.
proctocolectomy	The surgical removal of the entire colon and rectum.
proton pump inhibitors (PPIs)	A class of drugs that reduce the production of acid in the stomach but that are more potent than H2 blockers and, thus, promote healing of ulcers in a shorter period of time.
pyloric sphincter	The circular layer of muscle around the pyloric opening that regulates the passage of food into the intestines.
pylorus	The opening between the stomach and the small intestine.
rectum	A chamber that begins at the end of the large intestine, immediately following the sigmoid colon.
salivary glands	Glands around the mouth and throat that secrete saliva into the oral cavity, where it is mixed with food during the process of chewing.
sigmoid colon	The bottom part of the colon after the descending colon and before the rectum.
sigmoidoscopy	A shorter colonoscopic procedure used to investigate only the sigmoid colon.
small bowel	Another name for *small intestine*.
small-bowel resection	A procedure in which a diseased portion of bowel is removed and the two healthy ends are joined back together.
small intestine	A long tube that connects the stomach to the large intestine and is responsible for the actual digestion of food.
soft palate	The posterior part of the palate, or roof of the mouth, formed by soft tissue.
spider angiomas	Tiny clusters of red veins close to the surface of the skin.
splenic flexure	The name given to the turn of the colon next to the spleen.
steatorrhea	A condition in which the feces contain excessive fat, causing them to float and be very foul smelling.
stoma	An artificially created opening.
stomach	A muscular, saclike organ that receives food from the esophagus during digestion.
stool	Firm solid waste material excreted from the body.

Term	Meaning
stool culture	A test that checks for the presence of abnormal bacteria in the digestive tract.
stricture	A narrowing of part of the intestine.
stricturoplasty	A procedure used to widen narrowed areas of the intestines due to scarring.
sublingual (glands)	A pair of salivary glands located under the tongue.
submandibular (glands)	A pair of salivary glands located beneath the lower jaw (mandible).
syndrome	Another word for *a group of symptoms*.
tongue	A mobile mass of muscular tissue covered with mucous membrane, occupying the cavity of the mouth and forming part of its floor. It is the organ of taste and assists in the chewing and swallowing of food as well as articulating speech.
transjugular intrahepatic portosystemic shunt (TIPS)	A procedure used to treat bleeding from the esophagus or stomach and ascites in the abdomen caused by portal hypertension by inserting a stent to connect the portal veins to adjacent blood vessels that have lower pressure.
transverse colon	The top portion of the colon extending from the hepatic flexure to the splenic flexure.
ulcerative colitis	An ulcerated inflammation of the top layer of the large intestine.
upper gastrointestinal (GI) series, syn. barium swallow	An x-ray examination of the esophagus, stomach, and duodenum using contrast material.
uvula	A small piece of soft tissue hanging down from the soft palate over the back of the tongue, which is used primarily in speech production.
vagotomy	The surgical cutting of the vagus nerve adjacent to the esophagus in order to reduce acid secretions in the stomach.
vagus nerve	A nerve that helps control function of the esophagus, larynx, stomach, intestines, lungs, and heart.
vermiform appendix	A narrow, fingerlike tube attached to the cecum that has no real function.
viral hepatitis	An invasion of the liver by one of several hepatitis viruses that infect the liver and begin replicating, delineated by types (A, B, C, D, and E).
Whipple procedure, syn. pancreaticoduodenectomy	A surgical procedure that generally includes the removal of the head of the pancreas, the duodenum, a portion of the stomach, and other nearby tissues.
xanthomas	Small, fatty, yellow lumps that develop on the eyelids, hands, and elbows.

Add Your Own Terms and Definitions Here:

_____

_____

_____

_____

_____

_____

_____

REVIEW QUESTIONS

1. Name the three sections of the small intestine.
2. What is malabsorption?
3. Why is IBS a syndrome and not a disease?
4. What is the difference between open cholecystectomy and laparoscopic cholecystectomy?
5. What makes Barrett esophagus different from simple stomach irritation?
6. What are the two main types of inflammatory bowel disease and what is the difference between them?
7. Which type of hepatitis does not have a vaccination to treat the disease, and why?
8. What are xanthomas?
9. What is digestion?
10. What is the difference between a colonoscopy and sigmoidoscopy?

CHAPTER ACTIVITIES

Soundalike Word Choice

Circle the correct word in the following sentences.

1. The patient fell and suffered a fracture of his right (palate, patella).
2. Many medical transcriptionists confuse the terms (ilium, ileum), which is the lower portion of the small intestine, and (ilium, ileum), which is the flaring portion of the hip bone.
3. Due to the patient's recent stroke and subsequent (dysphagia, dysphasia), a percutaneous gastrostomy tube was placed for feeding purposes.
4. Ms. Cox's (MELT, MELD) score was high enough to place her at the top of the transplant list.
5. His stomach was so damaged by disease that a(n) (vitrectomy, antrectomy) had to be performed.
6. On postoperative day 1, the patient was afebrile, with no evidence of (ciliary, biliary) sepsis.
7. She was sent to the emergency room, where on examination she reported abdominal pain consistent with mild (constipation, lactation).
8. His (bile, bowel) obstruction was relieved with enemas given every 8 hours.
9. A prescription was provided for GoLYTELY in preparation for anticipated (colonoscopy, colposcopy) to evaluate the large intestine.
10. The family history is unremarkable for GI abnormalities except for the mother having gastroesophageal (reflex, reflux) during her pregnancy.

Medical Terminology Review

Circle the correct word in the following sentences.

1. The stomach turns food into (chyme, chemosis) before it enters the duodenum.
2. Visual examination of the digestive tract is called (ductoscopy, endoscopy).
3. A HIDA scan is also referred to as a (cholescintigraphy, cholecystectomy).
4. The presence of gallstones in the common bile duct is referred to (cholelithiasis, choledocholithiasis).
5. Palmar (edema, erythema) is a condition in which the palms of the hands may be reddish and blotchy.
6. An upper GI series uses (barium, balium) as a contrast material.
7. A scope can be used to examine the stomach only, called a (gastroduodenoscopy, gastroscopy).
8. (Genophils, genotypes) are hepatitis C genes that mutate into new variations.
9. Another name for the GI system is the (alimentary, augumentary) tract.
10. The (antrum, cardia) is the lower portion of the stomach.

Multiple Choice

Answer the following questions by circling the correct term in the Choices (right) column.

Question	Choices
1. What is another name for upper GI series?	barium enema, barium swallow, laparoscopy
2. What is the middle part of the small intestine?	ileum, antrum, jejunum
3. What is the opening at the end of the digestive tract?	anus, rectum, colon
4. What is bleeding in the stomach called?	hematemesis, melanoma, melena
5. What is the bacterium involved in gastritis?	*H pylori, H pylorus, H papillus*
6. What is a yellowish cast to the skin?	xanthoma, bilirubin, jaundice
7. What is the condition in which feces contain excessive fat?	steatohepatitis, steatorrhea, cirrhosis
8. What is the pouch at the beginning of the large intestine called?	cecum, colon, cardia
9. What is inflammation of the cells of the liver called?	pancreatitis, gastritis, hepatitis
10. What is another word for *hidden*?	occult, obtund, obese

Abbreviations Practice

Fill in the definition of the following abbreviations.

Abbreviation	Definition
1. EUS	_____
2. GI	_____
3. IBD	_____
4. GERD	_____
5. HCV	_____
6. PUD	_____
7. EGD	_____
8. IPAA	_____
9. GES	_____
10. NASH	_____

Anatomy Sort Exercise

Place the following in the correct order, starting with the mouth.

Term	Order
decending colon	1. mouth
esophageal sphincter	2.
anus	3.
cecum	4.
~~mouth~~	5.
transverse colon	6.
esophagus	7.
rectum	8.
pharynx	9.
ascending colon	10.
stomach	11.
pyloric sphincter	12.
small intestine	13.

Gastroenterology Puzzle

Complete the crossword puzzle by filling in the correct answers from the clues into the corresponding spaces on the puzzle grid.

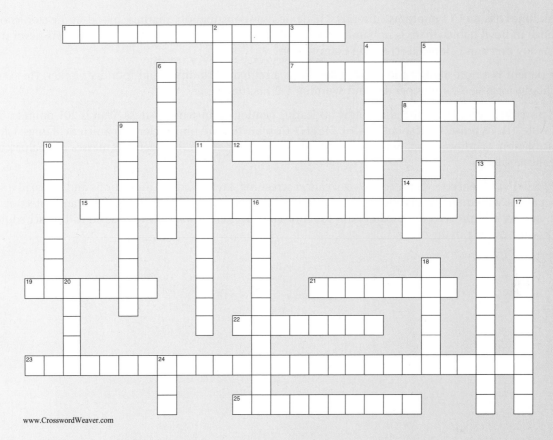

www.CrosswordWeaver.com

Across

1 Another name for ERCP.

7 The first part of the small intestine.

8 A sensation of a lump in the throat.

12 Inflammation of the lining of the stomach.

15 Evaluates speed at which food leaves the stomach.

19 Accumulation of fluid in the abdomen.

21 Cracks in the anal skin.

22 A yellowish cast to the skin.

23 NASH.

25 Examines the throat and esophagus.

Down

2 "Hidden."

3 Abbrev. for peptic ulcer disease.

4 An inflammation of liver cells.

5 An enzyme produced by the pancreas.

6 _____ ligament, divides the lobes of the liver.

9 Rocklike material in the gallbladder.

10 Abnormal tunnels.

11 Ulcerative colitis of the entire colon.

13 Inflammation of the gallbladder.

14 Abbrev. for endoscopic ultrasound.

16 Wavelike movements of muscle.

17 Vomiting of blood.

18 Black, tarry stools.

20 Another name for large intestine.

24 Abbrev. for hepatitis C.

Proofreading Exercise

Circle the errors in the following clinic report. Then retype the corrected report using the same format on a blank document screen. When finished, print one copy and save the corrected report as CHAPTER-14-NOTE.

John Jones has no CI symptoms currently. He denies any constipation, diarhea, blood in the stoole, or any change in bowl habits. there is no family history of colon cancer or colorecta polyps. He has never underwent any previous colorectal screening examination?

the patient is a non-smoker and nondrinker, He is a retired truck driver and foundry worker. He exercises regularly, jogging 6-7 miles per day and swiming 1-2 hrs. frequentcy.

On physical examination, she is a healthy-appearing gentleman in acute distress. Wait is 201 pounds, blood pressure 111-73 pulse 49, respirations 16. HEENT Conjunctiva are pink. Sclerae is anicteric. Lungs: Clear to auscultation. Cardiovascular, Normal S1, S2. Abdomen: Soft and nontender. No masses are palpated. No organomegaly.

IPRESSION: Patient referral for colonrectal cancer screening. I reviewed the indications and alternatives with the patient who understands and agrees. I discussed the risks of preforation, bleeding, and infection with her, and we will proceed to schedule him for colnscopy. If there is a lesion found: he will be scheduled to followup with me in the office.

TRANSCRIPTION PRACTICE

Open your word-processing software. Insert the student CD-ROM and locate the dictation for this chapter. For each of the words in the "listen for these terms" list for each report, use a medical dictionary or other resource to identify and write down a brief definition of the term on a separate sheet of paper to attach with your work. Then listen to the dictation and transcribe each report. Use the current date for each report where a date is indicated. Insert a heading into the document if the text falls to a second page.

At the end of each report, indicate the name of the dictating physician under the signature line and insert reference initials. For date dictated and transcribed and date of admission, use the current date. Proofread your work, print one copy for your instructor along with your term definitions, and save the completed report to your student disk.

Report #T14.1: Operative Report
Patient Name: Jorge Crespo
Medical Record No.: 8808922
Attending Physician: Eugene Richards, MD

Listen for these terms:
Optiview system
trocar
lumen
crura
Penrose (drain)
gastroepiploic arcade
Endo GIA 60 (stapler)
Endo bag
Maxon

Report #T14.2: SOAP Note
Patient Name: Lavonia Wilson
Medical Record No.: 5552311
Attending Physician: Andrea Biggs, MD

Listen for these terms:
borborygmi
NSAIDs
cruciferous vegetables

Report #T14.3: Procedure Note
Patient Name: Mildred Mangrum
Medical Record No.: MM-3352811
Attending Physician: Andrea Biggs, MD

Listen for these terms:
capsule endoscopy
iron deficiency anemia
gastric lumen
stigmata
AVM
erythematous gastropathy
antral ectasia

UROLOGY

INTRODUCTION

Urology is a medical specialty that deals with diseases and disorders of the male and female urinary systems as well as of the male reproductive organs. Although classified as a surgical subspecialty, urology focuses on both the surgical and medical management of diseases that affect this body system. The term **genitourinary** (GU) refers to both the parts of the body that play a role in reproduction (*genit/o-*) and those that dispose of liquid waste products (*urinary*). A **urologist** is a physician who

has specialized knowledge and skill regarding problems with both the urinary system and the male genital organs.

This chapter provides a fundamental understanding of the organs that comprise the genitourinary system as well as the terminology encountered in the diagnosis and treatment of urologic diseases and disorders. Because several disorders that affect male patients typically involve both the urinary tract and the reproductive system, a brief review of the male reproductive organs is included in this chapter.

ANATOMY OF THE GENITOURINARY SYSTEM

The **urinary system**, sometimes referred to as the **excretory system**, is like a water treatment plant in that it filters the blood and expels the resulting liquid waste products from the body. The organs that work together to clean and remove excess fluid and waste material from the body include the kidneys, ureters, bladder, and urethra, as shown in Figure 15.1.

Kidneys

Nephrology is the branch of medicine concerned with the kidneys. The term comes from the Greek word

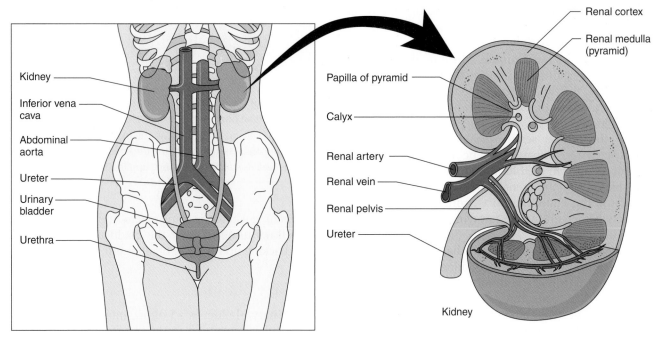

FIGURE 15.1. The Genitourinary System. The urinary tract includes the kidneys (enlargement at right), ureters, and bladder. Reprinted with permission from Willis, MC. *Medical Terminology: The Language of Healthcare.* Baltimore: Williams & Wilkins, 1996.

nephros and the suffix *–logy* (study). The term *renal* is an adjective referring to the kidneys and is derived from *ren*, the Latin word for kidney. All of the critical filtering operations take place in the **kidneys**. The two kidneys are fist-sized, bean-shaped organs lying on each side of the spinal column just behind the abdominal cavity. They serve to filter the blood to remove excess waste products and process them for excretion through other structures of the body. The kidneys have other functions as well, some of which are not directly related to the filtering of waste products from the blood. For example, the kidneys help regulate the body's blood pressure: when blood pressure is too high, they excrete excess sodium; when blood pressure is too low, the kidneys produce and secrete an enzyme called **renin**, which activates enzymes in the body that help raise blood pressure levels. In addition, the kidneys secrete other hormones that are vital to body function, including **erythropoietin**, which aids in the formation of red blood cells, and **calcitriol**, an active form of vitamin D that helps increase the absorption of calcium and phosphorus from the small intestine.

Enclosing each kidney is a tough, protective membrane called the **renal capsule**, which helps maintain the kidney's shape and protects it from infection. Surrounding each capsule is a cushion of fatty tissue and a layer of connective tissue called the **renal fascia**, which attaches each kidney to the abdominal wall. Atop each kidney lies an **adrenal gland**, which produces hormones that help control heart rate, blood pressure, and other important body functions (see Chapter 15 for more information about these and other glands that

make up the endocrine system). At the center of one side of each kidney is a concave indentation that leads into a hollow chamber called the **renal sinus**. The entrance to this chamber is the **renal hilum**, through which blood vessels, nerves, and a ureter pass.

The kidney is divided into three distinct regions. The outermost area is called the **renal cortex**, which contains blood-filtering mechanisms. The renal cortex surrounds a middle area called the **renal medulla**, which functions as a collecting chamber. It contains wedge-shaped masses of tissue called **renal pyramids**. The tip of each pyramid is called the **papilla**. The tissue of the renal cortex dips into the medulla between the renal pyramids, forming structures called **renal columns**. The cortex and medulla make up the **parenchyma**, or functional tissue, of the kidney. The third region is the **renal pelvis**, located in the renal sinus, which collects the urine as it is produced. Funnel-shaped extensions of the renal pelvis, called **calyces** (singular, **calyx**) enclose the papillae of the renal pyramids.

The cortex and the medulla contain **nephrons** that filter the blood and produce urine. Numbering over a million in each kidney, nephrons consist of two major components: a renal corpuscle and a renal tubule. The **renal corpuscle** contains a ball-shaped cluster of tiny capillaries, called a **glomerulus** (plural, **glomeruli**), surrounded by a hollow, saclike structure called a **glomerular capsule** (also called the **Bowman capsule**). These capillaries trap proteins and red and white blood cells that are too large to pass through the kidney's filtering system. These particles remain in the blood to circulate throughout the body, while the smaller particles (such as ions, sugars, and ammonia) pass through the membranes of the glomerulus into the Bowman capsule. The Bowman capsule is situated at the end of a U-shaped tubule called the **renal tubule**, which receives the fluid filtered by the glomerulus during the process of making urine. Thus, the fluid entering the tubule is identical to the blood, except that it contains no proteins or red or white blood cells.

In the tubule, semipermeable membranes allow selective passage of particles to be reabsorbed back into the blood or from the blood into the tubule. The particles that pass into the renal tubule empty into a collecting duct. The collecting ducts from all the nephrons merge together, ultimately emptying into the bladder as urine to be excreted.

The major source of blood to the kidneys is through the **renal arteries**, one for each kidney. The renal arteries branch off from the **abdominal aorta**, the portion of the aorta that passes through the general area of the abdomen. The renal artery for each kidney enters the renal hilum and branches into smaller arteries that eventually pass between the renal pyramids toward the renal cortex. Blood then flows into the various structures of the kidney to be filtered. After waste products have been removed, the cleaned blood exits the glomerulus through venules, which join the renal vein that exits from the kidney through the hilum. The renal vein joins the **inferior vena cava**, the major vein that returns blood from the kidneys back to the heart.

Urine is a waste product composed of water, certain electrolytes, and various soluble wastes manufactured by the kidneys during the process of cleaning and filtering the blood. As blood flows through the body, wastes resulting from the cells' metabolism of food are deposited in the bloodstream and must be disposed of in some way. The kidneys, particularly the nephrons, are responsible for a major portion of this filtering process. The main function of the nephrons is to control the composition of body fluids and remove wastes from the blood by filtering certain substances out of the blood and reabsorbing others back into the bloodstream. The substances that are not reabsorbed during this process then move from the kidneys to the bladder to be excreted from the body as urine.

Ureters

The **ureters**, one beginning in the renal pelvis of each kidney, are muscular tubes that pass urine from the kidneys to the bladder. The ureters contain smooth muscle that tightens and relaxes in a peristaltic motion that forces urine downward from the kidneys to the bladder. The presence of urine in the renal pelvis initiates these waves, the frequency of which keeps pace with the rate of urine formation. The ureters enter the posterior surface of the bladder at the **ureteral orifices**. A fold of mucous membrane called the **ureteral sphincter** covers

the opening where the urine enters, and acts like a valve that allows urine to enter the bladder but prevents it from backing up from the bladder into the ureter.

Urinary Bladder

The **urinary bladder** is a hollow, muscular sac located in the pelvic cavity that serves as a storage reservoir for urine until it is eliminated from the body. The walls of the bladder consist of layers of smooth muscles that expand when the bladder fills. The outermost layer of muscle is called the **detrusor muscle** or **muscularis propria**. Part of the detrusor muscle surrounds the bladder neck and forms the **internal urethral sphincter**. The smooth muscle fibers of this sphincter prevent the bladder from involuntarily emptying until urination occurs.

At the base of the bladder is a triangular area called the **trigone**, formed by three openings in the floor of the urinary bladder. Two of these openings are the ureters, which form the base of the trigone. The third opening is a short, funnel-shaped extension called the **bladder neck**, which contains the opening into the urethra. The trigone generally remains in a fixed position, although the rest of the bladder distends and contracts with the amount of urine drained into it by the ureters.

Urethra

The **urethra** is a tube that conveys urine from the bladder to the outside of the body. In women, the urethra is shorter than in men and runs anterior to the vagina. In men, the urethra is much longer and transports both urine and semen. The **external urethral sphincter** is a collective name for the muscles used to control the flow of urine from the bladder. These muscles envelop the urethra so that when they contract, the urethra closes. Working in conjunction with the internal urethral sphincter at the bladder neck, the external urethral sphincter expands to control when urine leaves the bladder.

Male Genital Organs

In males, the urinary tract passes through and is part of the structures of the male reproductive system. When

QUICK CHECK 15.1

Fill in the blanks with the correct answers.

1. The triangular area located at the base of the bladder is called the _____.

2. Each nephron consists of a _____ and a _____.

3. The _____ delivers blood to be filtered into the kidneys.

4. The _____ are structures that pass urine from the kidneys to the bladder.

5. What structure sits on top of each kidney? _____.

---

preparing reports for a genitourinary practice, a medical transcriptionist will encounter accounts of disorders in male patients involving both the urinary and reproductive systems. The male genital anatomy consists of the following main structures:

- **Penis.** The penis is the external male reproductive and urinary organ through which both semen and urine leave the body. It contains the urethra, which ends in an external swelling at the tip of the penis called the **glans penis**, sometimes dictated as simply *the glans*. The opening at the tip of the glans, which allows for urination and ejaculation is called the **meatus**. When the penis is erect during sex, the flow of urine is blocked from the urethra, allowing only semen to be ejaculated at orgasm.

- **Testicles.** The testicles, or **testes** (singular, **testis**), are the organs that produce sperm and male sex hormones, including testosterone. They are located at the base of the penis in a sac called the **scrotum**. Each testicle is connected to a coiled tube called the epididymis, where sperm are stored for as long as six weeks while they mature.

- **Epididymis.** The epididymis (plural, **epididymides**) is a comma-shaped tube that is coiled on the back side of each testicle. Within each epididymis, the sperm complete their maturation and are stored until ejaculation. Each epididymis is connected to the prostate gland by a pair of tubes called the vas deferens, which transport mature sperm to the urethra in preparation for ejaculation. Together, the epididymis and vas deferens make up the duct system of the male reproductive organs.

- **Seminal vesicles.** The paired seminal vesicles are saclike pouches that attach to the vas deferens near the base of the bladder. The seminal vesicles produce a fluid that helps with sperm motility and makes up most of the volume of a male's ejaculatory fluid.

- **Prostate.** The prostate is a firm, muscular gland located just below the bladder and in front of the rectum. It encircles the first inch of the urethra as it emerges from the bladder. The prostate secretes a protein called **prostate-specific antigen** (PSA) and an enzyme, prostatic acid phosphatase, which empty into the prostatic urethra and join the seminal fluid in helping to nourish the sperm. Because of its location, enlargement of the prostate causes difficulty with urination.

- **Bulbourethral glands.** These glands, also called **Cowper glands**, are pea-sized structures located on the sides of the urethra just below the prostate gland. They produce a clear, slippery fluid that empties directly into the urethra in order to lubricate the urethra and neutralize any acidity that may be present due to residual drops of urine in the urethra.

PROCESS OF URINATION

The kidneys form urine from blood; therefore, blood flow through the kidneys is a major factor in determining urine output. Urine formation begins with the process of filtration, selective only in terms of the size of materials that can be filtered through the glomeruli.

When blood enters the kidney, it contains both useful chemicals and dissolved waste materials. Because the capillaries of the glomerulus are thin and permeable, most of the blood, except the red and white blood cells and proteins, filters readily through the glomerulus and glomerular capsule into the tubule. The resulting clear, filtered fluid that is the precursor of urine is called **glomerular filtrate**. Glomerular filtrate consists primarily of water, excess salt, potassium, and urea. **Urea**, the most abundant of the waste products excreted by the kidneys, is a byproduct of the metabolic process in the liver and is a reflection of the amount of protein in the diet. The clear, filtered fluid enters the glomerular capsule and passes into the renal tubules.

The glomerular filtrate passes along the tubule where a network of capillaries reabsorbs water, glucose, and salts from the filtrate and secretes unwanted substances into the filtrate. This reabsorption process is selective in terms of usefulness, allowing only those useful substances from the filtrate to be returned to the blood. The remaining fluid containing waste products, now called urine, drains from the tubule into a collecting duct, eventually to be excreted from the body. Here the urine may continue as dilute urine or, if needed by the body, water can be absorbed from the urine and returned to the blood, making the urine more concentrated. **Antidiuretic hormone** (ADH), which is produced by the pituitary gland, is released when the amount of water in the body decreases. ADH and other hormones help the kidneys balance the volume of water and minerals in the body.

The urine drains from the collecting ducts of thousands of nephrons into the calyces. Each kidney has several calyces, all of which then drain into the renal pelvis and finally into the ureter. The ureter passes the urine into the bladder, where it is eventually excreted by the body via the urethra.

COMMON GENITOURINARY DISEASES AND TREATMENTS

Diseases of the urinary tract include problems with kidney function, urinary tract infections, obstructions along the urinary tract, and other abnormalities that can cause scarring to these structures, leading to kidney failure.

Urinary Tract Infections

A **urinary tract infection** (UTI) is an infection in the urinary tract caused by the invasion of disease-causing microorganisms. The most common cause of UTIs is tiny bacteria from the bowel and digestive tractthat enter the urethra and begin to multiply. They then cause an infection in the urethra (**urethritis**) or travel upward, causing infection in the bladder (cystitis, described below). If the infection is not treated promptly, bacteria may travel even farther up the ureters to infect the kidneys. In men, a UTI is often the result of an obstruction, such as a urinary stone or an enlarged prostate. Symptoms of a UTI include **polyuria** (excessive urination), **dysuria** (painful or difficult urination), **hematuria** (blood in the urine), **bacteruria** (bacteria in the urine), and **pyuria** (pus in the urine).

To diagnose a UTI, the patient may be asked to obtain what is called a **clean-catch** urine sample—that is, a sample obtained after washing the genital area and collecting a midstream sample of urine in a sterile container. After analyzing the urine for white and red blood cells and bacteria, a physician can determine the correct medical treatment to clear the infection.

UTIs are usually treated with antibiotics; the choice of drug and the treatment length are determined by the results of the urine tests that identify the offending bacteria. There are dozens of antibiotics available to treat these infections. Some of the most commonly used antibiotics for UTIs frequently encountered in transcription include the following:

- Fluoroquinolones (also dictated as *quinolones*): ciprofloxacin (Cipro); norfloxacin (Noroxin); levofloxacin (Levaquin); and gatifloxacin, also dictated as a shortened form, *gatti* (Tequin).
- Cephalosporins: cefuroxime (Ceftin), cefaclor (Ceclor), and cefotaxime (Claforan).
- Tetracyclines: tetracycline (Sumycin) or doxycycline (Doxycin).
- Other frequently-used antibiotics: amoxicillin (Amoxil), amoxicillin-clavulanate (Augmentin), trimethoprim-sulfamethoxazole (a combination of Bactrim, Cotrim, and Septra), nitrofurantoin (Macrodantin), vancomycin (Vancocin), and gentamicin (Gentak).

Although most UTIs clear up in a few days, some infections, such as kidney infections, may require several weeks of antibiotic treatment. Researchers are also working on a vaccine that helps patients build up their own immunity to fight against live organisms such as those that cause UTIs.

Kidney Disorders

Kidney disease may be caused by many factors such as injury, infections, or cancer; it can also be part of a more generalized disease affecting other parts of the body. Kidney disorders can affect one or both kidneys and may be of sudden onset or occur gradually over several years. If not treated, kidney disorders can cause the kidneys to lose their ability to filter wastes from the body.

Kidney Failure

When injury or illness prevents their removal from the blood, waste products can build up in the body at abnormally high levels. The kidneys' inability to filter waste from the body adequately is called **kidney failure**, or **renal failure**, and can become life-threatening if not treated. Kidney failure can be acute or chronic. **Acute renal failure** is the sudden loss of the kidneys' ability to

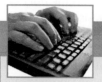

TRANSCRIPTION TIP:

Sometimes physicians will shorten the names of vancomycin, ampicillin, and gentamicin in dictation, respectively, as *vanc, amp, and gent*. As with other shortened forms of words, spell out these terms when transcribing the names of these medications.

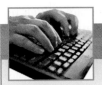

TRANSCRIPTION TIP:

When patients with chronic renal failure develop more acute symptoms, their physicians may diagnose *acute on chronic* renal failure. Do not transcribe this diagnosis as *acute and chronic.*

excrete wastes. This can be caused by injury, infection, or sudden shock to the kidneys. After the cause is identified and treated, the renal failure usually reverses. **Chronic renal failure**, on the other hand, is a long-term condition whereby the kidneys gradually and progressively lose their ability to function, affecting both blood pressure and the quality of blood because of their inability to filter wastes properly. Chronic kidney disease progresses over a number of years as the structures of the kidneys are damaged from long-term illnesses, such as hypertension or diabetes. As kidney function decreases, the kidneys are increasingly unable to regulate water and electrolyte balances, to clear excess fluids and waste products from the body, and to promote red blood cell production. Symptoms of kidney failure include edema, congestive heart failure, **hyperkalemia** (an excessive amount of potassium in the blood), heart arrhythmias, **uremia** (also called **azotemia**, which is an excess amount of urea and other nitrogenous waste in the blood), and lethargy.

Kidney failure is treated by **dialysis**, a filtering process that removes wastes from the blood when the kidneys are not able to do so naturally. There are two main types of dialysis: **hemodialysis** and **peritoneal dialysis**. In hemodialysis, blood is removed from a patient's artery and filtered outside of his or her body by means of special filtering tubes within a **dialysis machine**. This machine works in a similar fashion to the way real kidneys filter blood through the renal glomeruli and tubules. The blood flows from the patient's artery through a tube to the dialysis machine. It flows across a semipermeable membrane in the machine along with solutions that help remove the toxins from the blood. The purified blood is then returned to the patient's body through another tube situated in one of the patient's veins.

For hemodialysis to be successful there must be a way to remove the blood from the patient's body and return it to the body at a continuous high rate of flow to maximize the amount of blood cleansed during dialysis treatments. Normally blood flows from arteries through capillaries and back to the heart through the veins. When a method is created to bypass the capillaries, blood flows directly from an artery to a vein. The site on the body where blood will be removed and returned through an artery and vein during dialysis is referred to as **access**. The access for dialysis can be temporary or

permanent. In a temporary situation, such as in a situation where dialysis must be performed immediately without time to create a permanent access, a catheter that has two chambers to allow a two-way flow of blood is used. The catheter is inserted into a vein in the neck, chest, or leg near the groin and can suffice in short-term dialysis situations.

Long-term dialysis requires permanent access, which allows easier and more efficient removal and replacement of blood with fewer complications. This is obtained by tunneling a catheter under the skin to connect an artery directly to a vein for a two-way blood flow. Blood flows from the artery into the dialysis machine, and filtered blood flows back into the body through the vein. There are two types of long-term vascular access for dialysis, as shown in Figure 15.2: an **arteriovenous (AV) fistula** and an **arteriovenous (AV) graft**. Recall that a **fistula** is an opening or connection between two natural structures, such as a hole in the tissue that separates the bladder from the bowel. In this instance, a fistula is artificially created between an artery and a vein to provide adequate blood flow for dialysis. To create the AV fistula, a surgeon connects an artery directly to a vein, usually in the forearm, to make the vein larger and stronger for dialysis. Connecting the artery to the vein allows blood to bypass the capillaries, thereby allowing it to flow into the vein in bigger quantities and at a more rapid rate.

In a situation where an AV fistula is not possible, such as when a patient's veins are too small to allow it, an artificial connection to an artery, or an AV graft, can be placed. The AV graft acts like a natural vein and provides adequate blood flow for hemodialysis.

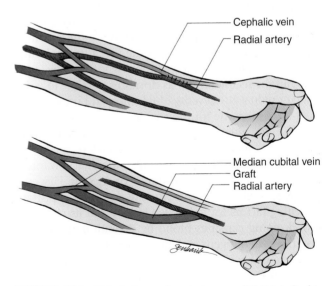

FIGURE 15.2. Dialysis Access. An arteriovenous (AV) fistula (top) is created by a side-to-side joining of an artery and vein. An arteriovenous (AV) graft (bottom) shows the graft establishing connection between the artery and vein. Reprinted with permission from Smeltzer SC, Bare BG. *Textbook of Medical-Surgical Nursing,* 9th ed. Philadelphia: Lippincott Williams & Wilkins, 2000.

Peritoneal dialysis is a technique in which the lining of the patient's abdominal cavity, called the **peritoneum**, is used as a dialysis membrane to filter the blood. The peritoneum lines the walls of the abdominal cavity like the lining of a coat and allows waste products and extra fluid to pass from the blood into the dialysis solution. The dialysis solution used contains a sugar called dextrose, which pulls wastes and extra fluid into the abdominal cavity. The fluid is injected through a dialysis catheter into the abdominal cavity. Wastes in the blood are then diffused through the peritoneum and into this fluid. The solution is allowed to absorb wastes for several hours, and then the waste-filled fluid is exchanged for a fresh batch of solution.

Kidney transplantation is the process of placing a healthy kidney from one person (the donor) into the body of another person (the recipient). A transplantation procedure may be a **living-related transplant**, where the donor is a living relative of the recipient, or a **cadaveric transplant**, where the donated kidney comes from a person who has died. In either case, the single donated kidney does the work previously done by the two failed kidneys.

The transplantation process consists of many steps. Clinic notes include not only the surgical procedure itself, but the details of preparing a patient for transplantation as well. A kidney transplant candidate begins by working with a transplant team, which considers various factors in matching donor kidneys with recipients. This process helps to determine whether a patient is a suitable transplant candidate and is documented in the clinic notes.

The ultimate goal in matching a donor kidney with a person seeking transplantation is to transplant an organ that will be tolerated indefinitely by the body of the recipient. The matching of tissues between organ donor and recipient avoids **rejection**, or the immune system's attack on foreign tissue or a transplanted organ. Physicians seek a donor whose tissue type matches the recipient type as closely as possible to eliminate or reduce the severity of rejection and improve the long-term outcome for the recipient.

The transplant team considers three factors in matching donor kidneys with potential recipients in order to help predict whether an individual's immune system will accept the new kidney or reject it. First, the patient's blood group and type are the most important matching factors for a donated kidney and its recipient. Blood typing classifies blood by determining the reaction between antigens and antibodies. The recipient and donor must have either the same blood type or compatible types. Blood groups are transcribed as single or dual letters, sometimes accompanied by a capital letter or number, with the word *group* in small letters. For example: group A, group A1, or group A1B. Blood types are written as a capital letter followed by the designation of being positive or negative. For example: B negative, A

positive. The words *negative* and *positive* are written out because the minus or plus sign can be easily overlooked.

A second test called **tissue typing** relates essentially to genetic matching between the donor and recipient. **Human leukocyte antigens** (HLAs) are antigens tolerated by the body that correspond to genes which govern immune responses. An **antigen** is any substance that causes the immune system to produce antibodies against it. Examples of antigens are chemicals, viruses, spores, or bacteria. **Antibodies** are a type of protein produced by the immune system in response to foreign substances that may be a threat to the body.

Human tissue is unique in its makeup. To be able to destroy invaders, the body must be able to distinguish them from self. The body makes this distinction because all cells have identification molecules on their surface. In humans, these molecules are HLAs. HLA molecules are called antigens because they can provoke an immune response in another person; they do not normally provoke an immune response in the person who has them. A cell with molecules on its surface that are not identical to those on the body's own cells is identified as being foreign.

The tissues of different individuals can sometimes share characteristics such as certain antigens, enabling the transplanted kidney to be compatible with the tissue of the recipient. HLA antigens are found on many cells of the body but are seen mostly on white blood cells. Each person has a unique set of HLAs, a total of six, three inherited from each parent; and these are the substances tested for a match to ensure the recipient's response to a transplanted kidney. Family members are most likely to have a match of these antigens, although they may not be a complete match. The closer the match, the better the chance that the recipient's body will not reject the transplanted kidney. The HLA status of the donor in a report is transcribed as being either an *HLA-identical* or *HLA-nonidentical* match.

Finally, a **crossmatching antigen test** is performed to define how a kidney transplant recipient may respond to particular cells or proteins of the donor kidney, even when the blood group and tissue type of a donor and recipient are found to be compatible. In this test, a sample of the donor's blood is mixed with a sample of the transplant candidate's blood to see if there is an adverse reaction between the properties of the two samples. If the cells attack one another, the test is called a **positive crossmatch**, meaning that the recipient's blood cells have responded to the donor's blood cells adversely and that the transplant should not be carried out. If no reaction occurs, the test is called a **negative crossmatch**, meaning that the recipient's blood cells havenot responded adversely to the donor's blood cellsand that the transplant operation can proceed. Although the language may seem a bit backwards, it should be remembered that a *positive* response to the recipient means that a rejection of the transplanted

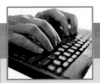

kidney *will* occur; a *negative* response means a rejection of the transplanted kidney *will not* occur.

During the transplantation surgery, a surgeon removes the damaged kidney from the lower abdomen and places the new kidney in its place. The artery and vein of the new kidney are then connected to the patient's renal artery and vein.

Nephritis

Nephritis is a broad term for any inflammation of one or both kidneys. It may involve the kidney's filtration units, the spaces within the kidney, or the main tissues that make up the kidney and renal pelvis.

Glomerulonephritis is an inflammation of the glomeruli, the clusters of capillaries that filter blood. As the result of the inflammation of the capillary loops in the glomeruli, the kidneys are unable to filter waste products from the blood. Red and white blood cells and protein are permitted to pass through the glomeruli and enter the fluid that becomes urine. Blood in the urine is called **hematuria**. Progressively damaged glomeruli are unable to filter metabolic waste products, which then accumulate in the blood. Fluid can accumulate outside the circulatory system and cause swelling in the face, hands, feet, or ankles.

Glomerulosclerosis is the scarring or hardening of the tiny blood vessels within the kidney. A significant symptom of glomerulosclerosis is **proteinuria**, or excessive amounts of protein in the urine. The loss of large amounts of protein could cause swelling in the ankles or accumulation of fluid in the abdomen. **Focal segmental glomerulosclerosis** (FSGS) results from scar tissue that forms in some segments of the glomeruli in the kidney. The term itself is descriptive:

- *Focal* means that only some of the glomeruli in the kidney become scarred while others remain normal.
- *Segmental* means that only part, or a segment, of an individual glomerulus is damaged.
- *Glomerul/o* is the combining form relating to the glomerulus of the kidney.
- *Sclerosis* is a term that means scarring.

The cause of FSGS is usually unknown. A small number of cases result from **reflux nephropathy**, a condition in which the kidneys are damaged by backward flow of urine into the kidney. Some other conditions that may increase the risk for FSGS include anemia, obesity, and infections such as human immunodeficiency virus (HIV). FSGS also results from other kidney diseases that damage the kidneys and causes scarring. Most patients with FSGS will progress to complete renal failure within 5 to 10 years.

There is no cure for FSGS, and treatment is usually focused on controlling symptoms of the disease. Corticosteroids may be prescribed to reduce inflammation. Medications to treat high blood pressure, such as angiotensin-converting enzyme (ACE) inhibitors, angiotensin receptor blockers, and diuretics, as discussed in Chapter 13, *Cardiology*, may help control symptoms such as high blood pressure and edema. Antibiotics are used to control infections.

Interstitial nephritis is an inflammation of the spaces between the renal tubules and may include inflammation of the tubules themselves (called **tubulointerstitial nephritis**). *Interstitial* means that the inflammation does not affect the blood vessels or filters in the kidney, but only the parts in between them. It is usually caused by the effects of various drugs or toxins on the kidney and is usually a temporary, reversible condition; the condition improves when the offending drug is discontinued or treatment of the underlying disease is effective, although some kidney scarring may occur.

Pyelonephritis is an inflammation of the renal pelvis as a result of a bacterial or viral infection. Some researchers believe that the bacteria that cause pyelonephritis may develop elsewhere in the body and travel through the bloodstream to the kidney; however, more commonly, the infection is the result of bacteria from outside the body traveling back up the urinary stream through the urethra to the bladder and eventually to the kidneys. Obstructions such as a stricture or scar tissue may cause an infection or inflammation in the urethra, enabling bacteria to enter and travel to the kidney. Finally, the insertion of catheters or other instruments can cause infection.

The treatment for acute pyelonephritis includes identification of the infecting organism by means of laboratory work and cultures as well as treatment with a broad-spectrum antibiotic. In some patients, surgery may be necessary to relieve an obstruction or correct an anatomic anomaly that can cause chronic obstructions. Chronic pyelonephritis can cause destruction of kidney tissue as a result of recurring or untreated bacterial infections, leading to kidney failure.

Polycystic Kidney Disease

Polycystic kidney disease (PKD) is a genetic disorder characterized by the growth of numerous fluid-filled cysts in the kidneys. The cysts grow out of the nephrons in the kidney, then separate from them and continue to enlarge, causing the kidney itself to enlarge. Finally the cysts, which can number in the thousands, replace much of the mass of the kidney, reducing its function and leading to chronic high blood pressure and kidney infections. Eventually the cysts lead to kidney failure. About half of all patients with PKD progress to kidney failure so far advanced that it cannot be reversed, a condition called **end-stage renal disease** (ESRD). When PKD causes the kidney to fail, dialysis or kidney transplantation is necessary.

Autosomal dominant polycystic kidney disease (ADPKD) is the most common inherited form of the disease, accounting for about 90% of all PKD cases. Children of parents with ADPKD have a 50% chance of acquiring the disorder.

PKD is most commonly diagnosed through ultrasound technology in which sound waves can visualize the cysts in the kidneys. Although a cure for PKD is not available, treatment of symptoms can offer relief and prolong life. Pain medication is often used to relieve pain in the back and flanks. Urinary tract infections, a problem often accompanying PKD, can be treated with antibiotics. Keeping blood pressure under control with medication and lifestyle changes can slow the effects of the disease. In severe cases, dialysis and/or kidney transplantation may be required. Kidney transplantation has become a common and successful solution for PKD patients, and a healthy transplanted kidney does not develop cysts.

Kidney Stones

A **kidney stone**, also called a **renal calculus** (plural, **calculi**) is a hard, solid piece of material that forms in the kidney from crystals that separate from the urine and build up on the inner surface of the kidney. The presence of stones in the kidneys is referred to as **nephrolithiasis**. The general term for a stone that develops anywhere in the urinary tract is called **urolithiasis**. A stone that forms in one or both ureters is called **ureterolithiasis**. If the crystals remain tiny enough, they pass through the urinary tract and out of the body without being noticed. Kidney stones cause problems when a stone breaks loose and begins to work its way through the urinary system. If a stone becomes large enough to block the flow of urine from the kidney, it can cause pressure, pain, and infection. If a stone moves out of the kidney with the flow of urine, it can cause severe pain as it moves through the ureters or gets stuck, causing an infection. An untreated kidney stone can even cause permanent damage to the kidneys.

Kidney stones form when the salts and minerals that are normally found in the urine become out of balance. Different types of stones are formed as a result of this imbalance:

- Calcium stones—The vast majority of kidney stones are calcium stones, which comprise calcium and oxalate, a compound occurring naturally in some fruits and vegetables. Calcium that is not used by the bones and muscles goes to the kidneys, which flushes the excess calcium out with the rest of the urine. In some people, however, the calcium remains in the kidneys, forming stones.
- Struvite stones—These stones are the result of chronic urinary tract infections. **Struvite** is a chemical compound created by the body that can form crystals in the kidney and bladder. These stones often have the shape of a stag's horn and can seriously damage the kidneys.
- Uric acid stones—These stones are composed of **uric acid**, a byproduct of the body's metabolism. Most of the uric acid is filtered out by the kidneys and passes out of the body in urine; the rest passes out of the body in stool. However, if too much uric acid is being produced or if the kidneys are not able to remove it from the blood properly, the level of uric acid in the blood increases and crystals develop.
- Cystine stones—These stones represent only a small percentage of kidney stones and are the result of a hereditary disorder that cause the kidneys to excrete excessive amounts of **cystine**, an organic building block that helps make up muscles, nerves, and other parts of the body.

Most kidney stones can pass through the urinary system with plenty of water to help move the stone along. To prevent another stone from forming, physicians may advise lifestyle changes, such as drinking more fluid and cutting back on foods, such as chocolate and coffee, that may increase the risk of stones forming. A physician may prescribe certain medications to prevent calcium and uric acid stones, such as allopurinol (Zyloprim), which controls the amount of acid or alkali in the urine, key factors in crystal formation. Diuretics, such as hydrochlorothiazide (Diuril), tend to decrease the amount of calcium released by the kidneys into the urine by favoring calcium retention in bone.

Surgical intervention may be warranted for patients who have stones that are resistant to medical therapy, stones that are too large to pass through the urinary tract, or anatomic abnormalities of the urinary tract that may prevent the passage of even small stones. Some common procedures that are used to break up or remove kidney stones are illustrated in Figure 15.3 and include the following:

- **Extracorporeal shock wave lithotripsy (ESWL).** ESWL is a noninvasive method of breaking kidney stones using high-energy shock waves. **Lithotripsy** comes from the root word *lith-*, meaning *stone*, and *-tripsy*, meaning *to crush*. In this procedure, the patient typically lies flat on a procedure table.

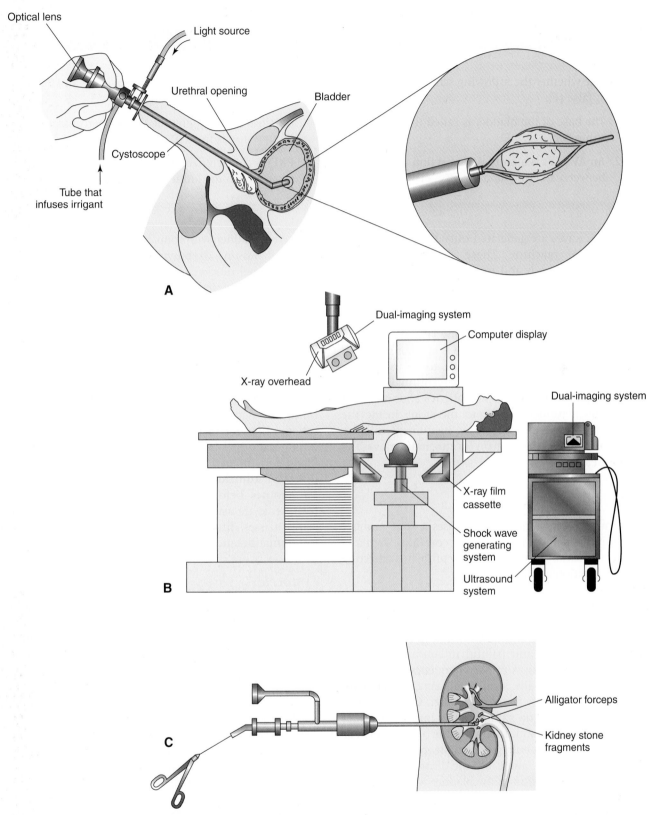

FIGURE 15.3. **Removal of Renal Stones.** **(A)** Cystoscopy with basket removal; **(B)** extracorporeal shock wave lithotripsy (ESWL) using shock waves focused over the area of the renal stone; **(C)** percutaneous nephrolithotomy. An incision is made in the abdomen to remove or destroy the stone with a nephroscope. Reprinted with permission from Smeltzer SC, Bare BG. *Textbook of Medical-Surgical Nursing,* 9th ed. Philadelphia: Lippincott Williams & Wilkins, 2000.

QUICK CHECK 15.2 ✓

Indicate whether the following sentences are true (T) or false (F).

1. The base of the bladder is called the urethral sphincter.   T   F

2. An AV graft is a natural connection created between an artery and a vein.   T   F

3. Family members are most likely to be an HLA match to a transplant candidate.   T   F

4. Calcium stones represent a small percentage of kidney stones treated.   T   F

5. PKD is characterized by fluid-filled cysts that grow within the kidney.   T   F

Shock waves are generated outside of the body by a special machine. These shock waves travel through the body and are focused directly onto the stone by x-ray guidance. The stone is pulverized into sandlike granules, which can then pass through the urinary system.

- **Percutaneous nephrolithotomy (PCN)**. This procedure is used when the stone is large or in a location that does not allow ESWL to be used effectively. In this procedure, the surgeon makes a tiny incision in the side of the patient's abdomen and creates a tunnel directly to the stone inside the kidney. Using an endoscopic instrument called a **nephroscope**, the surgeon locates and removes the stone.

Bladder Disorders

The term *bladder disorder* encompasses a large number of conditions ranging from the very common, such as a simple infection, to more serious problems affecting bladder function and overall health.

Interstitial Cystitis

Interstitial cystitis (IC), also called *painful bladder syndrome*, is a chronic and painful inflammation of the bladder wall that causes urinary frequency, hematuria, dysuria, and pelvic pain. Symptoms may clear up seemingly at random, only to resurface later. Cystitis is usually caused by bacteria gaining entry into the bladder via the urethra. Any abnormality in the bladder, such as an obstruction or an enlarged prostate, may hinder the normal flow of urine and cause the disorder. Diagnosis involves an examination of the bladder wall to look for hemorrhages or ulcers that might lead to a definitive diagnosis of this condition.

Scientists have not yet found a cure for IC; therefore, current treatments are aimed at relieving symptoms. Tricyclic antidepressants block pain arousal. Some of the most commonly used tricyclics are amitriptyline (Elavil), doxepin (Sinequan), and imipramine (Tofranil). Other drugs that may be used to treat the pain, burning, or overactive bladder symptoms of IC include phenazopyridine (Pyridium), oxybutynin chloride (Ditropan), calcium channel blockers such as nifedipine (Procardia), and gabapentin (Neurontin).

Surgical procedures may also help IC patients. A **bladder distention** is a procedure whereby the bladder is inflated with a liquid or gas, temporarily enlarging it and thus helping to reduce the frequency with which patients need to urinate. Used as both a diagnostic test and initial therapy, researchers believe that it may increase capacity and interfere with pain signals transmitted by nerves in the bladder. A similar procedure called a **bladder instillation** may also be used to ease inflammation of bladder walls. In this procedure, the bladder is inflated with a chemical compound called dimethyl sulfoxide (DMSO) that is retained for about 15 minutes before being expelled. Although several treatments are usually needed, doctors believe this substance passes directly into the bladder wall to reduce inflammation and block pain.

Cystocele

A **cystocele**, also referred to as *fallen bladder* or *bladder prolapse*, is a condition in women that occurs when the wall between the bladder and the vagina weakens, causing the bladder to drop or sag into the vagina. Under normal conditions, the bladder is held in a position by a hammocklike support of pelvic floor muscles and ligaments. When these muscles are stretched or weakened, the bladder can sag through them into the vagina. In severe cases, the sagging bladder will appear at the opening of the vagina and even protrude through it. This causes discomfort and incomplete emptying of the bladder. If left untreated, the problems with urinary retention can lead to kidney damage or infection.

The most common cause of cystocele is the weakening of pelvic muscles due to multiple childbirths, but it may also be caused by a chronic cough, obesity, or heavy lifting. It can also occur during the aging process as a result of decreased estrogen after menopause.

A cystocele can usually be corrected in a number of ways. **Kegel** exercises, a series of exercises which are done by squeezing the pelvic floor muscles, help strengthen the muscles in and around the vagina. A **pessary**, which is a plastic or rubber ring, may be placed in the vagina to push the bladder back into place. In severe cases, surgery may be required to move the bladder back to its normal position.

Neurogenic Bladder

Neurogenic bladder is a disorder resulting from damage to the nerves that govern the urinary tract. Various nerves converge in the area of the bladder. These nerves carry messages from the bladder to the brain. They also carry signals from the brain to the muscles of the bladder, enabling it to perform its major functions of storing and eliminating urine from the body. When these message-carrying nerves are damaged or the nervous system that signals the bladder to function does not work properly, problems with bladder capacity or malfunction of control results. The bladder can contract too quickly or frequently, leading to urinary frequency or loss of bladder control and leakage, called **urinary incontinence**. The bladder may not empty completely, leading to urine backing up into the ureters, a condition called **vesicoureteral reflux**. When urine is not disposed of properly by the bladder, an infection in the bladder or ureters can occur.

Common causes of this damage to nerves and nerve pathways from the bladder to the brain include accidents that injure the brain or spinal cord; diabetes; birth defects, including spinal cord and nerve abnormalities; and heavy metal poisoning.

Treatment for neurogenic bladder depends on the symptoms and cause of the nerve damage. For example, for urinary frequency and leakage, physicians may prescribe medications to help the bladder stay relaxed or antibiotics to treat an underlying infection causing the symptoms. In extreme cases, surgery may be needed to construct an alternate tube for emptying the bladder or to increase bladder size. If the bladder is unable to empty urine, a catheter may be used to regularly empty the bladder, or endoscopic surgery may be used to improve urine flow.

Bladder Cancer

Bladder cancer accounts for approximately 90% of all cancers of the urinary tract. It usually originates in the bladder lining, which consists of transitional cells and squamous cells. Cancer that originates in the transitional cells of the bladder is called **transitional cell carcinoma**, whereas cases that begin in the squamous cells are called **squamous cell carcinoma**. A tumor that forms in the bladder lining is called a superficial cancer, or a **carcinoma in situ**. *In situ* means *in its normal place* or *confined to the site of origin*. These cancers are superficial; that is, they usually do not spread to other areas of the bladder or nearby organs.

Bladder tumors almost always begin in the bladder's smooth lining. The cells grow abnormally fast and then form a growth that projects into the interior of the bladder cavity. When the tumor grows through the bladder lining and into the muscular wall of the bladder, it is known as **invasive cancer**. Invasive cancer may grow into a nearby organ, such as the uterus or vagina in women or the prostate gland in men. It may also invade the wall of the abdomen itself.

Patients with bladder cancer have several treatment options, depending on the type and severity of the tumor. High-energy radiation from x-rays is used to kill cancer cells and shrink tumors, whereas chemotherapy uses anticancer drugs to kill cancer cells. (See Chapter 20 for a more detailed discussion of how these modalities are used to treat this and other types of cancer.)

Removal of the tumor is the most common treatment for bladder cancer. A **transurethral resection of bladder tumor** (TURB) is a procedure used to treat superficial bladder cancers. **Resection** means the surgical removal of tissue or part or all of an organ. In this procedure, a **cystoscope**, which is an endoscopic instrument used to examine the bladder and urethra, is inserted into the bladder through the urethra to the location of the tumor. Using a small wire loop and electric current attached to the cystoscope, the tumor is removed and remaining cancer cells are burned away with a laser or with high-energy electricity, called **fulguration**. For invasive bladder cancer, the most common type of surgery is a **radical cystectomy**. In this procedure, the entire bladder is removed, along with part of the urethra and nearby organs and structures that may contain cancer cells. In some cases, only part of the bladder may be removed; this is called a **segmental cystectomy**.

When the entire bladder is removed, an alternative method for collecting urine is needed because the kidneys continue to excrete urine. Surgeons create a new urinary system from a portion of the patient's own intestinal segments to allow for the elimination of urine. In this procedure, called a **bladder reconstruction**, a section of bowel is made into a balloon-shaped sac and connected to the top of the urethra so that urine can be stored and drain from the body normally. In cases where the urinary system is severely damaged or not working, a **urostomy**, or **urinary diversion** procedure, is used to release urine from the body. In this procedure, a short segment of small intestine is removed, with the remaining sections of intestine reconnected to function normally. Then one end of the removed short segment of intestine is placed at the skin's surface to create a stoma, or opening, while the ureters are attached to the other end. The urine now travels through the newly formed connection, called an **ileal conduit**, through the stoma and out into an external collecting pouch, which can be emptied regularly by a small tap in the bottom of the bag, as shown in Figure 15.4.

Alternatively, patients can undergo lower urinary tract reconstruction by means of Koch bladder replacement.

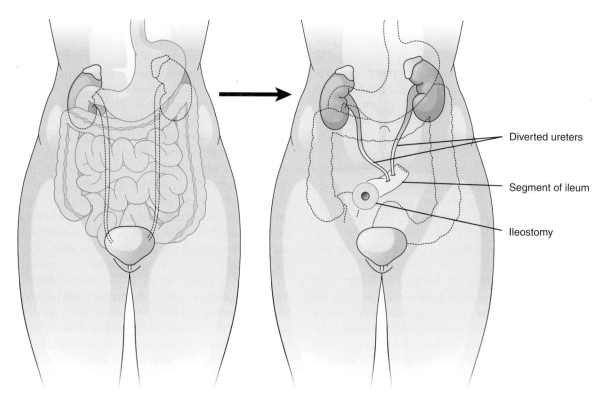

Diverted ureters

Segment of ileum

Ileostomy

FIGURE 15.4. Urinary Diversion. Urostomy with creation of ileal conduit. Reprinted with permission from Cohen BJ. *Medical Terminology,* 4th ed. Philadelphia. Lippincott Williams & Wilkins, 2003.

The **Koch pouch** (pronounced like *coke*), is created in a procedure similar to that of a urostomy, except the urinary pouch is placed inside the abdomen with a stoma created at the abdominal surface. A one-way valve, also made from the small intestine, is added to the pouch to prevent the flow of waste to the outside until a small tube is inserted by the patient to overcome the valve. The urine is emptied from the pouch by inserting a soft silicone catheter into the stoma several times per day.

QUICK CHECK 15.3 ✓

Circle the letter corresponding to the best answer to the following questions.

1. The presence of blood in the urine is called
   A. pyuria.
   B. anuria.
   C. melanuria.
   D. hematuria.

2. Dysuria means
   A. lack of urination.
   B. discolored urination.
   C. difficulty with urination.
   D. nighttime urination.

3. The formal name for *fallen bladder* is
   A. cystocele.
   B. cystogram.
   C. cystectomy.
   D. cyst bladder.

4. An inflammation of the bladder wall is referred to as
   A. interstitial cystitis.
   B. intrastitial cystocele.
   C. bladder distention.
   D. neurogenic bladder.

5. A pessary is used to
   A. kill cancer cells.
   B. push the bladder back into place.
   C. relax the bladder.
   D. kill invading bacteria.

Male Genitourinary Disorders

Several disorders of the urinary tract affect only males and involve the male reproductive organs. Disorders that affect males may involve the penis, urethra, or testes.

Hypospadias

Hypospadias is a birth defect found in boys in which the development of the penile urethra is abnormal. In hypospadias, the urinary tract opening is not located properly at the tip of the penis. Instead, the urethral opening (the meatus) develops at some point on the underside of the penis, interfering with normal voiding of urine. This malformation occurs during fetal development and its specific cause is unknown, although a number of theories suggest that hormones used during in vitro fertilization or environmental pollutants such as pesticides may play a role. Hypospadias may be accompanied by a downward curve of the shaft of the penis, a condition known as **chordee**.

Surgery is the sole treatment for hypospadias. The operation is usually performed when the child is between the age of 6 and 12 months and primarily involves creating a penis that is normal in both appearance and function. Although the surgery can be complicated, the development of new, more delicate and precise surgical techniques have made the operation highly successful.

Testicular Torsion

Testicular torsion is a twisting of the testicles and the **spermatic cord**, the structure that extends from the groin to the testicles, containing nerves, vessels, and the duct which carries sperm from the body. The torsion causes decreased blood flow to the testes, essentially strangling them by cutting off access to oxygen and nutrients. The condition can result from trauma to the scrotum or from incomplete attachment of the testes within the scrotum, a condition in which the testes have a wider-than-normal range of motion within the scrotum. Torsion can cause muscle wasting (**atrophy**), tissue death (**necrosis**), and can even require surgical removal of the testicles (**orchiectomy**) if not treated immediately to untwist the cord and save the testicle. Testicular torsion requires immediate intervention to avoid irreversible damage to the testes and to help prevent torsion from occurring again.

Prostate Disorders

Because of the prostate's location in the pelvis (at the base of the bladder, surrounding the urethra), the urinary symptoms caused by disorders of the prostate, discussed later, can be embarrassing and sometimes life-threatening. The three most common prostate problems involve infections, inflammations, and prostate cancer.

Prostatitis

Prostatitis is an inflammation of the prostate gland, causing diminished urine flow, swelling, pain between the scrotum and rectum, and sexual dysfunction. The pain can range from acute flare-ups to a long-term, chronic condition, with multiple recurrences of symptoms over time despite treatment.

Prostatitis is usually caused by a bacterial infection of the prostate gland. Bacteria that typically live in the bowel that cause urinary tract infections, such as *Escherichia coli*, *Klebsiella pneumoniae*, *Proteus mirabilis*, *Pseudomonas aeruginosa*, and *Staphylococcus aureus*, travel up the urethra to the prostate gland to cause infection even when other parts of the urinary tract do not become infected. Some sexually transmitted diseases (STDs) can also cause prostatitis. Even trauma to the prostate, such as passing a catheter into the bladder or a bladder obstruction, may sometimes allow bacteria to travel and infect the prostate.

Prostatitis commonly occurs along with inflammation of the urethra (urethritis), epididymides (**epididymitis**), or the testes (**orchitis**). Prostatitis usually clears after an identification of the bacteria is made and a course of antibiotics is started. In chronic cases, however, some patients fail to respond to antibiotics and experience recurrences.

Benign Prostatic Hyperplasia

When a man reaches middle age and beyond, the inner portion of the prostate begins to enlarge and may put pressure on the urethra. This enlargement of the prostate is called **benign prostatic hyperplasia** (BPH). Also called **benign prostatic hypertrophy**, it is the most common prostate disorder and an inevitable result of aging. Although there is no precise reason for prostatic enlargement, some experts believe the reason may be due to hormonal changes that occur during the aging process. An enlarged prostate puts pressure on the urethra, causing urinary difficulties such as incomplete emptying of the bladder and urinary frequency. If urine remains in the bladder, urine can flow back through the ureters to the kidney, resulting in kidney damage and uremia, a condition in which excessive amounts of urea and other waste products build up in the blood.

A physician can evaluate the size of the prostate with a **digital rectal examination** (DRE), in which a gloved finger is inserted into the rectum and presses on the prostate gland to check for enlargement. In addition, BPH can be diagnosed by checking the PSA level in the blood. Normally a small amount of PSA enters the blood from the prostate gland, but prostate abnormalities cause elevated levels of PSA in the bloodstream.

Treatment for prostatitis includes drugs that shrink the prostate by interfering with the function of hormones that cause prostate enlargement, and alpha-blockers, which relax the muscles within the prostate and bladder neck, allowing the flow of urine to improve. The most common of these drugs include terazosin (Hytrin), doxazosin (Cardura), tamsulosin (Flomax), and alfuzosin (Uroxatral).

A second family of drugs, 5-alpha reductase inhibitors, help to inhibit the conversion of testosterone to another, more active substance called **dihydroxy testosterone** (DHT), which is known to have a key role in prostate growth. To date, finasteride (Proscar) and dutasteride (Avodart) are used to help to reverse the condition to some extent and to shrink the prostate over time.

If surgery is necessary, a **transurethral resection of the prostate** (TURP, dictated as *terp*) is the most common method of removing excess tissue from an enlarged prostate. In this procedure, a thin, lighted tube called a **resectoscope** is inserted through the penis into the urethra. The resectoscope contains a light, valves for controlling irrigating fluid, and an electrical loop to remove the obstructing tissue and seal blood vessels. The surgeon removes the obstructing tissue that is pressing on the urethra, and the irrigating fluids carry the tissue to the bladder. This debris is removed by irrigation, and any remaining debris is eliminated in the urine over time. A TURP procedure removes only enough tissue to relieve urinary blockage. Unfortunately, in some cases, the prostate may continue to grow and urinary problems may return.

Prostate Cancer

Adenocarcinoma of the prostate, commonly called *prostate cancer*, is the growth of malignant cells in the prostate gland. Prostate cancer is the most common type of cancer in men in the United States, other than skin cancer, and is the second leading cause of cancer death in men, exceeded only by lung cancer. As prostate cancer grows, it may spread to the interior of the gland, to tissues near the prostate, to the seminal vesicles, and to distant parts of the body, such as the bones, liver, and lungs. As with other forms of cancer, the exact cause of prostate cancer is not known; age, family history, and lifestyle activities (such as a high-fat diet and smoking) are strong risk factors.

As with BPH, prostate cancer is detected through a rectal examination to measure prostate size, as well as through measurements of PSA. Multiple biopsies of the prostate may also be taken and analyzed to confirm the diagnosis. (See Chapter 20 for a discussion on how prostate cancer, as well as other cancers, are graded and staged for severity.)

Because prostate cancer tends to grow very slowly and takes years to spread, treatment is undertaken only if evidence indicates that the cancer is growing. When treatment becomes necessary, there are outpatient procedures and surgical options available.

Hormone therapy is the initial treatment for prostate cancer. The treatment is based on the fact that since hormones control the growth and activity of cells in the body, they also affect the growth of cancer cells. Prostate cancer depends on the male hormone testosterone, produced in the testicles, for its growth. By reducing the levels of testosterone in the body, the tumor's growth can be slowed and sometimes even be resolved completely. Two main classes of drugs are most often used to reduce testosterone levels and thereby shrink tumor growth. **Luteinizing hormone releasing hormone** (LHRH) agonists, such as goserelin (Zoladex), block the message from the pituitary gland for the testes to produce testosterone that enables the tumor to grow. **Antiandrogens**, also called **androgen agonists** in dictation, stop testosterone from the testicles from getting to the cancer cells and encouraging them to grow. Examples of antiandrogens include flutamide (Drogenil) and bicalutamide (Casodex).

Brachytherapy is an outpatient procedure in which very small radioactive seeds are implanted in the prostate. These small seeds (each about the size of a grain of rice) are placed into the prostate gland by using ultrasound to guide the passing of thin needles into the prostate gland through the skin between the scrotum and the rectum. As the needles penetrate through the prostate, the screen on the ultrasound machine helps guide their placement within the prostate. When each needle is in its correct position in the prostate, the individual seeds are injected into the prostate gland, and the needles are slowly withdrawn. The radioactive isotopes in the seeds give off low energy x-rays that destroy the cancer in the prostate, but leave the rest of the body unharmed.

Cryoablation (also sometimes dictated as *cryosurgery*) is a procedure in which extreme cold is used to destroy cancerous tissue. In this procedure, the surgeon inserts a warming catheter into the urethra to protect it from the freezing temperatures that will be used. Then an ultrasound transducer is inserted into the rectum and the prostate and surrounding tissue are viewed on a monitor. The image on the monitor is used to confirm placement of the **cryoprobe**, the instrument used to apply extreme cold to tissues. Very thin needles are inserted in the perineum and advanced to specific locations in the prostate tumor. Liquid nitrogen or argon gas is then injected through the probe to freeze the cancer cells to minus 40 °C. The targeted tissue freezes and icy crystals form, breaking up and destroying the cell structure. Once the sphere of tissue surrounding the cryoprobe is covered with ice, the liquid nitrogen or argon circulation is stopped and the area is allowed to thaw. The freeze-thaw cycle is repeated, and then the instruments are removed. This is an outpatient procedure, and it can be repeated if evidence of the cancer returns.

Laser therapy recently has been introduced to remove prostatic obstruction secondary to prostate cancer. In **photoselective vaporization prostatectomy** (PVP) or GreenLight laser therapy, a high-powered laser is used to produce a tissue-vaporization effect on prostatic adenomas and results in minimal bleeding and scar tissue. The procedure is done on an outpatient basis and is promising to be a safer alternative to more complicated prostate surgery.

If the prostate cannot be saved, total surgical removal of the prostate gland, the seminal vesicles, and part of the vas deferens (called a **radical prostatectomy**), along with removal of nearby lymph nodes (called **lymphadenectomy**) is the most definitive procedure to halt progression of the disease. If the surgeon accesses the prostate from the abdomen, the procedure is called a **radical retropubic prostatectomy** or **suprapubic prostatectomy**; if access is gained through the perineum, the procedure is called a **radical perineal prostatectomy**. After the surgery, radiation can be administered as an additional therapy in patients with high risk of recurrence.

Surgery to remove the testicles entirely is employed as a last resort when cancer has spread to the bone or spinal cord, or when other treatment modalities have failed. An orchiectomy (also called **orchidectomy**) is performed to help control the growth of prostate cancer by removing the testicles, the tumor's main source of testosterone that helps it live and grow. In this procedure, a small incision is made in the lower abdomen just below the belt line. The testicle is then pushed up from the scrotum through the incision and removed. After removal, the level of testosterone in the body falls dramatically and, in most cases, the tumor stops growing and actually shrinks.

Sexually Transmitted Diseases

(Note: Sexually transmitted diseases are also discussed in Chapter 16.)

A **sexually transmitted disease** (STD) is a disease caused by a pathogen (e.g., virus, bacterium, parasite, or fungus) that is spread from person to person, primarily through sexual contact. STDs were once called the outdated term **venereal diseases** after Venus, the goddess of love. Currently there are more than 20 types of STDs in existence that affect millions of men and women in the United States alone. STDs can be painful, irritating, debilitating, and life-threatening. The following are the most common STDs encountered by medical transcriptionists in the field of men's health, including causes and treatments:

Genital Herpes

Genital herpes is an STD caused by the herpes simplex virus (HSV). There are two kinds of herpes simplex virus, indicated as type 1 (HSV-1) and type 2 (HSV-2). HSV-1 and HSV-2 can be found in and released from the sores that the viruses cause, but they also are released between episodes from skin that does not appear to be broken or to have a sore. A person almost always gets HSV-2 infection during sexual contact with someone who has a genital HSV-2 infection, either during an outbreak of the infection or during a period with no symptoms. HSV-1 causes infections of the mouth and lips, so-called fever blisters. A person can get HSV-1 by coming into contact with the saliva of an infected person. HSV-1 infection of the genitals almost always is caused by oral-genital sexual contact with a person who has the oral HSV-1 infection, causing inflamed blisters and ulcers on the shaft of the penis or rectal area. Once infected, the virus remains in certain nerve cells of the body for life, causing periodic flares of small, painful, fluid-filled blisters.

Although there is no cure for genital herpes, there are oral medications available to treat symptoms and to help prevent future outbreaks which, in turn, can decrease the risk of passing herpes to sexual partners. Medicines to treat genital herpes include acyclovir (Zovirax), famciclovir (Famvir), and valacyclovir (Valtrex).

Gonorrhea

Gonorrhea, or gonococcus (GC), infection is a bacterial infection caused by the organism *Neisseria gonorrhoeae* that is transmitted by sexual contact and multiplies rapidly after it enters the body. It is usually transmitted by direct contact with an infected person during vaginal, anal, or oral sex, or during the birth process. Among men and women who are infected, up to one-half will also be infected with *Chlamydia trachomatis*, another type of bacteria that causes another STD, described in subsequent text. For men, symptoms include a burning sensation when urinating or a white, yellow, or green discharge from the penis. Sometimes men with gonorrhea get painful or swollen testicles.

In the past, the treatment of uncomplicated gonorrhea was a single injection of penicillin. Today, however, new strains of gonorrhea have become resistant to penicillin and are therefore more difficult to treat. Other drugs that have been developed to treat gonorrheal infections include the antibiotics cefixime (Suprax), ciprofloxacin (Cipro), ofloxacin (Floxin), and levofloxacin (Levaquin). Concurrent treatment for chlamydia is included since gonorrhea and chlamydia often exist together in the same person.

Chlamydia

Chlamydia is the most common bacterial STD in the United States today. It is caused by the bacterium *Chlamydia trachomatis* and can be transmitted during vaginal, oral, or anal sexual contact with an infected partner. In men, untreated chlamydia can affect the testicles, leading to swelling and pain. Related complications can lead to infertility.

There are many antibiotics that are effective against chlamydia, the most common is azithromycin (Zithromax), which often clears the infection in a single dose. Doxycycline can also be prescribed for seven days. Unlike the bacteria that cause gonorrhea, chlamydial organisms have not developed a significant resistance to antibiotics.

DIAGNOSTIC STUDIES AND PROCEDURES

Problems in the urinary system can be detected using a variety of laboratory and imaging techniques. These diagnostic studies help identify problems so treatment can begin promptly.

Laboratory Tests

Tests performed on samples of blood and urine are usually the first step in evaluating urinary tract problems. These tests can show how well the organs of the urinary system are functioning to eliminate excess fluids and waste.

Blood Studies

Blood tests are commonly used to help physicians determine if the kidneys are failing to remove wastes. The tests commonly used to analyze the function of the urinary tract include:

- **Glomerular filtration rate** (GFR). The glomerular filtration rate (GFR) refers to the rate at which wastes are filtered from the blood (per minute). This test measures how well the kidneys are removing excess fluid and waste from the blood. It is calculated with a formula considering the patient's age, weight, and body size. The result is a two-digit arabic number, with a normal value being 90 or higher.
- **Blood urea nitrogen** (BUN). Blood urea nitrogen (BUN) is produced from the breakdown of food protein and is a measure of the kidneys' ability to excrete urea. It is transcribed as a value of milligrams per deciliter, or mg/dL. A normal BUN level is between 7 and 20 mg/dL; higher numbers indicate decreased kidney function.
- Serum creatinine. **Creatinine** is a waste product from meat protein and from normal wear and tear on the body. As with BUN, it is transcribed as a value of milligrams per deciliter, or mg/dL. A normal creatinine level is between approximately 0.6 and 1.2 mg/dL; as kidney disease progresses, the level of creatinine in the blood increases.
- **Electrolytes**. The balances of these minerals that maintain **homeostasis** are often affected by kidney disease (see Chapter 8 for a more detailed discussion of the function of electrolytes).
- Complete blood count (CBC). Hemoglobin, measured as part of a complete blood count, may be indicative of kidney abnormalities. As the kidneys produce erythropoietin, a hormone that controls red blood cell production, a low hemoglobin value may indicate the onset of anemia due to kidney malfunction.

To diagnose prostate disorders, physicians check the blood for levels of PSA. Some diseases, including prostate cancer, cause the prostate to make a larger quantity of PSA, as discussed previously. By measuring PSA levels in the blood, doctors may be able to find prostate cancers in their early stages. A sample of blood is drawn from a vein, and the level of PSA in the blood is obtained in the laboratory, transcribed as nanograms per milliliter, or ng/mL. A normal PSA value is 4 ng/mL or less.

Urine Studies

Urine tests can show how quickly waste materials are being removed and can disclose evidence of abnormalities in the urinary system, even when there are no

TABLE 15.1   Abnormal Components of Urine

Characteristic	Formal Name	Meaning
Glucose	Glycosuria	The presence of glucose in the urine indicates that blood glucose is more than what the kidneys can absorb.
Protein	Proteinuria	Protein in the urine indicates that the glomeruli are not filtering blood properly.
Blood	Hematuria	Red blood cells may indicate bleeding in the urinary tract or improper filtration by the glomeruli.
Bacteria	Bacteriuria	Bacteria indicate an infection in the urinary tract.
Ketones	Ketonuria	Elevated levels of ketones indicate abnormal carbohydrate metabolism in the body.
White blood cells	Pyuria	White blood cells or pus in the urine usually signifies a urinary tract infection, such as cystitis, or renal disease.

significant signs or symptoms. Tests that evaluate the urine for genitourinary disorders include the following:

- Urinalysis and culture. Normal urine contains fluids, salts, and waste products; but it is free of bacteria, viruses, fungi, and other substances. A complete urinalysis includes a microscopic examination of a urine sample as well as a dipstick test. The presence of some substances that do not belong in urine may indicate abnormal kidney function or other problems such as diabetes, bladder infections, and kidney stones. Table 15.1 lists some abnormal substances that could be found in urine and possible reasons for each. A urine culture can identify the specific bacteria causing a urinary tract infection so that proper antibiotics can be administered.
- **Creatinine clearance**. This test is used to help evaluate the rate and efficiency of kidney filtration by the glomeruli. It compares the level of creatinine found in a 24-hour collection of urine to the creatinine level in the blood to measure how much creatinine is removed from the blood by the kidneys per minute, a value transcribed as milliliters per minute mL/min. A decrease in creatinine clearance indicates less creatinine is being excreted in the urine due to less blood flow to the kidneys; this can indicate disorders such as congestive heart failure, kidney obstruction, or kidney failure.

STD Cultures

A **culture** is a material or specimen obtained from the body and incubated with a nutrient medium to isolate organisms and determine the cause of an illness or infection. Specimens for STD cultures are obtained to look for signs of the bacteria that cause infection from

STDs, most commonly gonorrhea and chlamydia. In this procedure, a sample of the discharge that is present is obtained from the penis with a swab or small brush and sent to a laboratory. The sample is combined with substances that promote the growth of bacteria, and the cultures are left to grow for a couple of days. After this time, the sample that is cultured is examined under a microscope for the presence of the bacteria that cause gonorrhea and chlamydia. If bacteria are present in either culture, the test is said to be *positive*; if no bacteria are present, the test is *negative*.

Radiologic Studies

Physicians have used x-ray technology to diagnose diseases for more than 100 years. In the genitourinary system, x-rays can help highlight the location of kidney stones, show the size and shape of the prostate, and reveal blockages in the urinary tract.

Kidney, Ureter, and Bladder X-ray

A **kidney, ureter, and bladder x-ray** (KUB) is a supine x-ray of the abdomen, showing the kidneys (K), ureters (U), and bladder (B). Also called a *flat plate x-ray*, a KUB may be performed to diagnose the cause of abdominal pain, such as masses, perforations, or obstructions in the urinary tract. In addition, a KUB can supply basic information regarding the size, shape, and position of the kidneys, ureters, and bladder.

Intravenous Pyelogram

An **intravenous pyelogram** (IVP) is a series of x-rays taken of the kidneys, ureters, and bladder in order to locate a suspected obstruction to the flow of urine through the collecting system (such as a stone) and to define the degree of blockage caused by the obstruction. In this procedure, a contrast dye is injected into a patient's vein and a series of x-rays is taken as the dye moves through the kidneys, ureters, and bladder. The dye provides an outline of the entire urinary system and shows any narrowing or blockage in the urinary tract.

Voiding Cystourethrogram

A **voiding cystourethrogram** (VCUG) is another type of x-ray procedure that looks at the functioning of the bladder. In patients who have recurrent urinary tract infections, this test is used to locate a possible defect in the urinary tract as a cause of the problem. It can also show blockages from an enlarged prostate in men or abnormal bladder position in women. In this procedure, a catheter is inserted into the urethra and used to fill the bladder with contrast dye. The x-ray machine then captures images of the dye during urination. The dye shows whether urine is backing up into the ureters or whether urine outflow through the urethra is blocked.

Ultrasound Studies

An ultrasound study uses high-frequency radio waves to get a picture of the kidneys. It may be used to look for abnormalities in size or position of the kidneys or to look for obstructions such as stones or tumors. In this test, a technician holds a transducer that sends sound waves into the body; the waves bounce off internal body structures and create a picture on a monitor. A **transrectal ultrasound** is used to examine the prostate. The transducer is inserted into the rectum so that it lies next to the prostate. The ultrasound waves are directed at the prostate and the echo images create an image of the gland on a monitor. The image obtained shows the size and shape of the prostate and any irregularity that might be a tumor.

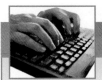

TRANSCRIPTION TIP:

When dictating urologic procedures, many physicians may use the abbreviated form *cysto* to describe the procedure. Do not expand this abbreviation unless you are absolutely sure the dictator is talking about a *cystoscopy* versus a *cystometry*.

Endoscopic Studies

As with other body systems, a flexible endoscope can be used to examine structures of the urinary system and to transmit those images to a television-type monitor. **Cystoscopy** is a procedure that uses a lighted scope called a cystoscope to view both the urethra (including the prostate in men) and the bladder. A cystoscope has extra attachments, such as a camera tip and extra tubes, to guide instruments for procedures to treat urinary problems. In this test, the cystoscope is inserted into the urethra and passed into the bladder to examine the urethra and interior lining of the bladder for tumors, obstructions, or other problems.

A **ureteroscopy** is a procedure used to locate and examine stones located in the lower portion of the ureter. An endoscopic instrument called a **ureteroscope** is inserted through the urethra and bladder to the location of the stone in the ureter. As with other endoscopic instruments, once a stone is located, it can be examined for its properties; or, using extra instruments attached to the ureteroscope, the stone can be removed using a small basket inserted through the ureteroscope or broken into fragments using a laser device attached to the ureteroscope.

Urodynamic Studies

Urodynamics is the study of the function or dysfunction of the lower urinary tract—bladder and urethra—using measurements such as urine pressure and flow

QUICK CHECK 15.5 ✓

Indicate whether each of the following is a (L) laboratory test, (R) radiologic test, (E) endoscopic procedure, or (U) urodynamic study.

1. KUB   _____

2. GFR   _____

3. VCUG   _____

4. UA   _____

5. CMG   _____

rates. **Urodynamic studies** are a series of tests that evaluate how the body stores and releases urine. These tests can show if the bladder empties steadily and completely or whether there are abnormal contractions that can cause leakage.

The first test in the procedure is called **uroflowmetry**, which is the measurement of urine speed and volume. Also dictated simply as a *uroflow*, this test measures the amount of urine expelled from the bladder as well as the flow rate, or how fast the urine is expelled. After the test is complete, a small catheter is placed inside the bladder to measure the amount of any remaining urine, called the **postvoid residual**, to check how well the bladder emptied. Following this measurement is a **cystometrogram** (CMG), or simply **cystometry**, which is a filling study to evaluate the function and stability of the bladder. This test measures how much the bladder can hold, how much pressure builds in the bladder as it stores urine, and how full it is when the patient feels the need to urinate. To obtain these values, a thin catheter with a pressure-measuring tube called a **cystometer** is placed into the bladder. The cystometer is used to fill the bladder slowly with warm water, measuring the pressure during various stages of filling (the volume of water and the bladder pressure when the patient feels the need to urinate). The cystometer also measures the extent to which the bladder muscle stretches during filling. Involuntary bladder contractions during the filling process can be identified and are used to measure how well the bladder stores fluid. Once all measuring of volumes and pressures is complete, the resulting measurements are analyzed to help the physician develop a treatment plan for a patient's individual bladder problem.

CHAPTER SUMMARY

Although classified as a surgical subspecialty, urology focuses on both the surgical and medical management of diseases of the male and female urinary tracts, as well as of the male reproductive organs. As a result, urology presents a wide spectrum of topics for medical transcription, ranging from office clinic notes to reports of minimally invasive outpatient procedures and complex surgical operations. With the aging population and the continued rise in the number of patients with urologic problems, urology is a rapidly expanding area of medicine, and advances in both diagnostic technology and treatment of urologic disorders ensure continued growth of this specialty field.

· I · N · S · I · G · H · T ·

A Simple Urine Test to Diagnose Autism?

Researchers from the Imperial College London and the University of South Australia have found that children diagnosed as autistic have a different chemical fingerprint in their urine than nonautistic children. This discovery will enable medical professionals to quickly identify the disorder in children and to provide care earlier in their development than is currently possible, thus greatly improving their progress. Although this chemical fingerprint is present a birth, currently autistic children are not diagnosed with the disorder until they start showing problems with communication and social skills, typically at anywhere from one to five years of age. The lengthy testing process currently in use includes evaluation in social interaction, communication, and imaginative skills testing; and even then, it is difficult to establish a definitive diagnosis.

The researchers discovered that children with autism spectrum disorder (ASD) have unusual microbes in their digestive systems that can be used to identify them as autism candidates as early as six months of age. By analyzing the chemical makeup of urine samples in groups of both autistic and nonaustistic children between ages three and nine, researchers found that children diagnosed with autism had a distinct metabolic fingerprint that was different from children who were not diagnosed with the disorder or those who were not diagnosed with the disorder but had an autistic sibling. The research is still in its early stages and more studies are needed; but the research is built on the known premise that, for some unknown reason, people with autism have a different makeup of bacteria in their GI systems than do nonautistic people. The goal of the research is to make it possible to distinguish between autistic and nonautistic children by looking at the byproducts of bacteria in the gut and the body's metabolic processes in the children's urine. If successful, this test would save families the trauma and expense of the countless psychological and medical tests currently used to pinpoint the disorder and would enable treatment to begin months or even years before the behavioral symptoms appear. Early diagnosis and treatment can greatly improve the quality of life of autistic children in years to come.

The next step in this research is to test a larger number of participants; but if continued trials demonstrate that the test works, it could be on the market within five years and cost as little as $10.

Common Soundalike Words

Word	Word Pronunciation	Soundalike	Soundalike Pronunciation
cystotome: In urology, an instrument used for incising. The term spelled with the letter "o" pertains to urology.	sis'tō-tōm	**cystitome**: In ophthalmology, an instrument used to open the capsule. The term spelled with the letter "i" pertains to the eye.	sis'ti-tōm
vesical: Relating to any bladder, but usually the urinary bladder.	ves'i-kăl	**vesicle**: A small sac containing liquid or gas.	ves'i-kăl
anuresis: A condition of inability to urinate. Total lack of urine.	an-yū'rē-sis	**enuresis**: Another word for bedwetting.	en-yū-rē'sis
prostate: Referring to the prostate gland.	pros'tāt	**prostrate**: Lying prone.	pros'-trāt
glans: A conical acorn-shaped structure (as in glans penis).	glanz	**glands**: An organized aggregation of cells functioning as a secretory or excretory organ.	glandz
dialysis: A method of artificial kidney function.	dī-al'i-sis	**diaphysis**: The long shaft of bone.	dī-af'i-sis
efflux: The process of flowing out, as in the flow of urine.	ē'flŭks	**reflux**: An abnormal backward flow, as of urine through the ureters.	rē'flŭks
ureteral: Pertaining to the ureter.	yū-rē'tĕr-ăl	**urethral**: Pertaining to the urethra.	yū-rē'thrăl
dilation: Expansion of an organ or vessel.	dī-lā'shŭn	**dilution**: Reducing the concentration of a substance by the addition of water or a thinner.	dī-lū'shŭn
creatinine: A component of urine.	krē-at'i-nēn	**creatine**: An amino acid found in the muscle tissue of vertebrates.	krē'ă-tēn

Combining Forms

Combining Form	Meaning	Combining Form	Meaning
albumin/o	protein	micturi/o	making urine
bacteri/o	bacteria	necr/o	death
balan/o	glans penis	nephr/o, ren/o	kidney
calcul/o	stone	noct/i	night
cali/o, calic/o	calyx	olig/o	little, few
cyst/o, vesic/o	urinary bladder	orch/o, orchi/o, orchid/o	testis or testicle
dialy/o	to separate	pelv/o, pyel/o	pelvis
epididym/o	epididymis	prostat/o	prostate
glomerul/o	glomerulus (little ball)	py/o	pus
gluc/o, glyc/o	sugar	sperm/o, spermat/o	sperm
inguin/o	groin	test/o	testis or testicle
ket/o, keton/o	ketones	trigon/o	trigone
leuk/o	white	ureter/o	ureter
lith/o	stone	urethr/o	urethra
meat/o	opening	ur/o, urin/o	urine
medull/o	medulla (inner region)	vas/o	vessel

Add Your Own Combining Forms Here:

_____

_____

_____

_____

_____

_____

ABBREVIATIONS

Abbreviation	Meaning	Abbreviation	Meaning
ADH	antidiuretic hormone	IVP	intravenous pyelogram
ADPKD	autosomal dominant polycystic kidney disease	KUB	kidney, ureter, and bladder (x-ray)
AV	arteriovenous	LHRH	luteinizing hormone releasing hormone
BPH	benign prostatic hyperplasia	PCN	percutaneous nephrolithotomy
BUN	blood urea nitrogen	PKD	polycystic kidney disease
CBC	complete blood count	PSA	prostate-specific antigen
CMG	cystometrogram	PVP	photoselective vaporization prostatectomy
DHT	dihydroxy testosterone		
DRE	digital rectal examination	STD	sexually transmitted disease
ESWL	extracorporeal shock wave lithotripsy	TURB	transurethral resection of bladder tumor
GFR	glomerular filtration rate	TURP	transurethral resection of the prostate
GU	genitourinary		
HLA	human leukocyte antigen	UTI	urinary tract infection
IC	interstitial cystitis	VCUG	voiding cystourethrogram

Add Your Own Abbreviations Here:

_____

_____

_____

_____

_____

_____

TERMINOLOGY

Term	Meaning
abdominal aorta	The portion of the aorta that passes through the general area of the stomach in the body.
access	The site on the body where blood will be removed and returned during dialysis.
acute renal failure	The sudden loss of the kidneys to excrete wastes.
adenocarcinoma of the prostate	Another name for *prostate cancer*.
adrenal gland	A small gland on top of each kidney that produces hormones which help control certain body functions.
androgen agonists	Another term for *antiandrogens*.
antiandrogens	A class of hormonal drugs used to stop testosterone from the testicles from getting to cancer cells and encouraging them to grow.
antibodies	A type of protein produced by the immune system in response to foreign substances that may be a threat to the body.
antidiuretic hormone (ADH)	A hormone that is released when the amount of water in the body decreases.
antigen	Any substance, such as chemicals, viruses, spores, or bacteria, which causes the immune system to produce antibodies against it.
arteriovenous (AV) fistula	An opening artificially created between an artery and vein to provide adequate blood flow for dialysis.
arteriovenous (AV) graft	A synthetic tube used as an artificial vein connected to an artery to provide adequate blood flow for dialysis.
atrophy	Muscle wasting.
autosomal dominant polycystic kidney disease (ADPKD)	An inherited form of polycystic kidney disease (PKD).
bacteruria	The presence of bacteria in the urine.
benign prostatic hyperplasia (BPH)	Enlargement of the prostate.
bladder distention	A procedure whereby the bladder is inflated with gas or liquid.
bladder instillation	A procedure whereby the bladder is inflated with the chemical compound DMSO to reduce inflammation and pain.
bladder neck	The opening from the trigone, which contains the opening into the urethra.
bladder reconstruction	A surgical procedure in which a section of bowel is made into a balloon-shaped sac and connected to the top of the urethra so that urine can be stored and drained from the body normally.
blood urea nitrogen (BUN)	A substance produced from the breakdown of food protein and a measure of the kidneys' ability to excrete urea.
Bowman capsule	Another name for *glomerular capsule*.
brachytherapy	An outpatient procedure in which tiny radioactive seeds are implanted into the prostate to help destroy cancer cells.
bulbourethral glands	Pea-sized structures that produce a clear fluid that empties directly into the urethra to lubricate the urethra and neutralize any acidity that may be present from residual urine.
cadaveric transplant	A transplantation procedure in which the donated kidney comes from a dead person.

Term	Meaning
calcitriol	An active form of vitamin D that helps increase the absorption of calcium and phosphorus from the small intestine.
calyx (plural, calyces)	Funnel-shaped extension of the renal pelvis.
carcinoma in situ	A cancer that has not spread to other areas of the body or nearby organs.
chlamydia	The most common type of sexually transmitted disease in the United States, named after the bacterium that causes the infection.
chordee	A downward curve of the shaft of the penis.
chronic kidney failure	A long-term condition in which the kidneys gradually and progressively lose their ability to function.
clean catch	The collection of a midstream sample of urine in a sterile container.
Cowper glands	Another name for the *bulbourethral glands*.
creatinine	A waste product from meat protein and from normal wear and tear on the body.
creatinine clearance	A test used to help evaluate the rate and efficiency of kidney filtration by the glomeruli.
crossmatching antigen test	A test that is performed to define how a kidney transplant recipient may respond to particular cells or proteins of the kidney donor.
cryoablation	A procedure in which extreme cold is used to destroy cancerous tissue.
cryoprobe	The instrument used to apply extreme cold to tissue.
culture	A material or specimen obtained from the body and incubated with a nutrient medium to isolate organisms and determine the cause of an illness or infection.
cystine	An organic building block that helps make up muscles, nerves, and other parts of the body.
cystocele	A condition that occurs when the wall between the bladder and the vagina weakens, causing the bladder to drop or sag into the vagina.
cystometer	An instrument that is used to study the pressure and filling capacity of the bladder.
cystometrogram (CMG)	A urodynamic study that measures the function and stability of the bladder.
cystometry	Another name for *cystometrogram*.
cystoscope	An endoscopic instrument used to examine the bladder and urethra.
cystoscopy	A procedure that examines structures of the urinary system.
detrusor muscle	The outermost layer of muscle of the bladder.
dialysis	The process of artificially removing wastes from the blood when the kidneys are not able to do so naturally.
dialysis machine	A machine that artificially filters blood similar to the way the kidneys filter blood in the renal glomeruli and tubules.
digital rectal examination (DRE)	A procedure whereby a gloved finger is inserted into the rectum and pressed on the prostate to check for enlargement.
dihydroxy testosterone (DHT)	A male hormone that is known to have a key role in prostate growth.
dysuria	Difficult or painful urination.
electrolytes	Minerals that regulate the body's balance of fluids.
end-stage renal disease (ESRD)	A name given to kidney failure that is so advanced that it cannot be reversed.
epididymis	A coiled tube in each testis that stores sperm until ejaculation.
epididymitis	An inflammation of the epididymis.

Term	*Meaning*
erythropoietin	A hormone that aids in the formation of red blood cells.
excretory system	Another name for the *urinary system*.
external urethral sphincter	A collective name for the muscles that expand and contract and work in conjunction with the internal urethral sphincter to control the flow of urine from the bladder.
extracorporeal shock wave lithotripsy (ESWL)	A procedure that uses highly focused impulses projected from outside the body to pulverize kidney stones.
fistula	An abnormal opening or connection between any two parts of the body which are usually separate.
focal segmental glomerulosclerosis	A condition resulting in scar tissue that forms some segments of the glomeruli in the kidney.
fulguration	Destroying tissue using an electric current.
genital herpes	A sexually transmitted disease caused by the herpes simplex virus.
genitourinary	Referring to both the organs of male reproduction and urination.
glans penis	The external swelling at the tip of the penis.
glomerular capsule	Also called *Bowman capsule*, a saclike structure surrounding the glomerulus of each nephron of the kidney which filters organic wastes, excess inorganic salts, and water from blood.
glomerular filtrate	The filtered fluid from the glomeruli.
glomerular filtration rate (GFR)	The rate at which wastes are filtered out of the blood per minute.
glomerulonephritis	An inflammation of the glomeruli.
glomerulosclerosis	The scarring or hardening of the tiny blood vessels within the kidney.
glomerulus (plural, glomeruli)	A ball-shaped cluster of tiny capillaries on a renal corpuscle, which is the area of blood filtering in the kidney.
gonorrhea	A sexually transmitted bacterial infection caused by the organism *Neisseria gonorrhoeae*.
hematuria	The presence of blood in the urine.
hemodialysis	A process of dialysis accomplished by the filtering of blood through a machine located outside the body.
human leukocyte antigens (HLAs)	Antigens tolerated by the body, corresponding to genes that govern immune responses.
hyperkalemia	An excessive amount of potassium in the blood.
hypospadias	A birth defect found in boys in which the opening to the urethra develops at a point under the penis instead of at the tip of the penis.
ileal conduit	A surgical connection in the abdomen that allows urine to bypass the bladder and exit into an external collecting pouch.
inferior vena cava	The major vein that returns deoxygenated blood from the kidneys back to the heart.
internal urethral sphincter	Part of the detrusor muscle that surrounds the bladder neck, which prevents the bladder from involuntarily emptying until urination occurs.
interstitial cystitis (IC)	An inflammation of the bladder wall.
interstitial nephritis	An inflammation of the spaces between the renal tubules.
intravenous pyelogram (IVP)	A series of x-rays taken of the kidneys, ureters, and bladder to locate obstructions to the flow of urine using contrast dye.

Term	Meaning
invasive cancer	A cancer that spreads beyond its site of origin to involve other tissues and organs.
Kegel exercises	A series of pelvic floor exercises that helps strengthen the muscles in and around the vagina.
kidney failure	The loss of the kidneys' ability to adequately filter waste from the body adequately.
kidney stone	A hard, solid piece of material that forms in the kidney from crystals that separate from the urine and build up on the inner surface of the kidney.
kidney transplantation	A surgical procedure in which a healthy kidney from a one person (the donor) is placed into the body of another person (the recipient).
kidney, ureter and bladder x-ray (KUB)	A supine x-ray of the kidney, ureters, and bladder.
kidneys	The paired organs of the genitourinary system responsible for the excretion of urine from the body.
Koch (pouch)	An internal pouch used to collect urine in a urostomy procedure.
lithotripsy	A method of breaking up urinary stones with a specialized tool and shock waves.
living-related transplant	A transplantation procedure in which the donor is a living relative of the recipient.
luteinizing hormone releasing hormone (LHRH) agonists	A class of drugs that block the message from the pituitary gland for the testes to produce testosterone that enables a tumor to grow.
lymphadenectomy	Surgical removal of lymph nodes.
meatus	The opening to the urethra.
muscularis propria	Another name for *detrusor muscle*.
necrosis	Tissue death.
negative crossmatch	A blood test result indicating that an organ transplantation should proceed.
nephritis	A broad term for any inflammation of one or both kidneys.
nephrolithiasis	The presence of stones in the kidneys.
nephrology	The branch of medicine concerned with the study of the kidney.
nephrons	The microscopic filtering units of the kidney.
nephroscope	An endoscopic instrument used to locate and remove kidney stones.
neurogenic bladder	A disorder resulting from damage to nerves that govern the urinary tract.
orchidectomy	Another term for *orchiectomy*.
orchiectomy	Surgical removal of the testicles.
orchitis	An inflammation of the testis.
papilla	The tip of the renal pyramid.
parenchyma	The functional tissue of the kidney.
penis	The external male urinary and reproductive organ.
percutaneous nephrolithotomy (PCN)	A procedure that uses a scope placed through an incision in the side of the abdomen to remove a kidney stone that is too big to pass.
peritoneal dialysis peritoneum	A process of dialysis that involves using the peritoneum as a dialysis filter with which to filter the blood. The membranous lining of the abdominal cavity.
pessary	A plastic or rubber ring placed in the vagina to push the bladder back into place.

Term	Meaning
photoselective vaporization prostatectomy	A procedure in which a high-power laser is used to vaporize prostatic adenomas.
polycystic kidney disease (PKD)	A genetic disorder characterized by the growth of numerous fluid-filled cysts in the kidneys.
polyuria	Excessive urination.
positive crossmatch	A blood test result indicating that an organ transplantation should not proceed.
postvoid residual	A urodynamic study that measures how well the bladder empties.
prostate	A gland in the male reproductive system just below the bladder that secretes PSA, which helps form part of semen.
prostate-specific antigen (PSA)	An enzyme secreted by the prostate that helps form part of semen.
prostatitis	An inflammation of the prostate gland.
proteinuria	Excessive amounts of protein in the urine.
pyelonephritis	An inflammation of the renal pelvis as a result of a bacterial or viral infection.
pyuria	The presence of pus in the urine.
radical cystectomy	A procedure in which the entire bladder is removed, along with part of the urethra and nearby organs and structures that may contain cancer cells.
radical perineal prostatectomy	A prostatectomy that is performed through the perineum.
radical prostatectomy	Total surgical removal of the prostate gland, the seminal vesicles, and part of the vas deferens.
radical retropubic (or suprapubic) prostatectomy	A prostatectomy that is performed through an abdominal approach.
reflux nephropathy	A condition in which the kidneys are damaged by backward flow of urine into the kidney.
rejection	A reaction in which the immune system attacks foreign tissue, including transplanted organs.
renal artery	The artery that branches off from the abdominal aorta, which is the major source of blood to the kidneys.
renal calculus (plural, calculi)	A hard, solid piece of material that forms in the kidney from crystals that separate from the urine and build up on the inner surface of the kidney.
renal capsule	The membrane that encapsulates each kidney.
renal columns	The tissue of the renal cortex in between the renal pyramids.
renal corpuscle	One of two major parts of a nephron of the kidney.
renal cortex	The outermost area of the kidney.
renal failure	Another name for *kidney failure*.
renal fascia	A layer of connective tissue that attaches the kidney to the abdominal wall.
renal hilum	The entrance on the medial border of the kidney through which blood vessels, nerves, and a ureter pass.
renal medulla	The middle area of the kidney that contains the renal pyramids.
renal pelvis	The large cavity formed by the expansion of the ureter within the kidney at the hilum that collects urine as it is produced.
renal pyramids	Wedge-shaped masses of tissues in the renal medulla.
renal sinus	The hollow cavity of the kidney.
renal tubule	One of two major parts of a nephron of the kidney.

Term	*Meaning*
renin	An enzyme that initiates other enzymes that help raise blood pressure levels.
resection	The surgical removal of tissue or part or all of an organ.
resectoscope	A thin, lighted tube inserted through the penis into the urethra used to remove obstructing tissue and seal blood vessels in the prostate gland.
scrotum	A sac at the base of the penis that holds the testicles.
segmental cystectomy	A procedure in which part of the bladder is removed.
seminal vesicles	Fluid-producing pouches that attach to the vas deferens near the base of the bladder, the fluid of which helps with sperm motility.
sexually transmitted disease (STD)	A disease caused by a pathogen that is spread from person to person, primarily through sexual contact.
spermatic cord	The structure that carries sperm from the body.
squamous cell carcinoma	A cancer that begins in the squamous cells of the bladder.
struvite	A chemical compound that can form crystals in the kidney and bladder.
testes (singular, testis)	Another name for *testicles*.
testicles	The organs that produce sperm and testosterone.
testicular torsion	A twisting of the testicles around the spermatic cord, resulting in decreased blood flow to the testes.
tissue typing	A test used to determine the genetic match between the donor of a transplanted organ and its recipient.
transitional cell carcinoma	A cancer that originates in the transitional cells of the bladder.
transrectal ultrasound	An ultrasound procedure used to examine the prostate.
transurethral resection of bladder (tumor) (TURB)	A surgical procedure in which a tumor is removed from the bladder through the urethra.
transurethral resection of the prostate (TURP)	A surgical procedure to remove tissue from the prostate using a lighted resectoscope inserted through the urethra.
trigone	The triangular area at the base of the bladder.
tubulointerstitial nephritis	An inflammation of the renal tubules and spaces between the tubules.
urea	A byproduct of the metabolic process in the liver.
uremia, syn. azotemia	An excess of urea and other nitrogenous waste in the blood.
ureter	A thin tube that carries urine from the kidney to the urinary bladder.
ureteral orifices	The openings from the ureters to the bladder.
ureteral sphincter	A muscular flap that covers the opening where the urine enters and acts like a valve which allows urine to enter the bladder but prevents it from backing up from the bladder into the ureter.
ureterolithiasis	The presence of stones in the ureter.
ureteroscope	An endoscopic instrument used to remove or break up stones located in the lower portion of the ureter.
ureteroscopy	A procedure used to remove or break up stones located in the lower portion of the ureter.
urethra	A tube that conveys urine from the bladder to the outside of the body.
urethritis	An inflammation of the urethra.
uric acid	A byproduct of metabolism that can cause crystals to develop in the kidneys.
urinary bladder	A hollow, muscular sac that stores urine before it is eliminated from the body.

Term	Meaning
urinary diversion	Another term for *urostomy*.
urinary incontinence	Loss of bladder control and leakage of urine.
urinary system	The body system that filters the blood and expels the resulting liquid waste products as urine.
urinary tract infection (UTI)	An infection in the urinary tract caused by disease-causing microorganisms.
urine	A waste product produced by the kidneys during the process of cleaning the blood.
urodynamic studies	A series of tests that evaluate how the body stores and releases urine.
urodynamics	The study of the function or dysfunction of the bladder and urethra.
uroflowmetry	A urodynamic study that measures urine speed and volume.
urolithiasis	Another name for *nephrolithiasis*.
urologist	A physician who has specialized knowledge and skill regarding problems with both the male and female urinary tracts and the male genital organs.
urology	The medical specialty that deals with disturbances of the male and female urinary tract system as well as the male reproductive organs.
urostomy	Another term for *urinary diversion*.
venereal diseases	An outdated term for *sexually transmitted diseases*.
vesicoureteral reflux	A condition where the urine backs up from the bladder into the ureters.
voiding cystourethrogram (VCUG)	An x-ray procedure using contrast dye that captures images of the bladder during urination.

Add Your Own Terms and Definitions Here:

_____

_____

_____

_____

_____

_____

_____

_____

REVIEW QUESTIONS

1. What are the three distinct regions of the kidney?
2. What openings form the bladder trigone?
3. Describe the difference between glomerulonephritis and focal segmental glomerulosclerosis.
4. Name the four types of kidney stones that form as a result of electrolyte imbalances.
5. What is PSA?
6. What do Cowper glands do?
7. What does GFR stand for and what does it measure?
8. Name three different functions of the kidneys.
9. What is the treatment for hypospadias?
10. How does BPH affect the urethra?

CHAPTER ACTIVITIES

Soundalike Word Choice

Circle the correct word in the following sentences.

1. We recommended Kegel exercises to help with her (cystocele/cystogram).
2. Enlargement of the prostate or (TURP/BPH) is a common disorder of aging.
3. The tube that carries urine from the kidney to the bladder is the (urethra/ureter).
4. The patient is scheduled to have her (cystectomy/cystocele) procedure next week.
5. PKD can cause cysts to interfere with (necrotic/nephron) function.
6. A kidney stone is also called a renal (calcium/calculus).
7. (BUN/BUS) is produced from the breakdown of food protein.
8. The lab work showed his (PSA/PKD) level had risen to 4.5 in the last month.
9. Physicians use (urodynamic/urethroscopic) studies to evaluate how the body stores and releases urine.
10. As kidney disease progresses, the level of (creatine/creatinine) in the blood increases.

Creating Medical Words

Search for and combine the following prefixes, suffixes, and combining forms in the following list to create medical words that best fit the definitions. Verify the spelling of the word you create with a medical dictionary.

-cele	-itis	orch-
-tripsy	necr/o	-metry
dys-	-sis	prostat-
nephr/o	hem/o	-logy
-iasis	dialy/o	-uria
-ectomy	cyst/o	aden/o
lith/o	-emia	-stasis
-sis	pyel/o	-lysis
ur/o	home/o	lymph-

Definitions

1. Difficult or painful urination. _____
2. A condition where the bladder falls into the vagina. _____
3. Inflammation of one or both kidneys. _____
4. An inflammation of the renal pelvis. _____
5. A state of balance in the body. _____
6. Blood in the urine. _____
7. A method of breaking up stones with shock waves. _____
8. Surgical removal of lymph nodes. _____
9. The study of the urinary tract system as well as male reproductive organs. _____
10. A study that measures the function and stability of the bladder. _____
11. Inflammation of the prostate gland. _____
12. An excess of urea and other nitrogenous waste in the blood. _____
13. Inflammation of one or both testes. _____
14. Tissue death. _____
15. The process of artificially removing wastes from the body when the kidneys cannot do so naturally. _____

True or False

Read each statement and indicate whether it is true or false. If false, rewrite the sentence in the Correction column to make the statement true.

Statement	True (T) or False (F)	Correction, if False
1. A Koch pouch is a pouch placed outside the abdomen.	_____	_____
2. The glomerular capsule is also called the Bowman capsule.	_____	_____
3. Urodynamics is the study of the function or dysfunction of the bladder and urethra.	_____	_____
4. A cystocele is an inflammation of the bladder.	_____	_____
5. The middle part of the kidney is called the renal medulla.	_____	_____
6. A patient's cross-matching antigen test is the most important matching factor to a donated kidney and its recipient.	_____	_____
7. ADH is a hormone that aids in the formation of red blood cells.	_____	_____
8. Urea is the most abundant of the waste products excreted by the kidneys.	_____	_____
9. The enlargement of the prostate is called PSA.	_____	_____
10. A cystocope is used to break up stones located in the lower portion of the ureter.	_____	_____

Understanding Medical Documents

Read the following excerpt from a procedure note and, using resource materials or the Internet to locate terms you do not know, answer the questions that follow.

The patient is postop percutaneous nephrolithotomy and shock wave lithotripsy. KUB today shows the same stent in the upper ureter that was present 3 weeks ago. We have, therefore, decided to perform a cystoscopy and remove the stent. The patient was placed in the lithotomy position. Of note, he did receive Zosyn antibiotic prior to the procedure. A 26-French resectoscope was placed through the urethra and into the bladder. The entire stent was visualized and was removed. The patient was given instructions to return for symptoms of renal colic and was given 2 days of antibiotics to take upon going home. We will see him again next week unless he is symptomatic before that.

1. What procedure is being described? What leads you to that conclusion?
2. What is a KUB?
3. What do the procedures indicated in the first line of the paragraph tell you about the type of procedure(s) the patient had previously undergone?
4. What is the lithotomy position?
5. What part of the urinary system would renal colic involve?
6. What is Zosyn? Why do you think the patient would receive this medication prior to the procedure?
7. What is a resectoscope?

Matching

Match following terms to the organ in which they belong. Some organs may be used more than once.

Term

1. _____ cystocele
2. _____ brachytherapy
3. _____ ADPKD
4. _____ hypospadias
5. _____ pessary
6. _____ torsion
7. _____ pyelonephritis
8. _____ BPH
9. _____ trigone
10. _____ meatus
11. _____ renin
12. _____ nephron
13. _____ detrusor
14. _____ ureteroscope
15. _____ transplant

Organ

A. Kidneys

B. Ureters

C. Bladder

D. Urethra

E. Prostate

F. Penis

G. Testicles

TRANSCRIPTION PRACTICE

Open your word-processing software. Insert the student CD-ROM and locate the dictation for this chapter. For each of the words in the "listen for these terms" list for each report, use a medical dictionary or other resources to identify and write down a brief definition of the term on a separate sheet of paper to attach with your work. Then listen to the dictation and transcribe each report. Use the current date for each report where a date is indicated. Insert a heading into the document if the text falls to a second page.

At the end of each report, indicate the name of the dictating physician under the signature line and insert reference initials. For date dictated and transcribed and date of admission, use the current date. Proofread your work, print one copy for your instructor along with your term definitions, and save the completed report to your student CD.

Report #T15.1: Consultation Letter
Patient Name: Jeremy Carter
Medical Record No.: CAR-3811
Attending Physician: Kamraan George, MD

Listen for these terms:
dysuria
hypospadias
inguinal hernia
hydrocele
deep tendon reflexes

Report #T15.2: Clinic Note
Patient Name: Eldridge Crawford
Medical Record No.: 990-47211
Attending Physician: Samuel Voorhees, MD

Listen for these terms:
Flomax
nocturia
DRE

Report #T15.3: Operative Report
Patient Name: Antonio Romero
Medical Record No.: 44-39012
Attending Physician: Aurelio Garza, MD
Assistant: Lena Kushner, MD

Listen for these terms:
congenital nephropathy
hockey-stick incision
extraperitoneal dissection
Prolene
revascularization
Lich technique
double-J stent
seromuscular
Dexon

16

OBSTETRICS AND GYNECOLOGY

INTRODUCTION

Obstetrics is the branch of medicine that deals with the care of women during pregnancy, childbirth, and the recuperative period following delivery. The term derives from the Latin word *obstetrix*, meaning midwife. An **obstetrician** is a physician who is a specialist in the management of pregnancy and childbirth.

Gynecology literally means *the science of women*, but in medicine, this specialty focuses on the female repro-

ductive system. The term *gynecology* derives from the Greek word *gune*, meaning woman. A **gynecologist** is a physician who has specialized education and training in the health issues of the female reproductive system, including the diagnosis and treatment of gynecologic disorders and diseases.

Typically, a physician's education and training for both fields occurs concurrently. Thus, an **obstetrician/ gynecologist** (OB/GYN) is a physician who provides medical and surgical care of gynecologic health and also has particular expertise in reproductive issues. An OB/GYN practice includes preventative GYN care; prenatal care, including complications of pregnancy; sexually transmitted diseases; gynecologic cancers; diseases and disorders of the female urinary tract; and family planning.

This chapter provides a basic introduction to the anatomy and physiology of the female reproductive system, as well as to the basic processes of fertilization, pregnancy, and delivery. This chapter also reviews common gynecologic diseases and disorders, and the typical laboratory and diagnostic studies used to evaluate and treat them.

ANATOMY OF THE FEMALE REPRODUCTIVE SYSTEM

The female reproductive system consists of the external and internal genital organs, as well as the breasts. The

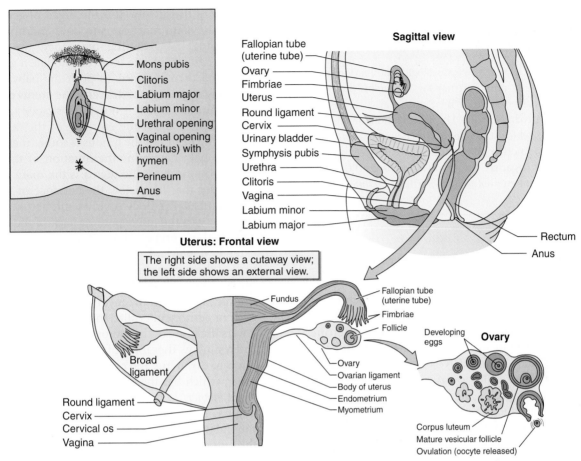

FIGURE 16.1. The Female Reproductive System. Reprinted with permission from Willis MC. *Medical Terminology: A Programmed Learning Approach to the Language of Health Care.* Baltimore: Lippincott Williams & Wilkins, 2002.

external and internal organs are illustrated in Figure 16.1.

External Genital Organs

The **external genital organs** are the genital structures found outside the body, which function to enable sperm to enter the body, to protect the internal genital organs from infectious organisms, and to provide sexual pleasure. The area containing these external organs is called the **vulva**. These structures consist of the following:

- **Clitoris.** This is a small mass of erectile tissue anterior to the opening of the urethra. Containing numerous sensory endings, its only function is sensory as it responds to sexual stimulation.
- **Bartholin glands.** These glands are located beside the vagina (discussed later). The secretions from these glands keep the mucosa moist and provide a lubricant for the vaginal opening during sexual intercourse.
- **Skene glands.** These are a pair of tiny glands located on each side of the lower end of the urethra. Named after physician Alexander Skene, who

described them first, these glands are the equivalent to the prostate gland in males. The Skene glands drain into the urethra and near the urethral opening and are believed to be the source of female ejaculation.

- **Labia.** The labia consist of two sets of skin folds that cover the external genital organs and tissues to protect them and to prevent drying of their mucosal membranes. The **labia majora**, comparable to the scrotum in males, is a pair of fleshy folds of skin that enclose and protect the other external genital organs. The **labia minora** is a pair of smaller folds of skin lying just inside the labia majora and surrounding the openings to the vagina and urethra.
- **Mons pubis.** This is a rounded mound of fatty tissue that covers the **pubic symphysis**, or pubic bone, one of three sections of the hip bone that form the front of the pelvis.

Internal Genital Organs

The **internal genital organs**, which are the structures involved in human reproduction, form a pathway called the **genital tract**. These structures consist of the following:

- **Ovaries**. The ovaries are small, oval structures attached to the uterus by ligaments. They produce hormones called **estrogen** and **progesterone**, which contribute to the development and function of the female reproductive organs and female sex characteristics. The ovaries also produce and release an egg cell, called an **ovum**, which if fertilized can produce an offspring. The ovaries contain thousands of fluid-filled sacs called **follicles**, each of which consists of an immature ovum, called an **oocyte**, surrounded by specialized secretory cells that produce female hormones. Every month one oocyte enlarges and develops to become an ovum, commonly referred to as an *egg*. At the appropriate time, the follicle discharges one ovum in a process called **ovulation**. The fimbriae guide the ovum into the fallopian tube for travel toward the uterus. A female infant is born with about a million eggs, which gradually degenerate and die, and all eggs are gone by the onset of menopause, as discussed later.

- **Fallopian tubes**. Although the formal term for each tube is **salpinx**, from the Greek word meaning *trumpeter*, the fallopian tubes are commonly referred to by the name of their discoverer, Gabriele Fallopius, a 16th-century anatomist who described them as *trumpets of the uterus*. The fallopian tubes are not connected to the ovaries. Instead, the end of each tube opens into a broad, flared end called the **infundibulum**, which overlies the ovary. The free edge of the infundibulum has several fingerlike extensions called **fimbriae**, which are draped over the ovary and guide a mature egg from the ovary to the opening of the fallopian tube during ovulation. Each fallopian tube connects to the upper edge of the uterus.

- The uterus and cervix. The **uterus**, also called the *womb*, is a thick-walled, pear-shaped organ located in the middle of the pelvis, behind the bladder and in front of the rectum. It is the organ of gestation; that is, its main function is to hold and nourish a developing baby. During pregnancy, the uterus expands greatly in size to accommodate a growing baby and then contracts to push the baby out of the body at the time of delivery. The uterus consists of the **fundus**, which is the dome-shaped top portion that lies above the entrance of the fallopian tubes. The height of the fundus is sometimes measured to help determine the duration of the pregnancy. The **body** of the uterus is the main part of the uterus that lies below the entrance of the fallopian tubes. The body narrows and becomes continuous with the lower part, or neck of the uterus, called the **cervix**. The tubular-shaped cervix extends downward to the top of the vagina. The wall of the uterus consists of three layers: the inner lining called the **endometrium**, a thick, muscular middle layer called the **myometrium**, and an outer layer of peritoneum called the **perimetrium**, which covers the body of the uterus and part of the cervix. Interestingly, the root of these terms, *metrium*, refers to the uterus and comes from the Greek word *meter*, which has the same meaning as the English word *mother*.

- **Vagina**. The vagina, also called the *birth canal*, is a muscular passageway that connects the uterus to the outside of the body. Located below and behind the urethra, the vagina is the entryway for the penis during sexual intercourse and the exit for menstrual blood and vaginal discharge as well as for a newborn infant. When stimulated, the Bartholin glands secrete a thick fluid that supplies lubrication for intercourse. The opening of the vagina is also referred to as the **introitus**.

Mammary Glands

The breasts are functionally related to the reproductive system because they contain the milk-producing organs for the nourishment of offspring. Glands located in the breasts, called **mammary glands**, prepare for milk production during pregnancy. The term **lactation** refers to the production of milk in the breast and comes from the word *lactos*, the Latin term for milk. In the third trimester of pregnancy, they produce **colostrum**, a substance that contains milk fat and immunoglobulins. After birth, induced by a lactation-stimulating hormone called **prolactin**, they produce true milk that nourishes the infant.

Menstrual Cycle

The **menstrual cycle**, a process involving a complex interaction of hormones, is the series of changes a woman's body goes through in order to make eggs available for fertilization in preparation for a possible pregnancy.

QUICK CHECK 16.1 ✓

Indicate whether the following terms in the first column refer to either an external (A) or internal (B) structure.

Term

1. _____ Bartholin
2. _____ cervix
3. _____ labia
4. _____ fimbriae
5. _____ ovaries
6. _____ body
7. _____ vagina
8. _____ endometrium
9. _____ follicles
10. _____ Skene

Structure

A. external

B. internal

Typically this cycle lasts approximately 28 days, occurring on a monthly basis from the early teen years until approximately age 50. During the menstrual cycle, the pituitary gland in the brain secretes **follicle stimulating hormone** (FSH) and **luteinizing hormone** (LH), whereas the ovaries secrete the hormones estrogen and progesterone. These hormones all work together to stimulate the growth of ovarian follicles and promote the growth and maturation of the ovum and endometrium in the event of a pregnancy. If no pregnancy occurs, the endometrium breaks down and is shed through the vagina, a process called **menstruation**.

By definition, the menstrual cycle starts with the onset of menstruation, which occupies approximately five days of the complete 28-day cycle. At the start of the menstrual cycle, cells begin to repair the endometrium and follicles in the ovary begin to form an ovum. As ovulation approaches at around day 14, the blood supply to the ovary increases and the ligaments around the ovary contract, pulling it closer to the fallopian tube in order to aid the ovum, once released from the ovary, in finding its way into the tube. As the ovum travels through the fallopian tube toward the uterus, LH stimulates the ruptured follicle to become a temporary endocrine gland called the **corpus luteum**. The corpus luteum produces progesterone during the second half of the menstrual cycle, which, along with estrogen, works to thicken and prepare the lining of the uterus for a fertilized egg.

If pregnancy does not occur, the corpus luteum decreases secretion of progesterone and the blood vessels in the uterus respond by cutting off the blood supply to all but the deepest parts of the endometrium. This results in tissue breakdown and bleeding, which leads to the onset of menstruation, also called **menses**.

The onset of **menopause** marks the end of the monthly cycle of ovulation and is usually identified, retrospectively, when a woman has not had a menstrual period for one full year. It can be thought of as a hormonal shift in a stage of one's life, similar to puberty. During this time, which can last anywhere from 5 to 15 years, hormone levels begin to fluctuate. The brain continues to send out hormones trying to stimulate the development of ovarian follicles. The ovaries may respond erratically, causing many of the symptoms of menopause, such as hot flashes or irregular bleeding. Eventually the ovaries are no longer able to develop an egg for ovulation, hormones are no longer produced, and monthly bleeding stops. **Postmenopause** begins when 12 full months have passed since the last menstrual period.

When preparing clinic notes and other reports outlining a patient's gynecologic history, part of the dictation will refer to the patient's history of her menstrual cycles. The first menstruation, called **menarche**, normally occurs between the ages of 10 and 16. The physician will document the patient's age of menarche, the length of the menstrual cycle, the length of menstruation, and any problems that the patient has encountered during the menstrual cycle. The physician will also document the onset of menopause, as well as bleeding or menstrual cycle irregularities experienced by the patient during the process of menopause. Uterine bleeding abnormalities such as excessively heavy bleeding (**menorrhagia**), bleeding that occurs both during menses and at irregular intervals (**menometrorrhagia**), difficult or painful menstruation (**dysmenorrhea**), or the absence of bleeding (**amenorrhea**) are usually investigated thoroughly, as any one of them may indicate a benign gynecologic disorder or a life-threatening disease of the uterus or other part of the body.

FUNDAMENTALS OF HUMAN REPRODUCTION

Pregnancy and delivery are natural processes that have been occurring for millennia, with physicians becoming involved only in the relatively recent past. Medical reports document many facets of pregnancy, fetal development, labor, and delivery; and you should be familiar with these processes and procedures and the terminology used to describe them.

Fertilization

Fertilization, or *conception*, occurs when the genetic packages of a sperm and an egg merge to form what will become a human individual. For fertilization to occur, a sperm must locate and penetrate the egg while it is located in the fallopian tube as it travels to the uterus. Whether or not fertilization occurs, the fertilized egg continues to travel through the fallopian tube to the uterus. If fertilization has occurred, on approximately the seventh day following fertilization, the fertilized egg attaches itself to the lining of the uterus.

The term **singleton** refers to a pregnancy with only one baby. Sometimes, however, two ovarian follicles each release an ovum simultaneously. If both are fertilized, the resulting eggs develop separately and are called **fraternal twins**. When a single sperm fertilizes an egg and then, at a very early stage, the fertilized egg divides into two halves and starts to form two babies, the result is known as **identical twins**. When transcribing reports regarding twins, a physician will delineate each twin as *twin A* and *twin B*, respectively.

An **ectopic pregnancy** occurs when a fertilized egg implants itself outside the uterus. The most common site for an ectopic pregnancy is within a fallopian tube; however, in rare cases, an ectopic pregnancy can occur in other areas, such as the ovary or cervix. This is usually caused by a condition that impedes the movement of a fertilized egg through the fallopian tube to the uterus, such as a physical blockage in the tube or scarring of the tube from a prior surgery or infection. Ectopic pregnancies are unable to survive because the embryo quickly outgrows the space and available blood supply and, if not removed, will rupture the tube. Laparoscopic surgery is performed to confirm the diagnosis of ectopic pregnancy, remove the embryo, stop blood loss (in the event of a rupture), and repair any tissue damage. Removal of the fallopian tube may be necessary if it is damaged.

Once the fertilized egg has become implanted in the uterus, the **placenta**, the tissue created to connect the mother and baby, will begin to form. A temporary organ that implants itself in the wall of the uterus, the placenta is the site through which the fetus receives nutrients and oxygen from the mother's blood and passes out waste. The placenta is connected to the fetus by the **umbilical cord**, which is composed of blood vessels and tissue. The cord begins at the umbilicus of the

QUICK CHECK 16.2

Indicate whether the following sentences are true (T) or false (F).

1. Menopause refers to the shedding of the endometrium.   T   F

2. A young girl's first menstruation is called menarche.   T   F

3. Amenorrhea means absence of bleeding.   T   F

4. The menstrual cycle starts with the onset of menstruation.   T   F

5. FSH stimulates menstruation.   T   F

fetus and inserts into the center of the placenta, transporting blood between the fetus and the placenta. When the infant is delivered, the placenta is expelled from the uterus shortly afterward, and the umbilical cord is cut from the infant.

An **embryo** is the name given to the developing baby from the time of implantation into the uterus until about the eighth week of gestation; thereafter, until the time of birth, it is referred to as a **fetus**. The **amnion** is a thin membrane that eventually surrounds the embryo and contains **amniotic fluid**, which provides a cushion for the fetus as the mother moves. This fluid also contains waste from the fetus's kidneys after they have developed as well as cells that have sloughed off the fetus; these cells can be analyzed to detect certain genetic or chromosomal abnormalities in a fetus of at least 16 weeks. See Figure 16.2, which illustrates a pregnant uterus with an intact fetus.

In a GYN or labor and delivery note, a physician will usually include the obstetric history of the patient using the terms **gravida**, **para**, and **abortus**. *Gravida* refers to a woman's total number of pregnancies, regardless of whether they were carried to term, with multiple gestations counting as one pregnancy. *Para* indicates the number of births of viable children, with multiple births counting, again, as one. *Abortus* (plural, *aborta*) refers to the number of pregnancy losses before the 20th week. An abbreviated form of these terms is called the **GPA system**, in which the letter G indicates gravida, P

for para, and A for abortus. This history is transcribed in small letters with arabic numerals.

Example:

G1 or gravida 1	one pregnancy
P2 or para 2	two deliveries of viable offspring
gravida 1, para 1	one pregnancy, one viable offspring
gravida 1, para 2,	one pregnancy, two viable offspring
aborta 2	two abortions

The **TPAL system** is also used to describe the obstetric history of a patient, with the letter T representing the number of term infants, P representing the number of premature infants, A representing the number of abortions, and L representing the number of living children. An obstetric history using this system is transcribed using arabic numerals separated by hyphens.

Example: Obstetrics History: 3-1-2-3.

Oftentimes GPA terminology is combined with TPAL terminology in reports; this is transcribed using capital letters and arabic numerals separated by hyphens:

Example:

The patient is a 28-year-old female, G4, P2-1-3-2.
or gravida 4, para 2-1-3-2.
or gravida 4, 2-1-3-2.

Other terms used to describe the patient's obstetric history include **nulligravida** (no pregnancies), **primigravida** (first pregnancy), **secundigravida** (second pregnancy), and **nullipara** (no deliveries of viable offspring).

The majority of women have normal, uncomplicated pregnancies and deliveries. However, complications can and do occur. Some of these may include:

- **Placenta previa**, a pregnancy in which the placenta is implanted in the lower part of the uterus instead of the upper part, causing it to partly or completely block the cervix. As the pregnancy progresses, the placenta usually moves higher in the uterus, away from the cervix. However, if it remains near or over the cervix, the mother is at risk for excessive bleeding as the cervix thins and opens during labor. For this reason, this type of pregnancy is usually delivered by cesarean section.

- **Placenta abruptio**, a complication in which the placenta breaks away, or abrupts, from the wall of the uterus too early, before the baby is born, causing premature birth or major blood loss in the mother.

- **Preeclampsia**, also called *toxemia*, is a condition in pregnant women marked by high blood pressure and a high level of protein in the urine. **Eclampsia** is the final and most severe phase of the condition if preeclampsia is left untreated, which can lead to seizures, coma, or even death of the mother and baby before, during, or after childbirth.

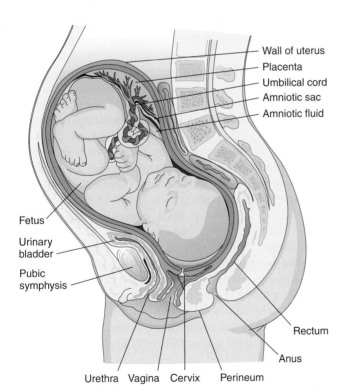

Wall of uterus
Placenta
Umbilical cord
Amniotic sac
Amniotic fluid

Fetus
Urinary bladder
Pubic symphysis

Rectum
Anus

Urethra   Vagina   Cervix   Perineum

FIGURE 16.2. Pregnant Uterus with Intact Fetus. Reprinted with permission from Cohen BJ, Wood DL. *Memmler's The Human Body in Health and Disease,* 9th ed. Philadelphia: Lippincott Williams & Wilkins, 2000.

- **Gestational diabetes**, a form of diabetes that develops during pregnancy. See Chapter 21, *Endocrinology*, for a further discussion about this and other types of diabetes.
- **Hyperemesis gravidarum**, a rare complication characterized by severe and excessive nausea and vomiting during pregnancy.
- **Rh factor incompatibility**, a situation which occurs when the mother has Rh-negative blood and the baby has Rh-positive blood. When routine bloodwork is taken during pregnancy, one of the results is the blood type of the mother and baby. These results are expressed as a letter and indicated as either positive ($+$) or negative ($-$). The positive or negative factor refers to the Rh system of blood testing. When the Rh factor is not compatible between mother and child, the body's immune system mistakenly identifies the baby's red blood cells as foreign and produces antibodies to destroy them (called **hemolysis**), leading to anemia and other symptoms in the infant. **RhoGAM** is the shortened name for *Rho immunoglobulin*, an injectable blood product used to protect an Rh-positive fetus from the antibodies produced by its Rh-negative mother. The injections are given at about 28 weeks of pregnancy and immediately after delivery, ensuring that the mother's immune system will not react to the baby's Rh-positive blood or that of any subsequent fetus.

Fertility Issues

Infertility is the inability of a couple to become pregnant, regardless of the cause. **In vitro fertilization** (IVF) is a method of helping a couple achieve pregnancy by artificial means, in which eggs from a woman are combined with sperm in a laboratory dish, where fertilization takes place. The resulting embryo is then transferred to the woman's uterus to implant and develop naturally. The term *test tube baby* was previously used to refer to this method of fertilization. Louise Joy Brown, the world's first child conceived as a result of this method, was born in Great Britain in 1978. IVF was first used successfully in the United States in 1981. Since then it has become a safe and successful treatment that may allow a woman with fertility issues, such as anatomical abnormalities, pathology of her reproductive organs, or problems with a partner's sperm (quantity or quality), to have a child biologically related to her and her partner.

The steps in a conventional IVF and embryo transfer procedure include the following:

- **Ovulation induction**, or the stimulation of development of eggs in the ovaries, which increases the chance that several mature eggs will develop in the ovaries (as opposed to the single egg which develops each month with ovulation). Stimulating and monitoring the development of eggs. Ovulation induction uses hormonal therapy. Sometimes referred to as "fertility drugs," these medications are designed to trick the ovaries into producing many eggs in a single cycle by stimulating the woman's hormones to perform their jobs more efficiently. Drugs currently in use to stimulate egg development include clomiphene (Clomid); human menopausal gonadotropin (hMG), a drug that combines FSH and LH; and leuprolide (Lupron). Other alternatives are follitropin beta (Follistim) and human chorionic gonadotropin (hCG), estrogen (Estrace), and progesterone (Prometrium). The egg development is monitored by blood tests that measure hormone levels, such as those of estrogen and LH. Estrogen increases as follicles develop; LH triggers ovulation.
- The harvesting of developed eggs. The eggs are retrieved using ultrasound imaging to guide a hollow needle through the vagina to the pelvic cavity to identify a mature follicle. The egg is then removed through the needle by a suction device, a process called **follicular aspiration**. The needle may also be guided through the abdominal wall if follicles are inaccessible through the vagina.
- Insemination and fertilization of the eggs. **Insemination** is the transfer of sperm to establish a pregnancy. The partner's sperm is collected and placed with each egg in a separate dish containing a culture medium that facilitates fertilization. Sometimes the physician may feel that the chance that the egg will be easily located and fertilized by the sperm is low. The sperm may, for example, have difficulty moving through the culture medium to locate the egg, in which case a procedure may be undertaken to manually assist with fertilization. In the procedure called **intracytoplastic sperm injection** (ICSI), very precise maneuvers are used to pick up a single live sperm from the dish and inject it directly into the center of the egg. The dish is placed in an incubator that is the same temperature as the woman's body. After 48 hours in the incubator, the fertilized eggs are ready to be implanted into the woman's uterus.
- Transfer of the embryos into the woman's uterus. The process of placing the fertilized eggs into the woman's uterus is known as **embryo transfer**. In this procedure, the patient lies on a table with her feet in stirrups. One or more embryos suspended in the IVF culture medium are drawn into a **transfer catheter**, a long, thin tube with a syringe on the end of it. The physician gently guides the catheter through the vagina and cervix and deposits the fluid into the uterine cavity. One or more embryos may be transferred during this procedure. In the days following the transfer, the patient is monitored for

early pregnancy symptoms. A blood test or an ultrasound can be used to determine if embryo implantation and pregnancy has occurred.

Sometimes physicians use a process called **assisted zonal hatching** to chemically thin the **zona pellucida**, or outer shell of a fertilized egg, prior to transferring it to the uterus. It is believed that this outer shell becomes thicker as eggs age in the uterus. As such, older women or women with problems involving the quality of the endometrium of the uterus may have a decreased chance of embryo implantation. Therefore, the physicians use a very fine needle to identify the wall of the egg and apply a diluted acidic solution to it in order to thin its outer shell, thereby enhancing the embryo's ability to *hatch*, or to implant successfully into the uterus after transfer.

In some cases, embryos that are transferred during the embryo transfer process of IVF have been previously frozen, a procedure called **cryopreservation**. If frozen embryos are used, the procedure is called a **frozen embryo transfer**. This is accomplished by first thawing the frozen embryo and then transferring it into an appropriately prepared uterus. In the past, the survival rate of embryos after thawing was not very high. In recent years, however, techniques in the cryopreservation of embryos at different stages of development have improved; and the survival rate is now very good. Embryos can be frozen and used to achieve pregnancies after as long as five years of storage. Donor sperm can also be cryopreserved for use at a later time.

Labor and Delivery

Labor is the term given to the process of giving birth to a child at the conclusion of a pregnancy. Labor consists of a series of rhythmic, progressive contractions of the uterus that cause effacement and dilation of the uterine cervix. On admission, a thorough physical and laboratory examination of the patient is performed, the account of which is transcribed in an initial history and physical. Some of the common procedures described in a report documenting an expectant mother's initial examination include the following:

- Assessment of amniotic fluid. The breaking of the patient's sac of amniotic fluid is referred to as **rupture of membranes** (ROM). **Premature rupture of membranes** (PROM) refers to the rupture of the amniotic fluid sac before the onset of labor. During a sterile vaginal examination, Nitrazine and fern tests are used to determine whether membranes have ruptured. In the **Nitrazine test**, paper test strips impregnated with Nitrazine determine the pH of the amniotic fluid. The fluid reacts with the paper strip, the result being positive or negative. In the **fern test**, when the fluid is applied to a microscope slide and allowed to dry, the estrogen in the amniotic fluid will show a fernlike pattern on the slide. Therefore, if the membranes have ruptured, the fluid will be indicated in the report as fern- and Nitrazine-positive.

- Effacement and dilation. **Effacement**, or thinning, of the cervix is the process by which the cervix prepares for delivery. As the baby drops closer to the cervix, the cervix gradually softens (called **ripening**) and becomes thinner. This value is measured in percentages, such as 25%, 50%, or 75%. When the cervix is completely effaced, it is said to be 100% effaced and ready to dilate. **Dilation** refers to the opening of the cervix during labor and is measured in centimeters (cm) from one to ten. A woman who is 1 or 2 cm dilated may be in early labor, whereas a woman who is 10 cm dilated is said to be ready to push the baby out. This information would be transcribed, for example, as: "The cervix was 50% effaced and 3 cm dilated."

- Station. The term **station** refers to the position of the baby's presenting part (face/chin, foot, shoulder, etc.) in the mother's pelvis relative to her ischial spine, located at the lower end of the spine. The ischial spine is indicated as 0 station, and above or below that point is measured in numbers from −4 (just entering the pelvis) to +4 (ready to be born).

- Fetal well-being. A main concern during labor is fetal well-being. The fetus is monitored to ensure that it is receiving enough blood and oxygen from the placenta during the birth process. This is assessed by the documentation of **fetal heart rate**, or **fetal heart tones**, and its comparison to the normal heart rate of a baby before birth. Increases in the fetal heart rate, called **accelerations** (which may be dictated as *accels*), are documented, as are **decelerations** (*decels*); and both are tracked against fetal movement. Uterine contractions are monitored with a **tocodynamometer** (*toco*); and an ultrasound transducer, which measures fetal heart rate, is attached to the mother's abdomen. Monitoring can also be done internally with an **intrauterine pressure catheter** (IUPC), a small catheter that is placed alongside the baby in the uterus and measures the strength and duration of uterine contractions. A **fetal scalp electrode** (FSE) is a device placed just under the skin of the baby's scalp that is used to monitor the baby's heartbeat while still in the uterus.

A baby may be injured by labor that is progressing too slowly. Labor may have to be hastened or augmented. **Oxytocin** is a natural hormone produced by the pituitary gland in the brain that causes uterine contractions. Pitocin is the synthetic form of oxytocin and is administered to make the uterus contract more frequently and forcefully. Other medications that can be

TRANSCRIPTION TIP:

Many women choose to attempt a vaginal birth after a cesarean section, and most succeed. This is referred to as a **vaginal birth after C-section** (VBAC), which sounds like *VEE-back* when dictated.

used include prostaglandin (Cervidil) and misoprostol (Cytotec). In the event that labor has to be slowed or delayed, terbutaline may be given to slow the rate of contractions.

A vaginal birth without complications is referred to as a **normal spontaneous vaginal delivery** (NSVD). Sometimes forceps may be used to assist in the delivery of the infant. **Forceps** are metal surgical instruments resembling tongs with rounded edges that fit around the baby's head. Forceps are occasionally required if the baby is in an abnormal position in the birth canal or if the patient is having difficulty pushing. A **vacuum extractor** can be used along with forceps to assist with delivery. It consists of a vacuum device with a small rubberlike cup attached to its end. The cup is inserted into the vagina and a gentle suction is used to help ease the baby through the birth canal. When dictated, physicians may describe the use of these tools as a *vacuum-assisted forceps delivery*.

Cesarean section, also called **C-section**, is the delivery of a newborn through a surgical incision in the abdomen and front wall of the uterus. The origin of the name of the procedure is not known; although, it was originally believed to have derived from the legend that Julius Caesar was born in this fashion, which was later determined to not be the case. The procedure is performed whenever abnormal conditions complicate labor and vaginal delivery, threatening the life or health of the mother or the baby. **Dystocia**, or difficult labor, is a common reason for C-sections, as is a **breech presentation**, in which the baby is positioned in the uterus buttocks or feet first as opposed to head first. In a cesarean section, a transverse incision, called a **Pfannenstiel incision**, is made in the lower part of the abdomen. It is named after German physician Hans Hermann Johannes Pfannenstiel who first employed the technique in the late 1800s. The uterus is opened, the amniotic fluid is drained, and the baby is delivered. The baby's mouth and nose are suctioned to clear them of fluids, and the umbilical cord is clamped and cut.

Whether delivered vaginally or by C-section, the newborn is handed to a pediatrician who attends the birth and examines the infant immediately after it is born. Part of the examination includes assigning an **Apgar score**. The Apgar test was designed to quickly evaluate a newborn's physical condition after delivery and to determine any immediate need for extra medical or emergency care. Developed in 1952 by anesthesiologist Virginia Apgar, the score evaluates pulse, breathing, color, tone, and reflex irritability. Each of these initial signs is rated 0, 1, or 2, at one and five minutes after birth. Each set of ratings is totaled, and both totals are reported. It is easy to remember what is being tested by thinking of the letters in the name "Apgar": **a**ctivity (muscle tone), **p**ulse (heart rate), **g**rimace (reflex response), **a**ppearance (color), and **r**espirations (breathing).

The Apgar score, when transcribed, is initially capped. The ratings and times are written in arabic numerals with the times, if given, written out in order to avoid confusion. For example: "The infant's Apgars were 7 and 9 at one and five minutes." Although the often-dictated brief form *Apgars* is often used, you should expand the term and transcribe this as *Apgar score* if your employer permits.

QUICK CHECK 16.3

Fill in the blanks with the correct answers.

1. When transcribing reports regarding twins, a physician will delineate each twin as Twin A and _____.

2. The term _____ indicates the number of births of viable children, with multiple births counting as one.

3. Thinning of the cervix in preparation for delivery is called _____.

4. A procedure used to assist with the manual fertilization of the egg in a culture medium is called _____.

5. A device placed just under the skin of the baby's scalp that is used to monitor the baby's heartbeat while still in the uterus is called a _____.

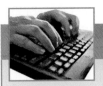

TRANSCRIPTION TIP:

Pediatricians are present during the birth of a baby to examine and care for the baby immediately after it is born. Dictators will often refer to these physicians as *peds* (pronounced like "peeds") and say, for example, "the infant was handed off to waiting *peds*." Use the word *pediatricians* when transcribing dictation that shortens this term.

COMMON GYNECOLOGIC DISEASES AND TREATMENTS

Disorders that affect the female reproductive system, including the breasts, are called **gynecologic disorders**. These gynecologic conditions can be simple or complex, but most of them can be treated successfully by a gynecologist or OB/GYN.

Sexually Transmitted Diseases

(Note: Sexually transmitted diseases are also discussed in Chapter 15, Urology.)

Sexually transmitted diseases (STDs) are diseases caused by a pathogen that are spread from person to person, primarily through sexual contact. STDs can have severe consequences for women if not treated promptly. Some STDs can lead to pelvic diseases that cause infertility, while others can prove fatal.

Human Papillomavirus

Human papillomavirus (HPV) is a group of viruses that produces genital warts, or **papillomas**, on the skin and mucous membranes. There are more than 60 known strains of HPV. The virus is transmitted by sexual contact and incubates in the body for approximately two months before warts appear. Studies show an association between some types of HPV and increased instances of cervical cancer in women, although, in most cases HPV does not lead to cancer.

Many cases of genital warts resolve spontaneously. Warts may also be removed by freezing the abnormal tissue with liquid nitrogen (**cryotherapy**), burning at high heat (**electrocautery**), laser removal, or surgical excision. Drug therapies include alpha interferon, which can be injected directly into the warts to eliminate or significantly reduce their size. Cream or gel treatments, such as podophyllin and trichloroacetic acid (TCA) are applied to external warts; over time, these therapies destroy the warts, as do self-applied prescription treatments such as imiquimod (Aldara) and podofilox (Condylox).

Pelvic Inflammatory Disease

Pelvic inflammatory disease (PID) is a general term that refers to the inflammation of the uterus (**endometritis**), fallopian tubes (**salpingitis**), and ovaries (**oophoritis**). It is a common and serious complication of some sexually transmitted diseases, particularly gonorrhea and chlamydia. PID is the result of disease-causing bacteria migrating through the vagina and cervix, invading and damaging the tissues of the upper genital tract. This eventually leads to inflammation and tissue damage of the internal genital organs. Without treatment, PID can cause permanent damage to the female reproductive organs. Infection-causing bacteria can silently invade the fallopian tubes, causing normal tissue to turn into scar tissue and increasing a woman's chances of infertility.

Prompt antibiotic treatment for PID can prevent severe damage to reproductive organs. Because PID is often caused by a combination of different types of bacteria, it is usually treated with a combination of antibiotics that are effective against a wide range of infectious agents. Treatment may be given by mouth or by injection. Some of the common regimens include ofloxacin (Floxin) or levofloxacin (Levaquin) with or without metronidazole (Flagyl); ceftriaxone (Rocephin) plus doxycycline (Vibramycin); or cefotaxime (Claforan) plus doxycycline (Vibramycin) with or without metronidazole (Flagyl).

Acquired Immunodeficiency Syndrome

Acquired immunodeficiency syndrome, or AIDS, is a sexually transmitted disease that was first reported in the United States in 1981 and has since become a major worldwide epidemic. The etymology of *AIDS* is as follows:

- *Acquired* means that the disease is not hereditary but develops after birth from contact with a disease-causing agent (in this case human immunodeficiency virus, or HIV).
- *Immunodeficiency* means that the disease is characterized by a weakening of the immune system.
- *Syndrome* refers to a group of symptoms that collectively indicate or characterize a disease. In the case of AIDS, this can include the development of certain infections and/or cancers, as well as a decrease in the number of certain cells in a person's immune system.

AIDS is caused by the **human immunodeficiency virus** (HIV). A healthy immune system includes special white blood cells, called CD4-positive T cells, which attack invading diseases. Any virus damages the cells into which it replicates, which is one of the things that cause a person to become ill. HIV seeks out these T cells and incorporates itself into them. It then either reproduces so quickly that it destroys the host cell, or it replicates itself in order to send out more virus particles to attack other T cells. Eventually the body's supply of T cells becomes depleted and the immune system becomes severely weakened and susceptible to diseases that previously could have been fought off easily.

As time goes by, an HIV-infected person is likely to become ill more and more often until a serious illness occurs and/or the number of immune system cells left in the body drops below a certain point. At this point, the person is said to have AIDS rather than HIV.

HIV may be passed from one person to another when infected blood, semen, or vaginal secretions come into contacted with an uninfected person's broken skin or mucous membranes. In addition, an infected pregnant woman can pass the disease to her baby during pregnancy or delivery, as well as through breastfeeding.

The **viral load** refers to the level, or concentration, of HIV in the blood. The viral load indicates how fast the virus is multiplying and also how well or how poorly the virus is being controlled by the immune system. Physicians also monitor the level of the CD4-positive T cell, commonly dictated as simply *the CD4 count*, to determine whether treatment is successful. The CD4 count indicates how strong the immune system is and helps determine how far HIV has advanced. Both the

CD4 count and viral load tests are ordered when a person is first diagnosed with HIV as part of a baseline measurement. In general, the CD4 count goes down as HIV disease progresses, whereas the viral load value increases. Both of these values are typically dictated. For example: "The patient's CD4 count was 450 with a viral load of 250,000."

Although there is no cure for HIV/AIDS at this time, a variety of medications, called **antiretroviral drugs**, are available, which work to reduce the amount of virus in the blood. This can slow the destruction of the immune system dramatically. Some common antiretroviral agents used include the combination of lopinavir and ritonavir (Kaletra), ritonavir (Norvir), abacavir (Ziagen); the combination abacavir, lamivudine, and zidovudine (Trizivir); atazanavir (Reyataz); tenofovir (Viread); the combination abacavir, lamivudine, and zidovudine (AZT or Retrovir); zidovudine and lamivudine (Combivir); indinavir (Crixivan); lamivudine (Epivir); saquinavir (Fortovase or Invirase); nelfinavir (Viracept); stavudine (Zerit); efavirenz (Sustiva); and amprenavir (Agenerase).

Cervical Dysplasia

Cervical dysplasia describes the development of abnormal cells in the lining of the cervix, which is sometimes, but not always, a precursor of cervical cancer.

The general term used to describe these abnormal cells in the lining of the cervix is a **squamous**

QUICK CHECK 16.4 ✓

Match the terms in the first column with the sexually transmitted disease it is associated with in the second column (some diseases will be used more than once).

Term

1. _____ CD4

2. _____ cryotherapy

3. _____ endometritis

4. _____ warts

5. _____ viral load

6. _____ infertility

7. _____ AZT

8. _____ TCA

9. _____ salpingitis

10. _____ T cell

Disease

A. acquired immunodeficiency syndrome

B. pelvic inflammatory disease

C. human papillomavirus

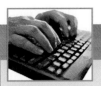

intraepithelial lesion (SIL). This term is broken down as follows:

- *squamous* means that the cells are the flat cells found on the surface of the cervix
- *intraepithelial* means within or among epithelial, or surface, cells; in this case, that the abnormal cells are present only in the surface layer of the cervix
- *lesion* refers to an area of abnormal tissue

SIL is further divided into two categories: **Low-grade SIL (LGSIL)** refers to early changes in the cells that form the surface of the cervix. **High-grade SIL (HGSIL)** means there are a large number of precancerous cells on the surface of the cervix.

Another scale physicians use to describe these precancerous changes is CIN. An alternative name for cervical dysplasia is **cervical intraepithelial neoplasia (CIN)**. This term is broken down as follows:

- *cervical* means pertaining to the cervix
- *intraepithelial* means that the abnormal cells are present only in the surface layer of the cervix
- *neoplasia* means new (neo-) growth (-plasia) and, in this case, a new growth on the cervix

Physicians use the abbreviation *CIN* to categorize the abnormal changes observed in cervical tissue. CIN levels are expressed with arabic numbers from grade 1 (minimal or low degree of abnormality) to grade 3 (high-grade or most severe). A hyphen is placed between the CIN and the numeral.

Example: CIN-1, CIN-2, or CIN-3
CIN grade 1, CIN grade 2, or CIN grade 3

In most cases, low-grade dysplasia will spontaneously revert to normal without treatment over a period of several years. However, if left untreated, these cells *may* be the first evidence of cervical cancer that develops later. Precancerous changes of the cervix usually do not cause pain and, in general, do not produce any symptoms. They are detected by a pelvic examination or a Pap test, described later in this chapter.

More than 90% of women who are diagnosed with cervical dysplasia and/or cervical cancer also carry HPV. Although physicians are not absolutely certain that HPV is the direct cause of cervical cancer, it is known that HPV causes or at the very least is strongly associated with cervical cancer. Women who are diagnosed with cervical dysplasia are usually tested and treated for HPV as well.

Endometriosis

Endometriosis is a disorder in which endometrial tissue that normally lines the uterus grows elsewhere in the abdominal cavity, such as in the ovaries, fallopian tubes, and abdominal wall. It is a chronic condition causing pain, heavy or prolonged menstrual periods, or infertility. The cause of this disorder is unclear, but one theory suggests that the endometrial cells loosened during menstruation may flow backward through the fallopian tubes and into the pelvis, where they implant and grow in the pelvic or abdominal cavities. As the disorder progresses, the misplaced endometrial tissue tends to gradually increase in size or spread to new locations, eventually causing bands of scarlike tissue called **adhesions** to form in the tubes and ovaries.

There is no cure for endometriosis, but there are many treatments for the pain and other symptoms it causes. Pain medications such as ibuprofen (Advil, Motrin) or naproxen (Aleve) are typically used for mild pain. Hormone suppression in the form of birth control pills blocks the effects of natural hormones on endometrial growth, forcing the disease into remission and relieving symptoms. Common hormonal therapies include the use of estrogen and progesterone, progesterone alone, or **gonadotropin releasing hormone (GnRH) agonists** such as leuprolide (Lupron).

Usually surgery is performed only on women with severe endometriosis, including those with adhesions or infertility problems. The goal of surgery is to remove or destroy all of the endometrial tissue and adhesions and to restore the pelvic area to as close to normal as possible. **Laparoscopy** can be used as both a diagnostic tool and treatment modality for mild forms of the disease. In this procedure, a surgeon uses a laparoscope inserted through small incisions in the abdomen to visualize the abdominal cavity. The laparoscope can locate and evaluate damaged tissue in the uterus, then remove growths and scar tissue without risking damage to surrounding tissue. **Laparotomy** is used for severe endometriosis, as the surgeon makes a much bigger incision in the abdomen in order to reach and remove growths of endometrial tissue that have invaded the abdominal cavity.

Some cases of endometriosis may require treatment by **hysterectomy**, which is the surgical removal of the uterus and, sometimes, the cervix. The Greek word *hystero* means *uterus*. Interestingly, it is also the root of another Greek word: *hysteria*. In ancient Greece, physicians had the notion that only women became extremely emotionally upset and attributed this perceived difference from men to the presence of a uterus.

This procedure can be performed through the vagina, called a **vaginal hysterectomy**, or through the abdomen, called an **abdominal hysterectomy**. A **total hysterectomy** is the removal of the uterus and part or all of the cervix. When only the uterus is removed, it is called a **partial hysterectomy**. A **total abdominal hysterectomy** (TAH) is performed through the abdomen and removes the uterus, including the cervix. Removal of a fallopian tube and ovary on either side is called a **salpingo-oophorectomy** (LSO for the left, and RSO for the right). The removal of both fallopian tubes and ovaries is called **bilateral salpingo-oophorectomies** (BSO). Removal of the uterus, cervix, fallopian tubes, and ovaries is referred to as a total abdominal hysterectomy with bilateral salpingo-oophorectomies (TAH/BSO).

Uterine Fibroids

Uterine fibroids, also called *myomas* or *leiomyomas*, are noncancerous growths composed of muscle and fibrous tissue that develop in the wall of the uterus, causing heavy or irregular vaginal bleeding, abdominal and back pain, and/or frequent urination. They can grow in tiny clusters or in large single knots, expanding to the size of a melon. In most cases, fibroids are benign tumors that will not develop into cancer. However, in rare cases, they can turn into a malignant cancer called a **leiomyosarcoma**. Although the cause of fibroid formation is unclear, it appears that they thrive on hormones like progesterone and estrogen. For example, fibroids often enlarge during pregnancy, when estrogen levels are high, and often shrink during menopause, when hormone levels decrease.

Fibroids are treated if symptoms worsen or if they enlarge substantially. Although no drug can permanently shrink a fibroid, nonsteroidal anti-inflammatory drugs (NSAIDs), given alone or with progestin, a drug similar to the male hormone progesterone, can reduce symptoms. As with endometriosis, GnRH agonists can shrink fibroids by causing the body to produce less estrogen.

Fibroids can be removed surgically in a process called a **myomectomy**, in which an incision is made in the abdomen and the fibroids are removed laparoscopically while leaving the uterus intact. Other procedures include **myolysis**, in which a probe is inserted through the cervix and into the uterus, and electric current is used to destroy the fibroid; or, in the case of **cryomyolysis**, liquid nitrogen is used to freeze and destroy fibroid tissue. **Endometrial ablation** involves the removal of only the lining of the uterus, which either reduces menstrual flow or ends it completely. The term **ablation** means *surgical removal* or *excision*, and it comes from Latin term *ablatum*, meaning *to carry away*. In this procedure, the uterine lining is surgically removed.

Uterine artery embolization is a procedure in which a catheter is used to inject small synthetic particles called **polyvinyl alcohol** (PVA) into the body under x-ray guidance through a small incision in the groin. These particles, each about the size of a grain of sand, travel to the small arteries supplying the fibroid and block the blood flow that feeds the fibroid, causing it to shrink.

Finally, a newer treatment, **focused ultrasound surgery** (FUS), is used to destroy rather than remove fibroids. In this procedure, the patient is placed into a magnetic resonance imaging (MRI) scanner to allow the physician to locate the fibroid and visualize the anatomy. The fibroid is then located by ultrasound guidance and destroyed with focused high-frequency sound waves.

Gynecologic Cancers

Cancers that occur in any part of the female reproductive system are called **gynecologic cancers**. As with other types of cancers, GYN cancers can invade nearby tissues and organs and spread to distant parts of the body. The following is a brief overview of the most common types of gynecologic cancer, along with various treatments available.

Ovarian Cancer

Ovarian cancer, also called **ovarian carcinoma**, occurs in the ovary and commonly affects women older than 60 years of age. More than 30 types of tumors can form in the cells of the ovaries, and they are grouped within three major categories, according to the type of cells from which they were formed:

- **Epithelial carcinomas**, which begin on the surface of the ovaries.
- **Germ cell tumors**, which start from germ cells, which are the cells that produce eggs in the ovaries.
- **Stromal cell tumors**, which begin in the cells of the fibrous tissue and ligaments, called **connective tissue**, which hold the ovaries together.

Ovarian cancer causes the affected ovary to enlarge. Although enlargement of an ovary in a younger woman is likely to be caused by benign cysts, in women who are older than age 50, an enlarged ovary is often a sign of ovarian cancer. Diagnosing this type of cancer in its early stages is often difficult because symptoms usually do not appear until the cancer is quite large or has spread beyond the ovaries.

Uterine Cancer

Uterine cancer originates in the body and muscle layers of the uterus. **Endometrial cancer** begins in the endometrium and accounts for about 90% of uterine cancers. **Uterine sarcoma** originates in the myometrium and accounts for less than 10% of all cases. Other types of cancer that can originate in the uterus or the ovary include **papillary serous carcinoma** and **clear cell carcinoma**. Abnormal uterine bleeding, including postmenopausal bleeding, or unusually heavy, irregular periods, is the most common early symptom of this disease.

Cervical Cancer

Cervical cancer develops in the lining of the cervix. There are two types of cells on the surface of the cervix: squamous cells and columnar cells. Most invasive cervical cancer develops in the squamous cells that line the cervix and is called **squamous cell carcinoma**, as illustrated in Figure 16.3. The cause of cervical cancer is unknown, but infection with HPV is strongly associated with cervical cancer and is the primary risk factor. HIV infection reduces the body's ability to fight infection, including HPV infection, and also increases the likelihood that precancerous cells will progress to cancer. Smoking is an additional risk factor for developing cervical cancer. The rate of development of cervical cancer is very slow, starting as cervical dysplasia, as discussed previously. Sometimes these precancerous changes can develop into cervical cancer and spread to the bladder, intestines, lungs, and liver. Patients with cervical cancer usually are not symptomatic until the cancer is advanced and has spread to other organs.

Cervical cancer, if caught early, can be cured by removing or destroying the precancerous or cancerous tissue. Procedures for removal include cryosurgery, which uses liquid nitrogen to freeze and remove abnormal cervical tissue, and laser surgery, which uses light to excise abnormal tissue. A **loop electrosurgical excision procedure** (LEEP) uses a thin wire loop with an electric current running through it to remove the abnormal tissue.

As with other cancers, treatment for cancer of the genital organs involves, primarily, removal of the cancerous tissue to stop the progression of the disease and tests to determine whether the cancer has spread to other organs. Surgery usually involves a total hysterectomy and bilateral salpingo-oophorectomies (TAH/BSO), with excision of the uterus and the cervix, as well as removal of the fallopian tubes and ovaries and other surrounding structures through which the cancer typically spreads, such as the omentum, which is the fatty tissue covering the bowel (omentectomy). In addition to surgery, concurrent treatments include chemotherapy and radiation therapy, along with hormone-blocking drugs, or a combination of these options (see Chapter 20, *Oncology*, for a more detailed discussion of chemotherapy and radiation treatments for cancer).

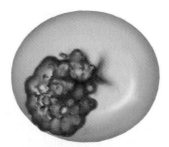

FIGURE 16.3. Carcinoma of the Cervix. In later stages, the cancer may look like an extensive, irregular, cauliflower-like growth on the cervix. Reprinted with permission from Bickley, LS and Szilagyi, P. *Bates' Guide to Physical Examination and History Taking*, 8th ed. Philadelphia: Lippincott Williams & Wilkins, 2003.

Breast Cancer

Breast cancer is a cancerous tumor of breast tissue. The disease occurs primarily in women, but men can get breast cancer too. Most breast cancers begin in the cells of the channels, called **ducts**, which carry breast milk to the nipple. Some begin in the glands that make breast milk, called **lobules**, and the rest in other breast tissue. The most common types of breast cancer include the following:

- **Carcinoma in situ.** This term refers to early-stage cancer that is confined to the place where it began.
- **Ductal carcinoma in situ (DCIS).** DCIS means that the cancer is confined to the ducts and has not spread into the tissue of the breast. It is the most common type of noninvasive breast cancer and nearly all patients with cancer at this stage can be cured.
- **Lobular carcinoma in situ (LCIS).** This type of cancer begins in the glands that make breast milk (lobules) but does not invade surrounding tissue.
- **Invasive (infiltrating) ductal carcinoma (IDC).** This type of cancer starts in a milk duct, breaks through the wall of the duct, and invades the tissue of the breast. From there it can spread to other parts of the body.
- **Invasive (infiltrating) lobular carcinoma (ILC).** This cancer starts in the milk glands and, like IDC, can spread to other parts of the body.

Most women with breast cancer will have some type of surgery to remove as much of the tumor as possible along with some normal tissue to provide the best chance of preventing cancer from recurring within the breast. Surgery can also be performed to determine whether the cancer has spread to other parts of the body. A **lumpectomy** involves removing only the tumor and some of the surrounding tissue. A **simple mastectomy** involves removal of one or both breasts but leaves the muscle under the breast and enough skin to cover the wound. A **modified radical mastectomy** involves removal of the entire breast as well as some of the surrounding tissues and structures. Concurrent treatments include chemotherapy and radiation therapy, along with hormone blocking drugs, or a combination of these options.

QUICK CHECK 16.5 ✓

Circle the letter corresponding to the best answer to the following questions.

1. A lumpectomy is a procedure commonly used in

   A. herpes.
   B. ovarian cancer.
   C. breast cancer.
   D. HPV.

2. HPV is strongly associated with

   A. ovarian cancer.
   B. HIV/AIDS.
   C. breast cancer.
   D. cervical cancer.

3. A _____ is a surgical procedure to remove the uterus and, sometimes, the cervix.

   A. mastectomy
   B. laparotomy
   C. hysterectomy
   D. myomectomy

4. The abbreviation BSO stands for

   A. bilateral salpingectomies.
   B. bilateral salpingo-oophorectomies.
   C. baseline sagittal oophorectomy.
   D. bilateral superior oophorectomies.

5. _____ refers to early stage cancer that is confined to the place where it began.

   A. Carcinoma in situ
   B. IDC
   C. Lobular carcinoma
   D. Ablative carcinoma

DIAGNOSTIC STUDIES AND PROCEDURES

OB/GYNs employ a variety of tests to diagnose conditions, ranging from pregnancy to cancer. Effective diagnostic testing is used to confirm the presence of a disease or eliminate it as a diagnostic option, to monitor the progress of a disease, and to evaluate the effectiveness of treatment. Diagnostic procedures for obstetric and gynecologic conditions may include imaging, laboratory tests, biopsies, and other testing.

Laboratory Studies

Laboratory tests measure levels of chemical components in body fluids and tissues using blood, urine, or samples of body tissue or other material. The following common laboratory tests are performed in obstetrics and gynecology.

Human Chorionic Gonadotropin Test

The hormone **human chorionic gonadotropin** (hCG) is a protein produced in the placenta of pregnant women. Blood or urine can be tested to detect the presence of hCG and confirm pregnancy; generally, hCG can first be detected by a blood test about 11 days after conception and by a urine test about 12 to 14 days after conception. There are two common types of hCG tests: A *qualitative* hCG test is used to confirm a pregnancy, with the result dictated as simply *positive* or *negative*. A *quantitative* hCG test (sometimes dictated as **beta hCG**) measures the amount of hCG actually present in the blood, with the result dictated as an arabic number. This test is used to more accurately monitor a pregnancy that may be failing (the hCG value will fall over time) or a miscarriage (the hCG value will be zero).

Pap Smear

A **smear** is generally defined as any type of laboratory study in which material is thinly spread over the surface of a microscope slide for examination. A **Pap test** (also called a *Pap smear*) involves the microscopic examination of cells collected from the vagina and cervix in order to detect abnormal changes that may lead to cancer or to show conditions such as infection or inflammation. Since the development of the Pap smear by Dr. George Papanicolaou in 1952, rates of cervical cancer in the United States and other industrialized nations have dropped by as much as 70%. HPV is most often detected on a Pap smear in females by checking for the presence of irregular cervical cells.

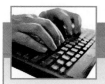

Wet Mount

A **wet mount** is a type of laboratory test commonly used to determine the cause of vaginal irritation and discharge. In this procedure, also called a **vaginal wet mount** or **vaginal smear**, a sample of vaginal discharge is placed on a glass microscope slide and mixed with a saline solution. The slide is then examined under a microscope for bacteria, yeast cells, and white blood cells that indicate an infection; it is also examined for **clue cells**, which are vaginal cells that appear fuzzy when coated with bacteria, indicating infection.

Cultures for Sexually Transmitted Diseases

Because a Pap smear does not test for STDs, many physicians obtain cultures for gonorrhea and chlamydia while taking a Pap smear. These tests are done separately, but the samples are collected at the same time. To obtain the culture, a sample of the discharge in the vagina and cervix is taken with a cotton swab. The sample is then sent to a lab and left to grow in a culture medium for two days. After this time, the sample will be examined under a microscope for the presence of bacteria, indicating a sexually transmitted infection such as gonorrhea or chlamydia.

Obstetrics Studies

Obstetricians employ a variety of tests. In addition to evaluating the cause of infertility of a couple attempting to become pregnant, they also evaluate fetal health on a regular basis to ensure early diagnosis and timely treatment of fetal disorders, including congenital heart diseases and chromosomal abnormalities.

Fertility Studies

Fertility tests are performed to help determine why a couple cannot become pregnant. The tests help determine whether the problem lies with the man's reproductive system, the woman's, or both. For women, further tests usually entail a closer examination of the reproductive anatomy, including the uterus, fallopian tubes, and ovaries.

A **hysterosalpingogram** (HSG) is an x-ray study of the uterus and fallopian tubes that enables a physician to determine if the fallopian tubes are open. In this test, a contrast dye is injected through the cervix and into the uterus and fallopian tubes. X-ray equipment is used to monitor the movement of the liquid as it progresses from the uterus to the tubes, which helps show the shape and structure of the uterine cavity and reveals whether the fallopian tubes are open or blocked.

A **hysteroscopy** is the visual examination of the interior of the uterus and fallopian tubes. In this procedure, a thin, lighted tube called a hysteroscope is inserted into the uterus through the cervix, enabling the physician to directly observe any sites of abnormal bleeding or other irregularities. The hysteroscope also has a separate channel through which instruments can be passed to retrieve a sample of the abnormal tissue or to seal off bleeding in the uterus or fallopian tubes with electrocautery or a laser.

A **sonohysterogram** (SHG) tests for defects in the lining of the uterus (from adhesions, fibroids, malformations, or polyps), which could prevent implantation of an embryo and thereby cause a miscarriage. This test is similar to HSG, described previously, but involves the use of an ultrasound to obtain a more detailed picture of the reproductive organs. In this procedure, an ultrasound probe is inserted into the vagina. Sterile saline solution is then injected into the uterus with a catheter, which helps to further expand the uterus, increasing visibility and allowing for a detailed look at the reproductive organs. The ultrasound probe emits sound waves that bounce off the walls of the uterus and produce images of the uterus on a monitor.

Amniocentesis

In **amniocentesis**, amniotic fluid is withdrawn from a woman's uterus to test for problems in the fetus, such as genetic defects, fetal infections, or fetal lung immaturity. Amniotic fluid contains live fetal skin cells that are normally shed during growth and other substances that provide important information about the baby's health before birth. After a sample of amniotic fluid is removed, the cells are grown in a laboratory for one to two weeks and then tested for chromosomal abnormalities and/or genetic birth defects.

Gynecologic Studies

Gynecologic studies enable a physician to evaluate the function of the internal reproductive organs as well as to diagnose and treat complex diseases and disorders of the GYN system. Although there are many diagnostic and therapeutic procedures available to evaluate and treat disorders of the female reproductive system, the following are the most common diagnostic studies encountered by medical transcriptionists in dictation.

Laparoscopy

Laparoscopy is used to directly visualize the uterus, fallopian tubes, and ovaries to determine the cause of pelvic pain, infertility, or other GYN disorders. In a laparoscopic procedure, a small incision is made in the skin below the navel. A special needle, called a **Veress needle**, is inserted into the incision. The Veress needle pumps carbon dioxide (CO_2) into the abdomen to separate the organs inside the abdominal cavity and make it easier for the physician to see the reproductive organs. The process of instilling the gas into the abdomen is called **insufflation**. The term **pneumoperitoneum** refers to the presence of gas or air in the abdominal cavity.

Once pneumoperitoneum is achieved, the Veress needle is removed and the laparoscope is inserted so that the pelvic organs can be viewed. A tiny camera attached to the laparoscope produces images that can be seen on a computer screen. Other instruments may be inserted through the laparoscope to obtain tissue samples or perform additional procedures. At the conclusion of the laparoscopy, the carbon dioxide gas is released and the incision is sutured.

Colposcopy

Colposcopy is a diagnostic procedure that uses an endoscopic instrument with magnifying lenses, called a **colposcope**, to evaluate abnormal areas in the vagina and cervix and to identify areas of cervical dysplasia in a patient with an abnormal Pap smear. Typically, the colposcope is used in combination with other instruments to obtain samples of tissue and fluid for further examination.

In preparation for the colposcopy, a **speculum** is inserted into the vagina to separate the vaginal walls, allowing for better visualization of the vagina and cervix. Then the cervix is cleaned with **acetic acid**, a vinegarlike solution that turns abnormal tissues white, making them more visible. The colposcope is inserted, and the bright light on the end of the instrument enables the physician to view the cervix, while special filters on the end of the colposcope cause blood vessels to stand out more clearly. This contrast makes it easier to identify abnormal tissue changes in the cervix and vagina. Abnormal changes in cervical tissue are seen as white areas on the surface of the cervix. In dictation, these white areas are referred to as **acetowhite lesions**, and their location is indicated using the clock method. For example: "Acetowhite lesions were noted at the 12 o'clock and 3 o'clock positions on the cervix." Biopsies or tissue samples are taken from these lesions with a spoon-shaped instrument called a **curet** (an alternative spelling is curette) in a procedure known as **endocervical curettage** (ECC). The collected tissue is sent to the lab for examination.

Cone Biopsy

A **cone biopsy** is a more extensive form of a conventional cervical biopsy. It refers to a surgical procedure in which a cone-shaped or cylinder-shaped piece of the cervix is removed and examined under a microscope. In a cone biopsy, a deeper, larger sample of abnormal tissue is removed than that obtained by conventional biopsy. The procedure is usually used to diagnose precancerous changes or to treat cancer. It not only provides a definitive diagnosis of an abnormal Pap smear but also may provide a cure for the problem at the same time if all of the diseased tissue is removed.

In a **cold knife cone biopsy**, a surgical scalpel is used to remove tissue. In this procedure, a small amount of normal tissue around the cone-shaped wedge of abnormal tissue is also removed so that a margin free of abnormal cells is left in the cervix; this may also serve as the treatment if all of the diseased tissue is

QUICK CHECK 16.6

Indicate whether the following sentences are true (T) or false (F).

1. Clue cells are lesions that appear white during colposcopy.   T   F

2. A hysterosalpingogram is an x-ray study of the uterus and fallopian tubes.   T   F

3. A cone biopsy is used to directly visualize the uterus, fallopian tubes, and ovaries.   T   F

4. An endocervical curettage refers to the removal of tissue from the inside of the cervix using a curet.   T   F

5. A beta hCG measures the amount of amniotic fluid in the uterus.   T   F

TABLE 16.1   The BI-RADS Coding System

BI-RADS Category	Finding	Meaning
0	Need additional imaging evaluation	The mammogram study is not yet complete because more information is needed to give a final report, such as additional mammography views or an ultrasound study.
1	Negative	There is nothing to comment on. The breasts are normal with no masses or calcifications present.
2	Benign finding	This is also a negative mammogram, but other findings, such as cysts, fibroadenomas, or lipomas are described in the report. The radiologist may make note of these items while still concluding that there is no mammographic evidence of cancer.
3	Probably benign finding; short interval followup suggested	A finding of an abnormality in this category is also probably benign and not expected to change during a followup examination, but the radiologist would prefer to establish this fact. The chance of breast cancer in this finding is approximately 2%.
4	Suspicious abnormality; biopsy should be considered	The findings in this category indicate that the lesions seen on the mammogram show suspicious changes, and the radiologist has sufficient concern to recommend a biopsy. However, less than half of women with category 4 mammograms end up having cancer.
5	Highly suggestive of malignancy; appropriate action should be taken	The lesions seen on the mammogram in this category show worrisome changes and have a high probability of being cancerous, and the radiologist has strongly recommended a biopsy. More than 90% of women with this category of mammogram will end up having cancer.

removed. Bleeding is controlled with the use of electrocautery or sutures. The tissue is then sent to the lab to determine the nature of the abnormal tissue and whether all abnormal tissue was removed.

Mammography

A **mammogram** is an x-ray picture of the breasts. It is used to detect tumors and cysts and to help differentiate malignant tumors from those that are benign. The test is also used to screen for breast cancer in healthy women with no symptoms. In this procedure, the x-ray technician positions the patient's breast on top of an x-ray plate. An adjustable cover is placed on top of the breast and pressed down, firmly compressing the breast against the plate so that a maximum amount of breast tissue can be imaged and examined. The plates are placed in different positions to obtain side views of breast as well. A radiologist later analyzes the images to evaluate them for signs of cancer in its early stages.

Mammogram results are documented using **BI-RADS,** pronounced in dictation like *BY-rads.* BI-RADS stands for Breast Imaging Reporting and Data System, and it was developed by the American College of Radi-

ology (ACR) as a means for radiologists to report mammogram results using a common language. This system ensures standardized reporting of results, reduced confusion in breast imaging interpretations, and better monitoring of results. In the BI-RADS system, radiologists outline a single-digit score ranging from 0 to 5 when the report of the mammogram is created, along with a final assessment that indicates a specific course of action improving the quality of patient care. Table 16.1 illustrates the BI-RADS assessment scale and the meaning of each code assigned.

CHAPTER SUMMARY

Each day brings advances in all areas of obstetrics and gynecology, including new trends in pregnancy and childbirth, computer-assisted evaluation and diagnosis of gynecologic disorders, and new medical and surgical techniques to treat them. Medical transcriptionists who work in this unique specialty will need to stay abreast of these trends and developments so that they will be familiar with the specialized vocabulary and terminology they will hear when transcribing OB/GYN documents and reports.

·I·N·S·I·G·H·T·

The Enigma of "Gorillapause"

It was conventionally thought that menopause was unique to the human species, but studies by primatologists suggest that menopause is not exclusively a human phenomenon. Research studies on gorillas in captivity may help to answer questions about the biological purpose of menopause and whether a woman's life span exceeding her reproductive years has some evolutionary benefit.

In a study funded by the National Institutes of Health, researchers monitored the hormonal levels and monthly sexual behavior cycles of 30 female gorillas in 16 zoos. They found that even though their lifespan is significantly less than that of humans, they seem to go not only through menopause like humans, but also through perimenopause, during which time they undergo hormonal changes and have a reduced likelihood of conception.

Gorilla research, in addition to helping scientists understand the physiological changes at menopause and suggesting ways to treat the health issues linked to the onset of menopause, may help decide why menopause evolved in the first place, an issue of long-standing debate among scientists. Why have some species evolved to live past their generative years while others have not? What is the biological purpose of menopause? Why is there no equivalent point for men at which their reproductive capacity ceases unquestionably?

The "grandmother theory," a view supported by physiologists, focuses on the societal roles that older mothers can play after their reproductive years end. It suggests that in ancient times, women who were past their reproductive prime contributed to the survival of the species by helping relatives grow and develop; they could devote more time to nurturing the young as they no longer had the burden of caring for their own infants. Anthropologists, on the other hand, believe that menopause may simply be the result of living longer due to advances in scientific knowledge, nutrition, and health care. In ancient societies, almost no one survived past the age of 45 or 50 to experience a decrease in fertility.

Research into postmenopausal health will become even more important as women's life spans lengthen. This type of study may help to solve the evolutionary mystery of menopause as well as to understand the physiological changes that occur with menopause and the health issues associated with the aging female population.

Common Soundalike Words

Word	Word Pronunciation	Soundalike	Soundalike Pronunciation
vulva: The external genitalia of the female.	vŭl′vă	**volvulus:** A twisting of the intestine that causes obstruction.	vol′vyu-lŭs
ectopic: In OB/GYN, a pregnancy occurring at a site other than the cavity of the uterus.	ek-top′ik	**atopic:** Relating to a state of hypersensitivity to environmental allergens.	ă-top′ik
cornua: The horns of the uterus, where the fallopian tubes join the uterine cavity.	kōr′-noo-ă	**cornea:** The transparent outer wall of the eye.	kōr′nē-ă
fetal: Relating to a fetus.	fē′tăl	**fecal:** Relating to feces.	fē′kăl
conization: Excision of a cone of tissue, such as from the mucosa of the cervix.	kō-nī-zā′shŭn	**colonization:** The growth of a group of cells on a solid nutrient surface, each arising from the multiplication of an individual cell; a clone.	kol′ŏ-ni-zā′shun
labial: Relating to the lips of the labia.	lā′bē-ăl	**labile:** Unstable; unpredictable.	lā′bīl
ECC: Abbreviation for endocervical curettage.	ECC	**ECG:** Abbreviation for electrocardiogram.	ECG
metrorrhagia: Irregular, acyclic bleeding from the uterus between periods.	mē′trō-rā′jē-ă	**menorrhagia:** Excessively prolonged or profuse menses.	men-ō-rā′jē-ă
perineum: A small area of the pelvis between the thighs of both males and females located between the anus and the overt genitals.	per-i-nē′ŭm	**peritoneum:** The serous membrane that lines the abdominal cavity and covers most of the organs contained therein.	per′i-tō-nē′ŭm
cervical: Relating to the cervix.	sĕr′vi-kăl	**surgical:** Relating to surgery.	sŭr′ji-kăl

Combining Forms

Combining Form	Meaning	Combining Form	Meaning
amni/o	amnion (fetal membrane)	hyster/o, metr/o, uter/o	uterus
bilirubin/o	bilirubin	mamm/o, mast/o	breast
cervic/o	cervix	men/o	menses
chorion/o	chorion (fetal membrane)	oophor/o, ovari/o	ovary
colp/o, vagin/o	vagina	ov/i, ov/o	egg
culd/o	cul-de-sac	salping/o	tube (as in fallopian tube)
embryon/o	embryo; immature form	spermato/o	sperm
episi/o	vulva	toc/o	labor or birth
galact/o, lact/o	milk	trachel/o	cervix
genit/o	genitalia	vulv/o	vulva
gynec/o	woman		

Add Your Own Combining Forms Here:

_____

_____

_____

_____

_____

_____

ABBREVIATIONS

Abbreviation	Meaning
AIDS	acquired immunodeficiency syndrome
BI-RADS	Breast Imaging Reporting and Data System
BSO	bilateral salpingo-oophorectomies
BUS	Bartholin, urethral, and Skene (glands)
CIN	cervical intraepithelial neoplasia
DCIS	ductal carcinoma in situ
ECC	endocervical curettage
EG/BUS	external genitalia/Bartholin, urethral, and Skene (glands)
FSE	fetal scalp electrode
FUS	focused ultrasound surgery
GnRH	gonadotropin releasing hormone
GPA	gravida, para, abortus
GYN	gynecology
hCG	human chorionic gonadotropin
HIV	human immunodeficiency virus
HPV	human papillomavirus
HSG	hysterosalpingogram
HSV	herpes simplex virus
ICSI	intracytoplasmic sperm injection
IDC	invasive (infiltrating) ductal carcinoma
ILC	invasive (infiltrating) lobular carcinoma

Abbreviation	Meaning
IUPC	intrauterine pressure catheter
IVF	in vitro fertilization
LCIS	lobular carcinoma in situ
LEEP	loop electrosurgical excision procedure
LSO	left salpingo-oophorectomy
NSAIDs	nonsteroidal anti-inflammatory drugs
NSVD	normal spontaneous vaginal delivery
OB/GYN	obstetrics/gynecology
PID	pelvic inflammatory disease
PROM	premature rupture of membranes
PVA	polyvinyl alcohol
ROM	rupture of membranes
RSO	right salpingo-oophorectomy
SHG	sonohysterogram
SIL	squamous intraepithelial lesion
STD	sexually transmitted disease
TAH	total abdominal hysterectomy
TIPAL	term infants, premature infants, abortions, living children
VBAC	vaginal birth after C-section

Add Your Own Abbreviations Here:

_____

_____

_____

_____

_____

_____

TERMINOLOGY

Term	Meaning
abdominal hysterectomy	A hysterectomy that is performed through access from the abdomen.
ablation	Surgical removal or excision.
abortus	The number of pregnancy losses before the 20th week.
accelerations	Increases in the fetal heart rate.
acetic acid	A vinegarlike solution spray applied to the cervix during colposcopy to make abnormal tissues turn white.
acetowhite lesions	Abnormal changes in the vagina and cervix that appear white after being sprayed with acetic acid.
acquired immunodeficiency syndrome (AIDS)	A sexually transmitted disease passed from one person to another through infected blood, semen, or vaginal secretions.
adhesions	Bands of fibrous scar tissue that form on organs.
adnexa (of the uterus)	Appendages or adjunct parts. The adnexa of the uterus consist of the fallopian tubes, ovaries, and the ligaments that hold them together.
amenorrhea	Absence of bleeding.
amniocentesis	A test in which amniotic fluid is withdrawn from the uterus to test for genetic defects, infections, or lung immaturity in a fetus.
amnion	A thin membrane that eventually surrounds the embryo.
amniotic fluid	A fluid that encases the fetus and provides a cushion for the fetus as the mother moves.
antiretroviral drugs	Medications that work to reduce the level of HIV in the blood which, in turn, can dramatically slow the destruction of the immune system.
Apgar score	The score of the Apgar test, which rates a newborn's physical condition immediately after birth.
assisted zonal hatching	The process of applying a diluted acidic solution to the wall of egg in order to thin its outer shell sufficiently for successful implantation in the uterus.
Bartholin glands	Glands that keep the vaginal mucosa moist and provide a lubricant for the vagina during sexual intercourse.
beta hCG	A hormone that is detected in a urine test to indicate pregnancy.
bilateral salpingo-oophorectomies (BSO)	The surgical removal of both fallopian tubes and ovaries.
BI-RADS	A system developed by radiologists to report mammogram results using a common language.
birth canal	Another word for *vagina*.
body	The upper part of the uterus that lies below the entrance to the fallopian tubes.
breast cancer	A cancerous tumor of breast tissue.
breech presentation	The baby's position in the uterus in which the baby is buttocks or feet first as opposed to head first.
carcinoma in situ	Early stage cancer that is confined to the place where it began.
cervical cancer	A cancer that develops in the lining of the cervix.
cervical dysplasia	The development of abnormal cells in the lining of the cervix.
cervical intraepithelial neoplasia (CIN)	An alternative name for cervical dysplasia and a method to categorize the abnormal changes observed in cervical tissue.

Term	Meaning
cervix	The tubular, lower portion of the uterus that opens into the vagina.
cesarean section	A method of delivery of a newborn through a surgical incision in the abdomen and front wall of the uterus.
clear cell carcinoma	A type of cancer that can originate in the uterus or the ovary.
clitoris	A small mass of erectile tissue in females that responds to sexual stimulation.
clue cells	Vaginal cells that appear fuzzy under a microscope when coated with bacteria, indicating infection.
cold knife cone biopsy	A procedure in which a section of abnormal tissue along with normal-appearing tissue is removed from the cervix with a surgical scalpel and examined under a microscope.
colostrum	A substance produced by the mammary glands that contains milk fat and immunoglobulins.
colposcope	A lighted instrument used to identify and evaluate abnormal areas in the vagina and cervix.
colposcopy	A procedure that uses a colposcope to view and evaluate abnormal areas in the vagina and cervix.
cone biopsy	A procedure in which a cone-shaped piece of abnormal tissue in the cervix is removed and examined under a microscope.
connective tissue	Tissue that connects, supports, binds, or separates other tissues or organs.
corpus luteum	A temporary endocrine gland formed from an ovarian follicle that has released an ovum, which secretes progesterone during the second half of the menstrual cycle.
cryomyolysis	A procedure in which liquid nitrogen is used to freeze and destroy a uterine fibroid.
cryopreservation	The process of freezing an embryo prior to IVF transfer.
cryotherapy	The freezing of diseased tissue with liquid nitrogen.
C-section	Another term for *cesarean section*.
curet	A spoon-shaped instrument with a cutting edge and handle used to remove tissue in the body.
decelerations	Decreases in the fetal heart rate.
dilation	The opening of the cervix during labor.
ductal carcinoma in situ (DCIS)	Cancer that is confined to the ducts of the breast that has not spread into the tissue of the breast.
ducts	The channels that carry breast milk to the nipple.
dysmenorrhea	Difficult or painful menstruation.
dystocia	Difficult labor.
eclampsia	The final and most severe phase of preeclampsia if left untreated, leading to seizures or coma in the mother or even death of the mother and baby before, during, or after childbirth.
ectopic pregnancy	A pregnancy that occurs when the egg implants itself outside the uterus.
effacement	Thinning of the cervix in preparation for delivery.
electrocautery	The burning of abnormal tissue by a device with a very hot tip, heated by electricity.

Term	Meaning
embryo	The name given to a developing baby from the time of implantation in the uterus until about the eighth week of gestation.
embryo transfer	The process of placing the fertilized eggs into a woman's uterus.
endocervical curettage (ECC)	The removal of tissue from the inside of the cervix using a curet.
endometrial ablation	A procedure in which the endometrial lining of the uterus is surgically removed.
endometrial cancer	A cancer that begins in the endometrium of the uterus.
endometriosis	A disorder in which endometrial tissue grows elsewhere in the abdominal cavity.
endometritis	Inflammation of the uterus.
endometrium	The inner lining of the uterus.
epithelial carcinoma	A cancer which begins on the surface of the ovary.
estrogen	A hormone produced by the ovaries.
external genital organs	Those genital structures found outside the body.
fallopian tubes	Tubular structures that extend from the upper edge of the uterus toward the ovaries.
fern test	A test used to determine whether membranes have ruptured.
fertilization, syn. conception	When sperm and egg form what will become a human individual.
fetal heart rate	The normal heart rate for a full-term infant.
fetal heart tones	Another term for *fetal heart rate*.
fetal scalp electrode (FSE)	A device placed just under the skin of the baby's scalp that is used to monitor the baby's heartbeat while still in the uterus.
fetus	The name given to a developing baby from the eighth week of gestation until delivery.
fimbriae	A number of fingerlike extensions of the fallopian tube that drape over the ovary.
focused ultrasound surgery (FUS)	A procedure that uses high-frequency sound waves to destroy uterine fibroids.
follicle stimulating hormone (FSH)	A hormone secreted by the pituitary gland to stimulate the growth of eggs in the ovaries.
follicles	Fluid-filled sacs in the ovaries, each containing an immature ovum.
follicular aspiration	The removal of a mature follicle by means of a suction device.
forceps	Metal surgical instruments resembling tongs with rounded edges that fit around the baby's head to assist with delivery.
fraternal twins	Twins produced by the simultaneous fertilization of two separate egg cells.
frozen embryo transfer	The process of using *cryopreserved* embryos during the in vitro fertilization (IVF) transfer process.
fundus	The dome-shaped top portion of the uterus that lies above the entrance of the fallopian tubes.
genital tract	Another word for *internal genital organs*.
germ cell tumor gonadotropin releasing hormone (GnRH) agonist	A cancer that starts from germ cells, the cells that produce eggs in the ovaries. A type of medication that tends to slow the growth of endometriosis and relieve symptoms.
gestational diabetes	A form of diabetes that develops during pregnancy.
GPA system	An abbreviated form of the terms gravida, para, and abortus used to indicate obstetric history.
gravida	The total number of pregnancies a woman has experienced.

Term	Meaning
gynecologic cancers	Cancers that occur in any part of the female reproductive system.
gynecologic disorders	Disorders that affect the female reproductive system.
gynecologist	A physician who has specialized education and training in the health, disorders, and treatment of the female reproductive system.
gynecology	The specialty of diseases of the female reproductive system.
hemolysis	The alteration, dissolution, or destruction of red blood cells.
high-grade SIL	Refers to a large number of precancerous cells on the surface of the cervix.
human immunodeficiency virus (HIV)	The virus that causes AIDS by destroying the blood cells in the body that help the human immune system to function properly.
human chorionic gonadotropin (hCG)	A protein produced in the placenta of pregnant women.
human papillomavirus (HPV)	A group of viruses that produce genital warts, transmitted through sexual contact, with some strains associated with increased instances of cervical and rectal cancer.
hyperemesis gravidarum	A complication of pregnancy characterized by severe and excessive nausea and vomiting.
hysterectomy	A surgery to remove the uterus and, sometimes, the cervix.
hysterosalpingogram (HSG)	An x-ray study with contrast dye of the uterus and fallopian tubes.
hysteroscopy	The visual examination of the interior of the uterus and fallopian tubes.
identical twins	Twins conceived from one egg.
in vitro fertilization (IVF)	A method of achieving pregnancy by artificial means.
infertility	The inability of a couple to become pregnant, regardless of the cause.
infundibulum	The part of the fallopian tube that overlies the ovary.
insemination	The transfer of sperm to establish a pregnancy.
insufflation	The process of instilling air or gas into a cavity (such as the abdomen).
internal genital organs	The structures involved in human reproduction.
intracytoplasmic sperm injection (ICSI)	A procedure that assists with fertilization by the manual injection of a single live sperm into an egg.
introitus	Another term for the opening of the vagina.
intrauterine pressure catheter (IUPC)	A small catheter for measuring the strength and duration of uterine contractions, which is placed alongside the baby in the uterus.
invasive (infiltrating) ductal carcinoma (IDC)	Cancer that starts in a milk duct of the breast and goes on to invade the tissue of the breast.
invasive (infiltrating) lobular carcinoma (ILC)	Cancer that starts in a lobule of the breast and goes on to invade the tissue of the breast.
labia	Two sets of skin folds that serve to cover the female external genital organs and tissues.
labia majora	A pair of prominent folds of skin from the mons pubis to the perineum that enclose and protect the other female external genital organs.
labia minora	A pair of smaller folds of skin lying just inside the labia majora that surround the openings to the vagina and urethra.
labor	The term given to the efforts of giving birth to a child at the conclusion of a pregnancy.
lactation	The production of milk in the breasts.

Term	Meaning
laparoscopy	Direct visualization of the abdominal cavity through a laparoscope, using a very small incision in the abdomen.
laparotomy	Direct visualization of the abdominal cavity through a laparoscope, using a much larger incision in the abdomen.
leiomyosarcoma	A malignant cancer of smooth-muscle cells.
luteinizing hormone (LH)	A hormone secreted by the pituitary gland to stimulate the growth of eggs in the ovaries.
lobular carcinoma in situ (LCIS)	Cancer that begins in the lobules of the breast but does not invade surrounding tissue.
lobules	The glands in the breast that make breast milk.
loop electrosurgical excision procedure (LEEP)	A procedure that uses a thin wire loop with an electric current running through it to remove cancerous tissue.
low-grade SIL	Refers to early precancerous changes in the cells of the lining of the cervix.
lumpectomy	A surgical procedure that involves removing only the tumor and some of the surrounding tissue of the breast.
mammary glands	Modified sweat glands located in the breasts that prepare for milk production during pregnancy.
mammogram	An x-ray of the breasts.
menarche	A young woman's first menstrual period.
menometrorrhagia	Bleeding that occurs both during menses and at irregular intervals.
menopause	The period preceding and following the last menstrual flow in a woman's life.
menorrhagia	Excessively heavy bleeding.
menses	The onset of menstruation.
menstrual cycle	The series of changes a woman's body goes through to make eggs available for fertilization in preparation for possible pregnancy.
menstruation	The periodic shedding of the uterine lining when no pregnancy occurs.
modified radical mastectomy	A surgical procedure that involves removing the entire breast as well as some of the surrounding tissues and structures.
mons pubis	A rounded mound of fatty tissue that covers the pubic bone.
myolysis	A procedure in which an electric current is used to destroy the blood supply leading to a uterine fibroid.
myomectomy	The surgical removal of a uterine fibroid.
myometrium	The thick, muscular middle layer of the uterus.
Nitrazine test	A test used to determine whether membranes have ruptured.
normal spontaneous vaginal delivery	A vaginal birth without complications.
nulligravida	Another term for *no pregnancies*.
nullipara	Another term indicating *no deliveries of viable offspring*.
obstetrician	A physician who is a specialist in the management of pregnancy and childbirth.
obstetrician/gynecologist (OB/GYN)	A physician who provides medical and surgical care regarding women's gynecological health and also has particular expertise in reproductive issues.
obstetrics	The branch of medicine that deals with the care of women during pregnancy, childbirth, and the recuperative period following delivery.

Term	*Meaning*
oocyte	An immature ovum contained in a follicle.
oophoritis	Inflammation of the ovaries.
ovarian cancer	A cancer that forms in the cells of the ovary.
ovarian carcinoma	Another word for *ovarian cancer*.
ovaries	A pair of oval structures attached to the uterus, which produce hormones and release eggs (ova).
ovulation	The process of discharging one ovum from an ovary.
ovulation induction	The use of hormone therapy to stimulate the development of mature eggs.
ovum	An egg cell in females that, if fertilized, can produce a human offspring.
oxytocin	A natural hormone produced by the pituitary gland that causes uterine contractions.
Pap smear	A test that involves the microscopic examination of cells collected from the cervix to evaluate for abnormal cell changes.
papillary serous carcinoma	A type of cancer that can originate in the uterus or the ovary.
papilloma	A benign epithelial tumor, such as a genital wart.
para	The number of births of viable offspring.
partial hysterectomy	The surgical removal of the uterus only.
pelvic inflammatory disease (PID)	A general term that refers to infection of the uterus, fallopian tubes, and ovaries.
perimetrium	The outer layer of the uterus that covers the body of the uterus and part of the cervix.
Pfannenstiel incision	A transverse incision made in the lower part of the abdomen during a cesarean section delivery.
placenta	A temporary organ implanted in the uterus from which the fetus receives nutrients and oxygen from the mother's blood and passes waste.
placenta abruptio	A complication of pregnancy in which the placenta breaks away, or abrupts, from the wall of the uterus too early, before the baby is born, causing premature birth or major blood loss in the mother.
placenta previa	A complication of pregnancy in which the placenta is implanted in the lower part of the uterus instead of the upper part, causing it to partly or completely block the cervix.
pneumoperitoneum	Air or gas in the abdominal cavity.
polyvinyl alcohol (PVA)	Small synthetic particles injected into the body which block the blood flow to a uterine fibroid, causing it to shrink.
postmenopause	The stage of menopause that begins when 12 full months have passed since the last menstrual period.
premature rupture of membranes (PROM)	Refers to the sac of amniotic fluid rupturing before labor actually begins.
preeclampsia, syn. toxemia	A condition in pregnant women marked by high blood pressure and a high level of protein in the urine.
primigravida	Another term for *first pregnancy*.
progesterone	A female steroid hormone produced by the ovaries.
prolactin	A lactation-stimulating hormone.
pubic symphysis, syn. pubic bone	One of three sections of the hipbone that form the front of the pelvis.

Term	Meaning
Rh factor incompatibility	A situation in pregnancy that occurs when the mother has Rh-negative blood and the Rh-positive blood, resulting in the mother's immune system producing antibodies to destroy the baby.
RhoGAM, syn. Rho immunoglobulin	An injectable blood product used to protect an Rh-positive fetus from the antibodies produced by its Rh-negative mother.
ripening	The term given to the softening of the cervix in preparation for delivery.
rupture of membranes	The loss of fluid from the amniotic sac.
salpingitis	Inflammation of the fallopian tube.
salpingo-oophorectomy	The surgical removal of a fallopian tube and ovary on either the left or the right side.
salpinx	The formal name for *fallopian tube*.
secundigravida	Another term for *second pregnancy*.
sexually transmitted disease (STD)	A disease caused by a pathogen that is spread from person to person primarily through sexual contact.
simple mastectomy	Excision of the breast including the nipple, areola, and some of the overlying skin.
singleton	A term that refers to a pregnancy with only one baby.
Skene glands	A pair of glands located on each side of the lower end of the urethra.
smear	Any type of laboratory study in which material is thinly spread over the surface of a microscope slide for examination.
sonohysterogram (SHG)	A visual study of the uterus and fallopian tubes using an ultrasound probe.
speculum	An instrument with a curved blade used to spread apart the vaginal walls, allowing better visualization of the vagina and cervix.
squamous cell carcinoma	An invasive type of cervical cancer that develops in the squamous cells that line the cervix.
squamous intraepithelial lesion (SIL)	A general term used to describe abnormal cells in the lining of the cervix.
station	The position of the baby's presenting part relative to the mother's ischial spine.
stromal cell tumor	A cancer that begins in the cells of the fibrous tissue and ligaments of the ovary.
tocodynamometer	An instrument used to measure the force of uterine contractions.
total abdominal hysterectomy	The surgical removal of the uterus and cervix by means of access from the abdomen.
total hysterectomy	The surgical removal of the uterus and part or all of the cervix.
TPAL system	A system used to describe the obstetric history of a patient.
transfer catheter	A catheter with a syringe that is used to transfer fertilized eggs into the woman's uterus.
umbilical cord	A cord composed of blood vessels and connective tissue that is connected to the fetus from the placenta.
urethra	The canal leading from the bladder that discharges the urine externally.
uterine artery embolization	A procedure that blocks the blood vessels that supply a uterine fibroid by injecting small particles of polyvinyl alcohol (PVA) into the arteries that supply it.
uterine cancer	Cancer that originates in the body and muscle layers of the uterus.
uterine fibroids, syn. myomas or leiomyomas	Noncancerous growths composed of muscle and fibrous tissue located in or on the uterus.

Term	Meaning
uterine sarcoma	A cancer that originates in the myometrium of the uterus.
uterus, syn. womb	A pear-shaped organ located in the middle of the pelvis that holds and nourishes a growing fetus.
vacuum extractor	A suction device used to assist with delivery.
vagina, syn. birth canal	A muscular tube projecting inside a female that connects the uterus to the outside of the body.
vaginal birth after C-section (VBAC)	A birth of a child by vaginal delivery after a previous cesarean section delivery.
vaginal hysterectomy	A hysterectomy performed by means of access through the vagina.
vaginal wet mount, syn. vaginal smear	A test performed on a sample of vaginal discharge to check for micro-organisms which may have caused an infection.
Veress needle	A special needle used to pump carbon dioxide (CO_2) into the abdomen to separate the organs inside the abdominal cavity during surgery.
viral load	The level of HIV in the circulating blood.
vulva	The area in which the female external genitalia organs are found.
wet mount	A test in which a sample of body fluid is examined under the microscope for the presence of micro-organisms.
zona pellucida	The outer shell of a fertilized egg.

Add Your Own Terms and Definitions Here:

_____

_____

_____

_____

_____

_____

_____

_____

REVIEW QUESTIONS

1. What structure enables an egg to travel from the ovary to the uterus?
2. When is an embryo considered a fetus?
3. What is the difference between carcinoma in situ and invasive carcinoma?
4. How is a fetus nourished during development?
5. How does HIV cause AIDS?
6. What is the purpose of the Bartholin gland?
7. Differentiate between the terms nulligravida, primigravida, and secundigravida.
8. Explain the difference between partial hysterectomy and total hysterectomy.
9. Name the three layers which comprise the wall of the uterus.
10. What is a Pfannenstiel skin incision?

CHAPTER ACTIVITIES

Soundalike Word Choice

Circle the correct word in the following sentences.

1. The patient complained that she was (neither/either) able to shower nor take a bath without pain.
2. She complained of abdominal pain and (amenorrhea/dysmenorrhea) each month with excessive bleeding around the time of her period.
3. She was to follow up next week (for/per) the ER report.
4. The diagnosis was a germ cell tumor; however, there was no pathology report (requiring/regarding) this finding.
5. On pelvic examination, there was no (uterine/urine) tenderness.
6. The patient underwent a (hysteroscopy/hysterectomy) to remove her uterus and cervix.
7. The patient was tried on a voiding (trail/trial) last month.
8. She was (infirmed/informed) that she could now start dressing changes.
9. Ms. Smith will return in 2 weeks for (postpartum/postmortem) care.
10. The patient states she is not on any form of birth control and, therefore, will remain (abstinent/absent) from sexual intercourse.
11. She states that lately her weight has made it difficult to (breathe/breath).
12. The patient came in today to have the (staples/stapes) removed from her incision.
13. I discussed with the couple the option of in (vitreous/vitro) fertilization.
14. The patient has undergone regular Lupron (injections/infections) to assist with fertilization.
15. The fibroid was visualized, but it was just (passed/past) the tip of the scope.

Matching

Match the following terms in the left column with their corresponding definitions in the right column.

Term

1. _____ SHG
2. _____ curet
3. _____ secundigravida
4. _____ lobules
5. _____ cryotherapy
6. _____ nullipara
7. _____ germ cell tumor
8. _____ PROM
9. _____ myometrium
10. _____ ovum
11. _____ endometritis
12. _____ salpinx
13. _____ menarche
14. _____ prolactin
15. _____ progesterone

Definition

a. Time of first menstruation.
b. Inflammation of the endometrium.
c. The middle layer of the uterus.
d. A female steroid hormone produced by the ovaries.
e. A lactation-stimulating hormone.
f. Another name for fallopian tube.
g. A spoon-shaped instrument.
h. Freezing diseased tissue with liquid nitrogen.
i. Another word for second pregnancy.
j. Sonohysterogram.
k. The glands that make breast milk.
l. No deliveries of viable offspring.
m. Premature rupture of membranes.
n. A cancer that begins in the cells that produce eggs in the ovaries.
o. An egg cell.

Converting Nouns to Adjectives

Convert each of the following OB/GYN nouns into its adjectival form.

1. cervix _____
2. adnexa _____
3. amnion _____
4. areola _____
5. vagina _____
6. endometrium _____
7. duct _____
8. fetus _____
9. gynecology _____
10. menopause _____
11. ovary _____
12. perineum _____
13. umbilicus _____
14. uterus _____
15. vestibule _____

Fill in the Blanks

Fill in the blanks of the following paragraph with the correct terms from the text.

For (1) _____ to occur, a sperm must locate and penetrate the awaiting egg while it is in the (2) _____. If two separate eggs are fertilized simultaneously, the resulting offspring are called (3) _____ twins. When a fertilized egg divides into two halves and starts to form two babies, the result is known as (4) _____ twins. An (5) _____ pregnancy occurs when a fertilized egg implants itself outside the uterus. From 8 weeks until delivery, the developing baby is known as a (6) _____. In the GPA system, the letter *G* stands for (7) _____, *P* for (8) _____, and *A* for (9) _____. The term (10) _____ means no pregnancies, whereas the term (11) _____ means one pregnancy. (12) _____ is the inability of a couple to become pregnant, regardless of the cause. In that instance, (13) _____ is a method of achieving pregnancy by artificial means.

Combining Forms Practice

For each of the following terms, circle the correct combining form that corresponds to the meaning given.

1. breast	mano/o	mamm/o	men/o
2. vulva	uvul/o	valv/o	vulv/o
3. uterus	unguin/o	uter/o	utiar/o
4. menses	mens/o	men/o	mann/o
5. ovary	oophor/o	over/o	ovilli/o
6. fallopian tube	fallop/o	tubor/o	salping/o
7. cervix	cervic/o	cervali/o	cerul/o
8. sperm	spimat/o	spermat/o	testic/o
9. labor or birth	toc/o	tachy/o	tac/o
10. vagina	virul/o	vagar/o	vagin/o

TRANSCRIPTION PRACTICE

Open your word-processing software. Insert the student CD-ROM and locate the dictation for this chapter. For each of the words in the "listen for these terms" list for each report, use a medical dictionary or other resources to identify and write down a brief definition of the term on a separate sheet of paper to attach with your work. Then listen to the dictation and transcribe each report. Use the current date for each report where a date is indicated. Insert a heading into the document if the text falls to a second page.

At the end of each report, indicate the name of the dictating physician under the signature line and insert reference initials. For date dictated and transcribed and date of admission, use the current date. Proofread your work, print one copy for your instructor along with your term definitions, and save the completed report to your student CD.

Report #T16.1: Discharge Summary
Patient Name: Dee Hampton
Medical Record No.: 21-07005
Attending Physician: Samuel Voorhees, MD

Listen for these terms:
salpingo-oophorectomy
enterolysis
fibroids
SCDs

Report #T16.2: Clinic Note
Patient Name: Tamara Becker
Medical Record No.: 00-323
Attending Physician: Andrea Biggs, MD

Listen for these terms:
abdominopelvic
circumscribed
adnexa

Report #T16.3: Operative Report
Patient Name: Holly Akins
Medical Record No.: 922-77400
Attending Physician: Andrea Biggs, MD
Assistant: Michael Josephs, MD

Listen for these terms:
Pfannenstiel skin incision
Mayo scissors
Kocher clamps
rectus muscles
bladder blade
vesicouterine peritoneum
footling breech
Dexon (sutures)

17

ORTHOPAEDICS

OBJECTIVES

After completing this chapter, you will be able to:

- Discuss the anatomy of bones and the organization and structure of the skeleton.
- Describe the types and composition of muscles and other structures that make up the musculoskeletal system.
- Recognize and define the terminology related to regions of the body and terms of movement.
- Describe common diseases and disorders affecting the musculoskeletal system, as well as the pharmacological and surgical methods used to treat them.
- Describe common laboratory tests and diagnostic procedures used to evaluate diseases and disorders involving the bones and muscles.

INTRODUCTION

The **musculoskeletal system** is a complex body system consisting of bones, muscles, tendons, ligaments, joints, and other connective tissue. These components all work together to provide form and support to the body, to protect delicate internal organs, and to enable the body to move. The study of bones is called **osteology**. How-ever, the science of diagnosis, treatment, rehabilitation, and prevention of diseases and abnormalities of the musculoskeletal system is called **orthopaedics**.

According to the American Academy of Orthopaedic Surgery, the proper spelling is *orthopaedic*, not *orthopedic*; although the alternative spelling, *orthopedic*, has become an accepted use. The term *orthopaedics* derives from the Greek roots *ortho* (straight) and *pais* (child), as much of the early work in orthopaedics involved treating children who had spine or limb deformities. Orthopaedic physicians continue to treat children with bone tumors and neuromuscular problems. They correct growth abnormalities such as unequal leg length and birth abnormalities such as club foot, hip dislocation, and abnormalities of fingers and toes. They also treat diseases prevalent in the elderly, such as osteoporosis.

An **orthopaedist** treats the special problems associated with the many components of the musculoskeletal system. In addition to injuries to bones such as fractures and dislocations, an orthopaedist treats disturbances in joints such as sprains or torn cartilages; back problems such as strains, ruptured disks, and curvatures; neck disorders; and inflammation of muscle or connective tissues. Some orthopaedists specialize in treating particular parts of the musculoskeletal system, such as the hands, feet, hips, or knees. Others specialize in sports medicine, treating injuries caused by athletic exertions. Orthopaedic surgeons employ a variety of mechanical devices, such as braces, splints, pins, screws, and nails, to repair skeletal injuries.

This chapter presents an overview of the body's skeletal structure, muscle structure, and the function of each; the common diseases and disorders treated by orthopaedists; and the diagnostic studies used to evaluate musculoskeletal disorders.

ANATOMY OF THE MUSCULOSKELETAL SYSTEM

Every movement of the body involves bones, muscles, and joints. Together, these components—along with tendons, ligaments, and cartilage—form the musculoskeletal system, which enables the body to support its own weight, to move, and to perform other functions essential to survival, such as chewing food and moving it through the digestive system.

Bones

The skeleton is the framework of the body and comprises hard endoskeletal tissue called **bone**.

Organization and Function

Bone is one of the hardest tissues in the human body (the hardest is tooth enamel). The 206 bones that make up the human skeleton provide support for the body against the pull of gravity, maintain its shape, and protect delicate vital organs. Bones provide a place to which muscles and supporting structures can attach and, with the movable joints, form a system of levers upon which muscles can act to produce body movements.

Bones also function as a storage site for minerals, primarily calcium and phosphorus, which are necessary for proper functioning of the muscles and nervous system. Approximately 99% of the calcium in the human body is stored in the bones. When the additional calcium is needed (such as during pregnancy or after menopause), the body uses stored calcium by taking what it needs from the bones. Therefore, individuals with calcium-deficient diets are at risk of losing bone mass and strength over time.

The bones are also the site for the formation of blood cells, a process called **hematopoiesis**. The spongy connective tissue that fills the cavities of the bones, called **marrow**, is the substance in which many of the blood elements—red blood cells, white blood cells, and platelets—are produced.

Bone is made up of two main types of tissues: **Compact bone** is tightly packed, hard material that makes up the outside surfaces of bones. **Spongy (or cancellous) bone** is less dense than compact bone. It is a latticelike structure of bony tissue that makes up the inner portion of bone. Spongy bone consists of thin, branching, bony plates called **trabeculae** and bars of bone that lie adjacent to small, irregular spaces that contain the tissue where hematopoiesis takes place. The trabeculae are organized to help support the body's weight and can realign if the direction of stress on the bone changes.

During youth bones grow in length and density. During the teen years maximum bone height is reached, but bones continue to grow more dense until about age 30 when peak bone density is attained. Once bone formation and density has peaked, bone mass is maintained by a process of reshaping, called **remodeling**. This process is one of continually building up and tearing down as the bone continues to grow. Two types of bone cells, called **osteocytes**, are involved in this process. **Osteoclasts** are cells that break down areas of old or damaged bone, while **osteoblasts** are cells that deposit new bone tissue in those areas. When it has reached its maximum size, as determined by genetics, the bone slows this process but continues to replenish old bone with the new. Remodeling is the process that occurs during the repair of broken bones.

Types of Bones

The human skeleton has four types of bones, and the names given to each type describe the general shape of the bones in each category.

Long bones are longer than they are wide. A long bone consists of a long shaft with two bulky ends or extremities. They are composed primarily of compact bone but may have a large amount of spongy bone near the inner edges. The major bones of the arms and legs are long bones.

The main features of the long bone are illustrated in Figure 17.1 and described as follows:

- The **diaphysis**, or shaft, is the tubular portion of the bone and is composed of compact bone tissue.
- The **epiphysis** (plural, epiphyses) is the expanded end of the bone.
- The **metaphysis** is the area where the diaphysis meets the epiphysis.
- The **medullary cavity**, or **marrow cavity**, is the open area within the diaphysis of the bone. It is filled with two types of marrow. **Red marrow** actively produces blood cells. **Yellow marrow** is bone marrow that does not have any blood-producing function but serves as a storage site for fat cells. During infancy and early childhood, all bone marrow is red; but as one grows older and less blood cell production is needed, the fat content of the marrow increases, forming more yellow and less red. This means that the elderly are more prone to infections and cancers because there are fewer lymphocytes being produced since the red bone marrow decreases. The medullary cavity functions as the storage site for fat cells.

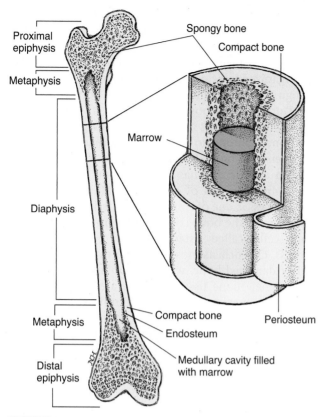

FIGURE 17.1. **Parts of a Long Bone and Composition of Compact Bone.** Reprinted with permission from *Stedman's Medical Dictionary,* 27th ed. Baltimore: Lippincott Williams & Wilkins, 2000.

- The **periosteum** is the membrane of dense connective tissue covering the outside of the diaphysis, as well as the epiphyses where articular cartilage is absent.
- The **endosteum** is the membrane that lines the marrow cavity.

Short bones are shorter than long bones and are shaped like cubes with vertical and horizontal dimensions approximately equal. They consist primarily of spongy bone, which is covered by a thin layer of compact bone. Short bones allow for flexibility; for example, the short bones of the finger allow the hand to be curled into a fist. Toes are also composed of short bones.

Flat bones are thin, platelike structures with broad surfaces, such as those found in the skull and ribs. Their function is protection; flat bones surround the vital parts of the body, such as the brain, heart, lungs, and reproductive organs.

Bones that do not fit into any of the categories described previously are classified as **irregular bones.** They have a variety of sizes and shapes and are distributed throughout the skeleton. The bones of the spine and some of the bones that make up the face in the skull are irregular bones.

Divisions of the Skeleton

The two major divisions of the human skeleton are the axial skeleton and the appendicular skeleton, as illustrated in Figure 17.2.

Axial Skeleton

The **axial skeleton** forms the vertical axis of the body. It includes the bones of the skull, the vertebral column, and the chest. See Table 17.1 for the bones of the axial skeleton.

- The **skull** provides protection for the brain and the organs of vision, taste, equilibrium, and smell. It consists of the **cranial bones,** (the top part of the skull that encloses the brain), the **mandible** (lower jawbone), and the **hyoid bone** at the base of the tongue (a horseshoe-shaped bone attached to muscles of the tongue and to the larynx). **Sutures** are immovable interlocking joints that join the skull bones together (not to be confused with sutures, or

TABLE 17.1	Bones of the Axial Skeleton
Region	*Name of Bone*
cranium (head)	frontal
	parietal
	temporal
	occipital
	sphenoid
	ethmoid
face	mandible
	maxilla
	zygomatic
	nasal bone
	lacrimal
	palatine
	inferior nasal concha
	vomer
auditory ossicles (ears)	malleus
	incus
	stapes
hyoid	hyoid
vertebrae (spine)	cervical vertebrae, C1-C7
	thoracic vertebrae, T1-T12
	lumbar vertebrae, L1-L5
	sacrum (5 fused), S1-S5
	coccyx
sternum	sternum: manubrium body of sternum xiphoid process
ribs	ribs (12 pairs)

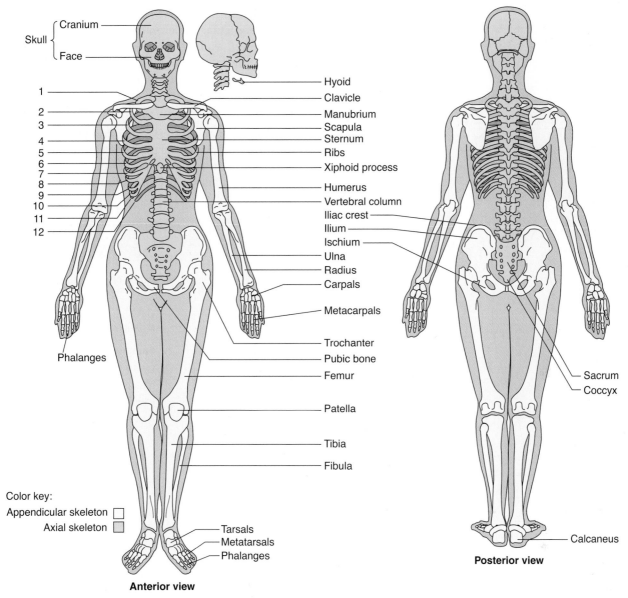

Color key:
Appendicular skeleton ☐
Axial skeleton ☐

FIGURE 17.2. **The Human Skeleton.** Anterior and posterior views of the human skeleton. Reprinted with permission from Willis MC. *Medical Terminology: A Programmed Learning Approach to the Language of Health Care.* Baltimore: Lippincott Williams & Wilkins, 2002.

stitches, that are used in surgery to sew a seam between two surfaces). **Fontanels** (also spelled *fontanelles*) are fibrous spaces between the cranial bones where the sutures are not yet closed. *Fontanel* derives from the French word that means *little fountain* and refers to any membrane-covered area between two bones. During birth, these spaces enable the soft bony plates of the skull to flex, allowing for better passage of the infant's head through the birth canal. As these sutures are not yet joined together, two fontanels, sometimes called *soft spots*, are present in the midline of the baby's skull, one near the front of the head and one near the back. The area in the front of the head is called the **anterior fontanel**, which usually closes between the ages of 10 and 18 months. The area in

the back of the head, called the **posterior fontanel**, usually closes by age two months. Many bones of the skull are hollow, which decreases the weight of the skull and provides resonance to the voice; the cavities inside the hollow bones are called **sinuses**.

● The **vertebral column**, also known as the *backbone* or *spine*, is made up of a stack of 24 small bones called **vertebrae** (singular, **vertebra**), the sacrum, and the coccyx, as illustrated in Figure 17.3. The **sacrum** is a group of fused vertebrae that join with the hip bones to form the most posterior part of the pelvis. The **coccyx** (commonly referred to as the *tail bone*) is a group of several smaller, fused vertebrae. The spine is divided into four regions, and the bones of the vertebral column are named according to their location along the length of the spinal

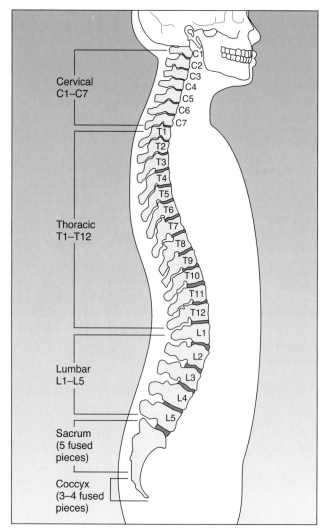

FIGURE 17.3. The Vertebral Column. The spinal column divided into four regions, and the bones are named according to their location along its length. Reprinted with permission from Willis MC. *Medical Terminology: A Programmed Learning Approach to the Language of Health Care.* Baltimore: Lippincott Williams & Wilkins, 2002.

column. There are seven **cervical** (neck) vertebrae, 12 **thoracic** (chest) vertebrae, and five **lumbar** (lower back) vertebrae. The sacrum and coccyx, which are vertebrae that have fused after puberty, consist of five and four vertebrae, respectively. All of the vertebrae form joints with one another on intervertebral **disks**, which are flexible pads of cartilage that separate the vertebrae from one another. Together the vertebrae and disks work in sequence to form a flexible backbone that supports the trunk and head.

- The **thoracic cage**, or chest, is made up of the 12 thoracic vertebrae, the sternum, the ribs, and the **costal cartilage**, which is the cartilage that occupies the spaces between the ribs and connects the ends of the ribs to the sternum. The rib cage protects the heart and lungs.

Appendicular Skeleton

The **appendicular skeleton** consists of the bones of the limbs as well as the bones that support and attach the limbs to the axial skeleton, called the **shoulder girdle** for the upper limbs and the **pelvic girdle** for the lower limbs. See Table 17.2 for the bones of the appendicular skeleton.

- The upper and lower limbs, along with their corresponding girdle structures, are similar in their composition. In the upper part of the body, each of the two shoulder, or **pectoral**, girdles attaches an arm

TABLE 17.2	Bones of the Appendicular Skeleton
Region	**Name of Bone**
shoulder girdles	clavicle
	scapula
upper extremities	humerus
	radius
	ulna
	carpals:
	scaphoid
	trapezium
	capitate
	trapezoid
	lunate
	triquetrum
	pisiform
	hamate
	metacarpals
	phalanges
pelvic girdle	two coxal (hip) bones:
	ilium
	ischium
	pubis
lower extremities	femur
	patella
	fibula
	tibia
	tarsal bones:
	talus
	calcaneus
	cuboid
	navicular
	medial cuneiform
	intermediate cuneiform
	lateral cuneiform
	metatarsals
	phalanges

to the axial skeleton. Each consists of a **scapula** (shoulder blade) and **clavicle** (collarbone). The scapula is a flat bone that anchors some of the muscles that move the upper arm. The clavicle is the bone that runs along the front of the shoulder to the breast bone and acts as a brace for the scapula and prevents the shoulder from coming too far forward. A shallow depression called the **glenoid fossa** forms the ball and socket joint with the **humerus**, or the long bone of the upper arm. The forearm consists of two thin bones: the **ulna**, on the little finger side; and the **radius**, on the thumb side. The **carpals** are eight small bones in the wrist that form joints with the distal ends of the ulna and radius and with the proximal ends of the **metacarpals**, which are the five bones of the hand. The **phalanges** are the bones of the fingers. Joints between the phalanges enable the fingers to move and grasp objects.

- Similarly, the pelvic girdle is fixed to the axial skeleton, where the two hip bones articulate with the sacrum at the base of the vertebral column. Each hip bone has three major parts: the **ilium**, **ischium**, and **pubis**. The **acetabulum** is the shallow depression in the hip bone that forms the ball and socket joint with the femur, or long bone of the thigh. The bones of the leg include the **femur** (the thigh bone); **patella** (kneecap); the two shin bones called the **tibia** and **fibula**; and the **tarsals**, the seven bones in the ankle. The heel bone is called the **calcaneus**, and the **talus** is the bone that transmits weight between the calcaneus and the tibia to form the ankle joint. The **metatarsals** are the five long bones of each foot, and the phalanges are the bones of the toes. As with the fingers, the phalanges enable the toes to move.

Joints

Arthrology is the branch of medicine that deals with joints and articulations. A **joint**, or **articulation**, is the point of connection between two or more bones, or between cartilage and bone. All bones, except for one (the hyoid bone in the neck), form a joint with another bone. Joints hold the bones together and allow the rigid skeleton to move.

Joints are classified by their range of movement. **Fibrous joints** are immobile. The sutures of the skull, for example, are fixed and do not allow for any movement in order to protect the brain. **Cartilaginous joints** can move only slightly. The joints between the vertebrae in the spine, each of which moves only slightly, are examples of cartilaginous joints. **Synovial joints** move in many directions. Most of the joints of the body—the hip, shoulder, elbow, knee, wrist, and ankle—are synovial joints. These joints contain **synovial fluid,** which acts as a lubricant to help the joints move easily.

Cartilage

Cartilage is fibrous, dense connective tissue that cushions and protects the ends of bones and permits smooth movement of joints. Cartilage also joins the ribs to the sternum. It is also found in the tip of the nose, in the external ear, in the walls of the trachea, and in the larynx, where it provides support and shape. As noted previously, the disks between the vertebrae of the spine are also made of cartilage.

The bones of the femur and the tibia join at the knee to form a single-hinge joint, which is protected by the patella. The knee joint is cushioned by two pieces of crescent-moon-shaped cartilaginous pads called **menisci** (singular, **meniscus**) that lie between the two joints formed by the femur and the tibia. The word *meniscus* means *a crescent-shaped structure*, and these pieces of cartilage are so named because of their crescent shape. The meniscus on the outer side of the knee joint is called the **lateral meniscus**. The meniscus on the inner side of the knee joint is called the **medial meniscus**. The menisci help distribute the load in the lower extremities during walking and also help keep the knee stable.

Ligaments

Ligaments are bands of fibrous connective tissue that contain both elastic fibers and a tough protein called **collagen**. They connect bones and other structures in the body to one another. They surround joints and bind them together, controlling range of motion of a joint and stabilizing it so that the bones move in only certain directions. If ligaments are stretched, either by injury, by excess strain on a joint, or by improper stretching techniques, the joint will become worn because the ligaments are not able to support it properly.

Muscles

Muscle is the body tissue responsible for the movement of the bones and joints. The human body has more than 650 muscles, which make up about half of a person's body weight. Their ability to contract not only enables the body to move, but provides the force that pushes substances, such as blood, food, and waste, through the body. Without the muscular system, none of the other organ systems would be able to function. Figure 17.4 illustrates the muscles of the human body.

Organization and Function

Muscles are composed of tiny, threadlike fibers bound together by connective tissue that contains blood vessels and nerves. When these fibers contract, they shorten and pull a bone to produce movement. Each individual muscle is made up of thousands of individual muscle

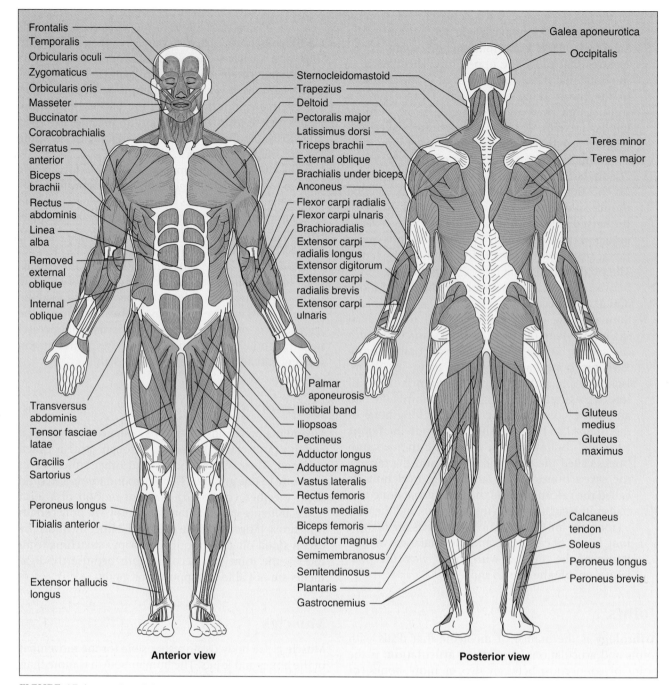

FIGURE 17.4. Muscles of the Body. Anterior and posterior view of skeletal muscles. Reprinted with permission from Willis MC. *Medical Terminology: A Programmed Learning Approach to the Language of Health Care.* Baltimore: Lippincott Williams & Wilkins, 2002.

cells, and, depending on the work a muscle is required to do, variable numbers of muscle fibers contract accordingly.

Movement of muscle is normally controlled by the brain. **Involuntary muscles** are those muscles whose movements are controlled by structures deep within the brainstem, which joins with the upper part of the spinal cord. Muscles throughout the body are in constant motion. Involuntary muscle movement enables the heart to beat, the lungs to breathe, and the blood vessels to help regulate the pressure and flow of blood through

the body. **Voluntary muscles** are those muscles whose movements are controlled by the parts of the brain known as the cerebral motor cortex and the cerebellum (see Chapter 18, *Neurology*, for a more detailed discussion of the brain anatomy). Voluntary muscle movement enables people to talk and to communicate, as well as to control the movements of their bodies in order to walk, run, swim, or ride a bicycle.

Muscles move by contracting and relaxing. When they contract, muscles pull on bones; but they cannot push them back to their original position. Therefore,

QUICK CHECK 17.1 ✓

Circle the letter corresponding to the best answer to the following questions.

1. The end of a long bone is called the
   A. medullary cavity.
   B. epiphysis.
   C. diaphysis.
   D. cartilage.

2. The skeleton that includes the arms and legs is called the
   A. appendicular skeleton.
   B. axial skeleton.
   C. body skeleton.
   D. muscular skeleton.

3. Blood cells are produced in the
   A. periosteum.
   B. joints.
   C. epiphysis.
   D. bone marrow.

4. Thin, platelike bones with broad surfaces are called
   A. long bones.
   B. short bones.
   C. flat bones.
   D. irregular bones.

5. Bones that support and attach the limbs to the axial skeleton are called
   A. axial bones.
   B. flat bones.
   C. girdles.
   D. thoracic bones.

they work in pairs of **flexors** and **extensors**. The flexor muscle contracts to bend a limb at a joint; then, after the flexor relaxes, the extensor muscle contracts to extend or straighten the limb at the same joint. For example, the biceps muscle, located in the anterior upper arm, is a flexor muscle, whereas the triceps, in the posterior upper arm, is an extensor muscle.

Types of Muscle

There are three types of muscles in the body, each with a different structure and purpose: Skeletal muscle, smooth muscle, and cardiac muscle.

Skeletal Muscle

Skeletal muscle is attached to bones of the skeleton at both ends by tendons and is the most prominent type of muscle in the body. These voluntary muscles are also called **striated muscles** because they are made up of fibers that appear to have horizontal stripes, or **striae**, when viewed under a microscope. Skeletal muscles provide form for the body and allow the body to move.

Most skeletal muscles are named according to some feature of the muscle. Often several features are combined into one name. Associating the muscle's characteristics with its name will help you to remember them. The following are some of the criteria used in naming muscles:

- Number of origins. Movement happens with one bone of the joint moving freely while the other

remains relatively stationary. All muscles have an origin and insertion. The **origin** is the part of the bone where the muscle attaches and which does not move when the muscle contracts. The **insertion** is the part of the bone where the muscle attaches and moves when the muscle contracts. Some muscles have multiple origins; that is, they have multiple locations of attachment to bone. A muscle's name may refer to the number of origins, such as biceps (two), triceps (three), or quadriceps (four) origins.

- Location of origin. A muscle may be named for the bone or body region near where it is located. For example, pectoralis (chest), brachii (arm), lateralis (lateral), supra- (above), infra- (below) or sub- (under or beneath).

- Shape. Muscles have names that describe their shape, such as deltoid (triangular), trapezius (like a trapezoid), rhomboid (like a rhombus), or latissimus (wide).

- Direction of muscle fibers. Muscles are named according to the direction of their fibers. For example, rectus (straight), transverse (across), oblique (diagonally), or orbicularis (circular).

- Size. Parts of muscle names refer to relative size, such as longus (long), minimus (small), maximus (large), or brevis (short).

- Action. Parts of muscle names may also refer to the movements generated. For example, flexor (contracting), extensor (extending), abductor (away from), adductor (toward), and levator (raise).

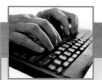

TRANSCRIPTION TIP:

Remember that the muscles biceps, triceps, and quadriceps are always spelled the same in the singular and plural forms. For example: The patient was diagnosed with a torn quadriceps femoris muscle.

Some names of muscles in the body, therefore, include the transverse abdominis, flexor hallucis brevis, extensor carpi radialis longus, latissimus dorsi, and internal oblique.

Smooth Muscle

Smooth, or involuntary, **muscle** is also made of fibers, but these muscles are smooth in appearance rather than striated. Smooth muscle movement cannot be controlled voluntarily but instead is controlled by the nervous system automatically. Smooth muscle is found in the digestive system (in the walls of the stomach and intestines to help move food through the gastrointestinal tract), in blood vessels to control the way blood flows through the circulatory system, and in some internal organs. Smooth muscle even increases or decreases the size of the pupils in response to light.

Cardiac Muscle

Cardiac muscle is muscle that is found only in the heart. The walls of the heart's chambers are composed almost entirely of cardiac muscle fibers. As discussed in Chapter 13, *Cardiology*, a heart muscle contraction originates with the sinoatrial node located within the heart itself. This node and the heart's electrical conducting system run through the cardiac muscles and control muscle movement.

Tendons

Tendons are tough, cordlike bands of connective tissue that attach each end of a muscle to a bone. They are surrounded by a thin **sheath**, or covering, which is lubricated to allow the tendons to move without disturbing the surrounding tissue. Tendons allow the muscles to pull on bones; an action which can be seen, for example, when you wiggle your fingers and the tendons on the back of the hand move back and forth. Tendons can be injured through repetitive action, such as in typing, with trauma, or by degeneration. Tendons can be strained as a result of over-stretching or tearing. Tendons that tear become inflamed and restrict movement, resulting in a condition called **tendonitis**.

Bursae

A **bursa** is a small, fluid-filled sac that lies under a tendon and eases the movement of a tendon over a bone. Bursae protect bones and tendons from injury or from rubbing against each other, causing wear and tear. **Bursitis** is an inflammation of a bursa that causes pain and swelling over the area involved. It often occurs in the shoulder, but it may also affect the knee, the elbow, or parts of the foot.

ANATOMIC REGIONS OF THE BODY

Table 17.3 illustrates terminology relating to specific regions of the body. Regional anatomy considers the organization of the human body as segments or major parts based on form and mass, and physicians often refer to these regions when dictating notes and procedures. Although these terms are used in many different contexts, they are helpful to remember when transcribing terms relating to the musculoskeletal system.

QUICK CHECK 17.2

Fill in the blanks with the correct answers.

1. Muscles that cause a joint to bend are called _____.

2. Skeletal muscles are joined to bone by tough connective tissue called _____.

3. A small, fluid-filled sac that eases movement of a tendon over a bone is called a _____.

4. Muscle tissue found only in the heart is called _____.

5. A muscle shaped like triangle is referred to as a _____ muscle.

TABLE 17.3	Anatomic Regions of the Body
Term	**Region**
axillary	armpit
brachial	shoulder to elbow
calcaneal	heel
carpal	wrist
cervical	neck
cubital	elbow
femoral	thigh
hallux	great toe
lumbar	lower back
metacarpal	hand
metatarsal	foot
nuchal	back of the neck
peroneal	lower leg or fibula
plantar	sole of the foot
popliteal	posterior knee
tarsal	ankle
thoracic	chest
volar	palm of the hand or the sole of the foot

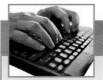

TRANSCRIPTION TIP:

To differentiate between the sounda-like terms *abduction* and *adduction*, many physicians will dictate these terms as A-B-duction and A-D-duction. Type these terms with their proper spelling, not as A-B-duction or A-D-duction.

ANATOMIC TERMS OF MOTION

Terms related to body movement commonly transcribed in orthopaedic reports are illustrated in Table 17.4. Physicians use these terms to describe the movement and direction of body parts, which occur at the joints. As with other terms relating to body plane and direction, these terms are based on the assumption that the body is in the anatomic position, as discussed in Chapter 3, *The Basics of Medical Terminology*.

COMMON MUSCULOSKELETAL DISEASES AND TREATMENTS

Musculoskeletal complaints account for more than 350 million outpatient visits per year. Many of these complaints involve pain from trauma or injury, or loss of function from overexertion or repetitive motion of muscles and their connective structures. Many of these conditions require minimal evaluation and symptomatic therapy. However, some urgent conditions, such as septic illnesses and some fractures, must be diagnosed promptly to avoid significant musculoskeletal deformity, organ shutdown, or even death. The following describes a few of the most common conditions that require orthopaedic intervention.

Sprains, Fractures, and Dislocations

A **sprain** is a stretch and/or tear of a ligament. Depending on the severity of the sprain, one or more ligaments can be involved, or the tear may be partial or complete. A sprain is different from a **strain**, which is an injury to either a muscle or a tendon. A sprain can result from a fall or a sudden twist that forces a joint out of its normal position and stretches or tears the ligament supporting that joint.

QUICK CHECK 17.3

Match each term in the left column with the region of the body it relates to in the right column.

Term

1. _____ metatarsal
2. _____ metacarpal
3. _____ axillary
4. _____ nuchal
5. _____ lumbar

Body Region

A. lower back
B. armpit
C. hand
D. foot
E. back of the neck

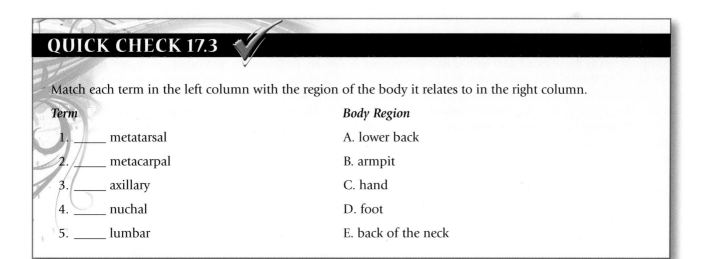

TABLE 17.4   Anatomic Terms of Movement

Term	Region	Example
flexion	Bending motion of a joint to decrease the angle between two adjacent segments.	Bending at the waist to touch the floor.
extension	Straightening motion of a joint to increase the angle between two adjacent segments.	Using your knee to kick a soccer ball.
circumduction	A circular movement of a body part.	Rotating the arm in a circle.
abduction	To move away from the midline.	Moving arms away from the body, straight out to the side.
adduction	To move closer to the midline.	Moving arms back toward the body, back to the side.
internal rotation	Movement of a joint around its long axis, toward the midline of the body.	Rotating the shoulder and turning the forearm inward.
external rotation	Movement of a joint around its long axis, away from the midline of the body.	Rotating the hip so that the feet point away from the body.
elevation	An upward movement.	Shrugging the shoulders.
depression	A downward movement.	Dropping the shoulders from an elevated position back to their normal position.
protraction	Moving a body part anteriorly.	Rounding the shoulders.
retraction	Moving a body part posteriorly.	Squeezing shoulder blades together.
supination	Rotation of the forearm to turn the palm up.	Holding a tray.
pronation	Rotation of the forearm to turn the palm down.	Typing.
opposition	Movement of the hand where the thumb touches the fifth digit.	Extending the thumb to touch the fifth digit of the hand.
inversion	Movement of the soles inward so they face each other and toes face outward.	Walking on the *outsides* of your feet.
eversion	Movement of the soles outward so they face away from each other and toes face inward.	Walking on the *insides* of your feet.
dorsiflexion	Movement of the foot upward toward the leg.	Pointing the foot upward.
plantar flexion	Movement of the foot downward, away from the leg.	Pointing the toes.

Typically, sprains occur when people fall and land on an outstretched arm, land on the side of their foot, or twist a knee while the foot is planted firmly on the ground.

Treatment for sprains and strains involves first reducing swelling and pain and then immobilizing the injured ligament or tendon. Physicians usually advise patients to follow a formula to treat a sprain: rest of the injured area, ice with cold packs or crushed ice in a plastic bag, compression of the affected area with elastic wraps, and elevation of the injured area above the heart to help decrease swelling. This treatment is often abbreviated as RICE (**r**est, **i**ce, **c**ompression, and **e**levation).

Over-the-counter pain relievers or nonsteroidal anti-inflammatory drugs (NSAIDs) may be used to reduce pain and inflammation. Then a cast or splint may be applied to help immobilize the ligament and allow for rest and healing. A cast is a molded bandage consisting of a firm covering, often made of plaster or fiberglass, which immobilizes the injured area while it heals. A splint is a partial cast that is usually held in place with an elastic bandage.

A **fracture** is a break or crack in the bone. Common fracture sites include the arm, wrist, hip, leg, and ankle. Fractures can happen in a variety of ways, although trauma or accident accounts for most of them. Osteoporosis, discussed later in this chapter, causes thinning of the bone, which can make it fragile and easily broken. Overuse, common among athletes, can also result in fractures.

There are several types of fractures that are treated by an orthopaedic physician; they are often named according to their appearance and characteristics, as indicated in Table 17.5.

The treatment of a fracture depends upon the type and location of the fracture when seen on an x-ray. The goal of treatment is to realign the bone into its normal position, and then to immobilize it so that the break can heal and the bone can function well. **Reduction** is the process of realigning bones into their normal position. This is accomplished to decrease pain, prevent deformity, and to allow use of the affected limb after it heals. There are two types of reduction procedures. An **open reduction** is a reduction of bone after an incision

TABLE 17.5	Types of Fractures
Type of Fracture	*Characteristics*
complete	The two parts of the bone are completely separated.
incomplete	The two parts of the bone are partially separated.
comminuted	The bone is shattered into two or more pieces.
greenstick	The bone is cracked on one side but simply bent on the other, such as can be seen when breaking a fresh, green stick of wood. Seen almost exclusively in children, as a child's bones are more pliable than an adult's, causing them to bend instead of break completely.
simple (closed)	The fracture does not protrude through the skin.
compound (open)	The fracture has broken the skin, causing tissue damage.
displaced	The pieces on either side of the break are out of line.
transverse	The fracture occurs perpendicular, or at a right angle to the long axis of the bone.
oblique	The fracture occurs at an angle to the axis of the bone.
compression (impact)	Generally occurs after a fall where the vertebral column is compressed and cracks or breaks under pressure.
spiral	The fracture line goes around, or spirals, the bone.
stress	A hairline break in the bone caused by overuse, such as in sports. The muscles become fatigued and are unable to absorb added shock. Eventually the fatigued muscle transfers the overload of stress to the bone, causing a tiny crack.

is made into the skin and muscle over a fracture site. An open reduction procedure is used if the bone is fragmented or difficult to reduce, and it may require the use of screws, rods, pins, or a plate to hold the pieces in place. The orthopaedic surgeon makes an incision in the skin to expose the bone fragments and, after moving the bone fragments back into their normal position, uses hardware to hold the realigned bones in place. A **closed reduction** is a procedure that aligns the broken bone manually without making an incision in the skin. A closed reduction is used when the bone has broken in only one place, has not broken the skin, and does not require pins or screws to hold the bone in place. In this procedure, the physician gently manipulates the bone back into its normal position under the skin.

In orthopaedics, the term **fixation** means the immobilization of the parts of a fractured bone through the use of hardware, such as screws, pins, or metal plating, to hold the bones in place while they heal. The common name for this procedure in medical reports is **open reduction and internal fixation** (ORIF). **Internal fixation** is the placement of instruments or hardware in the bone to correct the fracture underneath the skin. With **external fixation**, the pins or screws are connected to a metal bar outside the skin. This device acts like a frame to stabilize and hold the bone in the proper position until it heals.

Traction is a method used to align bones with a gentle, steady pulling action using a system of weights and pulleys. The force may be transmitted to the bone through skin tapes or a metal pin through the bone. The procedure involves the use of heavy weights to pull on a damaged bone, relieving pressure on the bone to maintain proper position and to facilitate healing. Traction may be necessary until the bone has healed and moved back into its normal and correct position.

Exercises called **physical therapy**, which are performed during the healing process and after the bone has healed, are often used to help restore normal muscle strength and joint motion and flexibility.

A **dislocation** is the displacement of a joint from its normal position, where the ends of the bones are forced out of their normal positions and cannot rest together naturally. A dislocation is usually caused by a blow, fall, or other trauma. In addition to displaced bones, there may be damage to the joint capsule and surrounding muscles, blood vessels, and nerves. The symptoms of a dislocation include loss of motion, swelling, and pain, and sometimes a joint visibly out of place. A shoulder dislocation, for example, is an injury that occurs when the top proximal end of the upper arm bone (humerus) is separated from the socket of the shoulder blade (scapula).

A **subluxation** is an incomplete or partial dislocation that separates the joint's movable surfaces. In this instance, the ball of the joint is not fully out of its socket but either is too mobile in the joint or is partly sitting outside the normal ball and socket alignment. Some dislocations reduce, or go back into place spontaneously. However, if the dislocation does not go back into place, the physician will attempt to place the joint back into its proper position manually so that it will heal. In some cases, surgery may be necessary to reposition the dislocation and repair and tighten the ligaments that hold the joint together.

Scoliosis

Scoliosis is the abnormal lateral curvature of the spinal column with rotation of the vertebrae within the curve, due to the vertebrae not being correctly aligned. The spine usually bulges toward the right when the curvature is in the upper back and to the left when it is in the lower back. The result is that one shoulder appears higher than the other, or one hip may be higher than the other. Scoliosis affects the muscles and ligaments connected to the spine and, if left untreated, can lead to deformities of the rib cage, which, in turn, can result in heart and lung problems. In most cases, the exact cause of scoliosis is not known. Scoliosis may begin in childhood but often is not noticed until the teenage years. The disorder affects more adolescent girls than boys.

In most cases, no treatment is needed, but the physician will monitor the curve with regular physical examinations. A corrective brace may be used to keep the spine from curving any further. If a brace does not stop the spine from curving, surgery may be needed. Surgery typically involves fusing together two or more vertebrae and holding them in place with metal rods or other devices, called implants. These implants, or rods, remain in the body after surgery to help keep the spine straight. A brace also may be required to stabilize the spine after surgery.

Avascular Necrosis

Avascular necrosis (AVN), also called **osteonecrosis**, is the death of bone or tissue due to a permanent loss of blood supply. The term derives from *osteo* (bone) and *necrosis* (death). The term *avascular* also means *without blood or lymphatic vessels*. Without blood vessels to deliver blood to the bone tissue, it dies; and, ultimately, the bone may collapse. If the process involves the bones near a joint, it often leads to collapse of the joint surface as well. Although it can happen in any bone, most commonly osteonecrosis affects the end (epiphysis) of the femur, the bone extending from the knee joint to the hip joint. Other common sites include the upper arm bones, knees, shoulders, and ankles.

In older people, AVN is usually caused by a hip fracture, but it may also be caused by disease that blocks the small blood vessels that supply the ends of the long bones. For example, fatty material may block blood vessels in people with alcohol-induced liver damage, or displaced fractures or dislocations may have torn or physically damaged the blood vessels that supply blood to the bone. Aside from injury, one of the most common causes of osteonecrosis is the use of corticosteroid medications such as prednisone. Corticosteroids are commonly used to treat inflammatory diseases, such as inflammatory bowel disease, severe asthma, and other disorders. Studies suggest that long-term use of corticosteroids is associated with nontraumatic osteonecrosis.

Simple treatment measures include NSAIDs or other analgesics for pain, reduced weightbearing on the affected joint, and range-of-motion exercises to help keep the joint mobile. However, most people with osteonecrosis will eventually need surgery. A number of surgical options are available:

- **Core decompression**. Core decompression (not *cord*, as is often mistranscribed) is a surgical procedure in which an inner cylinder of bone is removed, reducing the pressure within the bone, increasing blood flow to the bone, and allowing more blood vessels to form. Core decompression works best in people who are in the earliest stages of osteonecrosis, often before the collapse of the joint. This procedure sometimes reduces pain and slows the progression of bone and joint destruction.
- **Osteotomy**. This treatment involves the cutting and reshaping of a bone to reduce stress on the affected area. This procedure is most effective for patients with early-stage osteonecrosis or those with just a small area of affected bone.
- **Bone grafting**. In this procedure, bone tissue with blood vessels intact from elsewhere in the body is attached to the bone tissue and blood vessels near the affected area. The graft serves as an infrastructure from which the body forms new bone.
- **Total joint replacement**. Total joint replacement, also called **arthroplasty**, is the treatment of choice in late-stage osteonecrosis and when the joint is destroyed. Arthroplasty is often performed in the knees, called a **total knee arthroplasty** (TKA), or in the hips, called a **total hip arthroplasty** (THA). In this procedure, the diseased joint is replaced with long-lasting artificial components. Total joint replacement is often recommended for people for whom other efforts to preserve the joint have failed.

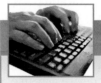

TRANSCRIPTION TIP:

Note the correct term for the group of medications called *corticosteroids*, not *cortical steroids*, as is commonly mistranscribed.

Osteoporosis

Osteoporosis literally means *porous bones*. Osteoporosis is a disorder in which bones gradually lose their density and become weak and brittle. The bone loss is greatest in bones containing a large amount of spongy bone, such as in the spine, the hips, and the wrists. These bones lose calcium and phosphorus as well as the connective tissue of the bone. As a result of severe bone loss, the bones become brittle and prone to fracture.

Recall that bone mass is maintained by a process called remodeling, involving osteoclasts, which break down damaged bone, and osteoblasts, which build up new bone. The problem with this process is in the give and take of bone mass; that is, the osteoblasts are less efficient at making bone than the osteoclasts are at removing it, causing an imbalance between the two types of bone cells. As a result, gradual loss of bone density occurs as a person ages, as osteoclasts remove more bone than can be replaced by osteoblasts. Any factor that causes a higher rate of bone remodeling will ultimately lead to a more rapid loss of bone density and, thus, more fragile bones. For example, heredity, diet, sex hormones, physical activity, lifestyle choices, and the use of certain medications can affect the rate of bone density loss. Men have larger, stronger bones than women, which explains, in part, why osteoporosis affects fewer men than women; however, if men live long enough, they are at risk for osteoporosis later in life as well.

Osteoporosis has no symptoms because bone density loss occurs gradually. Eventually, however, the patient loses height and becomes stooped. This condition, called **kyphosis** or **Dowager hump**, manifests as a forward curvature of the thoracic spine caused by compression fractures. Back pain from the collapse of spinal vertebrae can become severe, and fractures can occur without warning.

Treatment for osteoporosis is aimed at slowing down or stopping bone loss, preventing bone fractures by minimizing the risk of falls, and controlling pain associated with the disease. Regular exercise can reduce the likelihood of bone fractures associated with osteoporosis. Studies show that exercise requiring muscles to pull on bones causes the bones to retain and perhaps even gain density. A diet high in calcium and vitamin D, although not a cure for bone loss, will ensure that a supply of the materials the body uses for bone formation and maintenance is available.

There are a variety of drug treatments for osteoporosis. According to a study called the Women's Health Initiative Posthormonal Therapy Trials conducted by the National Institutes of Health (NIH), it was found that women who used estrogen, with or without progesterone, resulted in an increased risk of breast cancer, heart disease, and stroke. The Food and Drug Administration (FDA) did approve these products for women who are significant risk for osteoporosis (at the lowest dose and for the shortest duration possible)

as opposed to the prevention of heart disease. For women who are unable to take estrogen or choose not to, **selective estrogen receptor modulators** (SERMs) such as raloxifene (Evista) offer an alternative. SERMs have been designed with the goal of producing the same benefits that estrogen has on the bones and cholesterol levels without increasing the risk of hormone-related cancers, heart disease, or strokes.

Bisphosphonates (not *this phosphonate* or *disphosphonate*, as is commonly mistranscribed) are a nonhormonal family of drugs developed to inhibit bone breakdown, preserve bone mass, and even increase bone density in the spine and hip, thereby reducing the risk of fracture. These drugs work by slowing down the process of bone breakdown while allowing the production of new bone to proceed as normal. Bisphosphonates can strengthen existing bone and reduce the damage caused by osteoporosis. These drugs are commonly given orally in tablet form, the most common being alendronate (Fosamax), risedronate (Actonel), and ibandronate (Boniva).

In recent years, scientists have focused on drugs as well as stem cell technology that aim to build new bone. Researchers are also looking at the very nature of bone cells to help understand their structure and properties in order to one day replicate the balance of building up and breaking down bone that exists in healthy bones.

Meniscal Tears

The knee is essentially a hinge type of joint located between the thigh and the lower leg; it is one of the most important and complicated joints in the body. The bones that meet in this joint are the femur, or thigh bone; the tibia, one of the lower leg bones; and the patella, also known as the kneecap.

The anatomic makeup of the knee includes the two menisci located in each knee between the femur and the tibia, as discussed earlier. Called the *shock absorber of the knee*, each meniscus distributes weight across the knee joint, allowing for smooth, painless movement of the knee. In orthopaedic terminology, surgeons divide each meniscus into thirds, with three geographical zones: The front third is referred to as the **anterior horn**, the back third the **posterior horn**, and the middle third the **body**. The menisci, like other cartilage, are **avascular**; that is, they do not contain blood vessels, so they generally are unable to undergo a normal healing process when they are injured.

The menisci may be torn if they get caught between the tibia and the femur when the knee is forcibly rotated in a flexed or semiflexed position, such as when playing sports. A torn meniscus causes swelling, locking in the knee joint, and pain with any movement of the knee.

Meniscal tears are treated with a surgical procedure called **arthroscopy**. Arthroscopy is used to visualize, diagnose, and treat problems inside a joint. The word derives from the Greek words *arthro* (joint) and *skopein* (to look). The term literally means *to look within the joint*. In an arthroscopic examination, an orthopaedic surgeon makes a small incision in the patient's skin and then inserts an endoscopic instrument called an **arthroscope** to magnify and illuminate the structures inside the joints. Like an endoscope, the arthroscope contains a fiberoptic light and a small lens to view the knee and its structures. A miniature camera attached to the arthroscope allows the surgeon to see the interior of the joint with the images displayed on a television screen. In a knee arthroscopy, the surgeon can determine the extent of the meniscal tear and then correct the problem.

Removal of the tear, called a **meniscectomy**, requires special instruments that pass through the arthroscopic portals to cut and remove only the torn portions of the meniscus. The remaining meniscal rim is then trimmed and smoothed to provide a gradual tapered transition to the area that was removed in order to preserve its function as a shock-absorbing structure of the knee.

Osteoarthritis

Osteoarthritis, also known as **degenerative joint disease** (DJD), is a chronic disorder of joint cartilage, causing pain and stiffness of the joints. The term literally means *inflammation of a joint*, but the disease is characterized by

the progressive breakdown of the joint cartilage, as well as by the formation of bony outgrowths called **osteophytes** and growth of dense bone at the margins of the joint. It is the leading cause of disability in the United States, affecting most people to some degree by age 70. Osteoarthritis occurs in almost all animals with a backbone—even fish and birds—and features of osteoarthritis have even been found in skeletons of Neanderthal man.

Although the exact cause of osteoarthritis is unknown, it is commonly believed that with aging the water content of the cartilage increases and the protein makeup of cartilage degenerates. Repetitive use of the joints over the years irritates and inflames the cartilage, causing joint pain and swelling. Eventually, cartilage begins to degenerate by flaking or forming tiny crevasses. In some cases, there is a total loss of the cartilage between the bones and joints, causing friction between the bones and leading to pain and limitation of joint mobility. Inflammation of the cartilage can also stimulate bony outgrowths, or **spurs**, to form around the joints. Other researchers believe that the disease is caused by a genetic disorder causing microscopic changes in the structure and composition of the cartilage, regardless of age or the amount of wear and tear on the joints with use. Whatever the cause, the disease causes pain, stiffness, and loss of function. Figure 17.5

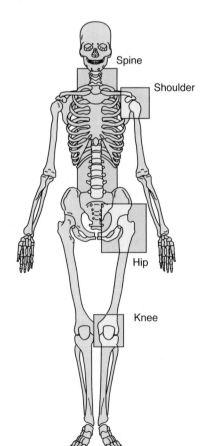

Spine

Shoulder

Hip

Knee

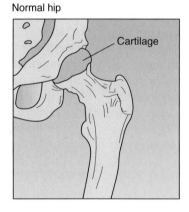

Normal hip

Cartilage

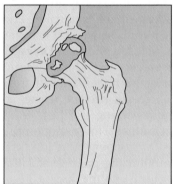

Hip with mild arthritis

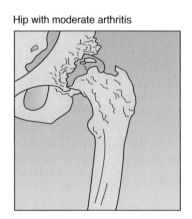

Hip with moderate arthritis

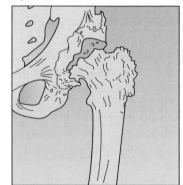

Hip with severe arthritis

FIGURE 17.5. **Osteoarthritis.** Common sites of osteoarthritis (left) and how osteoarthritis affects the hip (right). Reprinted with permission from Willis MC. *Medical Terminology: A Programmed Learning Approach to the Language of Health Care.* Baltimore: Lippincott Williams & Wilkins, 2002.

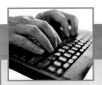

illustrates common sites of osteoarthritis as well as a representative example of how the disease affects the hip.

The degenerative damage to the joints is irreversible. There is no specific treatment to halt future cartilage degeneration or to repair damaged cartilage in osteoarthritis. The goal of treatment in osteoarthritis is to reduce joint pain and inflammation while improving and maintaining joint function. Conservative measures such as rest, exercise, weight reduction, physical and occupational therapy, and mechanical support devices offer some benefit in easing joint inflammation and stress. NSAIDs such as ibuprofen (Motrin), indomethacin (Indocin), and naproxen (Naprosyn) are used to reduce pain and inflammation in the joints. **Cyclooxygenase-2 (COX-2) inhibitors** are a class of NSAIDs used for inflammation that selectively block the COX-2 enzyme, which causes the pain and swelling of arthritis inflammation. However, because of problems that arose regarding cardiovascular safety with long-term use of these medications, the only COX-2 inhibitor currently approved by the U.S. Food and Drug Administration (FDA) to treat osteoarthritis is celecoxib (Celebrex).

In severe cases, surgery may be the option of last resort to relieve joint pain. The deteriorated joint may be replaced by arthroplasty or may be stiffened up with surgery or other artificial means, a procedure call **arthrodesis**.

Muscular Dystrophy

Muscular dystrophy (MD) is the name of a group of chronic hereditary disorders characterized by progres-

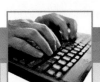

sive muscle wasting and weakness that begin with microscopic changes in the muscle. As muscles degenerate over time, the person's muscle strength declines.

Types of MD vary by body location and age of onset. The two most common forms of MD in children are **Duchenne muscular dystrophy** (DMD) and **Becker muscular dystrophy** (BMD), both of which primarily affect boys. DMD was first described by the French neurologist Guillaume Benjamin Amand Duchenne in the 1860s, whereas BMD is named after the German doctor Peter Emil Becker, who first described this variant of DMD in the 1950s. **Myotonic muscular dystrophy** is the disorder's most common adult form and is characterized by prolonged muscle spasms, cataracts, cardiac abnormalities, and hormonal disturbances.

DMD occurs when a particular gene on the X chromosome fails to make **dystrophin**, a protein that is vital to muscle function. People with BMD have some dystrophin, but not in sufficient volume or quality. Having some dystrophin protects the muscles of those with BMD from degenerating as badly or as quickly as those of people with DMD.

Boys affected with DMD, the most rapidly progressive form of the disease, begin to show signs of muscle weakness as early as age three. The disease gradually weakens the skeletal muscles; and by adolescence or even earlier, the heart and respiratory muscles also may be affected. BMD, a much milder form of the disease, usually occurs in the teens or early adulthood, and the course is slower and far less predictable than that of DMD.

In any case, MD is incurable and there is no specific treatment to stop or reverse any form of the disease. A physician may suspect MD if a child becomes weak and grows progressively weaker. Outward signs include enlargement of affected muscles, or **pseudohypertrophy**, which happens when muscle tissue is destroyed and replaced by fat. A muscle biopsy can also confirm the disease as, under a microscope, dead tissue and abnormally large muscle fibers are typically visible.

Treatment is purely supportive. Physical therapy can help maintain muscle strength; orthopaedic assistive devices such as braces and wheelchairs can provide support; and corrective orthopaedic surgery, in conjunction with physical therapy exercise, may improve mobility. Drug therapy includes corticosteroids to delay some damage to dying muscle cells.

Bone Tumors

A **tumor** is an abnormal growth of cells or tissues. A bone tumor is abnormal growth of cells in bones. A **sarcoma** is a cancer that starts in bone, muscle tissue, blood vessels, or fat tissues and can develop anywhere in the body. Bone tumors, like other forms of cancer, can be **benign** (noncancerous or harmless) or **malignant** (cancerous). The majority of bone tumors are benign.

The exact cause of most bone cancers is unknown. However, researchers have made great progress in recent years in understanding how certain changes in a person's DNA can cause bone cells to become cancerous. In addition, some bone cancers appear to be hereditary. Although some people believe an injury to a bone can cause cancer, most experts have not found any correlation between a bone fracture or other injury and a cancer developing in the same location.

Benign tumors do not spread to other tissues and organs and are not life-threatening. The most common form of benign bone tumors is **osteochondroma**, which accounts for nearly half of all benign bone tumors. An osteochondroma is a benign tumor that contains both bone and cartilage, usually occurring near the end of a long bone, which takes the form of a cartilage-capped bony spur or outgrowth on the surface of the bone. It actually is a developmental abnormality of bone. It occurs when part of the growth plate forms an outgrowth, or spur, on the end of long bones, especially the knees, ankles, hips, shoulders, and elbows. This bone outgrowth may or may not have a stalk. When a stalk is present, the tumor is said to be **pedunculated**; when no stalk is present and the outgrowth has a broad base of attachment, it is said to be **sessile**. Osteochondromas can be found at the ends of any long bones and along the pelvic and shoulder bones, but they can also be located under a tendon near a nerve or blood vessel, such as behind the knee. The most common symptom of an osteochondroma is a painless lump near the joints; but if the tumor presses on a nerve, it may cause numbness and tingling in the affected extremity.

Most of the time, benign tumors are simply observed by periodic x-rays and many simply disappear over time, especially benign tumors that occur in children. Surgery is considered if the tumor causes pain with activity or puts pressure on a nerve or blood vessel. If surgery is indicated, the osteochondroma is removed to the level of normal bone to lessen the likelihood of the tumor growing back.

Malignant tumors that arise in the bone itself are called **primary tumors**. Those that form as a result of cancer that has spread to the bone from other parts of the body are called **secondary tumors**. Primary bone cancer is rare; more commonly, bones are the site of tumors that result from the spread of cancer from another organ, such as the breasts, lungs, or prostate. Some common types of primary bone tumors include the following:

- **Osteosarcoma** is a fast-growing malignant tumor of the bone-forming cells and the most common of bone cancers. These tumors most often develop in the bones of the arms, legs, or pelvis and have a high mortality rate. Osteosarcoma commonly metastasizes to the lungs.
- **Ewing sarcoma** derives its name from Dr. James Ewing, the physician who first described it in 1921, and occurs primarily in children and adolescents. It tends to develop in the upper and lower legs, pelvis, upper arms and ribs, and like other sarcomas, Ewing's sarcoma can spread to other parts of the body.
- **Chondrosarcoma** is a large, slow-growing malignant tumor that most commonly occurs in adults and usually develops in the cartilage around the long bones of the body.
- **Multiple myeloma**. This is a malignant tumor of the plasma cells of the bone marrow, which can involve any bone in the body. It is a tumor that actually arises in bone, rather than to spread to bone. Myeloma is usually first found as a single tumor in a single bone, but most of the time it will go on to spread to the marrow of other bones.

The treatment goal for malignant tumors is to stop progression of the tumor and to preserve the function of the body as best as possible. Treatment depends on various factors, including whether the cancer has spread. One surgical option is **limb salvage surgery**, where the surgeon removes the cancerous section of bone but keeps nearby muscles, tendons, and other structures. The surgeon will remove a margin of healthy tissue around the tumor to help lessen the chance of it growing back. The excised bone is replaced with a metallic

QUICK CHECK 17.4 ✓

Indicate whether the following sentences are true (T) or false (F).

1. The degenerative damage to the joints in osteoarthritis is reversible.   T   F

2. A blockage of blood vessels to the ends of the long bones can cause AVN.   T   F

3. Muscular dystrophy can be cured with broad-spectrum antibiotics.   T   F

4. The realignment of bones back to their original position is called arthroscopy.   T   F

5. Scoliosis results in an abnormal curvature of the spinal column.   T   F

prosthesis, or a bone transplant. If the tumor is large, or if nerves or blood vessels are involved, the surgeon may perform an **amputation**, or removal of the entire limb.

Other treatment modalities used in conjunction with surgery, including radiation therapy and chemotherapy, are discussed in detail in Chapter 20, *Oncology*.

DIAGNOSTIC STUDIES AND PROCEDURES

Orthopaedic surgeons use a variety of diagnostic tests to help identify the specific nature of a musculoskeletal injury or condition in order to plan an appropriate course of treatment. The following are some frequently used diagnostic tests for musculoskeletal injuries and conditions.

Muscle and Flexibility Tests

Muscles are soft tissues; therefore, they do not appear on x-ray imaging. During a physical examination, an orthopedist will perform a variety of tests on the muscles to measure the extent and/or prognosis of a musculoskeletal condition. For example, muscle strength against resistance is tested by having the patient push or pull while the physician pushes or pulls in the opposite direction. Joints are tested using range of motion tests, also called flexibility tests, which measure how well joints can be moved or rotated. Weakness in a muscle may indicate injury to the nerves leading to the muscle, and range-of-motion difficulties may point to an abnormality in the joint or general weakness from trauma or degeneration of tissue. There are several different muscle and joint tests; each is geared to specific joints and muscles, and each is conducted differently. Table 17.6 indicates the names of some of the common tests encountered when transcribing orthopaedic reports.

Laboratory Tests

Laboratory analysis of blood, urine, joint (synovial) fluids, and body tissue are used to identify abnormal elevations of chemicals that may indicate an infection or a particular disease.

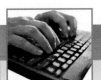

TRANSCRIPTION TIP:

Physicians refer to many specific orthopaedic tests when examining a patient. If you cannot locate the name of the test in a medical dictionary or word book, try searching under the headings *test, sign,* or *maneuver* for the specific name of the test.

TABLE 17.6	**Muscle and Flexibility Tests**
Part of Body Tested	*Name of Test*
head	Romberg
	cranial nerve examination
cervical spine	Spurling test
shoulder	Allen test
	anterior/posterior drawer test
	Apley scratch test
	lift-off test
	Neer impingement test
	Hawkins test
	O'Brien test
	Speed test
	Yergason test
arm	Tinel sign
	varus/valgus stress test
	Finkelstein test
	Murphy sign
	Phalen test
spine and hip	straight-leg-raise test
	Trendelenburg test
	Patrick test
	Faber test
	Ober test
leg	anterior/posterior drawer test
	Lachman test
	McMurray
	patellar grind test
	pivot shift test
	Homans sign
muscle groups	manual muscle test

Blood Tests

Blood tests can detect the presence of elevated blood levels or abnormal substances that may help identify a particular orthopaedic condition. Common blood tests ordered by orthopaedists include the following:

- Complete blood count (CBC). An elevated white blood cell count in a CBC can indicate the presence of an infection.
- **Erythrocyte sedimentation rate** (ESR) and/or **cAMP receptor protein** (CRP), also called C-reactive protein. ESR is a blood test that measures the speed at which red blood cells settle on the bottom of a tube of unclotted blood; a high sedimentation rate signals possible inflammatory disease. CRP measures the concentration of a special type of protein produced by the liver that is present during acute episodes of inflammation or infection.

- **Creatine phosphokinase (CPK) and aldolase**. CPK and aldolase tests measure the amount of muscle damage in the body. CPK is an enzyme that turns creatine into phosphate, which is burned as a quick source of energy for cells. When muscle is damaged, muscle cells break open and spill their contents into the bloodstream. Because most of the CPK in the body normally exists in muscle, a rise in the amount of CPK in the blood indicates that muscle damage has occurred, or is occurring. Similarly, aldolase is a substance found in the muscles. The amount of aldolase in the blood shows the extent of muscle damage. As the muscle damage becomes worse, the amount of aldolase in the muscle decreases over time. Muscle weakness can result from a neurological or a muscular problem; therefore, this test can determine the cause of the weakness. The aldolase level will not change when weakness is caused by a neurological problem.
- Liver enzyme tests, including aspartate amino-transferase (AST), alanine aminotransferase (ALT), bilirubin, and alkaline phosphatase, measure the degree of liver damage, as discussed in Chapter 8, *Laboratory Studies and Medical Imaging*. Some medications used to treat orthopaedic conditions can cause damage to the liver. In addition, alkaline phosphatase, produced by the bones and the liver, rises with increased activity in bone cells, which may indicate a bone disorder.
- Uric acid. This test measures the amount of uric acid in the blood and is primarily used to detect the presence of gout, an inflammatory joint condition.
- Rheumatoid factor (RF). This blood test is used to distinguish rheumatoid arthritis from other disorders (see Chapter 19, *Immunology*, for a discussion of rheumatoid arthritis).
- Serum calcium. This test measures the amount of calcium in the blood. Abnormally high levels are present in some bone disorders.

Cultures

Cultures are performed to identify organisms that cause infection. Fluids that are obtained for culture include blood, urine, and joint fluid. A sample of urine can be obtained with a clean-catch urine specimen, whereas a blood sample is usually obtained via venipuncture, which is the collection of a blood specimen from a vein, usually from the inside of the elbow or the back of the hand. In either case, the fluid is placed in a culture medium and incubated for isolation and identification of the organism causing an infection.

Joint aspiration, called **arthrocentesis**, is a procedure whereby a sterile needle and syringe are used to drain fluid from the joint for examination in the laboratory. Fluids in the joint can build up through inflammation or through injuries or arthritis. Removal of the fluid usually relieves the pressure and swelling, and a microscopic examination of the fluid may identify infections or inflammatory responses. In this procedure, a sterile needle with a syringe attached is inserted within the joint and fluid is pulled back, or aspirated, from the joint. As with urine and blood cultures, the fluid is placed in a culture medium container for the purpose of growing micro-organisms (bacteria, fungi, or viruses) in the laboratory.

While the fluid is incubating, a microbiologist in the laboratory inspects the cultures daily for growth. If microorganisms are detected, other tests may be initiated to identify the infectious agent and determine the susceptibility of the organisms to medications. Antibiotic therapy can then be determined on the basis of these results.

Biopsy

A biopsy is a procedure where tissue samples are obtained and examined under a microscope. A sample of the bone marrow, located in the medullary canals of the long bones, can be obtained. In this procedure, called a **bone marrow aspiration and biopsy**, a small incision is made and a biopsy needle is forced through the outer cortex of a flat bone—such as the sternum or iliac crest—where the bone marrow is located. The syringe is used to pull a small liquid sample of the bone marrow cells through the needle. Then a small solid piece of bone marrow, called a **core biopsy**, is obtained using a special hollow needle. The bone marrow samples are then sent to the laboratory for microscopic examination. This procedure is used to diagnose such conditions as avascular necrosis or myelofibrosis, a disorder in which bone marrow is replaced with scar tissue, leading to anemia.

Doppler Ultrasound

Doppler ultrasound is used to detect blockages in blood vessels. This is the same kind of test as a standard ultrasound examination, but with an added audio effect. As in a standard ultrasound, the Doppler uses high-frequency sound waves that echo off the body, creating a picture of the blood vessels, tissues, and organs as they function. In the Doppler ultrasound, the Doppler audio system detects and transmits the *whooshing* sound of the blood flow through the vessels, creating an image on a computer screen and allowing the physician to identify areas of blockage in muscles, tendons, joints, and soft tissue. Ultrasound technology can be useful in diagnosing tendon tears, abnormalities in the muscle anatomy, or bleeding and other fluid collections within the muscles and joints.

Imaging Studies

Imaging studies provide a view of the bones and the soft tissues, which comprise muscles, ligaments, cartilage, tendons, and blood vessels. A variety of orthopaedic imaging studies are used to evaluate musculoskeletal disorders.

Radiography

X-ray imaging is probably the most common diagnostic tool used by orthopaedists and is usually the first imaging study used to evaluate a musculoskeletal problem. X-rays can identify even fine hairline fractures or chips and can show how a fracture has healed after treatment. They also can detect damage to a bone or joint from other conditions such as arthritis or avascular necrosis. In an x-ray study, the part of the body being imaged is positioned between the x-ray machine and a plate of photographic film. The machine sends electromagnetic waves through the body, creating a picture of the structure, which is later read and evaluated by a radiologist.

Bone Densitometry

Bone densitometry, sometimes dictated as a *bone density test*, uses x-rays to measure bone mass, or the weight of the skeleton. Formally called **dual-energy x-ray absorptiometry** (DEXA), this test evaluates the amount of bone in the skeleton in order to determine how strong it is. It can monitor precise changes in bone density in patients with suspected osteoporosis even before a fracture occurs.

The DEXA scanner beams x-ray energy from two different sources toward the bone being examined (usually the lower spine or hip). Two different energies are used to distinguish between bone and soft tissue, giving an accurate measurement of bone density at these sites. A radiation detector device is slowly passed over the area of examination, producing images projected onto a monitor. A computer is then used to analyze the resulting images and calculate bone density based on the amount of radiation absorbed by the bone and tissues. The denser the bone, the more radiation it absorbs. Later these values are compared to normal values for people of the same age. Using these data, physicians can accurately design a treatment plan to prevent further loss of bone density or to restore bone density once it has been lost.

Bone Scan

A **bone scan**, also called a **radionuclide scan**, uses radioactive contrast material to detect abnormal processes occurring in the bone not identified on x-ray, such as bony metastasis, fractures, avascular necrosis, or infections. In this procedure, a radioactive tracer material called **technetium-99** is injected into the bloodstream through a vein. As the material is absorbed by the bones, a special camera slowly scans the body, capturing images of how much radiotracer collects in the bones. If bone tissue is healthy, the material will spread in a uniform fashion. Areas that show increased uptake, or accumulation of the material, appear black on the images. Areas where there is less uptake of the radiotracer appear light or white on the scan images.

Computerized Tomography

A **computerized tomography (CT) scan** is a type of x-ray procedure that uses hundreds of x-ray images to produce a detailed, three-dimensional view of specific parts of the body. Showing more details than a regular x-ray, a CT scan can produce images of any part of the body, including fractures or other trauma to bones and muscles. In this procedure, an x-ray tube slowly rotates around the patient, taking continuous pictures from many angles. The scanner's computer then processes the images, which can be stored, viewed on a computer screen, or printed on film or computer disk. In addition, three-dimensional models of organs can be created by stacking the individual images, called slices. These images are similar to slices of a loaf of bread, in that each image individually shows exact details of the inside of the body, allowing complete and remarkable visualization of the body area scanned from all angles.

Myelography

Nerve signals travel back and forth between the body and the brain through the spinal cord and its nerves. A **myelogram** is an x-ray examination of the spinal cord and the space around it, called the **subarachnoid space**. The spinal cord and nerves run within this central canal in the bones of the spinal column and are surrounded by a clear liquid material called **cerebrospinal fluid** (CSF), which cushions and protects the spinal cord from injury. The x-ray film is taken after injecting a contrast material into the CSF. After the contrast dye is injected, it appears on an x-ray screen, allowing the radiologist to view the spinal cord, subarachnoid space, and other surrounding structures more clearly than with standard x-rays of the spine.

In this procedure, the contrast dye is injected into the spinal canal by means of a lumbar puncture. A **lumbar puncture** (LP) is performed by inserting a hollow needle into the subarachnoid space in the lumbar area (lower back) of the spinal column in order to inject the contrast material. After the contrast material is injected, the x-ray table is slowly tilted. The table that is used for myelogram can be tilted so that contrast material will run up and down the spine and surround the nerve roots that enter and exit the spinal cord. During this time, the contrast is observed flowing into the spinal canal, cord, and nerve roots during imaging, and x-rays are taken as the contrast flows into each area. The contrast material outlines parts of the spine that usually are not visible on normal x-rays. The images produced show the best detail of the bony structures of the spine as well as the nerve structures, enabling a physician to better diagnose a patient's spine problem.

A CT scan is sometimes done immediately after a myelogram while contrast material is still present in the spinal canal. This blend of imaging studies is known as **CT myelogram**.

Magnetic Resonance Imaging

Magnetic resonance imaging (MRI) is a noninvasive procedure that uses magnets to produce cross-sectional views of the body's organs and tissues. The parts of the musculoskeletal system that are most often imaged with MRI are the hips, knees, and shoulders, although MRI has also been used to study almost every joint in the body. Unlike standard x-rays or CT scanning, MRI does not rely on radiation; rather, it uses radio waves and a strong magnetic field to create sharp pictures. MRI allows visualization and evaluation of body structures that may not be as visible with other imaging methods. Even different types of tissue within the same organ can be easily seen.

The patient is placed into an MRI scanner. A large magnet creates a magnetic field around the scanner. Pulse radio waves are directed into the magnetic field and absorbed by the hydrogen atoms in the body. The machine's computer creates images by measuring the emission of energy from the movement of hydrogen atoms within the body. The computer translates these radio waves into high-resolution, three-dimensional images of the body's internal structures and tissues. Because MRI can give such clear pictures of soft tissue structures near and around bones, orthopaedic surgeons find this useful for examination of the body's major joints, of the spine for disk disease, and even of tendons and muscles to reveal small tears and injuries.

Lumbar Diskography

Lumbar diskography, also called a **diskogram**, is an enhanced x-ray of the intervertebral disks, the cushioning pads that separate the bones of the spine. It specifically focuses on injuries or damage to the disks by determining whether they are the source of lower back pain. In this procedure, a small needle is inserted into the back and advanced into the disk. Then an x-ray machine is used to confirm proper placement of the needle. Once the needle is in the disk, a small amount of radiographic dye is injected. A dye injection will not cause pain in an uninjured disk. However if the patient's pain is coming from the disk, it is likely that the contrast injection will cause pain similar to that which the patient normally experiences. Discography is usually performed in the lumbar spine but can be done also in the cervical and thoracic spine.

Electromyography

Normally, electrical signals travel from the brain through the spinal cord and into the nerves that lead to the muscles, stimulating them to contract. However, if muscles are inflamed or abnormal, they may not be able to respond properly to a nerve impulse. In persons with muscle weakness, nerve impulses are usually able to reach the muscles without a problem, but the muscles are unable to respond in a normal way due to disease.

Electromyography (EMG) is a method of diagnosing the health of muscle tissue by measuring these electrical signals and their effect on the muscle. EMG can diagnose diseases that damage muscle tissue, nerves, or the junctions between the nerves and muscle. At rest, muscles are electrically silent, producing no electrical impulses; but when stimulated by the brain to contract, they generate an electrical current. In this test, an electrode that combines the reference point and a needle for recording the data is inserted into the specific muscle to be tested and attached by wires to a recording machine. Once the electrodes are in place, the electrical activity in that muscle is recorded while the muscle is at rest and when it is contracting. The electrical activity in the muscle is displayed as wavy and spiky lines on a special video monitor called an **oscilloscope**, and may also be

---

QUICK CHECK 17.5 ✓

Indicate whether the following sentences are true (T) or false (F).

1. Obtaining a small solid piece of bone marrow is called a core biopsy.   T   F

2. Another name for a bone densitometry test is a DEXA scan.   T   F

3. An MRI uses high-frequency x-rays to obtain images of the body.   T   F

4. Joint aspiration refers to a type of CT scanning.   T   F

5. An EMG is an x-ray examination of the spinal cord.   T   F

heard on a loudspeaker as machine gun-like popping sounds when the muscle is contracted.

EMG is often used in conjunction with **nerve-conduction studies** that measure the speed at which motor or sensory nerves conduct impulses. These studies are used to determine whether symptoms like muscle weakness are caused by a nerve disorder such as carpal tunnel syndrome, in which a nerve is pinched by ligaments in the wrist. Nerve and muscle disorders cause the muscles to react in abnormal ways.

During the procedure, the nerve being tested is stimulated with a small charge of electricity to trigger an impulse, and the time it takes for the muscle to contract in response to the electrical pulse is recorded. The speed of the response is called the **conduction velocity**. The nerve may be stimulated repeatedly to determine how well the connection between the nerve and muscle is functioning and to see if there is a progressively weaker response of the muscle.

Measuring the electrical activity in muscles and nerves can help detect the presence, location, and extent of diseases that can damage muscle tissue. EMG and nerve-conduction studies are usually done together to provide more complete information.

CHAPTER SUMMARY

Medical transcriptionists who work in the field of orthopaedics type documents containing a wide variety of medical, physical, and rehabilitative information regarding the musculoskeletal system. The future of orthopaedics will be influenced by several major trends, including an aging population with increasing numbers of fractures and reconstructive surgeries; tissue engineering to assist in the development of tissue transplants and resorbable materials to assist in healing; and continuing advancements in technology, gene therapy, and medical management of disease. A thorough understanding of the anatomy and physiology of the musculoskeletal system and the diagnosis and treatment protocols for the surgical and medical management of orthopaedic health issues can prepare you for challenging new career opportunities in this field.

· I · N · S · I · G · H · T ·

Biologics and Fracture Repair

A novel approach to treating fractures and breaks is the use of biodegradable polymer to hold broken bones together. Instead of using metal pins, plates, and screws that are surgically inserted inside the body to hold bones in place, the surgeon applies the polymer implants, either in the form of free-form putty or precast molds, directly to the fractured bone. First introduced in the mid-1990s, these polymer devices have become better over time and have generated an explosive interest in the field of orthopaedic surgery as a way to save costs and reduce the time it takes for a fracture to heal.

Orthopaedic surgeons find that this new technology has a lot of advantages. Absorbable fixation devices look more natural than metal fixation devices in radiographs, enabling the surgeon to see how accurately the bone is put together without pins, rods, and other metal fixation obstructing the view. The use of biologic fixation modalities that can be absorbed over time by the patient's body may be safer (and, in the end, more cost effective) than the use of the metal fixation devices traditionally used in surgery, as the biologic devices never require removal. Metal fixation devices, unlike absorbable fixation devices, must sometimes be removed during a second costly surgical procedure; in addition, they can become colonization sites for pathogens, possibly leading to infection.

As part of a clinical trial, researchers treated several patients with metacarpal fractures using absorbable fixation devices. Among those patients was a martial arts enthusiast who refractured his hand in a different area six months after an absorbable fixation device had been used in its repair. The researchers found that upon viewing the site of the first fracture, there was no evidence of injury; the body had literally absorbed the polymer fixation device.

Not all orthopaedic surgeons favor the new absorbable fixation-device technology. Many are waiting until more scientific data accumulate to prove that the absorbable fixation devices do disappear, to the benefit of the patient, and that money is saved through their use. However, most practitioners who have turned to absorbable fixation devices agree that their use will accelerate as the technology regulating the performance and cost effectiveness of this new treatment modality improves.

Common Soundalike Words

Word	Word Pronunciation	Soundalike	Soundalike Pronunciation
osteal: Relating to bone or to the skeleton.	os'tē-ăl	**ostial**: Relating to an orifice, or ostium.	os'tē-ăl
flexor: A muscle that flexes a joint.	flek'sŏr	**flexure**: The bent part of an organ or structure, as in *sigmoid flexure*.	flek'shŭr
malleolus: The rounded lateral projections of the bone at the ankle.	ma-lē'ō-lŭs	**malleus**: The outermost of three small bones in the ear.	mal'ē-ŭs
metacarpal: The bones of the hand.	met'ă-kar'păl	**metatarsal**: The bones of the foot.	met'ă-tar'săl
metaphysis: The wide part at the end of a long bone.	mĕ-taf'i-sis	**metastasis**: The spread of disease.	mĕ-tas'tă-sis
peroneal: Referring to the fibula or to the outer side of the leg and muscles related to it.	pĕr-ō-nē'ăl	**peritoneal**: Referring to the peritoneum, the serous membrane lining the abdominal and pelvic cavities.	per'i-tō-nē'ăl
		perineal: Referring to the perineum (the area between the scrotum and anus in the male, and between the vulva and anus in the female).	per-i-nē'ăl
humerus: The bone of the upper arm, joining with the shoulder above and the elbow below.	hyū'mĕr-ŭs	**humorous**: Something funny.	hyū'mor-ŭs
thecal: Relating to a sheath, especially a tendon sheath.	thē'kăl	**cecal**: Relating to the cecum, or the first part of the large intestine.	sē'kăl
		fecal: Relating to feces.	fē'kăl
valgus: A bending or twisting away from the midline of the body.	val'gŭs	**vagus**: A nerve that supplies the pharynx, larynx, lungs, heart, esophagus, stomach and most of the abdominal organs.	vă'gŭs

Combining Forms

Combining Form	Meaning	Combining Form	Meaning
ankyl/o	crooked or stiff	lei/o	smooth
arthr/o, articul/o	joint	lord/o	bent
brachi/o	arm	lumb/o	lower back
burs/o	sac	muscul/o, my/o, myos/o	muscle
carp/o	wrist	myel/o	bone marrow or spinal cord
cervic/o	neck		
chondr/o	cartilage	oste/o	bone
cost/o	rib	patell/o	knee cap
crani/o	skull	pelv/i, pelv/o	hip bone or pelvic cavity
dactyl/o	digit	phalang/o	phalanges (bones of fingers and toes)
fasci/o	fascia		
femor/o	femur	radi/o	radius
fibr/o	fiber	scoli/o	twisted
fibu/o	fibula	spondyl/o, vertebr/o	vertebra
ili/o	ilium (hip bone)	stern/o	sternum
ischi/o	hip	ten/o, tend/o, tendin/o	tendon
kyph/o	humped-back	thorac/o	chest
lamin/o	lamina (part of vertebra)	uln/o	ulna

Add Your Own Combining Forms Here:

_____

_____

_____

_____

_____

_____

ABBREVIATIONS

Abbreviation	Meaning	Abbreviation	Meaning
ALT	alanine aminotransferase	FDA	Food and Drug Administration
AST	aspartate aminotransferase	LP	lumbar puncture
AVN	avascular necrosis	MD	muscular dystrophy
BMD	Becker muscular dystrophy	MRI	magnetic resonance imaging
CBC	complete blood count	NSAID	nonsteroidal anti-inflammatory drug
COX-2	cyclooxygenase-2 (inhibitors)		
CPK	creatine phosphokinase	ORIF	open reduction and internal fixation
CRP	cAMP receptor protein		
CSF	cerebrospinal fluid	RF	rheumatoid factor
CT	computed tomography (scan)	RICE	rest, ice, compression, elevation
DEXA	dual-energy x-ray absorptiometry	SERM	selective estrogen receptor modulator
DJD	degenerative joint disease		
DMD	Duchenne muscular dystrophy	THA	total hip arthroplasty
EMG	electromyography	TKA	total knee arthroplasty
ESR	erythrocyte sedimentation rate		

Add Your Own Abbreviations Here:

_____

_____

_____

_____

_____

_____

TERMINOLOGY

Term	Meaning
acetabulum	The socket in the hip bone that forms the ball-and-socket joint with the femur.
aldolase	An enzyme tested to measure the amount of muscle damage in the body.
amputation	The removal of an entire limb.
anterior fontanel	The area, sometimes called a *soft spot*, located toward the front and at the top of an infant's head, between the growing skull bones.
anterior horn	The front third of the meniscus.
appendicular skeleton	The bones of the limbs as well as the shoulder and pelvic girdles of the skeleton.
arthrocentesis	The aspiration of fluid from a joint for examination in the laboratory.
arthrodesis	Surgical fusion of bones.
arthrology	The branch of medicine that deals with joints and articulations.
arthroscope	An endoscopic instrument used to magnify and illustrate the structures inside a joint.
arthroscopy	The endoscopic examination of the interior of a joint.
avascular	A term meaning *without blood or lymphatic vessels*.
avascular necrosis (AVN), syn. osteonecrosis	The death of bone tissue due to a permanent loss of blood supply.
axial skeleton	The skeleton that includes the bones of the skull, vertebral column, and chest.
Becker muscular dystrophy (BMD)	A common form of muscular dystrophy in children and a milder form of the disease.
benign	A term describing a tumor that is noncancerous or harmless.
bisphosphonates	A family of drugs developed to inhibit bone breakdown.
body	The middle third of the meniscus.
bone	Hard connective tissue that makes up the skeleton.
bone densitometry	A procedure that uses x-rays to measure the bone mass, or weight, of the skeleton.
bone grafting	A procedure in which bone tissue with the blood vessels intact from elsewhere in the body is attached to damaged bone tissue and blood vessels in order to serve as an infrastructure from which the body forms new bone.
bone marrow aspiration and biopsy	A procedure performed to obtain bone marrow for biopsy.
bone scan, syn. radionuclide scan	A test that uses radioactive contrast material to detect abnormal processes involving the bone.
bursa	A small, fluid-filled sac that lies under a tendon.
bursitis	An inflammation of a bursa.
cAMP receptor protein (CRP)	A protein produced by the liver that is present during acute episodes of inflammation or infection.
calcaneus	The heel bone of the foot.
cancellous	Denoting bone that has a latticelike or spongy structure.
cardiac muscle	Muscle that is found only in the heart.
carpals	The eight small bones of the wrist which articulate with the distal ends of the ulna and radius and with the proximal ends of the metacarpals.

Term	Meaning
cartilage	Dense, fibrous connective tissue that cushions and protects the ends of bones and permits smooth movement of joints.
cartilaginous joints	Joints that can only move slightly.
cerebrospinal fluid (CSF)	A clear fluid that flows in the cavities and around the surface of the brain as well as the spinal cord.
cervical	A term relating to the vertebrae of the neck.
chondrosarcoma	A large, slow-growing malignant tumor that usually develops in the cartilage around the long bones of the body.
clavicle	The bone that runs along the front of the shoulder to the breast bone (the collar-bone).
closed reduction	Reduction by manipulation of bone without incising the skin and muscle over the site of the fracture.
coccyx	The bottom of the spine, made up of four separate but fused vertebrae.
collagen	A major protein found in connective tissue, cartilage, and bone.
compact bone	Tightly packed, hard material that makes up the outside surface of bones.
computerized tomography (CT) scan	A type of x-ray procedure that uses hundreds of x-ray images to produce a detailed, three-dimensional view of specific parts of the body.
conduction velocity	The speed of the response of motor or sensory nerve impulses during nerve conduction studies.
core biopsy	The small piece of bone marrow obtained for microscopic examination.
core decompression	A surgical procedure used to increase blood flow to bone in patients with avascular necrosis (AVN).
coronal suture	The immobile joint that unites the frontal bone and two parietal bones of the skull.
costal cartilage	The cartilage that occupies the spaces between the ribs and connects the ends of the ribs to the sternum.
cranial bones	The top part of the skull that encloses the brain.
creatine phosphokinase (CPK)	An enzyme tested to measure the amount of muscle damage in the body.
CT myelogram	A myelogram used in conjunction with a CT scan to examine the spinal cord and subarachnoid space.
cyclooxygenase-2 (COX-2) inhibitors	A class of NSAIDs that block the enzyme that causes pain and swelling of joints.
diaphysis	The tubular shaft of a long bone.
disk	Flexible pads of cartilage that separate the vertebrae from one another.
dislocation	The displacement of a joint from its normal position.
Dowager hump	Another term for *kyphosis*.
dual-energy x-ray absorptiometry (DEXA)	The formal name for a *bone densitometry test*.
Duchenne muscular dystrophy (DMD)	A common form of muscular dystrophy in children and the most rapidly progressive form of the disease.
dystrophin	A protein vital to the function of muscle.
electromyography (EMG)	A method of evaluating the health of a muscle by measuring the electrical activity generated by muscles.
endosteum	The membrane that lines the marrow cavity of bone.

Term	*Meaning*
epiphysis	The expanded end of a long bone.
erythrocyte sedimentation rate (ESR)	A blood test that evaluates the extent of inflammatory disease.
Ewing sarcoma	A malignant tumor occurring primarily in children and adolescents that tends to develop in the upper and lower legs, pelvis, upper arms, and ribs.
extensor (muscle)	A muscle that contracts to extend or straighten a limb at the joint.
external fixation	The placement of instruments or hardware to a fracture on the outside of the skin.
femur	The long bone of the thigh.
fibrous joints	Joints that do not move.
fibula	One of the two lower leg bones.
fixation	The immobilization of the parts of a fractured bone.
flat bones	Thin, platelike bones with broad surfaces, such as those found in the skull and ribs.
flexor (muscle)	A muscle that contracts to bend a limb at the joint.
fontanels	Spaces between the cranial bones that are filled with fibrous membranes.
fracture	A break or crack in the bone.
girdles (shoulder and pelvic)	The bones that support and attach the limbs to the axial skeleton.
glenoid fossa	A shallow depression that forms the ball-and-socket joint of the shoulder with the humerus of the upper arm.
hematopoiesis	The process of formation and development of the blood cells.
humerus	The long bone of the upper arm.
hyoid bone	A horseshoe-shaped bone attached to muscles of the tongue and related structures, and to the larynx and related structures.
ilium	A major bony component of the pelvis.
insertion	The part of a muscle that attaches to a bone and moves when the muscle contracts.
internal fixation	The placement of instruments or hardware to a fracture underneath the skin.
involuntary muscle	A muscle whose movement is controlled by the brain stem and spinal cord.
irregular bones	Bones of varied shapes and sizes that are distributed throughout the skeleton.
ischium	A major bony component of the pelvis.
joint, syn. articulation	The point of connection between two or more bones, or between cartilage and bone.
kyphosis	A forward curvature of the thoracic spine caused by compression fractures.
lateral meniscus	The meniscus located on the outer side of the knee joint.
ligaments	Bands of fibrous connective tissue that contain both elastic fibers and collagen.
limb salvage surgery	A surgical procedure in which only the cancerous section of bone is removed but nearby muscles, tendons, and other structures remain intact.
long bones	Bones that consist of a long shaft with two bulky ends or extremities.
lumbar	A term relating to the vertebrae of the lower back.
lumbar discography, syn. discogram	An enhanced x-ray of the intervertebral disks of the lower spine to determine if they are the source of a patient's back pain.

Term	Meaning
lumbar puncture (LP)	A procedure in which a hollow needle is inserted into the subarachnoid space in the lumbar area (lower back) of the spinal column.
magnetic resonance imaging (MRI)	A noninvasive procedure that uses magnets to produce cross-sectional views of the body's organs and tissues.
malignant	Another term for *cancerous*.
mandible	The lower jawbone.
marrow	The spongy connective tissue within the cavities of the bones that produces many of the blood elements—red blood cells, white blood cells, and platelets—in the body.
medial meniscus	The meniscus located on the inner side of the knee joint.
medullary cavity, syn. marrow cavity	The central area of the bone shaft of a long bone that contains bone marrow.
meniscectomy	The surgical excision of meniscus, usually from a knee joint.
menisci (singular, meniscus)	Two crescent moon-shaped pieces of cartilage that lie between the two joints formed by the femur and the tibia.
metacarpals	The five bones of the hand.
metaphysis	The area where the diaphysis meets the epiphysis in a long bone.
metatarsals	The five long bones of the foot.
multiple myeloma	A malignant tumor of the plasma cells of the bone marrow.
muscle	A type of body tissue responsible for the movement of the bones and joints.
muscular dystrophy (MD)	A group of hereditary disorders characterized by progressive muscle wasting and weakness.
musculoskeletal system	The complex body system involving the body's muscles and skeleton, and including the joints, ligaments, tendons, and other connective tissue.
myelogram	An x-ray exam of the spinal cord and subarachnoid space.
myotonic muscular dystrophy	The most common adult form of muscular dystrophy, characterized by prolonged muscle spasms, cataracts, cardiac abnormalities, and hormonal disturbances.
nerve conduction studies	A test, used in conjunction with EMG, which measures the speed at which motor or sensory nerves conduct impulses.
open reduction	Reduction by manipulation of bone, after incision in the skin and muscle over the site of the fracture.
open reduction and internal fixation (ORIF)	The surgical repair of a fracture in which an incision is made to reduce the fracture, and instruments such as rods, screws, and plates, are used to stabilize the bone as it heals.
origin	The part of a muscle that attaches to a bone and does not move when the muscle contracts.
orthopaedics	The science of diagnosis, treatment, rehabilitation, and prevention of diseases and abnormalities of the musculoskeletal system.
orthopaedist	A physician who manages the special problems associated with the musculoskeletal system.
oscilloscope	A device that produces a visual trace of a voltage on a monitor during an EMG study.

Term	Meaning
osteoarthritis, syn. degenerative joint disease (DJD)	A disease characterized by the progressive breakdown of joint cartilage as well as by the formation of bony outgrowths and growth of dense bone at the margins of the joints.
osteoblasts	Bone cells (osteocytes) involved in the redepositing of new bone tissue in areas of old or damaged bone in the process of remodeling.
osteoclasts	Bone cells (osteocytes) that break down old or damaged bone in the process of remodeling.
osteocytes	A type of cell found in bone involved in the restructuring processes that regulate bone mass.
osteochondroma	A benign tumor that contains both bone and cartilage, usually occurring near the end of a long bone, which takes the form of a cartilage-capped bony spur or outgrowth on the surface of the bone.
osteology	The study of bones.
osteophytes	A bony outgrowth or protuberance.
osteoporosis	A disorder in which bones lose their density and become weak and brittle.
osteosarcoma	A fast-growing malignant tumor of the bone-forming cells and the most common of bone cancers.
osteotomy	A process of cutting and reshaping a bone to reduce stress on an affected area in patients with avascular necrosis (AVN).
patella	The kneecap.
pectoral girdles	The bones that attach the arms to the axial skeleton.
pedunculated	A term that describes something supported upon a stem or stalk.
pelvic girdle	The bones that attach the lower limbs to the axial skeleton.
periosteum	Dense connective tissue that covers the outer surface of bone diaphyses.
phalanges	The bones of the fingers and toes.
physical therapy	Exercises performed during the healing process and after the bone has healed, used to help restore normal muscle strength and joint motion and flexibility.
posterior fontanel	The area, sometimes called a *soft spot*, located towards the rear of the top of an infant's head between the growing skull bones.
posterior horn	The back third of the meniscus.
primary tumor	A tumor at the original site in which it first arose.
pseudohypertrophy	Enlargement of an organ or a part, due not to specific functional elements but to that of some other substance, such as fatty tissue.
pubis	A major bony component of the pelvis.
radius	One of two forearm bones, located on the thumb side of the arm.
red marrow	Bone marrow that actively produces blood cells.
reduction	The realignment of bones back into their normal position.
remodeling	A continuous growth and replacement process of bone.
sacrum	A curved triangular bone at the base of the spine, consisting of five vertebrae that have fused after puberty.
sarcoma	A cancer that starts in bone, muscle tissue, blood vessels, or fat tissues, and can develop anywhere in the body.
scapula, syn. shoulder blade	A flat bone that anchors some of the muscles that move the upper arm.

Term	Meaning
scoliosis	An abnormal lateral curvature of the spinal column with rotation of the vertebrae within the curve.
secondary tumors	Tumors that form as a result of cancer that has spread from other parts of the body.
selective estrogen receptor modulators (SERMs)	A drug that acts like estrogen on some tissues without increasing the risk of hormone-related cancers.
sessile	A term that describes something with a broad base of attachment; not pedunculated.
sheath	A thin covering that surrounds a tendon.
short bones	Short, cube-shaped bones important for flexibility, such as those in fingers and toes.
shoulder girdle	The bones that support and attach the arms to the axial skeleton.
sinuses	The air-filled spaces inside the hollow bones of the skull.
skeletal muscle	Muscle that is attached to the bones of the skeleton.
skull	The bony skeleton of the head.
smooth muscle	Muscle found in the digestive system, reproductive system, blood vessels, and some internal organs.
spongy bone	A latticelike structure of bony tissue that makes up the inner portion of bone.
sprain	A stretch and/or tear of a ligament.
spurs	Bony outgrowths, or projections, from bones.
strain	An injury to either a muscle or a tendon.
striae, syn. stripe or streak	Another term for *stripe* or *streak* when describing the appearance of muscle fibers.
striated muscles	Muscles composed of fibers that have horizontal stripes when viewed under a microscope.
subarachnoid space	The space through which cerebrospinal fluid (CSF) circulates in the spine.
subluxation	An incomplete or partial dislocation that separates a joint's movable surfaces.
sutures	Immovable interlocking joints that join the skull bones together.
synovial fluid	A lubricating fluid that helps the joints more easily move.
synovial joints	Joints that can move in many directions.
talus	The bone of the foot that articulates with the tibia and fibula to form the ankle joint.
tarsals	The bones that comprise the seven bones in the ankle.
technetium-99	A radioactive contrast used in bone scans.
tendonitis	An inflammation of a tendon.
tendons	Tough, cordlike bands of connective tissue that attach each end of a muscle to a bone.
thoracic	A term relating to the vertebrae of the chest.
thoracic cage	The bones of the chest.
tibia	One of the two lower leg bones.
total hip arthroplasty (THA)	A procedure in which a diseased joint in the hip is replaced with long-lasting artificial components.

Term	Meaning
total joint replacement, syn. arthroplasty	A surgical repair or replacement of a diseased joint.
total knee arthroplasty (TKA)	A procedure in which a diseased joint in the knee is replaced with long-lasting artificial components.
trabeculae	Thin bony plates that make up part of spongy bone.
traction	A process of aligning bone with the use a gentle, steady, pulling action.
tumor	An abnormal growth of cells or tissues.
ulna	One of two forearm bones, located on the little finger side of the arm.
vertebrae (singular, vertebra)	The bones of the spine.
vertebral column	The stack of small bones (vertebrae) that make up the spine.
voluntary muscle	A muscle whose movement is controlled by the cerebral motor cortex and the cerebellum of the brain.
yellow marrow	Bone marrow that does not have any blood-producing function but serves as a storage site for fat cells.

Add Your Own Terms and Definitions Here:

_____

_____

_____

_____

_____

_____

_____

_____

REVIEW QUESTIONS

1. Describe the four types of bone and give an example of each.
2. Name the three groups of bones that make up the axial skeleton.
3. What is cartilage?
4. What is the difference between ultrasound and Doppler ultrasound?
5. Why is smooth muscle referred to as involuntary muscle?
6. Name the two most common forms of muscular dystrophy that affect children and explain the difference between them.
7. What is "open reduction" and how is it different from "closed reduction"?
8. Describe three functions of bones.
9. What is the function of bone marrow?
10. What is the difference between a muscle sprain and a strain?

CHAPTER ACTIVITIES

Soundalike Word Choice

Circle the correct word in the following sentences.

1. The patient had recently undergone bipolar right hip (hemiarthroplasty, hemiapraxia).
2. The patient is a 12-year-old female with a history of a right ankle (malleolar, mallear) plate.
3. The patient went to the operating room to correct a metatarsal (vagus, valgus) deformity of the left foot.
4. Ms. Grant was diagnosed with a bunion on her right foot, requiring surgical correction of the first (metacarpophalangeal, metatarsophalangeal) joint last year.
5. The patient's (grid, grip) strength has improved, as she can now grab and hold onto a stair railing without difficulty.
6. Overall, strength is 5/5 on the right with the exception of the (gluteus, glutinous) medius muscle, which measures 4/5.
7. Part of the patient's operative procedure included a V-shaped (osteotomy, osteopathy) to repair the bone of her left foot.
8. Mr. Smithson is a 77-year-old gentleman who underwent a revision of posterior lumbar (fission, fusion) of L2-S1 with Dr. Renner.
9. Once she was tolerating (oral, oval) medication, she was placed back on her home medications.
10. As a result of years of repetitive typing on a computer, Sarah developed (tarsal, carpal) tunnel syndrome.

Multiple Choice

Circle the letter corresponding to the best answer to the following questions.

1. To which region of the body does the term *cervical* refer?
    A. chest
    B. leg
    C. neck
    D. wrist

2. To which region of the body does the term *metacarpal* refer?
    A. knee
    B. head
    C. foot
    D. hand

3. To which region of the body does the term *volar* refer?
    A. shoulder
    B. armpit
    C. ankle
    D. palm of the hand

4. To which region of the body does the term *femoral* refer?
    A. chest
    B. thigh
    C. ankle
    D. foot

5. To which region of the body does the term *metatarsal* refer?
    A. foot
    B. hand
    C. armpit
    D. heel

6. To which region of the body does the term *popliteal* refer?
    A. foot
    B. knee
    C. head
    D. lower back

7. To which region of the body does the term *peroneal* refer?
    A. lower leg (fibula)
    B. thigh
    C. lower back
    D. chest

8. To which region of the body does the term *brachial* refer?
    A. sole of the foot
    B. armpit
    C. shoulder to elbow
    D. ankle

9. To which region of the body does the term *thoracic* refer?
    A. elbow
    B. neck
    C. head
    D. chest

10. To which region of the body does the term *calcaneal* refer?
    A. great toe
    B. hand
    C. heel
    D. hand

Matching

Match each body movement term in the left column with its definition in the right column.

Body Movement Term   **Definition**

1. _____ flexion   A. Bending motion of a joint to decrease the angle between two adjacent segments.

2. _____ plantar flexion   B. Rotation of the forearm to turn the palm up.

3. _____ internal rotation   C. Movement of the hand where the thumb touches the fifth digit.

4. _____ abduction   D. Rotation of the forearm to turn the palm down.

5. _____ circumduction   E. Movement of the soles inward so they face each other and toes face outward.

6. _____ adduction   F. Movement of the soles outward so they face away from each other and toes face inward.

7. _____ extension   G. Straightening motion of a joint to increase the angle between two adjacent segments.

8. _____ inversion   H. Movement of the foot upward toward the leg.

9. _____ dorsiflexion   I. A circular movement of a body part.

10. _____ external rotation   J. Movement of the foot downward, away from the leg.

11. _____ supination   K. Movement of a joint around its long axis toward the midline of the body.

12. _____ opposition   L. To move toward the midline.

13. _____ pronation   M. A downward movement.

14. _____ depression   N. To move away from the midline.

15. _____ eversion   O. Movement of a joint around its long axis away from the midline of the body.

Abbreviations Practice

Circle the correct orthopaedic abbreviation in each group. Then define the abbreviation.

1. ORIF/ORMF/OFIR
   Definition: _____

2. DXD/DTD/DJD
   Definition: _____

3. DEXA/DZXA/DMXA
   Definition: _____

4. CXF/CSF/CMF
   Definition: _____

5. ROCE/RIIC/RICE
   Definition: _____

6. EOG/EMG/ELG
   Definition: _____

7. EVN/VVN/AVN
   Definition: _____

8. PSR/ESR/DSR
   Definition: _____

9. COX-2/COX-3/CX-2
   Definition: _____

10. FDD/FEA/FDA
    Definition: _____

Fill in the Blanks

Fill in the type of fracture with the brief characteristic clues given.

1. Break is *out of line.* _____
2. Bone is *shattered.* _____
3. Hairline break from *overuse.* _____
4. Fracture *does not break the skin.* _____
5. Two parts of bone are *completely separated.* _____
6. Breaks *like a fresh stick.* _____
7. Break occurs *at an angle.* _____
8. Vertebral column breaks *under pressure.* _____
9. Break occurs *across axis of the bone.* _____
10. Fracture is *exposed to the air.* _____

True or False

Read each statement and indicate whether it is true or false. If false, rewrite the sentence in the Correction column to make the statement true.

Statement	True (T) or False (F)	Correction, if False
1. An EMG uses electrical activity to measure muscle health.	_____	_____
2. Adduction means to move away from the midline.	_____	_____
3. The skeletal framework of the body is composed of bones.	_____	_____
4. A strain is a stretch or tear of a ligament.	_____	_____
5. Cord compression is a surgical treatment for AVN.	_____	_____
6. Osteoporosis literally means infected bone.	_____	_____
7. Muscular dystrophy is characterized by muscle wasting.	_____	_____
8. Dystrophin is an inflammation marker in blood.	_____	_____
9. The temporal bone is part of the cranium region of the axial skeleton.	_____	_____
10. A spur is a bony outgrowth.	_____	_____
11. Fixation refers to realigning bones back their normal position.	_____	_____
12. Shrugging your shoulders is an example of elevation in terms of body movement.	_____	_____
13. A myelogram is formally called a DEXA scan.	_____	_____
14. The patella is located in the shoulder girdle of the skeleton.	_____	_____
15. The term cubital refers to the posterior knee region of the body.	_____	_____

TRANSCRIPTION PRACTICE

Open your word-processing software. Insert the student CD-ROM and locate the dictation for this chapter. For each of the words in the "listen for these terms" list for each report, use a medical dictionary or other resources to identify and write down a brief definition of the term on a separate sheet of paper to attach with your work. Then listen to the dictation and transcribe each report. Use the current date for each report where a date is indicated. Insert a heading into the document if the text falls to a second page.

At the end of each report, indicate the name of the dictating physician under the signature line and insert reference initials. For date dictated and transcribed and date of admission, use the current date. Proofread your work, print one copy for your instructor along with your term definitions, and save the completed report to your student disk.

Report #T17.1: Discharge Summary
Patient Name: Grace Ellison
Medical Record No.: 000-543331
Attending Physician: Sabrina Scott, MD

Listen for these terms:
medial condyle
PCA
DVT
prophylaxis
SCDs
Foley

Report #T17.2: History & Physical
Patient Name: Tom Bauer
Medical Record No.: 99-57700
Attending Physician: Kamraan George, MD

Listen for these terms:
T12
extensor hallucis longus
quadriceps
hamstring
retropulsion

Report #T17.3: Operative Report
Patient Name: Lucille Durham
Medical Record No.: DUR-999
Attending Surgeon: Samuel Voorhees, MD
Assistant: Tonya Leach, MD

Listen for these terms:
intertrochanteric
greater trochanteric
fascia
Bennett retractor
C-arm
guidewire
purchase (as in dictation, *good purchase*)
Jackson bone clamp

18

NEUROLOGY

OBJECTIVES

After completing this chapter, you will be able to:

- Discuss the structures of the nervous system, including the brain, spinal cord, and nerves, and list the category to which each belongs.
- Identify and discuss the diseases and disorders associated with the nervous system and the treatment modalities related to them.
- Describe common laboratory tests and diagnostic procedures used to analyze, detect, and treat neurologic disorders and conditions.

INTRODUCTION

Tasting, smelling, seeing, hearing, thinking, dreaming, breathing, moving, talking, running, sleeping, laughing, singing, remembering, feeling happy or sad, feeling pain or pleasure, singing, painting, writing novels—we could not do any of these things without the nervous system. The nervous system, made up of the brain, spinal cord, and an enormous network of nerves that thread throughout the body, is an extraordinarily complex communication system that governs the functions of the entire body. Without the nervous system, we simply could not exist.

Neurology refers to the diagnosis and treatment of diseases and disorders of the nervous system, including the brain, spinal cord, and nerves. Neurologic disorders are common and run the gamut from relatively benign problems such as tension headaches to serious and debilitating problems such as brain tumors, strokes, seizure disorders, spinal cord paralysis, and motor diseases. Physicians specializing in this field of medicine are called **neurologists** and are trained to diagnose, treat, and manage patients with neurologic disorders. Most neurologists are trained to treat and diagnose disease in adults. Pediatric neurology, nearly always a subspecialty of pediatrics, is the study of neurologic disease in children. Neurologists examine the nerves of the head, neck, and spine as well as test reflexes and sensation. They evaluate memory, speech, language, and other cognitive abilities to help determine if a medical problem is caused by damage to the nervous system. Although neurologists can recommend surgery (because some neurologists are neurosurgeons, as described in subsequent text), most do not perform the surgery. That is the domain of the neurosurgeon.

Neurosurgery is, first and foremost, a surgical discipline, which means its practitioners are neurologists who operate on the nervous system. Most people give neurosurgeons the nickname *brain surgeons*. However, neurosurgeons, like neurologists, are medical specialists who diagnose and treat disorders of the entire nervous system. Of course, they do operate on the brain, but they actually spend most their time treating patients with spine and peripheral nerve problems, providing both surgical and nonsurgical care. Like the neurologist, a neurosurgeon is an expert in the diagnosis of neurologic disorders, who is capable of interpreting a variety of radiological studies such as CT scans, magnetic resonance images, and angiograms. However, unlike the neurologist, a neurosurgeon focuses on surgical approaches in the treatment of patients.

This chapter provides a general overview of the nervous system, its component anatomic structures, and functional processes as a whole. It also provides a description of common diseases and disorders that affect this delicate system, which is particularly vulnerable to injuries and other problems that can cause degeneration and damage. Finally, this chapter describes the diagnostic laboratory and imaging techniques used by physicians to detect, manage, and treat neurologic abnormalities.

ANATOMY OF THE NERVOUS SYSTEM

By definition, the **nervous system**—consisting of the brain, spinal cord, nerves, tissues, organs, and other structures—regulates the body's responses to internal and external stimuli. Simply put, the nervous system is the body's major system of control, regulation, and communication. It is the center of all mental activity including thought, learning, and memory. Every minute of every day, from birth to death, the nervous system continuously sends countless messages to the brain about what is happening both inside and outside the body; the brain interprets the signals it receives and makes adjustments where needed to allow for the smooth coordination of all body activities. Although the terminology related to this system seems to indicate that there are several different "nervous systems," it is important to recognize that these division names are used for description only; they are not actual divisions in the nervous system itself. The nervous system is composed of one overall system with subdivisions to create a single, highly integrated, interrelated system.

In a very general sense, the nervous system can be thought of as having three essential functions: sensory, integrative, and motor. The sensory component of the nervous system detects changes that occur both outside and inside the body. The integrative component of the nervous system interprets and processes the information that arrives from the sensory component. The motor component carries out changes based on the interpretation by the integrative component of the nervous system.

Nerve cells, or **neurons,** are unique cells that serve as the primary functional unit of the nervous system in that they respond to stimuli and transmit responses by means of electromechanical messages throughout the nervous system. Although there are several types of neurons, the job of all neurons is to pass messages from one part of the body to another. Billions of neurons run throughout the body like strings, sending electrical signals, called **impulses,** to each other and to other parts of the body. These impulses control the body's many functions and store information. Nerve cells in the brain receive messages from other nerve cells in every part of the body. The brain receives and processes these messages and sends responses back through other nerve cells. These subsystems of nerves all work together to control the motor, sensory, and cognitive functions of the body. A **nerve fiber** is a threadlike extension of a neuron that conducts electrical impulses; as bundles, they help form **nerves**.

The nervous system is commonly divided into two major parts, the components of which are described in more detail below: the central nervous system (CNS) and the peripheral nervous system (PNS).

Central Nervous System

The **central nervous system** (CNS) consists of the brain and the spinal cord and is the control center for the entire nervous system. Sensory information about the world around us is processed by this system, which interprets the information and determines the appropriate motor responses. The brain also performs more complicated human functions involving intellect, emotion, behavior, memory, and learning.

Brain

The **brain** is part of the CNS; it is contained in the skull and connected to the spinal cord through a large opening at the base of the skull where the spinal cord enters, called the **foramen magnum**. The brain is an amazing organ—weighing approximately four pounds and consisting of a trillion interconnected nerve cells, it controls every movement, thought, sensation, and emotion that comprise the human experience. Within the brain and spinal cord there are 10,000 distinct varieties of neurons, trillions of supportive cells, a few more trillion nerve connections, and miles of minuscule blood vessels. Ancient Egyptians believed the heart was the source of good and evil and the brain an unimportant organ to be discarded when mummifying corpses. Over two thousand years later, Hippocrates concluded that the brain was the seat of intelligence and emotion. Today it is common knowledge that the brain controls all vital functions; coordinates motor function and sensory information; and controls our thoughts, beliefs, memories, and moods. Figure 18.1 illustrates an overview of the brain's structures and lobes.

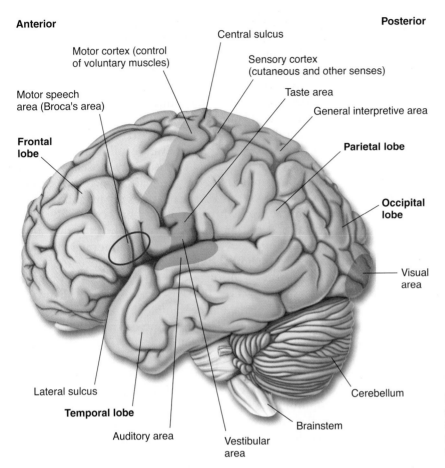

Anterior

Posterior

Central sulcus

Motor cortex (control of voluntary muscles)

Sensory cortex (cutaneous and other senses)

Motor speech area (Broca's area)

Taste area

General interpretive area

Frontal lobe

Parietal lobe

Occipital lobe

Visual area

Lateral sulcus

Cerebellum

Temporal lobe

Auditory area

Vestibular area

Brainstem

FIGURE 18.1. **The Structures and Lobes of the Brain.** Reprinted with permission from Bear M, Conner B, Paradiso M. *Neuroscience—Exploring the Brain*, 2nd ed. Baltimore: Lippincott Williams & Wilkins, 2000.

The brain is made up of billions of neurons as well as supporting cells, called **glia**. Messages throughout the brain are transmitted from one neuron to another through a delicate but complex network of nerve fibers, with some neurons commonly making 10,000 or more connections with other neurons. These messages are transported by routes called **pathways**, which can travel from one side of the brain to the other, from one structure to another, or from deeper regions of the brain to other regions of the CNS.

The brain consists of many component structures that function together as an integrated whole. These structures can be grouped into five major parts: the cerebrum, the limbic system, the brainstem, and the cerebellum, as well as the meninges and ventricles.

Cerebrum

The **cerebrum** is the uppermost and largest part of the brain, and is composed of dense, convoluted masses of tissue that encompass about two-thirds of the total brain mass. It lies over and around most of the remaining structures of the brain and is the site where the highest neural processing takes place, including language, memory, and cognitive function. It is what we usually visualize when we think of "the brain."

The cerebrum is divided into two parts: the **right hemisphere** and the **left hemisphere**, which are separated by a groove called the **great longitudinal fissure**. The hemispheres are joined by and communicate through a band of nerve fibers called the **corpus callosum**. The corpus callosum delivers messages from one half of the brain to the other, enabling each hemisphere to know the activity of the other. The right hemisphere controls voluntary muscle movements on the left side of the body, whereas the left hemisphere controls such movement on the right side of the body.

The surface of the cerebrum is covered by the **cerebral cortex** (often shortened to just *cortex*), a layer of billions of neurons and glia that carry out the many functions of the cerebrum. The cerebral cortex is referred to as *the thinking brain* and, because it appears grayish brown, it is often referred to as the **gray matter** of the brain. The surface area of the cortex is so great in humans (just over one square yard) that its tissue is formed into numerous folds in order to fit inside the skull. The folds are called **gyri** (singular, gyrus) and the grooves between them are called **sulci** (singular, sulcus). These folds permit the presence of millions more neurons in the cerebral cortex, enabling humans to read, speak, do long division, and perform functions that other animals, such as dogs and cats who have less cortex with very few grooves, cannot. (The insulting term *bird brain* derives from the fact that birds have virtually no cerebral cortex.)

Beneath the cerebral cortex, connecting fibers between neurons form a white-colored area referred to as **white matter**. The white matter of the brain does not do any real thinking or feeling but connects the lobes of the cerebrum to one another and to other parts of the brain. Embedded within the white matter are some islands of nerve-cell clusters known as the **basal ganglia**, which play a role in the control of movement and are affected in movement disorders such as Parkinson disease, described later in this chapter.

The left and right hemispheres are each divided into four interconnected areas, or **lobes,** which are named for the cranial bones under which they lie. Lying underneath the cerebral cortex, these lobes contain areas that, through very complex relationships with one another, serve very specific functions:

- **Frontal lobes**, located at the front of the brain, are the largest of the four lobes and control learned motor and speech skills. Through their connections with other lobes, they also participate in controlling intellectual processes such as personality, judgment, abstract reasoning, social behavior, language, expression, and movement.
- **Parietal lobes**, located behind the frontal lobes, interpret sensory information from the body such as temperature, pain, and touch. They also interpret size, shape, distance, and texture.
- **Temporal lobes**, located along the sides of the brain, are the auditory areas, which interpret hearing as well as language comprehension, and storage and recall of memories (although memories are stored in areas throughout the entire brain).
- **Occipital lobes**, the smaller lobes located at the base of the brain, are referred to as the visual processing centers of the brain. They receive and process visual stimuli and create visual memories from events. Other parts of the occipital lobes are concerned with spatial relationships, such as judging distance and perceiving colors, shapes, and motion.

Limbic System

The **limbic system** is a complex set of structures located in the cerebrum; it is part of the cerebral cortex, but it has a very different function. This set of more evolutionary primitive structures is often called *the feeling brain* because it is the brain's center of emotion and is involved in controlling the emotional response to a given situation.

The limbic system modulates specific functions that control such responses such as fear, anger, and emotions related to sexual behavior; it also controls feelings of pleasure such as those associated with eating and sex. Here specific mood functions are developed, such as the one that induces mothers to nurse and protect their offspring, or to develop playful behaviors. Emotions and feelings, like wrath, fright, passion, love, hate, joy, and sadness, all originate in the limbic system. This system is also responsible for some functions related to memory.

The limbic system controls certain behaviors that are necessary for the survival of all mammals. For example, if you stepped on a snake, your senses would gather information about the snake, which is passed to the limbic system. These structures organize the information and pass it on to the cerebral cortex, the analytical part of the brain. The cerebral cortex then tells the limbic system, "this is a snake, and it might be dangerous." The limbic system becomes alarmed and sends out a hormone through the endocrine system to make you jump. However, the senses continue to evaluate the snake. If the snake, for example, is made of plastic, it conveys the message to the limbic system that there is no danger. However, if you stepped on the snake and it rose up and rattled, the cerebral cortex would tell the limbic system, "be afraid." At that point, the limbic system would unleash chemicals to give you the power to run from the snake. However, a bird, who has no cerebral cortex, would be afraid of the snake even if were a plastic snake, not having the analytical reasoning (being a *bird brain*) to realize that plastic snakes do not bite.

The structures of the limbic system include the following:

- **Hippocampus**. Called *the brain's memory center*, the hippocampus is involved in the formation and retrieval of memories, transferring long-term memories to the cerebral cortex. It also governs the storage of dry facts, such as those retained in book learning. In patients with Alzheimer disease, the hippocampus is among the first areas of the brain to be damaged, which is why short-term memories are lost before long-term memories, which have already been transferred to the cerebral cortex.
- **Amygdala**. The amygdala controls the emotional impact of each thought and situation, although the cerebral cortex feeds intellectual information back to the amygdala and hippocampus in order for these structures to make intelligent choices about emotional responses.
- **Pituitary**. The pituitary is actually an endocrine gland, discussed in more detail in Chapter 21, *Endocrinology*. It produces hormones that control many functions of the other endocrine glands in the body. It receives messages from the hypothalamus and then helps the body produce the hormones it needs to respond to various situations.
- **Hypothalamus**. This small structure regulates automatic functions such as temperature control,

pituitary hormone production, sleep and wake cycles, and appetite.

- **Thalamus.** The thalamus serves as a relay station for almost all of the sensory impulses that come and go through the cerebral cortex. It picks up almost all of the incoming sensory messages, makes sense of them, and relays them to the appropriate processing centers in the brain.

Brainstem

The **brainstem** is the lower extension of the brain that connects the cerebrum to the spinal cord. The brainstem contains the major sensory nerves called cranial nerves, discussed later in this chapter. It is a major sensory and motor pathway for impulses running to and from the cerebral cortex. A system of nerve cells located in the brainstem regulates levels of consciousness and alertness, as well as automatically regulating critical vital functions such as heartbeat and respirations. Damage to the brainstem results in loss of consciousness, the cessation of automatic body functions, and death.

Cerebellum

The **cerebellum** is a cauliflowerlike structure attached to the brainstem. The term derives from the Latin word for *little brain* because, like the cerebral cortex, its surface is formed by a series of fold and grooves. The basic function of the cerebellum is to fine-tune the motor signals emanating from the cerebrum, and it performs these functions below the level of conscious thought. The cerebellum coordinates the brain's instructions for body movements (such as walking) and for maintaining balance and posture. For example, while the cerebrum sends the impulses for you to pick up a glass of water, the cerebellum modifies those impulses so that your arm and hand are coordinated and you do not reach past the glass or knock it over. The cerebellum fine-tunes the motor activity of fingers as they perform surgery or play a video game and helps the limbs move smoothly and accurately by adjusting muscle tone and posture. Damage to the cerebellum results in flailing limb movements or a gait that is uncoordinated and uncontrolled, called **ataxia**.

Meninges and Ventricles

The brain is covered by three protective, connective tissue layers collectively called the **meninges**. The thick, outermost layer of the meninges is the **dura mater**, which lines the skull and vertebral canal. The middle layer is the **arachnoid membrane**, which is made up of weblike strands of connective tissue. The space between the dura and the arachnoid membranes is called the **subdural space**. This closed area—commonly the site of hemorrhage after head trauma—offers no escape

route for blood accumulation. The layer of meninges closest to the surface of the brain is called the **pia mater**, which is a thin, delicate membrane with a rich blood supply that closely covers the brain's surface.

Beneath the surface of the brain lie four small chambers called **ventricles**, which are connected to the spinal cord. The ventricles are described as follows:

- **Lateral ventricles.** The lateral ventricles are a pair of long, C-shaped structures in the cerebral hemispheres. Each lateral ventricle consists of a triangular central body and four horns. The lateral ventricles communicate with the third ventricle through an opening between them called the **interventricular foramen**.
- **Third ventricle.** The ventricle is a narrow, slitlike structure located in the median (midline) cavity of the brain, bounded by the thalamus and hypothalamus on either side.
- **Fourth ventricle.** The fourth ventricle is tent-shaped and is the lowest of the four ventricles located near the brainstem.

The ventricles produce **cerebrospinal fluid** (CSF), a thin, watery substance that surrounds the brain. The CSF has several functions:

- It protects the brain from damage by cushioning it from injury.
- It gives the brain buoyancy, significantly reducing its weight in the skull.
- It carries potentially harmful metabolites, drugs, and other substances away from the brain to the bloodstream for disposal.
- It transports hormones from one area of the brain to another.

Most of the CSF is made by a vascular complex called the **choroid plexus** that lies on the floor of the lateral ventricles. After being formed in the ventricles, it flows in a specific pattern through the brain and spine and is eventually absorbed into the bloodstream. New CSF is formed by the ventricles to replace the old CSF several times a day.

Spinal Cord

The **spinal cord** is a long, tubelike column of nerve tissue that extends from the base of the skull to the level of the first lumbar vertebra near the bottom of the spine. It is the main pathway of communication between the brain and the rest of the body; like the brain, it is surrounded by a bony covering (the spinal vertebral column), meninges, and CSF.

Although portrayed as the main nerve connecting the brain to the rest of the body, the spinal cord is more than just a nerve. It is actually a complex organ consisting of gray and white matter, like the brain, as well as a system of nerves that enable it to possess an intelligence of its own. Emerging from the spinal cord between the vertebrae are the 31 pairs of spinal nerves, each named for the vertebra immediately below its exit point from the spinal cord, as discussed later. Figure 18.2 illustrates the spinal cord as it emerges from the midbrain along with its system of nerves.

Peripheral Nervous System

The **peripheral nervous system** (PNS) lies outside of the CNS. It consists mainly of nerves that connect the brain and spinal cord to sensory receptors, muscles, and glands. The PNS is generally responsible for delivering messages from the CNS to other nerves outside the CNS and from those nerves back to the CNS. Nerve fibers that carry sensory information *to* the CNS are referred to as **afferent nerves**. These nerves have receptors that detect information such as light, sound, touch, and temperature. They also allow the brain to have a sense or a perception—usually at a subconscious level—of the movements and position of the body, and especially its limbs, independent of vision but by input from sensory nerves (called **proprioception**), as well as the function of internal organs. Nerve fibers carrying information *from* the CNS to the periphery are referred to as **efferent nerves**. They carry motor information that affects structures such as skeletal muscle, cardiac muscle, smooth muscle of blood vessels and organs, and glands. Most nerves in the body consist of both afferent and efferent nerve fibers, but some are exclusively motor or exclusively sensory.

This system of nerves includes 12 pairs of cranial nerves that carry impulses to and from the brain, 31 pairs of spinal nerves that carry impulses to and from the spinal cord, and the autonomic nervous system.

Cranial Nerves

Nerves that carry sensory and motor messages to the face and neck are called **cranial nerves**. These 12 pairs of nerves are so named because they exit from the brain itself as opposed to the spinal cord. Many of them control the sensory and motor functions of the head and neck, although some cranial nerves reach beyond this area of the body. The impulses for the senses of smell, taste, sight, hearing, and equilibrium are carried on cranial nerves to their respective sensory areas in the brain. Some cranial nerves carry motor impulses to muscles of the face and eyes or to the salivary glands, whereas one

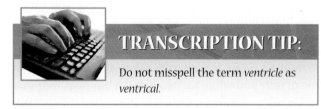

TRANSCRIPTION TIP:

Do not misspell the term *ventricle* as *ventrical*.

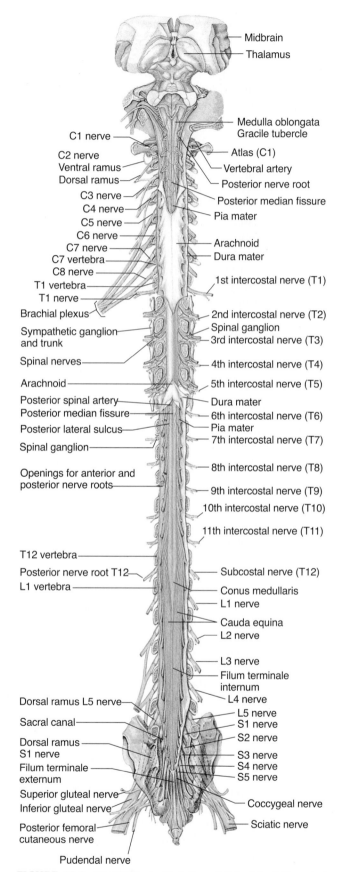

FIGURE 18.2. The Midbrain, Medulla, and Spinal Cord. The spinal cord runs inside the vertebral column and contains the spinal nerves that course through the body. Asset provided by Anatomical Chart Co.

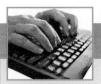

cranial nerve, the vagus nerve, branches to other parts of the body. Recall from Chapter 14, *Gastroenterology*, that the **vagus nerve** helps control function of the esophagus, larynx, stomach, intestines, lungs, and heart. Table 18.1 lists the cranial nerves and their functions.

Spinal Nerves

Nerves that connect the spinal cord with other parts of the body are called **spinal nerves**. The brain communicates with most of the body by use of the spinal nerves. There are 31 pairs of spinal nerves located between the vertebrae along the spine, each communicating with a different area in the body. At each segment, nerves that are responsible for specific parts of the body leave the cord, and nerves providing sensory information about those specific body parts enter the cord, carrying this sensory information to the brain. Many of these nerves end in a bundle of nerve roots extending beyond the end of the spinal cord, called the **cauda equina** (so named because of its horse-tail shape).

Each nerve emerges from the spinal cord as two short branches of nerve fibers called **nerve roots**: one at the front of the spinal cord and one at the back. Nerve roots at the front, which are **motor nerves**, carry commands from the brain and spinal cord to other parts of the body, such as the skeletal muscles. The nerve roots at the back are **sensory nerves** and carry sensory information (such as position, touch, temperature, and pain) to the brain from other parts of the body. These areas of the body are divided into specific regions called **dermatomes**, each of which is supplied by the sensory nerve fibers of a single nerve root. Sensory information from a specific dermatome is carried by sensory nerve fibers to the spinal nerve root of a specific vertebra. By noting where a person has weakness, paralysis, or other loss of function (and thus nerve damage), a neurologist can trace back and pinpoint where the spine is damaged. For example, the spinal nerves at level 1–2 of the cervical spine, located high and close to the skull, control breathing.

The sensory impulses to and from the spinal nerves can occur even without conscious effort. For example, many comatose or brain-dead patients have spontaneous movements (such as jerking of fingers or bending of toes) that can be disturbing to family members and healthcare professionals and even cause them to question the brain-death diagnosis. One of the most startling of these movements is called the **Lazarus sign**, named for the episode in the Bible where Lazarus is raised from the dead. It starts with the arms stretching out, then crossing and/or touching the chest, and finally falling alongside the torso. The living cells that order these muscles to move are not brain cells, but cells located in the spinal cord.

Autonomic Nervous System

The large autonomic nervous system supplies nerves to all the internal organs. These nerves are called **visceral nerves** because they relate to the **viscera**, which are the soft internal organs of the body, including the lungs, the heart, and the organs of the digestive, excretory, reproductive, and circulatory systems. These nerves carry messages from the brainstem and endocrine system to the viscera. They control the involuntary movements of smooth muscle, cardiac muscle, and secretions from the endocrine glands (a more thorough discussion of the endocrine system is described in Chapter 21, *Endocrinology*). This system is broken down further into subdivisions not discussed here, but in total, the autonomic nervous system works without our being aware of it, regulating such processes as temperature, digestion, and the proper amount of blood flow through vessels.

COMMON NEUROLOGIC DISEASES AND TREATMENTS

The brain is the most sophisticated and complex organ of the human body; it is also the most delicate in terms of survival. The brain needs constant nourishment of blood and oxygen to function. A loss of blood flow to the brain for more than 10 seconds can cause loss of consciousness; and it does not take much longer than that for serious malfunction to occur. A spinal injury can deprive the patient of all sensation and movement below the level of the injury. If the injury occurs very high in the neck, near the base of the skull, the muscles of respiration are affected and the patient usually dies before help arrives.

Meningitis

Meningitis is an infection causing inflammation in the meninges, the membranes that cover the brain and

TABLE 18.1   Cranial Nerves, Their Functions, and Testing Modalities

No.	Name	Function	Evaluation
I	olfactory nerve	Carries impulses for the sense of smell to the brain.	Patient is asked to identify smells with eyes closed.
II	optic nerve	Responsible for visual acuity.	Examiner shines a penlight into the patient's eyes to observe the optic nerve and check for equal constriction of both pupils. Visual fields are tested with the examiner's wiggling fingers while patient, focusing on another object, indicates if he/she can see the examiner's fingers.
III	occulomotor nerve	Responsible for carrying impulses to muscles around the eye, including the upper eyelid muscle (which raises the eyelid); the extraocular muscle (which moves the eye inward); and the pupillary muscle (which constricts the pupil).	This nerve is tested together with cranial nerves IV and VI. Extraocular movements of the eye are tested with the patient asked to follow the examiner's finger with his/her eyes, moving in all of the six directions that muscles move the eye.
IV	trochlear nerve	Controls extraocular eye movement. It is the only cranial nerve that arises from the back of the brainstem and thus follows the longest course within the skull of any of the cranial nerves.	This nerve is tested together with cranial nerves III and VI. Extraocular movements of the eye are tested with the patient being asked to follow the examiner's finger with his/her eyes, moving in all of the six directions that muscles move the eye.
V	trigeminal nerve	Functions both as the chief nerve of sensation for the face and the motor nerve controlling the muscles of mastication (chewing). The name derives from the Latin word *trigeminus*, meaning *threefold*, referring to the three divisions (ophthalmic, maxillary, and mandibular) of this nerve. Physicians refer to these three divisions in dictation as V1 (pronounced *vee-one*, even though the V is meant to refer to the roman numeral five, not the letter), V2, and V3.	The patient is asked to clench his/her jaw while examiner palpates, or feels, the jaw muscles. Facial sensation to light touch is when a sharp object (such as a sterile needle or broken end of wooden cotton swab) is touched to the forehead, cheeks, and chin on both sides of the face.
VI	abducens nerve	Supplies the muscle that moves the eye toward the side of the head and prevents inward turning of the eye, causing strabismus.	This nerve is tested together with cranial nerves III and IV. Extraocular movements of the eye are tested with the patient asked to follow the examiner's finger with his/her eyes, moving in all of the six directions that muscles move the eye.
VII	facial nerve	Supplies the muscles of facial expression and taste to the anterior two-thirds of the tongue.	To test the motor portion, the patient is asked to make faces such as grimacing, wrinkling the forehead, or frowning, to look for differences between the two sides of the face. To test the sensory portion, the patient is asked to taste items of different flavors (sweet, sour, salty, or bitter).
VIII	vestibulocochlear nerve	Responsible for the sense of hearing and also for the body's sense of balance.	Patient is asked if he/she hears the examiner's fingers rubbing near the ear.

TABLE 18.1   Cranial Nerves, Their Functions, and Testing Modalities (continued)

No.	Name	Function	Evaluation
IX	glossopharyngeal nerve	Controls swallowing movements, sensations of the throat, and taste in the posterior third of the tongue.	This nerve is tested together with cranial nerve X. The examiner presses a tongue blade firmly on the back third of the patient's tongue to elicit a gag reflex.
X	vagus nerve	Controls movement of the palate, swallowing, gag reflex, activity of the thoracic and abdominal viscera (heart, lungs, bronchi, and GI tract).	This nerve is tested together with cranial nerve X. The examiner presses a tongue blade firmly on the back third of the patient's tongue to elicit a gag reflex.
XI	accessory nerve	Controls shoulder movement and head rotation. The accessory nerve is so-called because, although it arises in the brain, it receives an additional (accessory) root from the upper part of the spinal cord.	With the examiner's hand on the patient's face from chin to ear, the patient is asked to push his/her head sideways against the examiner's hand (sternocleidomastoid muscle). To test the trapezius muscle, the examiner places both hands on the patient's shoulders and asks the patient to shrug.
XII	hypoglossal nerve	Supplies the motor function of the tongue.	The patient is asked to stick his/her tongue out and move it from side to side.

spinal cord. **Bacterial meningitis** is a rare but potentially fatal form of the disease. It is usually a complication of **bacteremia**, or the presence of bacteria in the blood from infections such as pneumonia, osteomyelitis, or endocarditis. The body's immune system is usually able to contain and defeat these bacteria during an infection. However, if the infection passes into the bloodstream, it can affect the nerves and travel to the brain and/or surrounding membranes, causing inflammation, brain damage, and even death. **Viral meningitis** is the most common form of meningitis in the United States. This form of meningitis is caused by **enterovirus**, a group of common viruses that cause the stomach flu. These viruses enter the body through the mouth, travel to the brain and surrounding tissues, and then multiply.

Immediate, aggressive treatment of bacterial meningitis is important, as the disease can progress quickly and has the potential to cause severe, irreversible neurologic damage. Strong doses of general antibiotics may be prescribed first, followed by intravenous antibiotics

QUICK CHECK 18.1

Fill in the blanks with the correct answers.

1. The folded outer covering of the brain is called the _____.

2. The central nervous system consists of the _____ and the _____.

3. The body's left side is controlled by the cerebrum's _____.

4. The cranial nerve responsible for controlling the sense of smell is the _____ nerve.

5. The brain and spinal cord are covered by three layers of connective tissue collectively known as the _____.

6. The brainstem connects the _____ with the _____.

7. The right and left hemispheres are linked by a bundle of neurons called the _____.

8. The largest and most prominent part of the brain is the _____.

9. The brain is protected by a bony covering called the _____.

10. The _____ is called *the brain's memory center.*

in more severe cases. Some antibiotics that are effective against the many bacteria that cause meningitis include ampicillin, penicillin, ciprofloxacin (Cipro), ceftriaxone (Rocephin), and gentamicin (Garamycin).

In addition, safe and effective vaccinations are available against some forms of meningitis. *Haemophilus influenzae* type b (Hib, pronounced like *hibb*) is the agent causing the most common form of life-threatening bacterial meningitis in the United States, but a vaccine developed in the 1990s and given to all children as part of their routine immunizations has drastically reduced the occurrence of the invasive disease caused by this bacterium. In addition, **Prevnar**, a vaccine developed in 2000, protects against the seven most common strains of the *Pneumococcus* bacteria that cause invasive diseases, including meningitis, and is also given to children as part of their routine vaccination record.

Unlike bacteria, viruses generally cannot be killed by antibiotics; therefore, patients with viral meningitis may be allowed to stay at home, although those who have a more serious infection may be hospitalized for supportive care. Viral meningitis is usually mild and often clears up on its own in 10 days or less.

Hydrocephalus

Hydrocephalus is a condition marked by excess fluid within the brain's ventricles. The term hydrocephalus is derived from the Greek words *hydro*, meaning water, and *cephalus*, meaning head. Although hydrocephalus was once known as *water on the brain*, the fluid that accumulates is the CSF that normally surrounds the brain and spinal cord. Hydrocephalus can be present at birth (**congenital hydrocephalus**) or can develop later (**acquired hydrocephalus**).

Recall that CSF is continuously created in the ventricles and absorbed into the bloodstream. This production of CSF is ceaseless, like a faucet that is never turned off. CSF flows through the ventricles by way of channels that connect one ventricle to another. Once CSF passes through the ventricles, it flows into spaces in the brain and spine and then is eventually absorbed into the bloodstream. Keeping the production, flow, and absorption of CSF in balance is important to maintain normal pressure inside the skull. **Noncommunicating hydrocephalus** is an obstructive form of the disorder and results from a blockage within the ventricular system of the brain that prevents the CSF from flowing between or out of them properly. A **stenosis**, or narrowing of a channel that connects two ventricles, is the most common cause of obstructive hydrocephalus. **Communicating hydrocephalus** is a nonobstructive form of the disorder and occurs when the CSF flows out of the ventricles into the spinal canal but is not absorbed normally by the bloodstream.

Any obstacle to the flow of CSF causes the fluid to accumulate, like a clog in a kitchen drain, and increases pressure on the brain. The excessive accumulation of CSF results in an abnormal dilation of the spaces in the ventricles which, in turn, causes potentially harmful pressure on the tissues of the brain. In adults, excess CSF enlarges the ventricles, increasing the pressure of the brain against the skull. In a small child, the growing skull is still pliable, with thin plates of bone designed to expand slowly during normal brain growth. Unchecked excess CSF fluid presses on these soft skull plates, inflating a child's head to abnormally large proportions and damaging delicate brain structures.

The cause of hydrocephalus is unknown. Genetic disposition or early developmental structural problems in the brain may be a factor in congenital hydrocephalus. A disease causing blood vessels in the brain to rupture or bleed may be a cause of acquired hydrocephalus; head injury is another possibility.

Treatment of hydrocephalus attempts to reestablish the balance between CSF production and reabsorption. Medications such as acetazolamide (Diamox) or furosemide (Lasix) can be used to temporarily reduce pressure from excess CSF. A lumbar puncture (LP) to measure CSF pressure and remove small samples of CSF for laboratory testing may be also used to relieve some of the extra pressure.

Surgery provides a long-term solution for both noncommunicating and communicating hydrocephalus. If the hydrocephalus is caused by an obstruction of flow between two ventricles, a **shunt** may be inserted to address both noncommunicating and communicating hydrocephalus. The insertion of this silicone rubber tube allows the CSF to flow away from the brain to other parts of the body where it can be absorbed. A common procedure is the placement of a **ventriculoperitoneal (VP) shunt** (often dictated as a *VP shunt procedure*). This involves placing one end of the shunt inside one of the ventricles of the brain and the other into the abdominal cavity. Shunt tubes are usually maintained for life, but infections or obstructions may require the shunt to be repaired or replaced, a procedure called a **shunt revision**. A **ventriculostomy** can also be performed, where an opening is made surgically between the ventricles, allowing CSF to flow unobstructed again.

Aneurysms

An **aneurysm** is an abnormal dilation of a blood vessel, usually an artery, caused by weakness in the vessel's wall. In the brain this dilation, called a **cerebral aneurysm**, appears as a saclike outpouching that can occur on the large arteries at the base of the brain, as shown in Figure 18.3. A weakness in the wall of an artery can slowly sprout into a thin-walled **bleb**, which is a blisterlike sac filled with blood, similar to a bulge in an old inner tube. The bulging aneurysm can put pressure on a nerve or surrounding brain tissue. It may also leak or rupture, spilling blood into the surrounding

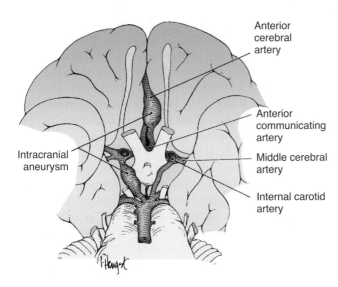

Anterior cerebral artery

Anterior communicating artery

Middle cerebral artery

Internal carotid artery

Intracranial aneurysm

FIGURE 18.3. Intracranial Aneurysms. Reprinted with permission from Smeltzer SC, Bare BG. *Textbook of Medical-Surgical Nursing,* 9th ed. Philadelphia: Lippincott Williams & Wilkins, 2000.

TRANSCRIPTION TIP:

When talking about aneurysms, physicians will often use abbreviated forms for two communicating arteries in the brain as the **anterior communicating artery** (AComA) and **posterior communicating artery** (PComA) in terms that sound like *A-COM* and *P-COM,* respectively. These abbreviations should not be transcribed with a hyphen.

tissue (called a **hemorrhage**). A **subarachnoid hemorrhage** (SAH) results from the rupture of a cerebral aneurysm into the space between the brain and the skull. Some causes of cerebral aneurysm include congenital defects, a degenerative process of the vessel or artery, and trauma.

Aneurysms usually cause no symptoms unless they rupture and bleed into the brain. Often, an aneurysm is found when a CT scan or MRI is performed for another reason. However, a larger aneurysm that is steadily growing may produce symptoms such as loss of feeling in the face or problems with the eyes. The rupture of an aneurysm can be a sudden, devastating event. The victim is felled immediately by a thunderclap-type headache. Meanwhile the body reacts to stem the hemorrhage by closing off the vessels feeding the aneurysm. This natural reaction forms a clot over the aneurysm but, unfortunately, cuts off oxygen and blood to the brain. This impeded blood supply results in brain damage and the death of large areas of the brain, called **stroke**. If a clot has not formed over the aneurysm and bleeding continues, death ensues.

Because symptoms often do not appear until bleeding occurs, a ruptured cerebral aneurysm is an emergency condition. **Microvascular clipping** involves cutting off the flow of blood to the aneurysm. An opening is made in the skull, called a **craniotomy**, and the aneurysm is located using an operating microscope. Then a tiny spring-loaded clip is placed across the aneurysm's **neck**, or at the point where it arises from the artery. Once the neck is clipped, the blood supply to the aneurysm is halted, and it is rendered harmless.

When aneurysms are discovered before rupture occurs, a noninvasive procedure called **coil embolization** may be performed. Unlike microvascular clipping, coiling does not require open surgery. Instead, physicians use **fluoroscopy**, or real-time x-ray technology, to visualize the aneurysm and treat it from inside. In this procedure, a catheter is placed into the femoral artery in the patient's leg, threaded through the vascular system, into the head, and finally into the aneurysm itself. Tiny platinum coils are then threaded through the catheter and deployed directly into the aneurysm. This blocks blood flow into the aneurysm, preventing rupture. The coils are made of platinum so they are visible on x-rays and are sufficiently flexible to conform to the aneurysm's shape.

Seizure Disorder/Epilepsy

A **seizure** is a condition caused by a sudden abnormal discharge of electrical activity in the brain that often causes unusual sensations, uncontrollable muscle spasms, and loss of consciousness. Seizures are not a diseasebut rather a symptom of many different disorders that can affect the brain. Some seizures are hardly noticeable, whereas others are totally disabling. Many people experience an **aura**, a subjective warning sign that occurs immediately before the onset of a seizure; the aura lasts for a few seconds and is generally characterized by nausea, distorted vision, or distinctive smells and tastes.

Seizures are classified into two main categories: partial and general.

Partial seizures are those that begin in a particular area of the brain. These include:

- **Simple partial seizures.** No change in consciousness occurs and the individual may experience numbness, weakness, twitching of the muscles or limbs, visual changes, or vertigo.
- **Complex partial seizures.** Consciousness is altered during this type of seizure. The individual may exhibit symptoms similar to simple partial seizures but with impaired awareness. He or she may exhibit autonomic repetitive behavior such as walking in a circle and smacking the lips together, as well as unusual thoughts, uncontrollable laughter, and visual or olfactory hallucinations.

Generalized seizures originate in several areas of the brain. Common types of generalized seizures include:

- **Tonic-clonic (grand mal) seizures.** This type of seizure is the most common form of generalized seizures. In a tonic-clonic seizure, the person loses consciousness, the body stiffens, and then falls to the ground. This is followed by jerking movements. After a minute or two, the jerking movements usually stop and consciousness slowly returns.
- **Absence (petit mal) seizures.** Absence seizures (not *absent* or *absense*, as commonly mistranscribed) are characterized by a brief loss of consciousness without associated twitching or jerking movements.
- **Myoclonic seizures.** These seizures are characterized by sudden and brief contractions of a single group of muscles or of the entire body. The patient may fall but does not experience a loss of consciousness.

Status epilepticus is a continuous, prolonged seizure state during which time the patient is unconscious. Status epilepticus can be **convulsive** (tonic-clonic or myoclonic seizures) or **nonconvulsive** (absence or complex partial seizures). This type of seizure is a medical emergency, which can result in death if not treated immediately.

Epilepsy is the name given to a group of neurologic disorders characterized by uncontrolled electrical discharge from the cerebral cortex and typically manifested by recurrent seizures with clouding of consciousness. It is usually diagnosed after a person has had at least two seizures that were not caused by some known medical condition like alcohol withdrawal or extremely low blood sugar.

Normal brain function requires an orderly, organized, coordinated discharge of electrical impulses. Nerve cells in the brain enable it to communicate with the spinal cord, nerves, and muscles as well as to enable different parts of the brain to communicate with each other. Epilepsy is a disturbance in the normal electrical function, resulting in a sudden burst of uncontrolled excess electrical activity in the brain.

Epilepsy is a disorder with many possible causes. Anything that disturbs the normal pattern of neuron activity—from illness to brain damage to abnormal brain development—can lead to seizures. Epilepsy may develop because of an abnormality in brain wiring, an imbalance of the nerve-signaling chemicals that send messages from one cell to another, called **neurotransmitters**, or some combination of these factors. There is often a family history of seizure disorders in patients with epilepsy.

Unless there is a reversible cause, epilepsy is considered a chronic, incurable condition. Once the condition is diagnosed, it is important to begin treatment as soon as possible. For most patients, seizures can be controlled with medications and surgical techniques.

There are numerous medications available to treat epilepsy. The choice of medication depends on the type of seizure, age of the patient, side effects, and other factors. Some oral anticonvulsants commonly mentioned by neurologists in medical reports include valproic acid (Depakene), divalproex sodium (Depakote), phenytoin (Dilantin), levetiracetam (Keppra), clonazepam (Klonopin), lamotrigine (Lamictal), gabapentin (Neurontin), topiramate (Topamax), carbamazepine (Tegretol), and oxcarbazepine (Trileptal).

Surgery is an alternative for some people whose seizures cannot be controlled by medications. The most common type of epilepsy surgery is a **temporal lobectomy**, or the removal of the portion of the temporal lobe, the part of the brain that is causing the seizures. Most patients who have temporal lobe surgery either become seizure-free or have a significant reduction in the number of seizures. If the portion of the brain that is causing seizures is too vital to remove, surgeons may make a series of cuts to help isolate that section of the brain. This procedure, called **subpial resection**, prevents seizures from moving into other parts of the brain. A third type of surgery, called a **corpus callosotomy**, severs the network of neural connections between the right and left hemispheres of the brain. This surgery is used primarily in patients who have severe seizures that start in one hemisphere and spread to the other side.

Parkinson Disease

First described in 1817 by the British physician James Parkinson, **Parkinson disease** (PD) is a motor-system disorder that results when nerve cells in the area of the brain that controls body movement begin to deteriorate, resulting in gradual progressive muscle rigidity, tremors, and clumsiness. Genes, brain injury, or environmental toxins may trigger the disease in some people, but in most cases its cause is unknown. It is one of the most common neurologic disorders of the elderly.

Parkinson disease begins when nerve cells in a part of the midbrain die or are impaired. These nerve cells produce **dopamine**, a primary neurotransmitter that controls body movement. Dopamine production commonly declines as people age, which accounts for the loss of coordination and muscular control that elderly people almost always experience. However, a gross deficit of dopamine causes the extreme loss of muscular control that is identified in PD. As these dopamine-secreting cells die over time, the other movement-control centers in the brain slowly become deregulated, causing the motor symptoms of PD: tremor or trembling of the arms, jaw, legs, and face; stiffness or rigidity of the limbs and trunk; slowness of movement (**bradykinesia**); postural instability, or impaired balance and coordination.

There is no cure for PD, but symptoms can be relieved or controlled by medications that work to increase levels of dopamine in the brain. Most patients are given levodopa combined with carbidopa. Nerve cells can use levodopa to make dopamine and replenish the brain's dwindling supply. Carbidopa delays the conversion of levodopa into dopamine until it reaches the brain. Dopamine agonists are drugs that do not change into dopamine in the body; rather, they mimic the effects of dopamine in the brain and cause neurons to act as though sufficient amounts of dopamine were present. Some common dopamine agonists include bromocriptine (Parlodel), pergolide (Permax), pramipexole (Mirapex), and ropinirole (Requip). Other drugs that provide relief for PD symptoms include selegiline (Eldepryl), amantadine (Endantadine), and coenzyme Q10, a supplement based on a compound that is made naturally in the body. In 2006, the U.S. Food and Drug Administration (FDA) approved rasagiline (Azilect) to be used along with levodopa for patients with advanced PD or as a single-drug treatment for early PD.

For patients who do not respond to drugs, **deep brain stimulation** (DBS) may prove effective. This involves the implantation of a device to deliver mild electrical stimulation to block the brain signals that cause tremors in PD patients. A thin, insulated wire lead with an electrode at the tip is surgically implanted into the thalamus area of the brain. The lead is connected by an extension wire passed under the skin to a battery-operated pulse generator implanted near the collarbone. The generator is programmed to send continuous electrical pulses to the brain, though the patient can turn the device on or off by swiping a special magnet over the generator. The stimulator battery lasts for about five years with 16 hours of use a day. When the battery needs to be replaced, the pulse generator is replaced, usually under local anesthesia in an outpatient procedure. This procedure has been successful in helping patients lead active and fulfilling lives and reducing or eliminating the need for antitremor medications.

Multiple Sclerosis

Multiple sclerosis (MS) is an inflammatory disease of the nervous system that disrupts communication between the brain and other parts of the body. MS affects the neurons of the brain and spinal cord. Surrounding and protecting some of these neurons is an insulating sheath made of a material called **myelin**. Myelin helps neurons conduct electrical signals. MS causes gradual destruction of the myelin, called **demyelination**, and the formation of plaques on portions of the neurons throughout the brain and spinal cord. The name *multiple sclerosis* refers to the multiple areas of hardening, or scars, on the myelin sheaths covering the neurons. This scarring interrupts signals from the neurons and results in such symptoms as changes in sensation, visual problems, muscle weakness, difficulties with coordination and speech, and pain.

MS is capricious in that it strikes quickly, and then follows an unpredictable course of waxing and waning over a patient's lifetime. The patient may be disabled for months, then recover and remain unaffected for years until another episode occurs. This form of the disease is called **relapsing-remitting multiple sclerosis**, which affects 85% of those diagnosed. About one-half of those patients diagnosed with relapsing-remitting MS will progress to a secondary phase of the disease in which there are less periods of stability and increased periods of active MS, making this form more difficult to treat.

At this time, there is no cure for MS. Treatment is primarily aimed at controlling how the disease progresses and to modify its course, if possible. There are currently several disease-modifying drugs for patients with relapsing-remitting disease that are approved by the FDA. Antineoplastic drugs, such as mitoxantrone, work on the immune system by suppressing the activity of T cells, B cells, and macrophages that are thought to lead the attack on the myelin sheath. Natalizumab is a drug designed to hamper the movement of potentially damaging immune cells from the bloodstream into the brain and spinal cord. See Chapter 19, *Immunology*, for a further discussion about cell types related to the immune system. Other interferon-type drugs are designed to delay the time between flare-ups, reduce the number of active lesions, and possibly lessen the severity of the flare-ups. Finally, antispastic drugs such as tizanidine (Zanaflex) or baclofen (Lioresal) are used to reduce painful muscle spasms and improve ambulation due to stiffness. Other immune-suppressing drugs are currently being tested that seem to offer longer periods of time (up to five years in some cases) of relapses of the disease.

Physical therapy may be used to strengthen muscles and preserve mobility in conjunction with occupational therapy and devices to help patients with their activities of daily living (ADLs). In addition, pain medications and medications for depression or bladder or bowel-control problems may also be used if indicated.

Plasmapheresis, or plasma exchange, is a recent approach for patients with sudden, severe attacks of MS that do not seem to respond to high doses of medication. Plasmapheresis involves the removal of blood and mechanical separation of the blood cells from the fluid (plasma). Blood cells then are mixed with a replacement solution, typically a synthetic solution or albumin. The solution with the blood cells is then returned to the body. It is not clear why plasma exchange seems to reduce symptoms of neurologic disorders, but some researchers believe that removing plasma removes all the antibodies, immune complexes, and immune messenger chemicals in the blood, thereby taming destructive autoimmune activity. Although the treatment is controversial, preliminary studies showed that plasma exchange benefits some people with acute onsets of MS attacks, relieving symptoms for months when the procedure is successful.

Bell Palsy

Bell palsy is an attack on the facial nerve. Named after Sir Charles Bell, the 19th century Scottish surgeon who first discovered it, this condition causes sudden weakness or paralysis of the muscles on one side of the face due to the malfunction of cranial nerve VII, which stimulates the facial muscles. Facial weakness can occur suddenly and range from mild weakness to complete paralysis. Only one side of the face is affected.

The disorder comes on suddenly and peaks within about 48 hours. The individual loses the ability to contract the muscles controlling the forehead, mouth, or cheek, making the mouth droop and the face appear distorted. Bell palsy may interfere with eye closure on the affected side, causing the eye to become dry and resulting in pain or damage. The disease may also interfere with the production of saliva, the sensation of taste in the front part of the tongue, or the ability to produce tears. Sounds on the affected side may seem abnormally loud (called **hyperacusis**) because the muscle in the inner ear that adjusts the tympanic membrane to sound is paralyzed.

The cause of Bell palsy is unknown, but most scientists believe that a viral infection, such as viral meningitis or the common cold sore virus, herpes simplex virus type 1 (HSV-1), causes the disorder when the facial nerve swells and becomes inflamed in reaction to the infection. Swelling causes the nerve to be compressed and its blood supply to be reduced.

There is no cure or standard course of treatment for Bell palsy, but many physicians approach the problem as if it were an HSV infection. The antiviral drug acyclovir is given to prevent the virus from replicating. Corticosteroids, such as prednisone, reduce swelling of the facial nerve. Eyedrops such as Artificial Tears are used to provide moisture to the eye until it can close completely. The extent of nerve damage determines the extent of recovery from Bell palsy; but with or without treatment, most individuals begin to get better within two weeks after the initial onset of symptoms and recover completely within three to six months.

Trigeminal Neuralgia

Trigeminal neuralgia (TN), also called **tic douloureux**, is a disorder of the trigeminal nerve (cranial nerve V), which is the main sensory nerve in the face. This nerve carries sensory information from the face to the brain and controls the muscles involved in chewing. TN causes sudden, short bursts of excruciating pain on one side of the face, in one of the areas supplied by the trigeminal nerve, usually along the second nerve divisions, which supply the lower face and jaw. The pain

can be set off by touching a sensitive area of the face, called a trigger point, or by certain movements of the jaw while speaking, chewing, or swallowing. The pain typically begins with a sensation of electrical shocks and culminates in less than 20 seconds with an excruciating, stabbing pain. The pain often leaves patients with uncontrollable facial twitching, which is why the disorder is also known as *tic douloureux*. TN attacks rarely occur when the sufferer is asleep, but may be worsened or alleviated by leaning or lying in a specific position.

This disorder is sometimes associated with compression of the nerve by an artery, which may be relieved by surgery; but in most cases, the cause is unknown. Because the bouts of pain are brief and recurrent, analgesics are usually not helpful, but many patients have found relief with the use of anticonvulsant medications that stabilize nerve membranes. Common drugs prescribed to help relieve the pain of trigeminal neuralgia include carbamazepine (Tegretol), phenytoin (Dilantin), oxcarbazepine (Trileptal), and gabapentin (Neurontin). Baclofen (Lioresal), a drug used to reduce muscle spasms, can also be helpful. Treatment is usually initiated with a single drug, increasing the dose as needed and as tolerated. If any single drug proves ineffective, another drug is tried alone; if this is not successful, treatment progresses to combinations of these drugs.

Neurosurgical interventions are considered when medical therapy proves ineffective in controlling TN pain. There are several surgical options available, the most common of which include:

- **Microvascular decompression**, which involves microsurgical exposure of the trigeminal nerve root, identification of a blood vessel that may be compressing the nerve, gentle displacement of the vessel or nerve away from the point of compression, and allowing the trigeminal nerve to recover and return to a more normal, pain-free condition.
- **Percutaneous stereotactic rhizotomy**, which destroys the part of the nerve that causes pain by applying a heating current that destroys some of the nerve fibers.
- **Stereotactic radiosurgery**, which delivers a single highly concentrated dose of ionizing radiation to a small, precise target at the trigeminal nerve root. Over a period of time and as a result of radiation exposure, the slow formation of a lesion in the nerve interrupts transmission of pain signals to the brain.

Brain Tumors

Recall that a tumor is an abnormal growth of cells or tissues. A **brain tumor** is a mass of abnormal cells growing in the brain. Brain tumors, like other tumors, are described by physicians as being **benign** or **malignant**, terms which refer to the aggressiveness of the tumor. A benign tumor does not contain cancer cells, and the cells in the tumor grow very slowly and rarely spread. This type of tumor can be removed and is not likely to recur. A malignant brain tumor contains cancer cells. It usually grows rapidly, interferes with vital functions, and is life-threatening. A malignant tumor is likely to invade the tissue around it, putting out roots that grow into healthy brain or spine tissue, although it rarely spreads to other parts of the body. The term **metastasis** refers to the spread of a disease process from one part of the body to another; and a tumor that originates elsewhere in the body and then travels to the brain via the bloodstream is called a **metastatic brain tumor**.

A tumor that originates in brain tissue is called a **primary brain tumor**. A **secondary brain tumor** is a brain tumor caused by a cancer that originates in another part of the body. The most common type of brain tumor is that which begins in the glial (supportive) tissue, called a **glioma**. Some common types of gliomas include:

- **Astrocytomas**, which arise from small, star-shaped cells called **astrocytes**. They may grow anywhere in the brain or spinal cord, but most often occur in the cerebrum. The most serious type of astrocytoma is called **glioblastoma multiforme**. Gliomas that occur in the brainstem are referred to as **high-grade astrocytomas**.
- **Ependymomas**, which usually develop in the lining of the ventricles.
- **Oligodendrogliomas**, which arise in the oligodendrocytes. An **oligodendrocyte** is a type of cell in the central nervous system that is responsible for making and supporting myelin, the material that covers and protects neurons. These tumors usually begin in the cerebrum, grow slowly, and usually do not spread into surrounding brain tissue.

There are other types of brain tumors that do not begin in glial tissue. The following are some of the most common:

- **Medulloblastomas** develop from the **primitive** (developing) nerve cells that normally do not remain in the body after birth. For this reason, medulloblastomas are sometimes called **primitive neuroectodermal tumors** (PNETs, pronounced in dictation like "PEE-nets"). Most medulloblastomas arise in the cerebellum; however, they may occur in other areas as well.
- **Meningiomas** grow from the meninges. They are usually benign and grow so slowly that they often grow quite large before causing symptoms.
- **Schwannomas** are benign tumors that begin in Schwann cells, which produce the myelin that protects the acoustic nerve.
- **Craniopharyngiomas** develop in the region of the pituitary gland near the hypothalamus. They are usually benign; however, they can press on or damage the hypothalamus and affect vital functions.

The cause of brain tumors is not well known. However, exposure to some types of radiation, head injuries, and hormone replacement therapy may be risk factors, as may some inherited genetic factors. In addition, researchers have found that some chemicals may change the structure of a gene that protects the body from diseases and cancer. Workers in oil refining and rubber manufacturing have a higher incidence of certain types of tumors. Which, if any, chemical toxin is related to this increase in tumors is unknown at this time.

Treating a brain tumor involves reducing the size of the tumor as much as possible or removing it entirely. Some brain tumors can be removed with little or no damage to the brain. Surgery sometimes causes damage to other vital areas of the brain, but removing the tumor is essential if its growth threatens important brain structures. In addition, surgery may be useful to reduce the tumor's size, relieve symptoms, and help doctors determine whether further treatments are necessary.

Some of the surgical options available to treat a brain tumor include the following:

- **Craniotomy**. A craniotomy, mentioned above, is the most common type of surgery performed to remove a brain tumor. In this procedure, an incision is made into the skin and membranous tissue covering the top of the head, called the **scalp**. The scalp tissue is then folded back to expose the skull bone. Using a high-speed drill, the surgeon drills a pattern of holes through the skull and uses a fine wire saw to connect the holes until a segment of bone, called a **bone flap**, can be removed. This gives the surgeon access to the inside of the skull and allows him to proceed with surgery inside the brain. After the surgical procedure is completed, the bone flap is replaced and secured into position with soft wire.
- **Craniectomy**. A craniectomy is similar to a craniotomy except that the bone removed for access to the brain is not put back before closing the incision. Recall the suffix *-otomy* means *cutting into*, whereas the suffix *-ectomy* means *removal*. This procedure may be performed if swelling occurs following the surgery or if the skull bone is not reusable. If the bone is not reusable, a prosthetic plate replaces the skull bone that is not put back in place.
- **Debulking**. The term *debulk* means to surgically reduce the size of a tumor that cannot be completely removed by removing as much of it as possible.
- Transsphenoidal surgery. This approach is often used with tumors located in the pituitary gland. The term **transsphenoidal** comes from the prefix *trans-*, meaning *through or across*, and the root word *sphenoid*, referring to the sphenoid bone that forms the central base of the cranium. The entry point is

QUICK CHECK 18.2 ✓

Circle the letter corresponding to the best answer to the following questions.

1. A silicone rubber tube implanted in the brain to relieve CSF accumulation is called a(n)

    A. bleb.
    B. tic.
    C. shunt.
    D. electrode.

2. The condition that causes sudden weakness or paralysis on one side of the face is called

    A. epilepsy.
    B. Parkinson disease.
    C. tic douloureux.
    D. Bell palsy.

3. Microvascular clipping is used as a treatment for

    A. multiple sclerosis.
    B. trigeminal neuralgia.
    C. an aneurysm.
    D. seizure disorder.

4. An inflammation of the membranes that cover the brain and spinal cord is called

    A. folliculitis.
    B. meningitis.
    C. subarachnoid hemorrhage.
    D. status epilepticus.

5. The motor system disorder characterized by tremors and clumsiness is called

    A. Parkinson disease.
    B. seizure disorder.
    C. Bell palsy.
    D. normal pressure hydrocephalus.

6. Slowness of movement is called

    A. bradykinesia.
    B. dysphasia.
    C. dyskinesia.
    D. ataxia.

7. A VP shunt is used to treat

    A. myoclonic seizures.
    B. meningitis.
    C. hydrocephalus.
    D. relapsing-remitting MS.

8. The symptom of uncontrollable facial twitching characteristic of trigeminal neuralgia is often referred to as

    A. tic neuralgia.
    B. tic douloureux.
    C. petit mal seizures.
    D. status epilepticus.

9. A blisterlike sac filled with blood is referred to as a

    A. tumor.
    B. bulla.
    C. blog.
    D. bleb.

10. The type of seizure that most people visualize when they think of a seizure is really called a(n)

    A. myoclonic seizure.
    B. partial complex seizure.
    C. tonic-clonic seizure.
    D. absence seizure.

through an incision made under the upper lip and over the teeth, or directly through the nostril.

- **Photodynamic therapy** (PDT). This procedure uses a light-sensitive drug called Photofrin and laser light to kill cancer cells. The drug is injected into the patient and concentrates on tumors. Photofrin remains inactive until it is combined with laser light. The light activates the drug, which reacts with oxygen to produce a chemical that destroys tumor tissue. PDT may also work by destroying the blood vessels that feed the cancer cells and by helping the immune system to attack the cancer.

Additional treatments, such as the use of chemotherapy and radiation therapy, are discussed in more detail in Chapter 20, *Oncology*.

DIAGNOSTIC STUDIES AND PROCEDURES

Neurologists use a variety of assessments, laboratory studies, and imaging tests to help identify and diagnose the specific nature of neurologic conditions and disorders. Some are performed in specialized settings, whereas others are performed in a physician's office or outpatient testing facility. The results of these tests help physicians plan appropriate courses of treatment. The following are some of the most frequently performed diagnostic tests used by neurosurgeons.

Neurologic Assessment

The **neurologic assessment** is a series of tests used to assess brain function of a patient as well as to evaluate for possible neurologic damage. While neurologic imaging studies look at the structural and physical condition of the brain, the neurologic assessment is used to examine brain *function*. These tests cover the range of mental processes from level of consciousness to simple motor and sensory performance, speech, cognitive function, and cranial nerve response. Some of this testing includes the following issues:

- Level of consciousness. The **Glasgow coma scale** (GCS) is the scoring system used most widely to quantify a patient's level of consciousness following a brain injury. It is used routinely by medical personnel to objectively describe a patient's neurologic status. A patient's responses to motor, verbal, and eye-opening cues establish a GCS score in the range of three to 15. Patients with a score of three to eight are said to be in a coma.

- Mental status. The physician asks a series of questions to determine if a patient's thought processes are normal. To determine a patient's orientation to person, place, and time, the physician might ask the patient to state his/her name, city, county, or hospital location as well as the time (month, date). The physician may ask other questions to assess the patient's mental status, such as the name of the current President of the United States, the name of his/her mother, how old he/she is, and what the patient had for breakfast. The results are dictated using all three parameters. For example, the dictator may say, "The patient was oriented to person, place, and time," or "The patient was oriented to person and time but not to place."

- Cranial nerve assessment. The cranial nerve assessment reveals valuable information about the condition of the CNS, especially the brainstem. Cranial nerves are commonly affected by disease, whether it is disease of the nerve itself or as part of another process (such as a hemorrhage or tumor formation) in the CNS. These small, slender nerves are commonly damaged in patients with head trauma, and they may also be damaged as part of a disease process such as cancer. For these reasons, a systematic examination of the cranial nerves is part of every patient's neurologic assessment. See Table 18.1 for a list of the cranial nerves and how they are evaluated.

- Motor examination. The motor assessment aids evaluation of the cerebral cortex and its initiation of

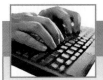

TRANSCRIPTION TIP:

Dictators may describe a *paucity of ideas* or a *paucity of speech*, meaning that the patient seems to have few ideas or limited speech. Do not mistranscribe this term as *posity or aposity*.

motor activity, the cerebellum's ability to coordinate and fine-tune movements, and the muscles and their capacity to carry out motor commands. The terms *motor* and *strength* are used interchangeably when testing extremity joints. The patient is asked to flex and extend the upper and lower extremities against resistance. The results are graded from one to five, with five showing full strength of the joint. These values are transcribed in the form of a fraction using arabic numbers. For example, "Strength in the right lower extremity was five out of five," would be transcribed as follows: "Strength in the right lower extremity was 5/5." Sometimes physicians use the plus (+) or minus (−) signs to more accurately indicate joint strength, such as "4 plus" or "5 minus," which should likewise be used when transcribing the fraction value. For example, "Strength in the right lower extremity was four plus out of five," would be transcribed, "Strength in the right lower extremity was 4+/5." The pronator drift test is another evaluation of muscle strength. Recall that a **pronator muscle** is a muscle that returns a part into the prone position from supine. The pronator drift test detects subtle weakness in the upper extremities, which can indicate an abnormality in the motor-nerve system. In the pronator drift test, the patient stands for 20–30 seconds with both arms straight forward, palms up, and eyes closed. The examiner then taps the palms briskly downward. In an abnormal finding, the patient will not be able to maintain extension and supination and the arm will drift back into pronation, or palm side down, indicating possible disease.

- Sensory examination. The patient's reaction to various sensations is tested to evaluate for nerve dysfunction. Terms dictated to relate a patient's sensation often include *light touch*, *temperature*, *vibration*, and *pinprick*.

- Cerebellar function. This series of tests is used to evaluate the patient's coordination and balance. The results of all of these tests are indicated as either positive or negative. In the gait test, the patient is asked to walk in a straight line so that the physician may note whether the gait is normal or **antalgic**, or limping. Next, in the **Romberg** test, the patient is asked to stand with feet together and eyes closed to test for falling. The result might be dictated, "The Romberg test was negative," or

"Romberg was negative," or "Negative Romberg," which should all be transcribed as dictated. In the finger-to-nose test, the patient is asked, with eyes closed, to first extend his/her hand out to the side, and next touch his nose with the tip of his finger without touching or pointing past it. The past-pointing test is primarily a test of proprioception, and it involves having the patient repeatedly bring his finger to a remembered position with his/her eyes closed. Patients with a CNS problem may point more to the side of the nose. Finally, in the heel-to-shin test, the patient, while lying down, is asked to place the right heel on the left knee (or vice versa) and slowly move the heel downward toward the foot to test the patient's ability to judge distance, power, and speed of a movement. Inability to judge these factors is called **dysmetria**.

- Reflex testing. A **reflex** is an automatic response to a stimulus. A stimulus, such as a light tap with a rubber hammer, causes sensory neurons to send signals to the spinal cord, which are then transmitted to the brain and to nerves that control muscles affected by the stimulation. Reflexes are tested to diagnose the presence and/or location of a spinal cord injury, damage to the peripheral nervous system (the nerves outside the spinal cord) called **peripheral neuropathy**, or a muscle disease. The deep tendons are those that attach the deep muscles (the muscles lying next to the bones) to the bones themselves. Testing of the reflexes of these tendons, called **deep tendon reflexes** (DTRs), can indicate pressure on or injury to the spinal cord. In this test, the examiner uses a rubber mallet to strike different points on the patient's body with a short, sharp blow and observes the response. The reflex tested by tapping just below the knee at the patellar tendon is referred to as a **knee jerk** in dictation, whereas the reflex tested by tapping the Achilles tendon of the foot is called an **ankle jerk**. The **Babinski test** is a reflex test that involves the gentle stroking of the sole of the foot with a sharp object to assess proper development of the spine and cerebral cortex. The normal response in adults and children is for the toes to curl downward, whereas in people with a neurologic problem, the big toe moves upward. The results are dictated as being negative or positive, but also can be dictated using the direction of the toes. For example, the dictator may say, "Babinski was positive (or negative)." or "Toes were upgoing (or downgoing)."

Laboratory Tests

Laboratory screening tests of blood and other substances are used to help diagnose disease, to monitor a disease process, and to evaluate the effects of therapeutic drugs on the body. Some tests are ordered as part of a regular checkup, whereas others are used to identify specific health concerns. Although a blood or urine test in itself

TRANSCRIPTION TIP:

In neurologic evaluations, physicians may describe the results of a pronator drift test with phrases such as, "Pronator drift is…Past-pointing is…" Too often medical transcriptionists leave the word *pronator* blank and mistakenly type the phrase *pass pointing*. Also remember that the term *past-pointing* is hyphenated.

cannot diagnose a neurologic disorder, blood tests are commonly used to check for vitamin deficiencies, toxic elements, and evidence of an abnormal immune response, which could identify potentially treatable causes of a neurologic problem. For example, genetic testing of DNA extracted from white blood cells in the blood can help diagnose congenital neurologic diseases before birth. A high white blood cell count may also indicate an infection in the brain or spinal cord, whereas a low red blood cell count may indicate an inadequate supply of oxygen to the brain. Blood tests can detect bone marrow disease or blood vessel damage. They can also be used to monitor levels of drugs used to treat epilepsy and other chronic neurologic disorders.

Biopsy

Recall that a biopsy is the removal and examination of a small piece of tissue from the body. Muscle or nerve biopsies are used to diagnose abnormal nerve anatomy or muscular disorders that can reveal if a person is a carrier of a defective gene that might be passed on to children. A biopsy of abnormal tissue located in the spine or brain can be used to diagnose a brain tumor or a plaque or lesion associated with a neurologic disorder, such as multiple sclerosis. It also can indicate the type and amount of damage done, whether the tumor is growing, and at what rate. As with a conventional biopsy, an incision is made in the skin; a small piece of nerve, muscle, or tissue is removed from the body; and the wound is sutured closed. The sample is then sent to the laboratory to be examined under a microscope.

Lumbar Puncture

A **lumbar puncture** (LP), also called a **spinal tap**, is a procedure used to evaluate the CSF from the space

TRANSCRIPTION TIP:

In a neurologic examination, the dictator may state that "Babinski is equivocal," or that any test is equivocal, meaning that the results are not clear.

surrounding the spinal cord. The fluid is tested to detect bleeding, brain hemorrhages, or infection in the brain or spinal cord; it is tested to measure pressure in the brain when evaluating hydrocephalus, and also can be used in some cases to diagnose other neurologic conditions such as multiple sclerosis.

A lumbar puncture is performed with the patient lying on his/her side in a fetal position. A puncture site is located between two vertebrae and the site is cleaned and a local anesthetic administered. A special needle is inserted into the subarachnoid space to remove a sample of the CSF from the spinal canal. The fluid sample is then sent to the laboratory for analysis.

Neurosonography

Neurosonography is an ultrasound examination of the brain and spinal column. Like conventional ultrasound, neurosonography uses high-frequency sound waves to obtain images of blood flow in the brain. It is commonly used in cases of possible stroke, inflammatory processes causing pain, buildup of CSF in the brain in cases of hydrocephalus, and soft tissue masses or tears in the ligaments or tendons in the back. In this test, the patient lies on an imaging table and a gel-like lubricant is applied to the area being examined. The transducer, which both sends and receives sound waves, is passed over the body. The sound wave echoes are recorded and display real-time visual images of the structure or tissue being examined on a monitor. The images are later analyzed by the physician to help diagnose a patient's neurologic condition.

Imaging Studies

Physicians may order one or more imaging studies to determine the specific nature of a neurologic disorder or injury. These tests use a variety of modalities, including small amounts of radioactive materials, magnets, or electrical charges, to study the anatomic structures of the brain and spinal cord. The following are some of the more common tests used to help diagnose a neurologic condition.

Cerebral Angiogram

Angiography is a type of x-ray examination used to detect blockages in blood vessels using radioactive contrast. A **cerebral angiogram** is used to detect an obstruction in a blood vessel in the brain, head, or neck; it can be used to diagnose a stroke or to determine the size and location of a brain tumor or aneurysm. In this procedure, a catheter is inserted into the femoral artery in the leg, located near the groin. The catheter is threaded through the body and into an artery in the neck. Once the catheter is in place, radioactive dye is injected into the artery and x-rays are taken while the dye moves through the artery. The x-rays show where the artery is blocked or narrowed and the amount of blockage, narrowing, or deformity that exists.

Computed Tomography

A computed tomography (CT) scan uses an x-ray to produce rapid, clear, two-dimensional images of organs, bones, and tissues, with the information displayed in cross-sections or slices of body tissue. In neurology, CT scans are focused on the head and spine. This type of imaging can detect tissue density (determined by the amount of contrast absorption), stenosis of the spinal canal, brain damage from a head injury or stroke, and other disorders. Because many neurologic disorders share certain symptoms and characteristics, a CT scan can be used to assist in narrowing the diagnosis by identifying the area of the brain affected by the disorder.

As with other CT scans, the patient lies still on an imaging table while x-rays pass through the body at various angles. Multiple pictures are taken at a fast pace and then are processed by a computer scanner and displayed as cross-sectional images on a monitor. Radioactive dye may also be used with a CT scan to highlight different tissues in the brain or spinal cord nerve roots. Dye cannot enter normal brain tissue, as it is unable to penetrate the system of capillaries called the **blood-brain barrier**, which acts as a shield and protects the delicate brain and spinal cord from all but the most essential nutrients. Portions of the brain where the barrier has been destroyed by infection, trauma, or other problem, enhance, or turn white, on the CT images.

With or without contrast-dye enhancement, a CT scan can display the detail of even the smallest bones in the body as well as surrounding blood vessels and tissues. This makes it an invaluable tool for diagnosing cranial and spinal problems.

Magnetic Resonance Imaging and Magnetic Resonance Angiography

Magnetic resonance imaging (MRI) and **magnetic resonance angiography** (MRA) are used separately or together to produce three-dimensional images of body structures, including tissues, organs, blood vessels, and nerves. These procedures involve the combination of large magnet, radiofrequencies, and computer technology. The images result from the different levels of water concentrations in the various tissues. An MRI can give clear pictures of soft tissue structures in and around bones, whereas an MRA is used to illuminate blood vessels in the neck and brain. Both tests use computer-generated radio waves and a powerful magnetic field (as opposed to radiation) to obtain images of body structures that can aid in the diagnosis of brain and spinal cord tumors, inflammation, infection, or blood vessel irregularities that may lead to a stroke or aneurysm. In addition, both MRI and MRA images can document brain injury from trauma.

A physician may refer to these tests in dictation as simply MR, MR imaging, MR angiography, MRI, MRA, or both abbreviations together. When both MRI and

MRA are indicated, they are transcribed together, divided by a slash: MRI/MRA.

The patient is placed in the MRI scanner. The scanning equipment creates a magnetic field around the body strong enough to temporarily realign water molecules in the tissues. Pulses of radio waves are sent from the scanner to detect the molecules as they realign back into their proper position and trigger a resonance signal at different angles within the body. These signals are received by a computer that analyzes and converts them to an image of the part of the body being examined, which appears on a viewing monitor. An MRA uses the same technology and testing method to detect, diagnose, and aid the treatment of stroke and other blood vessel diseases. Like an MRI, MRA provides detailed images of blood vessels without using any contrast material.

A **functional MRI** is sometimes used to look at how the brain is actually functioning by identifying regions of increased brain activity. In this procedure, the patient performs a particular task, such as tapping the thumb of one hand against each of the fingers in that hand, while the imaging is taking place. The patient's performance of specific tasks that correspond to different functions allows physicians to locate the area of the brain that governs that function. This information can be used, for example, to help a neurosurgeon avoid those important areas during surgery.

Positron Emission Tomography

A **positron emission tomography** (PET) scan is a nuclear diagnostic test that provides two- and three-dimensional images of brain activity by detecting how quickly tissues consume radioactive isotopes injected into the bloodstream. A PET scan can be used to highlight diseased tissue and cerebral dysfunction associated with tumors, seizure disorders, and Alzheimer disease.

In this procedure, a technician administers a biochemical substance, such as glucose, that is attached, or *tagged*, with isotopes, which act as tracers. The contrast material emits positrons that combine with negatively charged electrons in tissue cells to create gamma rays as it collects in the specific area of the body being tested. A ring-shaped machine is positioned over the target area, which picks up the gamma rays emitted from body tissues containing the contrast material. A computer translates the information into patterns that are displayed on a video monitor or on film. These patterns reflect cerebral blood flow, blood volume, and neuron activity in the brain.

Single Photon Emission Computed Tomography

A **single photon emission computed tomography** (SPECT) scan is a nuclear image of blood flow to tissues, which is used to evaluate how well an organ, such as the brain, is functioning. It can be used in patients with epilepsy to help pinpoint the area in the brain involved with seizure production and also can help identify certain types of tumors or infections. As with a PET scan, a radioactive contrast material, which binds to chemicals that flow to the brain, is injected intravenously into the patient and circulates through the blood. Areas of increased blood flow collect more of the contrast material. A special camera rotates around the head and records where the material has traveled. The information is converted by a computer to cross-sectional images that can be stacked to produce a three-dimensional picture of blood flow and activity within the brain.

Electroencephalography

Electroencephalography (EEG) is a test that monitors brain activity through the skull. EEG is used to record evidence of abnormal electrical discharges, which can occur with seizure disorders, brain damage from head injuries, inflammation, or degenerative disorders that affect the brain. It is also used to monitor brain activity when a patient loses consciousness and to confirm brain death.

This procedure uses electrodes, or leads, which are small devices attached to wires that carry the electrical energy of the brain to a machine. The machine creates a tracing of the brain activity using basic waveforms called alpha, beta, theta, and delta rhythms. Each rhythm type is associated with different brain activity, such as when the patient is awake, is experiencing anxiety, depression, or is responding to outside stimuli, such as light or noise. A series of electrodes are placed on the patient's scalp, and brain activity is recorded under normal conditions. The patient is then exposed to various stimuli, such as bright or flashing lights or noises. The patient is asked to open and close his/her eyes or change breathing patterns. The electrodes record the changes in brain wave patterns, which are displayed on the tracing, as shown in Figure 18.4.

A **video EEG**, also called continuous video EEG monitoring, is used to record seizures as they occur. In this test, a patient's seizure medications are reduced or temporarily stopped so that seizures may occur. The patient is admitted to the hospital and the EEG test is administered while the patient is continuously videotaped to record seizures as they occur. The correlation of the changes on the EEG with the patient's videotaped body movements during a

TRANSCRIPTION TIP:

When transcribing EEG reports, some of the terms you may hear include *alpha, beta* (or *fast activity*), *delta, theta* (or *slow activity*), *photic stimulation, epileptiform discharges, Hz, K complexes, spike-and-wave pattern, attenuation, symmetric sleep spindles,* and *amplitude.*

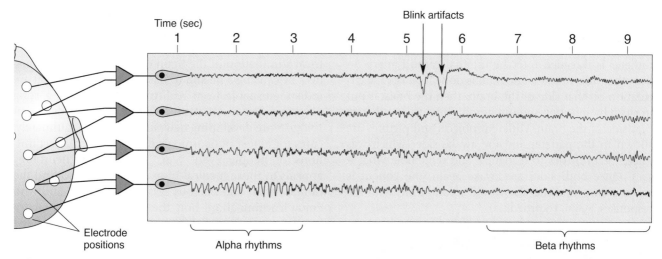

FIGURE 18.4. Normal EEG. In this EEG, the subject is awake and quiet, and recording sites are indicated at the left. The first few seconds show normal alpha activity. About halfway through the recording, the subject opened his eyes, signaled by the large blink artifacts on the top traces (arrows), and alpha rhythms were suppressed. Reprinted with permission from Bear MF, Connors BW, and Parasido, MA. *Neuroscience—Exploring the Brain,* 2nd ed. Philadelphia: Lippincott Williams & Wilkins, 2001.

seizure helps pinpoint the area of the brain in which the abnormal activity is occurring.

Wada Test

Most epilepsy patients considering surgery undergo the **Wada test**. This test, developed in 1949 by Dr. Juhn Wada, was originally created to determine which side of the brain controlled speech ability. Now it is used to test memory as well as language functions. It is a valuable tool in the evaluation of patients who are being considered for epilepsy surgery, as it is the only known way to examine the independent functions of the side of the brain that is targeted for surgery.

The test is performed on each side of the brain. As an initial step before the Wada test on each side, a cerebral angiogram is done, as described previously. The

angiogram looks at blood flow within the brain to make sure that there are no obstacles to performing the Wada. Once the angiogram is done, the catheter will stay in place for the Wada test on that side.

One side of the brain is anesthetized by injecting a barbiturate, sodium amobarbital, into the carotid artery. The side of the brain that is put to sleep cannot communicate with the other side. This allows the doctor and neuropsychologist to test each side of the brain for speech and memory separately. Once the physicians are sure that one side of the brain is asleep, the neuropsychologist will show the patient objects and pictures. The awake side of the brain tries to recognize and remember what it sees. After a few minutes, the sodium amobarbital wears off and soon both sides of the brain are fully awake. The neuropsychologist then questions the patient to see if he/she remembers what

QUICK CHECK 18.3

Indicate whether the following sentences are true (T) or false (F).

1. The Wada test is performed prior to epilepsy surgery.   T   F

2. A neurologic assessment is used to assess brain structure.   T   F

3. The narrowing of the spinal canal is called stenosis.   T   F

4. MRA stands for magnetic resonance angiography.   T   F

5. An EEG uses high-resolution x-rays.   T   F

6. Deep tendon reflexes are used to test a patient's mental status.   T   F

7. Angiography uses radioactive contrast to detect blockages in blood vessels.   T   F

8. The Babinski test is a type of motor examination.   T   F

9. A PET scan is used to record seizures as they occur.   T   F

10. Another name for a lumbar puncture is a DNA test.   T   F

was seen before, with the responses recorded word-for-word.

Then the other side of the brain is tested. The catheter is threaded into the internal carotid artery on the other side. A new angiogram is done to check the circulation on that side of the brain; then the brain is put to sleep by injecting sodium amobarbital to anesthetize that side of the brain. Different objects and pictures are shown to the patient, and the awake side (which was asleep before) tries to recognize and remember what it sees. Once both sides are awake again, the patient is asked about what was shown the second time, with the responses, again, recorded.

CHAPTER SUMMARY

In recent years, neurologic research has greatly advanced our understanding of the brain and nervous system. Using functional MRI and other technology, neuroscientists can almost read people's thoughts from the blood flow imagery in their brains, for example, distinguishing whether a person is thinking about a face, a place, or even an inanimate object such as a shoe. Electrical stimulation of the brain can even alter consciousness by causing a person to have hallucinations that are indistinguishable from reality, such as that of a song playing in the room. Armed with this knowledge, neurologists are developing new treatments and, ultimately, cures for a host of neurologic diseases which affect millions of people every year. The field of neurology appeals to those medical transcriptionists who find the human brain and nervous system fascinating and who enjoy learning about how the physicians who practice in this specialized field correct abnormalities of the nervous system. An understanding of the anatomic structure and function of the nervous system provides the foundation for the appreciation of the delicate balance between the skills and activities we take for granted and our vulnerability to injuries and other problems that can cause irreversible damage and can change the course of our daily lives.

· I · N · S · I · G · H · T ·

More to Magic Than Meets the Eye

The mechanisms that govern the brain's visual perception are only partly understood by scientists; in fact, much of what we know about how the human visual system works stems from investigations into our susceptibility to visual illusions. Although scientists have used knowledge of illusions to further our understanding of the mind, magicians have learned to master the art of deception for entertainment purposes. Researchers have studied the power of magicians to facilitate illusion and have uncovered the ways in which particular types of information—cues from the magicians—influence some aspects of the brain's processing of images while other components of the visual system remain unaffected.

According to Gustav Kuhn of the University of Durham (UK) and Michael Land of the University of Sussex (UK), whose findings were reported in *Current Biology*, our perception of an event is often significantly modulated by our past experiences and expectations. The researchers used a magic trick (the "vanishing ball" illusion) to demonstrate how magicians can distort our perception in an everyday situation by manipulating our expectations; the researchers then went on to investigate the mechanisms behind this deception.

The researchers found that when a magician performed the illusion, in which a ball was seen to disappear in the air after a fake throw, 68% of observers perceived the ball leaving the magician's hand, move upward, and disappear—this despite the fact that the ball did not leave the magician's hand. Experimental manipulations of the trick revealed that the observers' perception of the ball was determined by particular cues—namely the magician's head direction—that were indicative of the ball's intended location, rather than the actual location of the ball.

By measuring the eye movements of the observers, the researchers showed that rather than merely tracking the ball, most people looked at the magician's face prior to tracking the ball—consistent with the brain's visual system utilizing so-called social cues, such as the magician's head direction and gaze, to help form a perception of the ball's location. However, once the ball was no longer physically present in the course of the illusion, observers did not look at the area where they claimed to have seen the ball, suggesting that the oculomotor system, which governs motor control of the eyes, was not fooled by the illusion.

The study's findings show that although visual perception was strongly influenced by expectations, the oculomotor system itself was largely driven by "bottom up," visual information from the ball itself. The findings are also consistent with recent evidence from other studies suggesting that two separate neural pathways exist for perception and visuomotor control.

From: Medical News Today, www.medicalnewstoday.com

Common Soundalike Words

Word	Word Pronunciation	Soundalike	Soundalike Pronunciation
tic: A habitual spasmodic motion of particular muscles, especially the face.	tik′	**tick**: A bloodsucking arachnid.	tik′
consciousness: The state of awareness.	kon′shŭ -nes	**conscience**: A sense of right and wrong.	kon′shŭns
electroencephalogram (EEG): A test that measures and records the electrical activity of the brain.	ē-lek′trō-en-sef′ă-lō-gram	**electrocardiogram (EKG)**: A graphic record of cardiac action currents obtained with the electrocardiograph.	ē-lek-trō-kar′dē-ō-gram
basal: Relating to the base of a structure.	bā′săl	**basil**: A spice used in cooking.	bā′sil
cranial: Relating to the cranium or head.	krā′nē-ăl	**corneal**: Relating to the cornea of the eye.	kōr′nē-ăl
cord: A ropelike structure (such as the spine).	kōrd	**chord**: A combination of musical notes.	Kōrd
endorphin: A natural substance produced in the brain.	ĕn-dōr′fín	**endocrine**: The internal or hormonal secretion of a ductless gland.	en′dō-krin
paralysis: Loss of power of voluntary movement in a muscle through injury to or disease of its nerve supply.	pă-ral′i-sis	**peristalsis**: The wavelike movement of the intestine or other tubular structure.	per-i-stal′sis
absence: A type of seizure that usually can be brought on by hyperventilation.	ab′sens	**absent**: Not present.	ab′sent
axis: A straight line joining two opposing poles of a spheric body.	ak′sis	**abscess**: A circumscribed collection of purulent fluid appearing in an acute or chronic localized infection.	ab′ses

Combining Forms

Combining Form	Definition	Combining Form	Definition
arachn/o	spider, spider web	myel/o	the bone marrow; the spinal cord and medulla oblongata; the myelin sheath of nerve fibers
astr/o	starlike structure		
autonom/o	independent; self-governing		
cephal/o, encephal/o	brain	neur/o, nerv/o	nerve, nerve tissue, the nervous system
cerebell/o	cerebellum		
cerebr/o	cerebrum	occipit/o	back of the head
cortic/o	outer layer or covering	phren/o, psych/o	mind
crani/o	skull	rhiz/o	spinal nerve root
dendr/o	branching structure	scler/o	hard
esthesi/o	sensation	spin/o	spinal cord
gangli/o	ganglion (knot)	spondyl/o	vertebra
gemin/o	twins; set or group	sten/o	narrowness; constriction
gen/o	arising or produced by	tax/o	coordination
gli/o	glue	tempor/o	side of the head
hem/o	blood	thalam/o	thalamus
hydr/o	water	thym/o	thymus
kin/o	movement	ton/o	tension
megal/o	large	vascul/o	blood vessel
mening/o	meninges (membrane)	ventricul/o	ventricle
muscul/o, my/o	muscle	vertebr/o	vertebra
myelin/o	myelin		

Add Your Own Combining Forms Here:

_____

_____

_____

_____

_____

_____

ABBREVIATIONS

Abbreviation	Meaning	Abbreviation	Meaning
AComA	anterior communicating artery	MRI	magnetic resonance imaging
ADLs	activities of daily living	MS	multiple sclerosis
CNS	central nervous system	PComA	posterior communicating artery
CSF	cerebrospinal fluid	PD	Parkinson disease
CT	computed tomography (scan)	PDT	photodynamic therapy
DBS	deep brain stimulation	PET	positron emission tomography (scan)
DTRs	deep tendon reflexes		
EEG	electroencephalogram	PNS	peripheral nervous system
EEG	electroencephalography	SAH	subarachnoid hemorrhage
GCS	Glasgow coma scale	SPECT	single photon emission computed tomography (scan)
HSV-1	herpes simplex virus-1		
LP	lumbar puncture	TN	trigeminal neuralgia
MRA	magnetic resonance angiography		

Add Your Own Abbreviations Here:

_____

_____

_____

_____

_____

_____

TERMINOLOGY

Term	Meaning
absence seizure, syn. petit mal seizure	A type of generalized seizure characterized by a brief loss of consciousness without associated motor symptoms.
acquired hydrocephalus	Hydrocephalus that can occur at any time after birth.
afferent nerves	Nerve fibers that carry sensory information from the peripheral nervous system to the central nervous system.
amygdala	The part of the limbic system that controls emotional reaction to a given situation.
aneurysm	An abnormal dilation of a blood vessel caused by a weakness in the vessel's wall.

Term	Meaning
angiography	A type of x-ray used to detect blockages in blood vessels using radioactive contrast.
ankle jerk	The reflex tested by the tapping of the Achilles tendon of the foot with a short, sharp blow to the tendon with a tendon hammer.
antalgic (gait)	A limping-type gait.
anterior communicating artery (AComA)	A short artery that joins the two anterior cerebral arteries in the brain.
arachnoid membrane	The weblike middle layer of the meninges.
astrocytes	Small, star-shaped cells.
astrocytoma	A tumor that arises from small, star-shaped cells called astrocytes.
ataxia	Uncontrolled gait; inability to control and coordinate muscle activity.
aura	A subjective warning sign that occurs immediately before the onset of a seizure.
Babinski test	A type of reflex test that involves gently stroking the sole of the foot to assess proper development of the spine and cerebral cortex.
bacterial meningitis	An infection by bacteria causing inflammation of the meninges.
bacteremia	The presence of bacteria in the blood.
basal ganglia	Islands of nerve cell clusters embedded in the white matter of the brain.
Bell palsy	An idiopathic attack on the facial nerve, causing sudden weakness or paralysis of the muscles on one side of the face.
benign	Refers to the mild character of a tumor, such as a tumor that does not contain cancer cells.
bleb	A blisterlike sac filled with blood.
blood-brain barrier	A system of central nervous system (CNS) capillaries that prevent many substances from entering the brain and/or spinal cord, acting as a selective filter to limit harmful substances into the brain.
bone flap	A portion of the skull that is temporarily removed during a surgical procedure and replaced when the procedure is completed.
bradykinesia	Slowness of body movement.
brain	The part of the nervous system that is enclosed in the skull and connected to the spinal cord that includes all the body's higher nervous centers.
brain tumor	A mass of abnormal cells growing in the brain.
brainstem	The lower extension of the brain that controls levels of consciousness and automatically regulates critical vital functions such as heartbeat and respirations.
cauda equina	A bundle of nerves that extend beyond the end of the spinal cord.
central nervous system (CNS)	The division of the nervous system consisting of the brain and spinal cord.
cerebellum	The structure attached to the brainstem that fine-tunes the motor signals emanating from the cerebrum below the level of conscious thought, such as the coordination of the brain's instructions for body movements.
cerebral aneurysm	A saclike outpouching that can occur in the large arteries at the base of the brain.
cerebral angiogram	A test used to detect an obstruction in a blood vessel or in the brain, head, or neck.
cerebral cortex	A layer of millions of neurons and glia on the surface of the brain that carry out the many functions of the cerebrum.

Term	Meaning
cerebrospinal fluid (CSF)	A thin, watery substance that surrounds the brain and spinal cord.
cerebrum	The uppermost and largest part of the brain.
choroid plexus	The vascular complex that lays along the floor of the lateral ventricles where CSF is produced.
coil embolization	A procedure whereby tiny platinum coils are placed directly into an aneurysm to block blood flow and prevent rupture.
communicating hydrocephalus	A type of hydrocephalus that results from an actual problem with the actual production of CSF or absorption of CSF.
complex partial seizures	A type of partial seizure in which consciousness is altered during the seizure event.
computed tomography (CT) scan	A type of imaging study that uses an x-ray to produce rapid, clear, two-dimensional images of organs, bones, and tissues, with the information displayed in cross-sections or slices of body tissue.
congenital hydrocephalus	Hydrocephalus that is present at birth.
convulsive (seizure)	Relating to a type of seizure in which the body stiffens briefly, and then begins jerking movements.
corpus callosotomy	A procedure that severs the network of neural connections between the right and left hemispheres of the brain as a treatment for seizures.
corpus callosum	A band of nerve fibers that connect the left and right hemisphere of the cerebrum.
cranial nerves	Nerves that exit from the brain, which connect the brain with the eyes, ears, nose, and throat and with various parts of the head, neck, and trunk.
craniectomy	A surgical removal of a portion of the skull.
craniopharyngioma	A tumor that develops in the region of the pituitary gland.
craniotomy	A surgical opening made in the skull.
debulking	A procedure that involves surgically reducing as much as possible the size of a tumor that cannot be completely removed.
deep brain stimulation (DBS)	A procedure that involves implanting a device to deliver mild electrical stimulation to block the brain signals that cause tremors in patients with Parkinson disease.
deep tendon reflexes (DTRs)	A test of the deep tendons that can indicate pressure on or injury to the spinal cord.
demyelination	A gradual destruction of the myelin that surrounds and protects neurons.
dermatomes	Specific regions of the body which are supplied by the sensory nerve fibers of a single nerve root.
dopamine	An important chemical that helps transmit the nerve signals that cause the muscles to make smooth, controlled movements.
dura mater	The thick, outermost layer of the meninges.
dysmetria	The inability to judge distance, power, and speed of a movement.
efferent nerves	Nerve fibers that carry sensory information from the central nervous system to the peripheral nervous system.
electroencephalography (EEG)	A test that monitors abnormal electrical discharges in the brain.
enterovirus	A group of common viruses that is a common cause of viral meningitis.
epilepsy	The neurologic disorder characterized by recurrent seizures.

Term	Meaning
ependymoma	A tumor that develops in the lining of the ventricles.
fluoroscopy	An x-ray study of moving body structures.
foramen magnum	The large opening at the base of the skull where the spinal cord enters.
fourth ventricle	One of four ventricles located near the brainstem.
frontal lobes	The largest of the four lobes, located at the front of the brain.
functional MRI	An MRI imaging study that obtains images of the brain while it is actually functioning or performing a task.
generalized seizures	One of two main categories of seizures involving larger areas of the brain and often both hemispheres.
Glasgow coma scale (GCS)	A scoring system used to quantify a patient's level of consciousness following a brain injury.
glia	Non-neural (supporting) cells of the central and peripheral nervous system.
glioblastoma multiforme	The most serious type of astrocytoma.
glioma	A tumor that begins in the glial (supportive) tissue of the brain.
gray matter	Another name for cerebral cortex because of its appearance.
great longitudinal fissure	The groove that separates the left and right hemispheres of the cerebrum.
gyri (singular, gyrus)	The name given to the folds of the cerebral cortex.
Hemorrhage	A leak of blood, or bleeding, from a vessel.
high-grade astrocytoma	A glioma that occurs in the brainstem.
hippocampus	The part of the limbic system involved in the formation and retrieval of memories and storage of dry facts.
hydrocephalus	A condition in which excess CSF fluid builds up in the brain.
hyperacusis	Heightened auditory acuity; the ear's hearing of abnormally loud sounds.
hypothalamus	The part of the limbic system that regulates automatic functions such as appetite, thirst, and temperature.
impulse	An electrical signal or action potential of a nerve fiber.
interventricular foramen	The opening through which the lateral ventricles of the brain communicate with the third ventricle.
knee jerk	The reflex tested by tapping the patellar tendon of the knee with a short, sharp blow to the tendon with a tendon hammer.
lateral ventricles	A pair of ventricles in the brain where CSF is produced.
Lazarus sign	A complex spontaneous movement by nerves in the spinal cord without conscious effort of the patient (such as after a patient is comatose or brain-dead).
left hemisphere	One of two halves of the cerebrum that processes information.
limbic system	A complex set of structures located in the cerebrum that are involved in emotions, moods, and some functions of memory.
lobes	Interconnected areas in the left and right hemispheres of the cerebrum that serve specific functions.
lumbar puncture (LP), syn. spinal tap	A procedure used to evaluate the CSF from the space surrounding the spinal cord.
magnetic resonance angiography (MRA)	A test that uses a combination of a large magnet, radiofrequencies, and computer technology to obtain images of blood vessels in and around the neck and brain.

Term	Meaning
magnetic resonance imaging (MRI)	A test that uses a combination of a large magnet, radiofrequencies, and computer technology to obtain images of body tissues in and around bones.
malignant	The characteristic of having the properties of locally invasive and destructive growth, such as a tumor that contains cancer cells.
medulloblastoma, syn. primitive neuroectodermal tumor (PNET)	A tumor that develops from the primitive (developing) nerve cells that normally do not remain in the body after birth.
meninges	A three-layer system of membranes that cover the brain and spinal cord.
meningioma	A tumor that grows from the meninges.
meningitis	An infection causing inflammation of the meninges.
metastasis	A term that refers to the spread of a disease process from one part of the body to another.
metastatic brain tumor	A tumor that originates elsewhere in the body and then travels to the brain via the bloodstream.
microvascular clipping	A procedure that involves cutting off the flow of blood supply to an aneurysm with the use of a spring-loaded clip.
microvascular decompression	A microsurgical displacement of a blood vessel causing compression of the nerve root of the trigeminal nerve.
motor nerves	Nerves which carry commands from the brain and spinal cord to other parts of the body.
multiple sclerosis	An inflammatory disease of the nervous system that disrupts communication between the brain and other parts of the body.
myelin	The material that envelopes neurons and helps neurons conduct electrical signals.
myoclonic seizures	A type of generalized seizure characterized by repeated jerking contractions of one or more muscle groups.
neck	In aneurysms, the point where the aneurysm arises from the artery.
nerve fiber	A threadlike extension of a neuron that conducts electrical impulses.
nerve roots	Two short branches of nerve fibers that emerge from the spinal cord that carry commands from the brain and spinal cord to other parts of the body and vice versa.
nerves	Structures of bundled neurons that conduct electrical impulses throughout the body.
nervous system	The system of cells consisting of the brain, spinal cord, nerves, tissues, organs, and other structures that regulates the body's responses to internal and external stimuli.
neurologic assessment	A series of tests used to assess brain function of a patient and to evaluate for possible neurologic damage.
neurologist	A physician who specializes in the field of neurology.
neurology	The medical specialty that deals with the diagnosis and treatment of diseases and disorders of the nervous system.
neurons	Nerve cells that carry messages to and from the central nervous system.
neurosonography	An ultrasound examination of the brain and spinal column.
neurosurgery	The discipline in medicine that focuses on the diagnosis and treatment of the nervous system.

Term	Meaning
neurotransmitters	Nerve-signaling chemicals that send messages from one nerve cell to another.
noncommunicating hydrocephalus	A type of hydrocephalus that results from an obstruction within the ventricular system of the brain that prevents the CSF from flowing normally within the brain.
nonconvulsive (seizure)	Relating to a type of seizure in which the body does not stiffen or begin jerking movements.
occipital lobes	Lobes located at the base of the brain that receive and process visual information and process events into visual memories.
oligodendrocyte	A type of cell in the central nervous system that is responsible for making and supporting myelin, the material that covers and protects neurons.
oligodendroglioma	A tumor that arises in the cells that produce myelin that cover and protect nerves.
parietal lobes	The lobes located behind the frontal lobes, which interpret sensory information from the body associated with somatosensory functions, sense of direction, and problem-solving skills.
Parkinson disease	A motor system disorder caused by deterioration of nerve cells in the brain that control body movement.
partial seizures	One of two main categories of seizures that begin in a particular area of the brain.
pathways	Routes taken by neurons to transport messages throughout the central nervous system.
percutaneous stereotactic rhizotomy	A procedure in which the part of the trigeminal nerve that causes pain is destroyed with a heating current.
peripheral nervous system (PNS)	The division of the nervous system outside of the brain and spinal cord, consisting of the cranial nerves, the spinal nerves, and the branches of those nerves.
peripheral neuropathy	Damage to the peripheral nervous system (the nerves outside the spinal cord).
photodynamic therapy (PDT)	A procedure that uses a photosensitizing agent, which is activated by exposure to light in order to destroy cancer cells.
pia mater	The thin, delicate membrane layer of the meninges that is closest to the surface of the brain and spinal cord.
pituitary	An endocrine gland located in the limbic system, which produces hormones that control many functions of other endocrine glands in the body.
plasmapheresis	A procedure of plasma exchange in patients with sudden, severe attacks of multiple sclerosis.
positron emission tomography (PET)	A nuclear diagnostic test that provides images of brain activity using radioactive isotopes injected into the bloodstream.
posterior communicating artery (PComA)	One of a pair of right-sided and left-sided arteries that connects the three cerebral arteries of the same side in the brain.
Prevnar	A vaccine that protects against the seven most common strains of pneumococcal bacteria that cause invasive disease.
primary brain tumor	A tumor that originates in brain tissue.
primitive	Another word for *developing*.
pronator muscle	A muscle that returns a part into the prone position from supine.
proprioception	A sense or a perception, usually at a subconscious level, of the movements and position of the body and especially its limbs, independent of vision but by input from sensory nerves.

Term	Meaning
reflex	A simple nerve circuit.
relapsing-remitting multiple sclerosis	A form of multiple sclerosis characterized by periods of flares of symptoms, followed by periods of remission.
right hemisphere	One of two halves of the cerebrum that processes information.
Romberg test	A type of test used to evaluate a patient's coordination and equilibrium.
scalp	The skin and membranous tissue covering the top of the head.
schwannoma	A tumor that begins in Schwann cells, which produce the myelin that protects the acoustic nerve.
secondary brain tumor	A brain tumor caused by a cancer that originates in another part of the body.
seizure	A sudden abnormal discharge of electrical activity in the brain.
sensory nerves	Spinal nerve roots that carry sensory information to the brain from other parts of the body.
shunt	A silicone rubber tube used to divert CSF flow away from the brain to elsewhere in the body.
shunt revision	A procedure that involves repairing or replacing a shunt.
simple partial seizures	A type of partial seizure where there is no change in consciousness of the patient.
single photon emission computed tomography (SPECT)	A nuclear diagnostic test that obtains images of blood flow to tissues.
spinal cord	A long, tubelike column of nervous tissue that extends from the base of the skull to near the bottom of the spine, which carries both incoming and outgoing messages between the brain and the rest of the body.
spinal nerves	Nerves that connect the spinal cord with other parts of the body.
status epilepticus	A prolonged seizure or series of seizures that last for more than 30 minutes, during which time the patient is unconscious.
stenosis	Narrowing of a channel.
stereotactic radiosurgery	A procedure that involves delivering a single highly concentrated dose of ionizing radiation to a target at the trigeminal nerve root.
stroke	An impeded blood supply in the brain, resulting in damage and death of large areas of the brain.
subarachnoid hemorrhage	A leak of blood into the space between the brain and the skull.
subdural space	The space between the dura mater and the arachnoid membrane of the meninges.
subpial resection	A series of surgical cuts to help isolate the area of the brain that is causing seizures.
sulci (singular, sulcus)	The name given to the grooves between the folds of the cerebral cortex.
temporal lobectomy	The removal of a portion of the temporal lobe that causes seizures.
temporal lobes	Lobes located on the side of the brain that process memory, language, and music.
thalamus	The part of the limbic system that relays information that comes through the cerebral cortex.
third ventricle	One of four ventricles located in the median cavity of the brain.
tonic-clonic seizure, syn. grand mal seizure	A type of generalized seizure characterized by a stiffening of the body and jerking body movements and sometimes loss of consciousness.

Term	Meaning
Transsphenoidal	Refers to a path going through the sphenoid bone located under the eyes and over the nose that a surgeon uses to gain access to the pituitary gland.
trigeminal neuralgia, syn. tic douloureux	A disorder of the trigeminal nerve causing sudden attacks of pain on one side of the face.
vagus nerve	The cranial nerve that helps control function of the esophagus, larynx, stomach, intestines, lungs, and heart.
ventricles	A network of four chambers in the brain that produce cerebrospinal fluid (CSF).
ventriculoperitoneal (VP) shunt	A shunt placed inside one of the ventricles of the brain; its other end is placed into the abdominal cavity.
ventriculostomy	A surgical opening made between two ventricles to allow flow of CSF to be unobstructed.
video EEG	An EEG test used to record seizures as they occur.
viral meningitis	A virus infection that causes inflammation of the meninges.
viscera	A term relating to the soft internal organs of the body, including the lungs, the heart, and the organs of the digestive, excretory, reproductive, and circulatory systems.
visceral nerves	The nerves of the autonomic nervous system which carry messages from the brainstem and endocrine system to the viscera.
Wada test	A test that is used to evaluate memory and language functions in patients who are considering surgery for epilepsy.
white matter	The white-colored area of connecting fibers between neurons beneath the cerebral cortex.

Add Your Own Terms and Definitions Here:

_____

_____

_____

_____

_____

_____

_____

_____

REVIEW QUESTIONS

1. Name the two divisions of the nervous system and the components of each.
2. How does microvascular decompression relieve the pain of trigeminal neuralgia?
3. What is the difference between neurology and neurosurgery?
4. What is the purpose of the thalamus?
5. Name the four lobes of each cerebral hemisphere.
6. Why is a Wada test performed?
7. What is the Glasgow Coma Scale?
8. What is the procedure used to obtain and evaluate cerebrospinal fluid?
9. What is meningitis?
10. Describe the corpus callosum and its function.

CHAPTER ACTIVITIES

Soundalike Word Choice

Circle the correct word in the following sentences.

1. The patient was involved in a motor vehicle accident that damaged his spinal (core, cord).
2. This is a Hispanic female who has been previously diagnosed with trigeminal (arthralgia, neuralgia) on the right side.
3. Her CT scan showed (vesicular, ventricular) brain abnormalities consistent with a mild stroke.
4. The child was admitted to the hospital where a workup eventually diagnosed (absent, absence) seizures.
5. HEENT examination revealed extraocular movements to be intact with no (nystagmus, nystatin) and no diplopia.
6. (Electroencephalogram, Electrocardiogram) revealed background activity seen in the posterior regions of the brain, which was responsive to eye opening and eye closure.
7. Ms. Dolan was found to have a mass in the (basil, basal) ganglia.
8. Unfortunately, the patient sustained a left (thalamic, thymic) infarct after his cardiac catheterization last month.
9. The bundle of nerves at the base of the spine is called the cauda (equation, equina).
10. Sensations are grossly intact, and deep tendon (reflexes, refluxes) are symmetric.

Creating Neurology Words

Search for and combine the prefixes, suffixes, and combining forms in the following list to create medical words that best fit the definition. Verify the spelling of the word you create with a medical dictionary. The first answer is provided for you.

scler/o	cerebr/o	meningi/o	-al, -ar	kin/o
-rrhage	-ic	-ia	-esia	con-
rhiz/o	gemin/o	sten/o	crani/o	hem/o
cephal/o	brady-	neur/o	-us	vascul/o
-itis	gen/o	-osis	tri-	micro-
-logy	hydro-	myo-	-tomy	my/o

1. Uncoordinated and uncontrolled gait. _ataxia_
2. The medical specialty dealing with the diagnosis and treatment of diseases and disorders of the nervous system, including the brain, spinal cord, nerves. and muscles. _____
3. Pertaining to the head. _____
4. Inflammation of the membranes that cover the brain and spinal cord. _____
5. A cranial nerve composed of the ophthalmic nerve, the maxillary nerve, and the mandibular nerve. _____
6. A hardening of a structure within the nervous system, especially in the brain or spinal cord. _____
7. A surgical cutting of the spinal nerve roots for the relief of spasticity. _____
8. A narrowing of a canal or channel. _____
9. Pertaining to the cerebrum of the brain. _____
10. Bleeding, or blood flow, through a vessel wall. _____
11. Abnormally small head. _____
12. The slowing down of voluntary movement. _____
13. Existing at birth. _____
14. An accumulation of cerebrospinal fluid in the brain. _____
15. Referring to the small blood vessels. _____

Matching

Match the abbreviation on the left with its definition on the right.

Abbreviation

1. _____ CNS
2. _____ SPECT
3. _____ MS
4. _____ VP
5. _____ PNS
6. _____ PET
7. _____ LP
8. _____ MRI
9. _____ CSF
10. _____ CT
11. _____ PD
12. _____ TN
13. _____ GCS
14. _____ MRA
15. _____ EEG

Definition

A. A motor system disorder caused by deterioration of nerve cells in the brain that control body movement.

B. The division of the nervous system outside of the brain and spinal cord, consisting of the cranial nerves, the spinal nerves, and the branches of those nerves.

C. A thin, watery substance that surrounds the brain and spinal cord.

D. The division of the nervous system consisting of the brain and spinal cord.

E. A scoring system used to quantify a patient's level of consciousness following a brain injury.

F. A test that uses a combination of a large magnet, radiofrequencies, and computer technology to obtain images of blood vessels in and around the neck and brain.

G. A test that monitors abnormal electrical discharges in the brain.

H. A nuclear diagnostic test that obtains images of blood flow to tissues.

I. A type of imaging study that uses an x-ray to produce rapid, clear, two-dimensional images of organs, bones, and tissues, with the information displayed in cross-sections or slices of body tissue.

J. A procedure used to evaluate the CSF from the space surrounding the spinal cord.

K. Referring to one of the ventricles of the brain.

L. A test that uses a combination of a large magnet, radiofrequencies, and computer technology to obtain images of body tissues in and around bones.

M. A disorder of the trigeminal nerve causing sudden attacks of pain on one side of the face.

N. A nuclear diagnostic test that provides images of brain activity using radioactive isotopes injected into the bloodstream.

O. An inflammatory disease of the nervous system that disrupts communication between the brain and other parts of the body.

Proofreading Practice 18.1

*Circle the errors in the following clinic report. Then retype the corrected report using the same format on a blank document screen. When finished, print one copy and save the corrected report as **CHAPTER-18-NOTE1**.*

Today I had the pelasure of seeing Kelly in the pediatric neurosurgery outpatient Clinic. She is a 10 year old female who presented with a posterior fossa tumore (pylocitic astriocytoma). Therefore, a suboccipital cranitomy was done when the tumor was complete resected. He had an excellent postoperative course with no neurologic deficits and she had none subjective symptoms. She is here with both parents who denuies any history of vomiting seizures or lethargy. M-R-I was done which showed no evidence of recurrent.

Neurologic examination shows that she is alert and fully oriented. Cranial nerve exam are all within normal limits without any vocal neurologic signs. There is no papilloedema. There is no Nystagmus, and no cerebella dysfunction. Dark tendon reflexes are all within normal limits.

I reviewed the radiologists findings of the progress on MRI.

I am very pleased with her continuous progress. and I would like to see her in 6 months at the outpatient clinic with a repeat MRI with and without contrst.

Proofreading Practice 18.2

*Circle the errors in the following clinic report. Then retype the corrected report using the same format on a blank document screen. When finished, print one copy and save the corrected report as **CHAPTER-18-NOTE2**.*

Ms Jones is a 46-years-old african american woman who presented to us with a subarachnid hemorrhage from a ruptured right superior hypophysial artery aneurysm which was successfully coiled. The patient was also discovered to have three other aneurysms—a left superior hypophysial artery aneurysm which may be amenable to coiling, giving clinical indications, a 6.500 mmm anterior communicating artery aneurysm fueling from the left side which is not amenable to vascular treatment; and she also has a small submilimmeter carot terminus aneurysm which is not amenable to endovascular treatment. Today she comes to clinic for a discussion of treatment options.

We discussed with the patient two major options. One is leaving things alone, and the other is proceeding with the surgery. I explained that given the fact that one of the aneurysms already ruptured, she is probably already likely to have a large, 6.5 millimeter anterior communicating artery aneurysm ruptured during her lifetime. However I informed her that this decision is completely up to her.

The patient had a discussion with the family in my presence? and they elected to proceed with the operation. The patient did understand the general risks of the operation, which included but are not limited to, death, paralysis stroke dvt, pneumoniae and risks specific to surgery which may result from injury to the vessles. I asked her if she understood all the risk and what exactly we were going to do, and she verbalized understanding as well as the rest of the family.

We will make appropriate arrangements for the patient; to have the aneurysms clipped at her earliest convenience and we will put her on the schedule today.

Fill in the Blanks

Fill in the blanks of the following paragraph with the correct terms from the text. Some terms may be used more than once.

The brain is an amazing organ. It is divided into four major parts: The _____, _____, _____, and _____.

The largest and uppermost part of the brain is called the _____. It is divided into two parts called the _____ and _____ hemispheres. They are joined by a band of fibers called the _____. The _____ beneath the cerebral cortex does not do any real thinking or feeling.

The _____ structures are often called the "feeling brain" because they are involved in emotions. One of these structures, called the _____, serves as a relay station for the cerebral cortex. Another structure, called the _____, regulates automatic functions like eating and drinking.

The _____ comes from the Latin word for *little brain*. Disruptions in the function of this part of the brain results in motor problems such as an unsteady gait, called _____.

The _____ is a tubelike column of tissue that connects the brain to the rest of the body. The reflexes of this part of the body can cause limbs to move, even when a patient is comatose, a phenomenon called the _____.

Crossword Puzzle

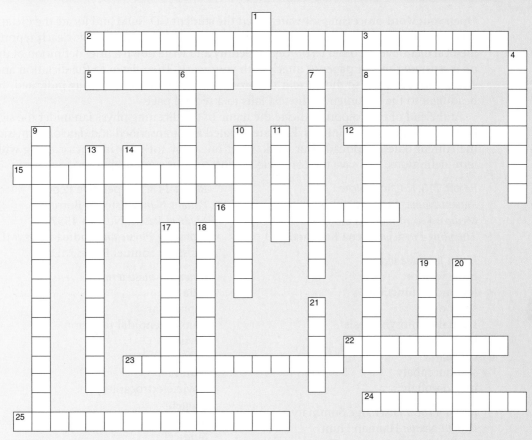

www.Crossword Weaver.com

Across

2 Hydrocephalus present at birth.
5 Narrowing of a channel.
8 A simple nerve circuit.
12 Another name for the cerebral cortex.
15 Nerves that exit from the brain.
16 An inflammation of the meninges.
22 An endocrine gland located in the brain.
23 The "feeling brain."
24 The outermost layer of the meninges.
25 A surgical opening made between two ventricles.

Down

1 Supporting cells of the nervous system.
3 Watery substance that surrounds the brain and spinal cord.
4 An abnormal dilation of a blood vessel.
6 A sudden abnormal discharge of electrical activity in the brain.
7 One who specializes in the field of neurology.
9 A motor system disorder.
10 The inability to judge distance, power, and speed of movement.
11 Uncontrolled gait.
13 Another name for trigeminal neuralgia.
14 A blisterlike sac.
17 The uppermost and largest part of the brain.
18 Common cause of viral meningitis.
19 The grooves between the folds of the cerebral cortex.
20 Another term for "lumbar puncture."
21 Interconnected areas in the left and right hemispheres of the cerebrum.

TRANSCRIPTION PRACTICE

Open your word-processing software. Insert the student CD-ROM and locate the dictation for this chapter. For each of the words in the "listen for these terms" list for each report, use a medical dictionary or other resources to identify and write down a brief definition of the term on a separate sheet of paper to attach with your work. Then listen to the dictation and transcribe each report. Use the current date for each report where a date is indicated. Insert a heading into the document if the text falls to a second page.

At the end of each report, indicate the name of the dictating physician under the signature line and insert reference initials. For date dictated and transcribed and date of admission, use the current date. Proofread your work, print one copy for your instructor along with your term definitions, and save the completed report to your student disk.

Report T18.1: Clinic Note
Patient Name: Matthew Olson
Medical Record No.: OLS-0090
Attending Physician: Lena Kushner, MD

Listen for these terms:
bone window
locomotor function
scaphoid
sagittal craniosynostosis
bi-lambdoid
coronal
scaphocephaly
plagiocephaly

Report T18.2: Discharge Summary
Patient Name: Hannah Hunt
Medical Record No.: 80045711
Attending Physician: Kamraan George, MD

Listen for these terms:
obstructive hydrocephalus
colloid cyst
percutaneous endoscopic gastrostomy
PICC line
cerebral palsy
foramina of Monro
lethargy
dysphagia
nectar-thick liquids
fenestration
septum pellucidum
ventriculoperitoneal shunt
PEG
Jevity

Report T18.3: Operative Report
Patient Name: Estevan Borrero
Medical Record No.: 00-4557
Attending Physician: Andrea Biggs, MD
Assistant: Samuel Black, MD

Listen for these terms:
sellar
suprasellar
transsphenoidal resection
clivus
optic chiasm
DuraPrep
Bovie electrocautery
rongeur
Kerrison rongeur
Surgicel
Dexon suture
Steri-Strips
DuraSeal
Merocel pack

19

IMMUNOLOGY

OBJECTIVES

After completing this chapter, you will be able to:

- Present an overview of the function of the immune system.
- Discuss the structures of the lymphatic system and the function of each.
- Describe common diseases and disorders associated with the immune system and the treatment modalities related to each.
- Describe common laboratory tests and diagnostic procedures used to analyze, detect, and treat immune disorders and conditions.

INTRODUCTION

Immunology is the study of the human immune system and the treatment of diseases of that system. The **immune system** is a complex network of specialized cells and organs that has evolved to defend the body against attacks by infections and foreign substances. When functioning properly, it fights off infections by agents such as bacteria, viruses, fungi, and parasites. When it malfunctions, however, it causes disease.

An **immunologist** is a physician who specializes in the field of immunology. Immunologists work in many different areas of health care as well as in biomedical research and environmental monitoring. Many diseases result from an immune system that behaves incorrectly, and immunologists try to understand how and why this system malfunctions and causes disease. They also conduct research to develop better ways of diagnosing and treating many immunologic conditions.

The success of the immune system in defending the body relies on an incredibly elaborate communications network among millions of cells, which pass information back and forth like clouds of bees swarming around a hive. This activity results in a system of checks and balances that is prompt, appropriate, and effective in keeping the body protected from infection. This chapter illustrates the many facets of this complex system by describing the structure and function of a normal immune system. It also provides an overview of common immunologic disorders and diseases in order to enhance an understanding of how a malfunctioning immune system affects the body. Finally, this chapter explains the testing modalities used to diagnose immune disorders, and also examines the latest medical and surgical treatments that help to maintain and stabilize an out-of-control immune system without disabling its basic function of protecting the body from toxic invaders.

OVERVIEW OF THE IMMUNE SYSTEM

The immune system works around the clock to defend the body from infection. This built-in protection takes many forms:

- The skin outside the body and other lining tissues inside form a barrier.
- Mucous lining of the gut and lungs traps invading bacteria, and the action of coughing moves the trapped debris out of the lungs.
- Stomach acid kills bacteria that have been swallowed.
- Helpful bacteria growing in the bowel prevent other bacteria from taking over.
- Urine flow flushes bacteria out of the bladder and urethra.
- White blood cells called neutrophils find and kill bacteria and other infectious agents.

The body is most vulnerable to infection where infection has a gateway in. In a person without wounds or broken skin, that means the mouth, eyes, nose, ears, and genitals all provide an opening for bacteria to enter. However, there are other ways in which the body's natural protection mechanisms can be compromised, causing an attack on the immune system:

- Breaks in the skin barrier, such as a cut or an open wound from surgery.
- Medications and long-term drug therapies, such as chemotherapy or radiation treatment for cancer, damage the lining of the intestines or the hairs and mucous membranes of the lungs.
- Catheter insertion into the body allows bacteria to enter through the catheter and cause an infection.

The immune system works silently, each day of our lives, protecting the body from billions of viruses, bacteria, parasites, pollutants, and other foreign materials the body is exposed to every day. We notice our immune system at work when we feel the side effects of its activity. For example, when you get a splinter in your foot, the immune system responds and eliminates incoming invaders while the skin heals itself and seals the puncture. A mosquito bite causes a red, itchy bump—another visible sign of the immune system at work.

The immune system has a multilayered system of defense. The first layer of defense from outside invaders is the skin and mucous membranes. As noted previously, this layer can be breached by organisms that can enter the body through a cut or wound.

Once inside the body, a foreign invader must face the second line of defense: the **innate immune system**, which triggers an acute response by the body in the form of cells and mechanisms that provide an immediate defense against infection by other organisms. When a foreign invader is detected, the bloodstream is flooded with illness-fighting specialized blood cells, called **macrophages** and **neutrophils**. The term *macrophage* comes from the Latin terms *macro*, meaning *big*, and *phage*, meaning *to eat*; thus macrophages are the gobblers of the immune system, grabbing bacteria, chewing them up into little pieces, and destroying them. The leftover crumbs of the meal signal other immune cells to join in the fray to destroy the invader. In the process, macrophages produce chemicals that cause inflammation, which also helps to heal the body. Neutrophils are a type of white blood cell that serve as "first responders," quickly appearing at the site of infection to ingest and destroy foreign particles.

The third layer of the immune system is called the **adaptive immune system** and is composed of highly specialized systemic cells that can recognize what belongs in the body and what does not. The adaptive immune system also has the ability to remember specific pathogens in order to mount stronger attacks each time the pathogen is encountered in the future, a concept called **self and nonself**.

SELF AND NONSELF

Central to the workings of the immune system is its ability to distinguish between what is the body's own cells (self) and foreign cells (nonself). Every cell in the body carries distinctive marker molecules called human leukocyte antigen (HLA) that distinguish it as self. Anything that the immune system finds that does not have these markers (or has the wrong markers) is considered to be nonself and fair game to be eliminated. When foreign, or *nonself*, molecules enter the body in the form of toxins or foreign invaders such as bacteria, fungi, or other harmful substances, they are known as **antigens**, which means, literally, *against self*, which trigger the immune system to launch an attack. This coordinated effort between the blood and the lymphatic system to destroy invading microorganisms is called the **immune response**.

Anything can trigger an immune response. It can be the detection of an invading organism or even part of an organism. Microorganisms such as bacteria, viruses, fungi, or yeast that cause disease are known as **pathogens**. Viruses and bacteria are by far the most common pathogens that cause illness for most people. Bacteria are single-celled organisms that are perhaps 1/100th the size of a human cell, yet they are completely independent organisms able to reproduce very quickly. In fact, one harmful bacterium can reproduce into millions in just a few hours. A virus, on the other hand, is not a living organism but a fragment of DNA in a protective coat. The virus comes in contact with a cell, attaches itself to the cell wall, and injects its DNA into the cell. The DNA uses the living cell to reproduce a new virus. Eventually the hijacked cell dies and bursts, freeing the new virus particles to search for new living cells; therefore, a living cell is a kind of factory for a virus.

The remarkable thing about immune cells is their ability to remember. They can recognize foreign substances the body was exposed to previously, called **active immunity**. Active immunity refers to the body's response and defense against pathogens it has encountered before. For example, after catching chickenpox at an early age, a person will never acquire it again. Exposure to the disease organism can occur through infection with the actual disease or through the introduction of a killed or weakened form of the disease organism through vaccination. In either case, if an immune person comes into contact with that disease in the future, the body's immune system will recognize it and immediately produce the antibodies needed to fight it. **Passive immunity** refers to the immunity provided when a person is given antibodies to a disease rather than producing them through his or her own immune system. For example, a newborn baby acquires passive immunity from its mother through the placenta. A person can also get passive immunity through antibody-containing blood products or a vaccine that may be given when immediate protection from a specific disease is needed. However, passive immunity lasts only for a few weeks or months. Only active immunity is life-long.

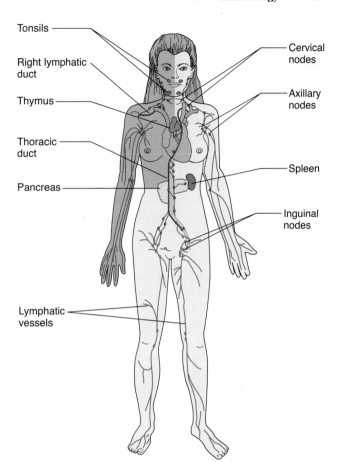

FIGURE 19.1. The Lymphatic System. Reprinted with permission from Willis MC. *Medical Terminology: A Programmed Learning Approach to the Language of Health Care.* Baltimore: Lippincott Williams & Wilkins, 2002.

ANATOMY OF THE IMMUNE SYSTEM

The immune system, also referred to as the **lymphatic system**, consists of a network of vessels and nodes, along with a few specialized structures that include the bone marrow, thymus, and spleen, as illustrated in Figure 19.1. These structures are generally referred to as **lymphoid organs** because they are concerned with the growth, development, and deployment of **lymphocytes**, the white blood cells that reside in the lymphatic system and blood-forming organs and help the body fight infection. The lymphoid organs are connected by a network of lymphatic vessels that course throughout the body in a circulatory system that is separate from the blood vessels.

Lymphatic Vessels and Nodes

The **lymphatic vessels** are a circulatory system of vessels that closely parallel the body's veins and arteries. The main difference between the blood flowing in the circulatory system and the fluid flowing in the lymphatic system is that the blood in the circulatory system is pressurized by the heart, whereas the fluid flow in the lymphatic system is passive. This relationship is analogous to that of a water and sewer system in a neighborhood. Water (blood) is actively pressurized and moves faster in the system, whereas sewage (lymph) is not pressurized and flows by gravity.

Cells and fluids are exchanged between blood vessels and lymphatic vessels, enabling the immune system to monitor the body for invading microbes. Tissue fluid enters the lymphatic vessels and becomes a clear fluid called **lymph**, which contains immune cells and bathes the tissues throughout the body. Lymph consists of blood plasma, the liquid that makes up blood (without the red and white blood cells). The lymphatic capillaries have openings that allow protein and waste products of the cells to be carried away by the lymph. The lymph also absorbs foreign materials and microorganisms from the bloodstream. These materials, along with the lymph, move along the lymphatic system by normal muscle and body motion to the lymph nodes. Once filtered, the cleaned lymph enters the lymphatic vessels again to patrol for foreign antigens and eventually is transported back into the lymph nodes to be filtered again.

The **lymph nodes** are small bean-shaped structures that are found periodically along the lymphatic vessels,

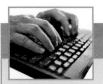

with clusters in the neck, armpits, abdomen, and groin. Their primary function is to collect and destroy the foreign invaders collected by the lymph. Each lymph node contains specialized compartments that act as filters, collecting bacteria or cancer cells that may travel through the lymphatic system. Cell activity in these areas, primarily fighting foreign substances, results in a swollen lymph node; this is a reliable sign that an infection exists.

Bone Marrow

The blood cells destined to become immune cells, like other blood cells, are produced in the **bone marrow** located in the spongy tissue of long bones, as discussed in Chapter 17, *Orthopaedics*. **Stem cells**, which are immature cells that grow into many different types of cells, are produced in the bone marrow. The most important of the immune cells produced here are the white blood cells; there are many varieties of these cells, including lymphocytes, the blood cells that help the body fight infection. The two major classes of lymphocytes are **B cells**, which mature in the bone marrow, and **T cells**, which migrate to the thymus to complete their maturity. B cells and T cells are just two of the types of cells used by the immune system to fight disease.

Thymus

The **thymus** is a gland found in the thorax under the breastbone. The function of the thymus is to produce

mature lymphoid cells called T cells, described later in this chapter. The thymus receives lymphocytes that migrate from the bone marrow. After maturity, the T cells are then released into the bloodstream. This process occurs for several months after birth; then the thymus gradually atrophies until adulthood, by which time only a remnant of the gland exists. Removal of the thymus in adults as a treatment for certain diseases does not have serious effects because the T cells have already been distributed throughout the body.

Spleen

The **spleen** is located at the upper left portion of the abdomen and is the largest of the lymphoid organs. Like the lymph nodes, it contains specialized compartments where immune cells gather and work, and it serves as a meeting ground where immune system cells confront foreign microbes. The spleen plays a vital role in the immune system by storing lymphocytes that assist the body in fighting infections, especially pneumonia and meningitis. Although people can live without a spleen lost to damage by trauma or disease, without the spleen, they are highly susceptible to infection. Therefore, vaccinations are given to these individuals to boost the body's immunity against such infections.

Lymphoid Tissues

Clumps of lymphoid tissue are found in many parts of the body, especially in the linings of the digestive tract, the airways and lungs—territories that serve as gateways to the body. The lymphoid tissue contains lymphocytes that defend against pathogens entering the body via the mucosa. Types and locations of lymphoid tissue include the following:

- **Tonsils**, located at the back of the throat;
- **Adenoids**, two glands located at the back of the nasal passage;
- **Peyer patches**, located in the mucosa of the small intestine; and
- **Appendix**, a small pouch that extends off the large intestine. Once thought to be a remnant of evolution, scientists now believe the lymphoid tissue inside the appendix may be useful in fighting infection.

Cells and Their Products

The immune system keeps a huge volume and variety of cells at its disposal to defend the body against invading organisms. Some immune cells take on all foreign invaders, whereas others pursue specific targets. To work effectively, immune cells need the cooperation of their comrades. Sometimes immune cells communicate directly by physical contact with an antigen; at other

QUICK CHECK 19.1 ✓

Fill in the blanks with the correct answers.

1. The _____ on a T cell receives signals from antigens, stimulating the T cell to initiate an immune response.

2. The largest of the lymphoid organs is the _____.

3. The immune system functions by its ability to distinguish _____ from _____.

4. T cells migrate from the bone marrow to the _____ where they mature.

5. B cells make proteins called _____ that locate and destroy foreign invaders.

times, they release chemical messengers. The immune system stores just a few of each kind of cell needed to recognize millions of possible enemies. When an antigen is detected, those few matching cells multiply into a full-scale army. After their job is done, they leave a few sentry cells behind to watch for future attacks.

B cells react against invading bacteria or viruses by producing Y-shaped proteins called **antibodies**, also called **immunoglobulins**, which are secreted into the body's fluids to locate and destroy bacteria, viruses, or other harmful toxins. Antibodies mark a pathogen so it can be recognized and destroyed by other cells, and each has a special section (at the tips of the two branches of the Y) that is sensitive to a specific antigen. This binding generally disables the chemical action of the toxin. By binding to the outer coat of a virus or the cell wall of a bacterium, the antibody can stop the movement of a virus or bacterium through the cell walls, disabling its ability to reproduce further. A large number of antibodies can also bind to an invader and signal other cells in the body that the invader needs to be removed. Different types of immunoglobulins play different roles in the immune system, as follows:

- Immunoglobulin G, or IgG, forms the body's basic active immunity.
- IgM is the largest immunoglobulin and is effective at killing bacteria.

TRANSCRIPTION TIP:

When a physician dictates abbreviations like "I-G-M" or "I-G-A" in a medical document, he/she is talking about an antibody, and this abbreviation is transcribed using a combination of capital and small letters, as indicated in this chapter.

- IgA is present in body fluids, such as tears, saliva, and secretions of the respiratory and digestive tracts.
- IgE protects against parasitic infections and is also responsible for causing the inflammatory response that signals an allergic reaction.
- IgD remains attached to B cells and helps initiate an early B-cell response to an antigen.

Like B cells, T cells travel through the body patrolling for foreign invaders. Although a B cell clones itself and produces antibodies designed to eliminate the germ, a T cell actually bumps up against the foreign cell and destroys it. On the surface of each T cell is a **receptor**, a kind of antenna that receives signals from molecules sitting on the surface of an antigen. When a T cell detects a foreign invader, it stimulates the B cells to secrete antibodies and calls other T cells into action to strike out at the antigen directly. In fact, it is T cells that are largely responsible for the rejection of tissue grafts and transplanted organs. We encounter millions of antigens during our lifetime, and the body possesses a vast array of T cells capable of recognizing, responding to, and remembering these antigens.

Different types of T cells have certain functions in the immune response:

- **Helper T cells** coordinate immune responses by communicating with other cells through chemical messengers called **cytokines** to organize and destroy the foreign invader.
- **Memory T cells** are created when a helper T cell is exposed to a pathogen. These T cells are inactive until the next time the pathogen enters the body, at which time they remember the pathogen and reactivate to destroy it.
- **Killer T cells** engulf and destroy the body's own cells that have been infected by a pathogen in order to prevent the organism from reproducing in the cell and then infecting other cells.

COMMON IMMUNOLOGIC DISEASES AND TREATMENTS

Diseases caused by improper functioning of the immune system include allergies, immunodeficiency disorders, and autoimmune disorders.

Allergies

An **allergy** is an abnormal reaction to a specific environmental antigen called an **allergen**. Allergens are substances that are typically harmless to most people and can be inhaled (dust, pet dander, or pollen), ingested (foods or medications), injected (medicine or venom), or brought into contact with the skin (cleaning fluids or plant toxins). An allergic reaction occurs when the immune system mistakenly believes that this substance is harmful to the body. In an attempt to protect the body, the immune system produces IgE antibodies to that allergen. The antibodies then cause the body to release chemicals into the bloodstream; one of these chemicals, **histamine**, causes symptoms in the eyes, nose, throat, lungs, skin, and gastrointestinal tract. Future exposure to that same allergen will trigger this antibody response again.

Allergies tend to run in families but are also affected by environmental factors. They develop by exposure to substances through a process called sensitization that can occur upon first contact or upon repeated exposure during the course of several years. During this period, the immune system is activated to react against the substance, even though it is harmless.

Once an allergy to a specific antigen is confirmed, several methods are used to treat the condition. Avoiding the offending allergen or making changes to the environment, such as filtering the air or managing pet dander, can help prevent allergy attacks. Medications, both over-the-counter and by prescription, are also used to treat allergy symptoms. These include the following:

- Antihistamines. These drugs have been used for years to treat allergy symptoms by blocking the histamine receptors that cause redness, swelling, itching, and changes in secretions. Common antihistamines prescribed by physicians to treat patients include desloratadine (Clarinex), fexofenadine (Allegra), and cetirizine (Zyrtec).
- Decongestants. These drugs relieve congestion and are often prescribed along with antihistamines. During an allergic reaction, tissues in the nose swell in response to contact with the allergen, producing fluid and mucus. Blood vessels swell, causing itching and redness. Decongestants shrink swollen nasal tissues and blood vessels to relieve these symptoms. Some examples of decongestants include loratadine plus pseudoephedrine (Claritin-D), fexofenadine plus pseudoephedrine (Allegra-D), and cetirizine plus pseudoephedrine (Zyrtec-D). Each of these medications combine a decongestant with the baseline allergy medication.
- Corticosteroids. These drugs reduce inflammation associated with allergies and can also decrease inflammation and swelling from other types of allergic reactions. A physician may prescribe a corticosteroid in addition to other allergy medications. Some common nasal corticosteroids include beclomethasone (Beconase), budesonide (Rhinocort), fluticasone (Flonase), mometasone (Nasonex), and triamcinolone (Nasacort), which are used to treat nasal allergy symptoms. Inhaled medications such as budesonide (Pulmicort), fluticasone (Flovent), and triamcinolone (Azmacort) are used to treat lung symptoms. Advair is an inhaled drug that combines a corticosteroid fluticasone propionate (Flovent) with salmeterol (Serevent), a drug used to treat asthma.
- Bronchodilators. These inhaled medicines are used to control asthma symptoms. A short-acting bronchodilator is used to provide quick relief for breathing difficulties during an attack. Long-acting bronchodilators provide up to 12 hours of relief from symptoms, which is helpful to people who have nighttime allergic symptoms. Bronchodilators relax the muscle bands that tighten around the airways, allowing more air in and out of the lungs, thereby improving breathing. Some types of bronchodilators typically prescribed include albuterol (Ventolin), levalbuterol (Xopenex), metaproterenol (Alupent), and pirbuterol (Maxair).
- Leukotriene modifiers. These drugs are used to treat nasal allergy symptoms. Leukotriene modifiers block the effects of leukotrienes, chemicals produced in the body in response to an allergy. The common drugs prescribed in this category include zafirlukast (Accolate) and montelukast (Singulair).
- Finally, allergy injections may be used for individuals with severe allergies or those with allergies for more than three months of the year. The injections

TRANSCRIPTION TIP:

Dark, bluish under-eye circles, resembling black eyes, seen frequently in children, are referred to in a physical exam as **allergic shiners**. The circles are not caused by a specific allergy but by any allergy affecting the sinuses and come from the blood vessels that are close to the surface of the skin. An **allergic salute** describes the upward motion of the hand against the nose, as opposed to rubbing side to side, to relieve nasal itching.

gradually increase the levels of the offending allergen to help the immune system build a tolerance to it.

Immunodeficiency Diseases

Immunodeficiency is a condition that is caused when the immune system fails to respond effectively to foreign bodies or is absent entirely. Immunodeficiency results in persistent or recurrent infections; opportunistic infections, caused by microorganisms that are usually controlled by a healthy immune system; severe infections by organisms that normally cause mild responses; incomplete recovery from illness or poor response to treatment; or an increased incidence of cancer or other tumors. In most cases, an immunodeficiency disorder can be either inherited or acquired. Temporary immune deficiencies can also develop in the wake of common viral infections, such as influenza, mononucleosis, and measles.

An inherited immunodeficiency disorder will result in a genetic abnormality. Some children are born with poorly functioning immune systems in that the B-cell system cannot produce antibodies. Other congenital disorders result when the thymus is either missing or small and abnormal, lacking sufficient T cells. Very rarely, infants are born lacking all of the major immune defenses, a condition called **severe combined immunodeficiency disease** (SCID).

An immunodeficiency disorder can be acquired as a result of a disease that affects the immune system. **Acquired immunodeficiency syndrome** (AIDS) is a disease caused by the virus **human immunodeficiency virus** (HIV) that infects the immune cells. First reported in the United States in 1981, AIDS has since become a major worldwide epidemic.

Recall that a virus attaches itself to the cell wall, injects its DNA into the cell, and then uses the living cell to reproduce new virus cells. HIV attacks and destroys the T cells that protect the body from disease, and it multiplies, disabling the body's immune system and paving the way for a variety of unusual, often life-threatening infections and cancers to develop in the body. The virus is spread by intimate sexual contact, transfer of the virus from mother to infant during pregnancy, or direct blood contamination. The virus will multiply in the body for a time, ranging from a few weeks to months, before the immune system responds. When a response is initiated, the immune system will start to make antibodies against the virus. At this point, the individual is said to be positive for HIV.

Often, people who are HIV-positive will stay healthy for many years. During this time, however, HIV is damaging the immune system by progressively destroying the body's ability to fight infections and cancers. A person is officially diagnosed as having AIDS when he/she meets one of several criteria developed by

the U.S. Centers for Disease Control and Prevention (CDC), the government agency responsible for tracking the spread of AIDS in the United States. The CDC's definition of AIDS includes all HIV-infected people who have fewer than 200 CD4+ T cells, a type of helper T cell, per cubic millimeter of blood (healthy adults usually have CD4+ T-cell counts of 1000 or more). In addition, the definition includes 26 clinical conditions that affect people with advanced HIV disease. Most of these conditions are opportunistic infections that generally do not affect healthy people. In people with AIDS, these infections are often severe and sometimes fatal because the immune system is so ravaged by HIV that the body cannot fight off certain bacteria, viruses, fungi, parasites, and other microbes.

When AIDS first surfaced in the United States in the early 1980s, there were no medicines to combat the underlying immunodeficiency disorder, and few treatments existed for the opportunistic diseases that resulted. Today, however, many drugs are available to fight both the HIV infection and its associated infections and cancers. One group of drugs, called **nucleoside reverse transcriptase inhibitors**, interrupts the ability of the HIV virus to make copies of itself in the early stages of infection. Common drugs of this type include azidothymidine (AZT), lamivudine (3TC, Epivir), abacavir (Ziagen), tenofovir (Viread), nevirapine (Viramune), and efavirenz (Sustiva).

Another class of drugs used to treat HIV infection, called **protease inhibitors**, interrupts the ability of the virus to make copies of itself at a later stage of the infection. These drugs commonly include ritonavir (Norvir), saquinavir (Invirase), indinavir (Crixivan), amprenavir (Agenerase), nelfinavir (Viracept), lopinavir (Kaletra), and atazanavir (Reyataz).

A third, newer class of drugs, called **fusion inhibitors**, work by interfering with the ability of HIV to enter the body's healthy immune cells by blocking the merging of the virus with the cell membranes. The first of these drugs approved by the U.S. Food and Drug Administration (FDA), enfuvirtide or T-20 (Fuzeon), is designed for use in combination with other anti-HIV treatments. It reduces the level of HIV infection in the blood and may be effective against HIV that has become resistant to current antiviral treatment regimens.

Because HIV can become resistant to any of these drugs when used alone, physicians often use a combination approach to effectively suppress the virus. The use of multiple drugs (three or more) in combination is referred to as **highly active antiretroviral therapy** (HAART, pronounced like *heart* in dictation); HAART can be used by people who are newly infected with HIV as well as by people with AIDS. Although HAART is not a cure for AIDS, it has greatly improved the health of many people with AIDS, as it reduces the amount of virus circulating in the blood to nearly undetectable levels. However, research has shown that HIV does remain present in places such as the lymph nodes, brain, testes, and retina of the eye, even in people who have been treated.

Autoimmune Diseases

Autoimmunity is an abnormal condition in which the immune system confuses normal body tissue (self) for foreign tissue (nonself) and attacks the tissues of the body it was created to protect, causing pain and loss of function. The word *autoimmune* derives from the prefix *auto-*, meaning *self*, and the suffix *-immune*, meaning *immune response*. This group of diseases is sometimes referred to as *collagen vascular diseases* because the soft tissues and blood vessels are frequently attacked. These confused antibodies, produced against the body's own tissues, are called **autoantibodies** because they turn against healthy tissue and cause many adverse conditions that fall under the category of autoimmune disease.

What causes the immune system to attack itself? Because the immune system is so complicated, researchers have found it difficult to pinpoint a single cause for autoimmune disease. Sometimes an antigen so closely resembles healthy self-tissue that when the immune system unleashes antibodies against the foreign cells, they mistakenly attack and destroy good cells as well. For example, the makeup of a certain strain of *Streptococcus* bacteria so closely mimics the tissues of the mitral valve of the heart that when the antibodies attack a streptococcal infection, they unwittingly attack the heart tissue as well, leading to a disease called **rheumatic fever**. An error in one's genetic code may play a role in autoimmune diseases, and more than one gene may be to blame for a single disease. Finally, a person may encounter some sort of trigger, such as an infection or a virus, which causes an abnormal reaction of T cells. For example, studies have tied exposure to **Epstein-Barr Virus (EBV)**, which causes infectious mononucleosis, to the autoimmune disease lupus, described later.

Amazingly, the consequence of a simple cell going awry is more than 80 different autoimmune disorders, each of which acts upon the body in a different way. Sometimes a single organ is selected for attack, such as the liver in autoimmune hepatitis; at other times, multiple organs are targeted. Hormones may also be involved, as many autoimmune diseases are more common among women.

The following are some common autoimmune disorders and the treatment protocol for each.

Systemic Lupus Erythematosus

Systemic lupus erythematosus (SLE), or simply **lupus**, is a multisystem disease characterized by such symptoms as achy joints (**arthralgia**); unexplained rashes on the face, neck, or scalp; inflammation of the kidneys, inflammation of the fibrous tissue surrounding the pericardium; as well as other problems. The term *lupus* comes from the Latin term for *wolf*; as like a wolf, the disease can stalk silently over years or strike suddenly without warning, attacking the skin of the face and vital organs. The term "lupus" has been used since the 1200s to describe this disease because the rash on the face and effects of the disease made the afflicted person resemble a wolf.

In lupus, like other autoimmune disorders, the immune system produces autoantibodies against the body's healthy cells and tissues. These autoantibodies contribute to the inflammation of various parts of the body and can cause damage to organs and tissues. The most common type of autoantibody that develops in people with lupus is called an **antinuclear antibody (ANA)** because it reacts with parts of the cell's nucleus, or command center. However, unlike other autoimmune diseases that target a single organ, such as thyroid disease, lupus can affect just about any organ or tissue in the body, including the joints, the kidneys, the heart, the lungs, the blood, and even the nervous system. Therefore, a patient diagnosed with lupus may need not only an immunologist, but also the specialists who treat the many symptoms of the disease. Lupus patients typically consult:

- A family doctor.
- A rheumatologist to treat joint problems.
- A nephrologist to treat kidney disease brought on by lupus.
- A hematologist, or blood disorder specialist, to treat blood abnormalities caused by lupus.
- A dermatologist to treat the skin manifestations of lupus.
- A neurologist to treat problems with the nervous system as a result of lupus.
- A psychologist or psychiatrist to treat the emotional aspects of lupus.

The cause of lupus is unknown, but there are environmental and genetic factors involved. Although scientists believe there is a genetic predisposition to the disease, it is known that environmental factors also play a critical role in triggering lupus. Some of the environmental factors that may trigger the disease are exposure to infections, antibiotics (especially those containing sulfa or penicillin), ultraviolet light, extreme stress, certain drugs, and hormones.

Lupus, like other autoimmune disorders, manifests in periods of acute disease activity, called **flares**, followed by periods of remission in which the disease is "quiet." This fluctuating pattern varies from one person to the next; in dictation, the acute phase is referred to as a **lupus flare**. Flares can have a number of triggers, including emotional stress, exposure to sunlight, infections, or certain medications. During a lupus flare, physicians measure the *activity* of disease; that is, the symptoms involving the physical changes that may be accompanied by abnormalities in a patient's blood workup. This degree of activity is quantified in a medical report by a scoring system called the **SLE Disease Activity Index** (SLEDAI, pronounced like *SLEE-day* in dictation), which lists the various physical findings and blood test results obtained during the flare: new or recurrent facial rash, sensitivity to light (**photosensitivity**), mouth ulcers, fatigue, joint swelling, unexplained fevers, or (through blood work) other organ involvement. The SLEDAI is the total of the number of problems, with a higher value denoting more disease activity.

Physicians often have difficulty definitively diagnosing lupus in its early stages because of its ability to mimic other disorders. For example, joint pain and stiffness may be diagnosed as arthritis; fatigue and depression may be attributed erroneously to major depression. Currently, no single laboratory test can determine whether a person has lupus; diagnosis is usually made by a careful review of a person's entire medical history, coupled with an analysis of the results obtained in routine laboratory tests and some specialized tests related to immune status.

Once diagnosed, symptoms can be treated using different medical therapies, as described later, to prevent flares, treat the symptoms of flares when they do occur, and reduce organ damage and other problems. Oral medications like those described at the end of this section, prescribed for lupus as well as other autoimmune disorders, provide relief from pain, inflammation of joints and tissues, skin rashes, and blood-clotting abnormalities; they also serve to suppress the immune system to reduce disease activity.

Rheumatoid Arthritis

Rheumatoid arthritis (RA) is a chronic autoimmune disorder in which the immune system attacks, and causes inflammation of, the joints and surrounding tissues of the body. It is the most prevalent of the autoimmune diseases, striking millions of people in the United States; most of the individuals afflicted with RA are women. RA can express itself in a variety of ways: For example, it can be **articular**, strikingly only the joints; or it can be **extra-articular**, meaning it can affect areas outside the joints as well, including nerves, organs such as the heart or lungs, and blood vessel walls. When autoimmune cells invade the cartilage and bone within a joint, the surrounding muscles, ligaments, and tendons become weak and are not able to function normally, leading to pain and deformity. Scar tissue eventually replaces the damaged tissue, and the spaces in the joints narrow and movements become limited.

The symptoms that distinguish rheumatoid arthritis from other forms of arthritis are inflammation and soft-tissue swelling of many joints at the same time, called **polyarthritis**, as illustrated in Figure 19.2. The pain is generally decreased with use of the affected joints, and there is usually stiffness of all joints in the morning that

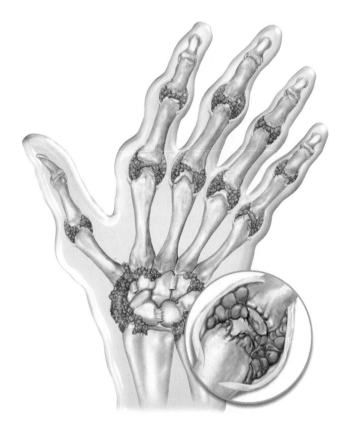

FIGURE 19.2. **Rheumatoid Arthritis**. This illustrates multiple joints affected in the hand and wrist. Asset provided by Anatomical Chart Co.

lasts for a period and then gets better as the day progresses. Therefore, the pain of rheumatoid arthritis is usually worse in the morning compared to the classic pain of osteoarthritis, which worsens over the day as the joints are used. Some people develop **nodules**, or bumps under the skin, which are found close to the joints. In addition, the disease manifests itself by flares of worsening symptoms that signal increased disease activity followed by periods of calm, characterized by a decrease in symptoms for an unpredictable amount of time until the disease flares again.

As with other autoimmune disorders, it is difficult to isolate a cause for RA. Investigators have developed important links to the disease, such as genetics, viruses, environmental triggers, and even malaria, but none have been proven to be the definitive source. With four times as many women as men diagnosed with the disorder, it appears that hormonal factors may also be involved.

Like other autoimmune disorders, RA is incurable; treatment is focused on alleviating pain and keeping the process of the disorder at bay. Medications that diminish the anti-inflammatory symptoms of most autoimmune disorders offer patients with RA pain relief and aid in joint mobility.

Arthroplasty (also called joint replacement) is the most frequently performed surgical treatment for RA, and just about any joint can be replaced with artificial parts made of metal and ceramic materials. Like other joint replacement surgeries discussed previously in Chapter 17, *Orthopaedics*, the diseased joint is replaced with long-lasting artificial parts affixed with cement. With newer materials and techniques, these replaced joints can not only improve functional mobility for a longer period but also make the joints, especially in the hands, look better.

Other surgical procedures used to treat RA include **tendon reconstruction**, which is a procedure used when RA damages or ruptures the tendons that attach muscle to bones. Tendon reconstruction is used primarily on the hands and involves the attachment of an intact tendon to a damaged one. This procedure helps to restore some hand function, especially if the tendon has not completely ruptured. As part of a tendon reconstruction, removal of inflamed synovial tissue, called **synovectomy**, may also be performed.

Autoimmune Thyroid Diseases

The **thyroid** is a butterfly-shaped gland located in the neck, just below the larynx. Thyroid hormones regulate **metabolism**, the rate at which the body converts food into energy. The thyroid is part of the endocrine system, described in more detail in Chapter 21, *Endocrinology*, but it also plays a role in autoimmune disorders. Thyroid disease is the most common of all autoimmune diseases, affecting more than 10 million people, primarily women.

Thyroglobulin is a protein produced by normal thyroid tissue. This protein is needed to carry molecules of thyroid hormone throughout the blood circulation. Cells inside the thyroid gland produce and store thyroglobulin, breaking it down when needed into the thyroid hormones **thyroxine** (T4) and **triiodothyronine** (T3), both of which work to regulate the body's metabolism. The production of these hormones and their release into the bloodstream is stimulated by **thyroid stimulating hormone** (TSH), a hormone produced by the pituitary gland in the brain. In autoimmune disease, antithyroglobulin antibodies are produced to replace thyroglobulin, thereby interfering with the function of the thyroid gland.

Graves Disease

A common autoimmune thyroid disease, **Graves disease**, is caused by overactivity of the thyroid gland, a condition called **hyperthyroidism**. When the thyroid is too active, it makes more thyroid hormones than the body needs. High levels of thyroid hormones can cause side effects such as weight loss, rapid heart rate, and nervousness. TSH produced by the pituitary gland enters the bloodstream and travels to the thyroid gland where it binds to special structures called receptors. This binding process stimulates the thyroid gland to take up iodine to produce thyroid hormone, which is then released into the bloodstream. In turn, thyroid hormone in the bloodstream travels to the pituitary gland where it acts to regulate the release of TSH. In Graves disease, a malfunction in the immune system releases abnormal antibodies that mimic TSH. Spurred by these false signals to produce, the thyroid's hormone factories work overtime and exceed their normal quota.

Exactly why the immune system begins to produce these abnormal antibodies is unclear. Heredity and other characteristics seem to play a role in determining susceptibility. Studies show, for example, that if one identical twin contracts Graves disease, there is a 20% likelihood that the other twin will get it as well. In addition, women are more likely than men to develop the disease. Smokers who develop Graves disease are more prone to eye problems than nonsmokers with the disease.

People with Graves disease experience a number of symptoms, some of which are obvious to a physician's examination, as shown in Figure 19.3. **Goiter**, the term used to describe a mass on the neck, is actually an enlarged, inflamed thyroid gland. Eye protrusion, called **exophthalmos**, describes eyes that are bulging in appearance as a result of water retention. Individuals with Graves disease may also experience darkening of the skin around the eyes, heat intolerance, and weight loss despite increased appetite. For unknown reasons, women seem to be affected with this disease in far greater numbers than men; however, men can have the disease as well, and one of the best known sufferers is former president George H.W. Bush. Interestingly, former first lady Barbara Bush had been diagnosed with Graves disease only two years earlier; in addition, even their dog, Millie, had lupus.

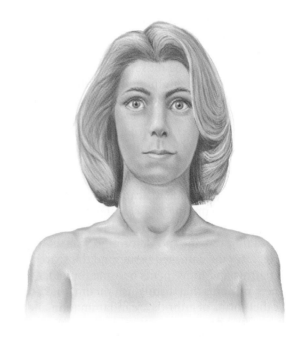

FIGURE 19.3. Graves Disease. A patient with Graves disease may show symptoms of an enlarged thyroid (goiter) and protrusion of one or both eyeballs (exophthalmos). Asset provided by Anatomical Chart Co.

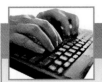

Treatments for Graves disease include drugs that can block the runaway production of thyroid hormone. The most common of these medications is levothyroxine (Levophed), or L-thyroxine. Radioactive iodine (commonly called radioiodine) is a form of iodine that gives off radiation that causes the thyroid gland to slow thyroid production. Given as a capsule or as a tasteless solution in water, radioiodine that is not retained by the thyroid gland is secreted rapidly by the body (within two or three days), primarily through the kidneys into the urine. Surgical options include a thyroidectomy, where all of the thyroid gland is removed. In most cases, people who have surgery for Graves disease will develop an underactive thyroid (hypothyroidism, described later) and must take thyroid replacement hormones for the rest of their lives.

Hashimoto Thyroiditis

Hashimoto thyroiditis, often referred to as simply **thyroiditis**, occurs when antibodies attack the thyroid gland directly, severely affecting its function. Ultimately, this leads to an insufficient production of thyroid hormone, a condition called **hypothyroidism**. The onset of the disease is usually slow—a person's thyroid laboratory tests may show up as intermittently abnormal with an overall years-long pattern of normal results. Other symptoms that eventually appear include weight gain, muscle weakness, difficulty concentrating or thinking, mood swings, cold intolerance, and overall fatigue. Again, this disorder strikes a disproportionate number of women as compared to men and appears to be prevalent in people with a family history of thyroid disease, but researchers cannot find a definite cause for the disorder.

Physicians work to regulate the thyroid's production of thyroid hormones to get thyroid levels back to normal. The most common medication to treat hypothyroidism is thyroxine (Synthroid), given in a pill form. Again, patients with the disorder usually must take the medication for the rest of their lives.

Vasculitis

Vasculitis is an inflammation of blood vessels, and different disorders can affect every type of blood vessel from the major arteries and veins to the tiny capillaries and venules.

Vasculitis can weaken a section of a blood vessel wall, causing it to stretch and bulge (**aneurysm**). In other cases, the inflamed vessel can become narrow and restrict blood flow (**ischemia**). A blood vessel may even close off entirely (**occlusion**), causing a blockage of blood flow altogether. Sometimes the body will compensate for the restricted blood flow by rerouting blood to other healthy blood vessels (**collateral vessels**); but if the collateral flow is not sufficient, the affected tissue around the diseased vessel dies (**infarction**). Every vessel in the cardiovascular system is fair game for these antibodies, which means that every vessel in the body is open to attack.

Vasculitis can affect one organ, such as the kidney, or it can affect several organ systems at once, called systemic vasculitis. Other forms of vasculitis include **giant cell arteritis** (GCA, also called **temporal arteritis**), an inflammation of the arteries that primarily supply the head, and **Wegener granulomatosis**, which affects primarily the lungs, kidneys, and upper respiratory tract. A third form of the disease, **Takayasu arteritis**, affects the aorta, which distributes blood from the heart.

Vasculitis occurs when the immune system mistakenly identifies blood vessels or parts of a blood vessel as foreign and attacks them. Cells of the immune system surround and infiltrate the affected vessels, damaging them and possibly damaging the tissues and organs they supply as well. Symptoms result from the direct damage to the blood vessels or from indirect damage to tissues (such as nerves or organs) whose blood supply has been disrupted. The swelling associated with vasculitis occurs when the damaged blood vessels leak. The inflamed area is red, tender, and feels hot to the touch. A person might also bleed from blood vessels under the skin, causing red or purple discolorations called **purpura**. The term *purpura* comes from the Greek word for purple, *porphyra*. Purpura includes both **petechiae** (singular, **petechia**), which are pinpoint spots of bleeding that appear as tiny dots on the skin, and **ecchymoses** (singular, **ecchymosis**), which are larger blotches. Patients with temporal (giant cell) arteritis may have severe headaches, blindness, and stroke, caused by vasculitis of the arteries in the brain and head. Vasculitis associated with Takayasu arteritis affects the large arteries, specifically those around the heart, which results in symptoms ranging from difficulty finding a pulse in locations where it can usually be felt to a heart attack.

Definitive triggers for vasculitis are unknown, but certain infections and reactions to certain drugs and vaccines may play a part. In addition, the disease is difficult to diagnose because no blood test can confirm it. Physicians usually suspect the disease when a combination of symptoms, such as unexplained patchy numbness or paralysis in a previously healthy individual, and laboratory results cannot be explained any other way.

Treatment of vasculitis is generally the same no matter what organ or tissue is involved. The goal is to decrease the immune system's production of autoanti-bodies, usually with medications called corticosteroids, described later, which relieve the symptoms of the disease and help to slow or stop its progression. Narrowed arteries, such as in Takayasu's, may be treated with **angioplasty**, in which a balloon-tipped catheter is threaded into the blood vessel to widen narrowed arteries. In some cases, damage from severe inflammation can require vessel bypass procedures or aortic valve replacement.

Sjögren Syndrome

Sjögren syndrome is actually the second most common autoimmune rheumatic disease after rheumatoid arthritis. It affects up to four million people, the vast majority of whom are women. This autoimmune disorder is an inflammatory condition in which the immune system attacks and destroys cells in the exocrine glands, most commonly the tear and salivary glands, resulting in lack of saliva and tears. Other areas of the body are also affected. Characteristically, the mucous membranes—any or all of them—dry up. Symptoms include a severely dry mouth; gritty, irritated eyes; difficulty swallowing; and dry vaginal mucosa and nasal passages.

There is no known cure for Sjögren syndrome and no specific treatment to restore gland secretion. Treatment is generally symptomatic and supportive, including moisture-replacement medications to help ease symptoms of dryness. Refresh Tears, Pred Forte, and other over-the-counter lubricating eye drops are prescribed to temporarily reduce inflammation and relieve symptoms of dry eyes. Pilocarpine hydrochloride (Salagen) and cevimeline (Evoxac) are commonly prescribed oral medications that stimulate saliva production, helping patients chew, swallow, and speak more easily. Nonsteroidal anti-inflammatory drugs may be used to treat musculoskeletal symptoms.

Scleroderma

Scleroderma is a chronic autoimmune disease that affects the connective tissues, which support the skin and internal organs, causing skin to harden and scar. In scleroderma, the immune system attacks and damages cells that produce **collagen**, the substance that makes skin elastic and supports other connective tissues inside the body such as joints, ligaments, and organ coverings. The attack leaves behind scar tissue, or **fibrosis**, which leads to degenerative changes in the skin, blood vessels, and skeletal muscle. As the disease progresses, scar tissue builds up and causes normally soft tissue to harden. To illustrate, the scab that appears on a wound is the same fibrotic material that builds up within the skin or organs of the body of a person with scleroderma. Literally, the disorder gets its name from the Greek words *sklero*, meaning *hard*, and *derma*, meaning *skin*, but in some cases it affects blood vessels and organs such as the heart, lungs, and kidneys. There are two main types of scleroderma: localized and systemic. **Localized scleroderma** usually affects only the skin, causing hard patches to form on the skin or streaks of thickened skin to form on various areas of the body. **Systemic scleroderma** affects many areas of the body, initially affecting the skin and then gradually involving the esophagus, lungs, intestines, or other organs, causing them to function abnormally. For example, lung cells are unable to exchange carbon dioxide for oxygen because scar tissue has formed over the thin membrane where this exchange takes place.

Symptoms of scleroderma include those that affect the blood vessels. Tiny blood vessels in the fingers and other areas of the body become narrowed and dysfunctional. In the hands, diminished blood supply makes fingers extremely sensitive to cold, causing a condition called **Raynaud phenomenon**; and the reduced blood circulation causes fingers to become pale, waxy-white, or purple in cold temperatures. **Sclerodactyly**, another well-known symptom of scleroderma, is a condition in which the skin of the fingers becomes thickened and tight from the loss of subcutaneous tissue, making it hard to bend or straighten the digits. This condition can affect the skin across the body in small or large areas, including the torso, back, and the upper and lower legs.

It is not known what triggers the immune reaction that causes scleroderma. Some theories explored include having a genetic predisposition to the condition or contracting a virus. In addition, many people who are exposed to certain chemicals such as arsenic or coal dust have been known to develop scleroderma.

As with other autoimmune disorders, there is no cure for scleroderma, but there are a number of treatments used by physicians for the various conditions associated with the disease. Along with the standard autoimmune drug therapies listed later in this chapter, medications used most often to treat symptoms of Raynaud phenomenon include **vasodilators**, which are drugs that improve blood flow to the small vessels in the fingers by causing the blood vessels to dilate, or expand. These include nifedipine (Procardia), diltiazem (Cardizem), losartan (Cozaar), and amlodipine (Norvasc). Gastroesophageal problems can be controlled with proton pump inhibitors (discussed in Chapter 14, *Gastroenterology*) such as esomeprazole (Nexium), pantoprazole (Protonix), or lansoprazole (Prevacid), which help to reduce acid production and reflux. Problems involving the lungs, heart, and kidneys are treated pharmacologically in a similar manner as discussed in Chapters 12, *Pulmonology*; 13, *Cardiology*; and 15 *Urology*, respectively.

High-dose chemotherapy with stem cell rescue is a newer treatment that involves harvesting stem cells, purifying and freezing them, and then destroying a patient's abnormal immune system with high doses of chemotherapy. The high-dose therapy portion of the procedure utilizes high doses of agents like chemotherapy and/or radiation to destroy cancer cells. However, these high doses also destroy normal cells, especially the blood-producing stem cells in the bone marrow, resulting in complications such as anemia, infection, and bleeding. The stem cell transplantation portion of the procedure is an attempt to restore the blood-producing stem cells after high-dose therapy has reduced them to dangerously low levels. During a stem cell transplant, the patient's own stem cells are collected from circulating blood before chemotherapy treatment, frozen, and then infused back into the patient after treatment to "rescue" the bone marrow.

Medications Used to Treat Autoimmune Disorders

Because most autoimmune diseases, including those described previously, are chronic, most patients must be monitored and treated for life. There is no cure at present for these disorders; therefore, treatment is aimed at lessening the severity of symptoms and slowing the immune system's destruction of the affected organs or tissues. The following drugs are commonly used for managing most types of autoimmune diseases and syndromes, including those disorders discussed previously:

- Nonsteroidal antiinflammatory drugs (NSAIDs) such as aspirin, ibuprofen (Motrin), naproxen (Naprosyn), indomethacin (Indocin), and nabumetone (Relafen) relieve inflammation and keep fever at bay. Cyclooxygenase 2 (COX-2) inhibitors, such as celecoxib (Celebrex), discussed in previous chapters, are also effective in reducing inflammation.
- Corticosteroids are used to suppress the immune system in an effort to harness overactivity. The most commonly prescribed corticosteroids include prednisone (Deltasone), dexamethasone (Decadron), and methylprednisolone (Medrol).
- Antimalarials are drugs that were originally used to treat malaria, which also suppress the inflammation leading to skin rashes, joint pain, hair loss, and fatigue in lupus. These drugs include chloroquine (Aralen) and hydroxychloroquine (Plaquenil). Plaquenil is the most commonly prescribed, and recent studies have suggested that this drug may also have a positive effect on bone mass, preventing bone loss at the hip and spine.
- Tumor necrosis factor (TNF) inhibitors, also referred to as biological response modifiers (BRMs), are a type of drug that blocks levels of TNF, a protein that is present in larger quantities than normal in people with inflammatory conditions, resulting in pain and tissue damage. Administered by injection or infusion, these drugs bolster or restore a person's immune responses, resulting in decreased joint pain and increased mobility. The most common TNF blockers currently used include etanercept (Enbrel), infliximab (Remicade), and adalimumab (Humira).
- Cyclosporine is an immunosuppressive drug that inhibits the transmission of messages between the various cells of the immune system and thereby reduces autoimmune activity.
- Immunomodulating drugs belong to a class of drugs called cytotoxic, or cell-killing drugs, that help suppress the immune system by reducing populations of immune cells. These drugs include azathioprine (Imuran), methotrexate (Rheumatrex), cyclophosphamide (Cytoxan), and mycophenolate mofetil (CellCept).
- Anticoagulants are prescribed for patients with clotting abnormalities to prevent blood clots in the leg veins, called **deep venous thrombosis** (DVT), or in the lungs or coronary arteries. Warfarin (Coumadin) and heparin are the most common blood-thinning medications used for this purpose.

Intravenous immunoglobulin (IVIG) is not a drug regimen but a pooled solution of antibodies compiled from the blood of many people, sterilized, and then administered to a patient with an autoimmune disorder. For immunodeficiency where the body does not make enough antibodies, IVIG supplies them. It slows down the autoimmune process by blocking other antibodies. It curtails inflammation, thereby providing temporary relief from autoimmune-related symptoms. IVIG is given in large doses of up to 4 g/kg (dosed according to the weight of the patient), administered over several hours and sometimes over several days.

Cancer of the Immune System

The cells of the immune system, like other cells, can grow uncontrollably, resulting in cancer. When normal cells turn to cancer cells, some of the antigens on their surface may change. If the immune system notices the foreign antigens, it launches an attack against them. However, the immune system cannot patrol everywhere

TRANSCRIPTION TIP:

Drugs that slow the progression of autoimmune disease, such as those listed previously, are collectively referred to as **disease-modifying antirheumatic drugs** (DMARDs). DMARDs include any drug that actually reverses the disease process, as opposed to just treating symptoms. Physicians frequently use this term when describing these drugs; in dictation, the term sounds like *DEE-mardz*.

to flush and eliminate all cells that become cancerous. A tumor develops when the immune system breaks down or is overwhelmed and cancer cells flourish.

Lymphoma is a general term for a group of cancers that originate in the lymphatic system from the uncontrolled growth of lymphocytes (T cells or B cells), causing tumors to grow. Recall that lymphocytes move about to all parts of the body through the bloodstream and lymphatic vessels. Lymph nodes scattered throughout the network of lymphatic vessels house collections of lymphocytes. Lymphomas result when a lymphocyte undergoes a malignant change and begins to multiply, eventually crowding out healthy cells and creating tumors that enlarge in the lymph nodes or other parts of the immune system. The lymphocytes that become cancerous, called **lymphoma cells**, may remain confined to a single lymph node or may spread to the bone marrow, the spleen, or virtually any other organ.

Lymphomas are divided into two main categories: Hodgkin lymphoma and all other lymphomas, called **non-Hodgkin lymphomas**. **Hodgkin lymphoma**, also referred to as **Hodgkin disease**, is named for Thomas Hodgkin, an English physician who first diagnosed the disease in 1832. Generally, Hodgkin lymphoma is uncommon, accounting for less than 1% of all cancers that occur in the United States yearly. The microscopic appearance of this disease is different from other lymphomas, which allows it to be diagnosed by examination of a tissue sample. This clinical difference is the presence of **Reed-Sternberg cells**, a kind of cell specific to Hodgkin lymphoma, which is found in the cancerous area. Under a microscope, these cells look different from cells of non-Hodgkin lymphomas and other cancers. Most scientists now believe that Reed-Sternberg cells are a type of malignant B cells.

Because lymphatic tissue is present in many parts of the body, Hodgkin lymphoma can start almost anywhere, but most often it starts in the lymph nodes in the upper part of the body, such as in the chest, neck, or under the arms. The tissue in these areas becomes enlarged, which can put pressure on important structures. The disease then progressively extends from one group of nodes to the next, with later involvement of the spleen and other tissues, including the liver and lungs.

As is true of most tumors, the cause of Hodgkin lymphoma is not known, and physicians can seldom explain why one person gets the disease and another does not. However, by studying the patterns of cancer in the general population, researchers have learned that the disease occurs more in men than in women, and that those with a family history of the disease have a higher-than-average chance of developing the disease. In addition, Epstein-Barr virus (EBV) may contribute to the emergence of the disease.

Hodgkin lymphoma is often treated with radiation therapy and/or chemotherapy. Radiation therapy consists

TRANSCRIPTION TIP:

Do not use the possessive form of eponyms (for example, Hodgkin disease, *not* Hodgkin's disease). However, in awkward constructions, such as when the noun following the eponym is omitted, the possessive form can be used (for example, "The patient suffers from Hodgkin's," not "The patient suffers from Hodgkin").

of the use of targeted radiation to kill cancer cells, while avoiding nearby healthy tissue. Chemotherapy is the use of drugs to kill cancer cells and shrink tumors. These drugs can be taken orally, in pill form, or put into the body by infusion into a vein. (These methods are used to treat a variety of cancers and are more thoroughly discussed in Chapter 20, *Oncology*.)

In Hodgkin lymphoma, the mainstream chemotherapy regimen consists of a combination of four drugs: doxorubicin (Adriamycin), bleomycin (Blenoxane), vinblastine (Velban), and dacarbazine (DTIC), collectively known by the acronym ABVD. For disease that is resistant to other treatments, the drug combination of mechlorethamine (Mustargen), vincristine (Oncovin), prednisone (Deltasone), and procarbazine (Matulane), collectively known as MOPP; or the drug combination of cyclophosphamide (Cytoxan), vincristine (Oncovin), prednisone (Deltasone), and procarbazine (Matulane), called COPP, may prove effective. All of these drug regimens can be used alone or can be alternated with each other. Modern combination chemotherapy controls the disease in a great majority of cases, and a substantial proportion of patients with this disease can expect to be cured.

A **bone marrow transplant** (BMT) is used to treat patients who relapse from standard chemotherapy treatments or in cases where high doses of chemotherapy may destroy the patient's bone marrow. In this procedure, marrow is taken from the bones before treatment. The marrow is then frozen and the patient is given high-dose chemotherapy as a first-line treatment, with or without radiation therapy, to treat the cancer. The stored marrow is then thawed and put back into the patient through a needle in a vein to replace the marrow that was destroyed. This type of transplant is called an **autologous bone marrow transplant**. If the bone marrow is taken from another person, the transplant is called an **allogeneic bone marrow transplant**.

Another type of transplant used in the treatment of lymphomas such as Hodgkin's is called a **peripheral blood stem cell transplant**. In this procedure, the patient's blood is passed through a machine that removes the stem cells, (which, as discussed previously, are immature cells in the bone marrow from which all

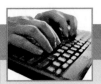

TRANSCRIPTION TIP:

Chemotherapy combination treatments are sometimes referred to as *regimens* or *protocols* in dictation. Listen carefully and always verify the combination dictated, as it is easy to confuse many regimens used for different diseases. For example, the protocol ABVD is not the same chemical combination as AVDP or EBVP. In addition, physicians will dictate some regimens as words instead of letters. For example, MOPP is often dictated as *mop*, and COPP is dictated as *cop*.

blood cells develop), a process called **apheresis**. The stem cells are treated with drugs to kill any cancer cells and then frozen until they are transplanted back into the patient.

Scientists are also experimenting with **immunotherapy**, which is a type of biological therapy to treat autoimmune disorders. Biological therapies use natural body substances or drugs made from natural body substances to treat diseases. Immunotherapies are treatments that boost the immune system. Current research involves genetically engineered viruses created in the laboratory. These viruses are combined with the patient's own lymphocytes as a new anticancer weapon to attack and destroy tumors.

Many chemicals used in the immune response can now be made in the laboratory. **Monoclonal antibodies** are produced in the laboratory to target specific antigens. They are called *monoclonal* because they are produced by the identical offspring of a single, cloned antibody-producing cell. Different antibodies have to be made for different types of immune disorders. For example, the drug rituximab (Rituxan) is a type of monoclonal antibody used in cancer detection or therapy that is commonly used to treat non-Hodgkin lymphoma, discussed previously.

Monoclonal antibodies can react against specific antigens on cancer cells such as those found in Hodgkin's and may enhance the patient's immune response. They can be programmed to act against cell growth factors, thereby blocking cell growth, and by linking monoclonal antibodies to anticancer drugs or other biologic response modifiers they can deliver their load of toxin directly to the tumor without harming healthy cells. More studies are being conducted to see how monoclonal antibodies can be used in imaging tests to detect or locate small groups of cancer cells.

Other researchers are testing therapeutic cancer vaccines, the goal of which is to improve on the natural anticancer response by stimulating strong T-cell responses against a tumor. These differ from traditional

QUICK CHECK 19.2 ✓

Circle the letter corresponding to the best answer to the following questions.

1. The most common type of antibody that develops in people with lupus is called
   A. SLE-70.
   B. antinuclear antibody.
   C. antiphospholipids.
   D. rheumatoid factor.

2. A bump under the skin in patients with RA is called a(n)
   A. nodule.
   B. lymph node.
   C. antibody.
   D. antigen.

3. The type of cells specific to Hodgkin lymphoma are called
   A. Anti-La cells.
   B. Ro-Sternberg cells.
   C. Reid-Steinberg cells.
   D. Reed-Sternberg cells.

4. Chemicals that can be produced in the laboratory to fight autoimmune diseases are called
   A. leukotriene receptors.
   B. disease modifying.
   C. intravenous immunoglobin.
   D. monoclonal antibodies.

5. The autoimmune disease characterized by hardening and scarring of the skin is called
   A. lupus.
   B. Sjögren syndrome.
   C. scleroderma.
   D. Hashimoto thyroiditis.

vaccines in that they are administered after the cancer has developed and are designed to help the immune system fight off the tumor. Although these new therapies are generally not able to destroy a tumor on their own, it is hoped that they can be effective partners if administered along with other traditional forms of cancer treatment.

DIAGNOSTIC STUDIES AND PROCEDURES

The diagnosis of an immune disorder is based on an individual's symptoms, findings from a physical examination, and results from laboratory tests. Diseases of the immune system are difficult to diagnose, especially in the early stages of the disease. Therefore, information is required from multiple sources (rather than a single laboratory test) to accurately diagnose specific immune system disorders.

Laboratory Tests

Laboratory and diagnostic investigations of immunologic disorders focus primarily on the detection and measurement of abnormalities in the cells used by the body for an immune response. These tests can help identify the exact immune disorder, the extent of damage already done, and the extent of other organ involvement, such as that of the liver and kidneys.

Allergy Skin Testing

An allergy skin test is used to identify the substances that are causing allergy symptoms. An extract of an allergen is applied to the skin, the skin is scratched or pricked to allow exposure (or is applied to a patch that is worn on the skin for a period of time), and then the skin's reaction is evaluated.

Blood Tests

Blood tests are a standard part of any autoimmune workup; and since no single test can determine whether a person has an immune disorder, several laboratory tests are available to help a physician make a definitive diagnosis. The most useful of these tests identify certain autoantibodies often present in the blood of individuals with these types of disorders. Some tests are used to identify antibodies specific to certain immune disorders, whereas others are used to evaluate organ function and to monitor the effect on the body of medications used to treat these disorders. The following are common blood tests used to evaluate and diagnose immune disorders:

- **Comprehensive metabolic panel** (CMP). A CMP measures counts of white blood cells, red blood cells, and platelets, as well as kidney and liver function. In an immune disorder workup, this panel can detect problems such as abnormally low levels of red blood cells (**anemia**), white blood cells (**leukopenia**), or platelets (**thrombocytopenia**). In addition, blood tests can measure the key number of neutrophils, a type of white blood cell that destroys invading bacteria and viruses. In some immune disorders, such as rheumatoid arthritis, these cells are overactive and are elevated on complete blood count (CBC) results. In others, neutrophils may be depleted (**neutropenia**), causing a risk of infection. Other parts of the CMP can be used to assess organ dysfunction resulting from coexisting diseases. For example, a CMP can detect abnormal calcium in the blood (**hypercalcemia**), and liver and kidney function tests can be used to monitor the effects of medications used to treat autoimmune disorders that may be toxic to the liver and kidneys, impairing their ability to function.

- **Rheumatoid factor** (RF). This antibody is found in the blood of most patients with RA, although it may not be easily detected in the early stages of the diseases. The test is used to diagnose rheumatoid arthritis and to distinguish it from other forms of arthritis and other conditions that cause similar symptoms of joint pain, inflammation, and stiffness. High levels of RF are associated with more severe rheumatoid disease and a higher tendency to develop nonjoint manifestations of rheumatoid disease, such as respiratory problems.

- Antinuclear antibody (ANA). The ANA is a common test used to look for antibodies that react against the nuclear material of cells. ANA test results are dictated as a **titer**, which is a concentration or strength of these antibodies in the blood. The number is based on how many times an individual's blood must be diluted to get a sample free of ANA. This figure is transcribed as a ratio, with a colon placed between the arabic numbers. For example, a titer of 1:640 shows a greater concentration of ANA than a titer of 1:320. This would be dictated as *1 to 640 (or six hundred and forty)* or *1 to 320, or three hundred and twenty*, respectively, but always transcribed in ratio form as *1:640* or *1:320*.

- **Anti-double-stranded DNA**. These antibodies bind to DNA, which contains the genetic instructions in every cell. A positive anti-double-stranded DNA test is considered highly specific for some immune diseases such as lupus. These antibodies also appear to track lupus activity, with levels waxing and waning with lupus flares. Therefore, this test is performed frequently in patients with lupus in an attempt to predict disease flares.

- **Anti-Ro, Anti-La, and Anti-Sm**. These are more specific individual types of autoantibodies which help to narrow down a diagnosis of a particular autoimmune disorder. They are named after the first two letters of the patients in which they were discovered, and the results are indicated as being positive or negative.

- Thyroid function tests. This test measures thyroid function by measuring the amount of thyroid stimulating hormone (TSH) in the blood. TSH causes the thyroid gland to produce two hormones: triiodothyronine (T3) and **free thyroxine** (T4), both of which help regulate the body's metabolism. The TSH level is elevated in patients with an underactive thyroid gland, such as in hypothyroidism (Hashimoto thyroiditis), and is low or undetectable in patients with an overactive thyroid, such as with hyperthyroidism (Graves disease).

- Immunoglobulins. Recall that immunoglobulins are released into the bloodstream in response to infections. A blood test called **immunoelectrophoresis** identifies immunoglobulins—IgG, IgA, and IgM—in a blood sample. As IgG, IgA, and IgM levels change in various disorders, these values can indicate the presence of immune disorders such as myelomas, leukemia, rheumatoid arthritis, and lupus.

- **Erythrocyte sedimentation rate** (ESR). This screening test, often called simply the **sed rate**, is the determination of the rate of speed at which red blood cells settle in a glass tube specimen of unclotted blood. ESR is often increased when proteins, produced in response to inflammation, interfere with the ability of red blood cells, or erythrocytes, to remain suspended in the blood.

- **Antiphospholipid antibodies** (APLs). This antibody, specifically **anticardiolipin** (aCL) and **lupus anticoagulant** (LA), can cause damage to blood vessels and act against proteins in the blood to promote clotting problems. Elevated levels of these antibodies can be suggestive of **antiphospholipid syndrome** (APS), a disorder in which autoantibodies promote blood clots that can cause unrelated problems such as miscarriages and strokes.

- The **Venereal Disease Research Laboratory** (VDRL) **test** is used to diagnose syphilis but also used to test for lupus. The antibodies produced in lupus may interact with chemicals used to test for other diseases, sometimes showing a false-positive reading for this disease. In this case, the VDRL does not mean that the person has syphilis; rather, it aids in diagnosing lupus in that it indicates the presence of anticardiolipin antibodies.

- **Complement** levels. Complement is a collective term for a system of at least 15 serum proteins designed to destroy foreign cells and help remove foreign materials. Complement levels can increase susceptibility to infection and predispose an individual to other diseases. Decreased levels are characteristic in such conditions as lupus, and the

TRANSCRIPTION TIP:

In dictation, the antibodies anti-Ro and anti-La sound like *anti-ROW* and *anti-LAH*, respectively. Anti-Sm, or anti-Smith antibody, is dictated as *anti-SMITH*, although this term is always transcribed as *anti-Sm*.

results of two specific components, C3 and C4, are often dictated in rheumatologic notes.

- SCL-70 is a blood test that isolates the scleroderma antibody. This antibody in and of itself is not the cause of scleroderma, but if it appears in the blood it is suggestive of the disease.

Urine Tests

A urine dipstick is used to measure abnormal levels of chemicals or bacteria in the urine to indicate a disease process. A microscopic examination of the urine can reveal abnormalities such as the presence of white or red blood cells or excessive protein in the urine, which may indicate kidney dysfunction.

Biopsy

A **biopsy** is a procedure whereby a small sample of tissue is removed from the body for examination under a microscope. Biopsies are often used to diagnose immune disorders. A biopsy can look for markers of inflammation and the degree of disease present in the body. For example, a skin biopsy is frequently ordered for patients with symptoms of a rash, sometimes a sign of lupus. A liver biopsy, in which a tiny sample of the liver is examined under the microscope, can help to identify autoimmune hepatitis, a disease in which the body's immune system attacks liver cells.

Types of biopsies used to evaluate immune disorders include **fine-needle aspiration** (FNA), which is a biopsy used to obtain samples of a small amount of tissue or fluid from a joint or nodule to investigate the type and extent of disease. For example, an FNA is used

TRANSCRIPTION TIP:

Dictators talk about *complements*, which is a collective term for serum proteins that destroy foreign cells and help the body remove foreign materials. Note the spelling—do not spell this term as *compliment*, which is a remark of praise or admiration.

to obtain a sample of a suspicious nodule in the thyroid when investigating autoimmune thyroid disease. In this procedure, a small needle is inserted into the nodule to withdraw a small amount of material for analysis. A fine-needle procedure may also be used to aspirate material from a lymph node to help determine the cause of lymph node enlargement and also whether a tumor in the lymph node is cancerous or noncancerous. This method almost always provides enough tissue to make a diagnosis of the type of Hodgkin disease (Hodgkin's or non-Hodgkin's). In trying to confirm a diagnosis of Hodgkin lymphoma, a pathologist examines the size and shape of the cells under the microscope and determines whether any of them are characteristic Reed-Sternberg cells. An FNA of synovial fluid may be examined for white blood cells, commonly found in patients with rheumatoid arthritis. To obtain a specimen, the physician inserts a needle into the joint to withdraw the synovial fluid into a syringe. The procedure is formally called **arthrocentesis** (or *joint aspiration*), as discussed in Chapter 17, *Orthopaedics.*

A node or nodule may be removed in its entirety for analysis by performing an **excisional biopsy**. In this procedure, the skin over the biopsy site is cleansed, a small incision is made, and the lymph node or part of the node is removed. The incision is closed with sutures and bandaged, and the sample is then sent to the laboratory for examination.

Imaging Studies

Imaging studies are used to produce a picture of internal body structures. Imaging tests are performed using sound waves, radioactive particles, magnetic fields, or x-rays that are detected and converted into images after passing through body tissues. Dyes are sometimes used as contrast agents with x-ray tests so that organs or tissues not seen with conventional x-rays can be enhanced. These studies are used to detect an immune disorder in its early stages or to determine the extent of damage of

an existing disease or to see how a given treatment is affecting the disease. As such, these studies represent crucial tools for the diagnosis and management of immune diseases. Refer to Chapter 8, *Laboratory Studies and Medical Imaging*, for a more detailed explanation of imaging studies used.

X-rays are used to look for signs of bone loss and joint destruction caused by inflammation of the joint space in immune disorders. For example, an x-ray can show damage to the bones, loss of cartilage, and distortion of the joints. Baseline x-rays are usually taken to provide a comparison with future progression of disease and to help assess the effectiveness of disease-modifying agents. In initial stages of diseases such as arthritis, the joints may appear normal on x-ray except for signs of soft tissue swelling and thinning of the bone around the joints, called osteopenia. Eventually signs of bone erosion and other destructive processes can be seen on x-ray, assisting in a more definitive diagnosis of a particular disease, such as rheumatoid arthritis.

X-rays are used with contrast medium to pinpoint damage to the gastrointestinal tract caused by autoimmune disease. For example, a barium swallow, or upper gastrointestinal series, discussed in Chapter 14, *Gastroenterology*, may be used to see whether there is scarring in the esophagus caused by scleroderma.

X-rays provide an image of the bones, but they do not show cartilage, muscles, and ligaments. Other noninvasive imaging methods such as computed tomography (CT), magnetic resonance imaging (MRI), and magnetic resonance angiography (MRA) are used to evaluate changes in bones, joints, and organs and to look for pathologic changes in tissues or spread of disease. For example, an MRI can show evidence of the start of bone erosion in areas close to a joint in rheumatoid arthritis as early as six weeks from the onset of disease. An MRA is the primary diagnostic test for vasculitis because it can show thickening of the aortic wall and other large blood vessel damage. A positron emission tomography (PET) scan can pinpoint hotspots of cellular activity present in many immune disorders. Finally, ultrasound imaging is used to create pictures of nodules, such as those found in the thyroid, using sound waves.

CHAPTER SUMMARY

The immune system acts as the body's built-in sentry and, when working normally, defends it against invading microorganisms. Abnormalities in the reactivity of this delicate system are so genetically complex and diverse that understanding and treating them is a challenge. Disorders of the immune system can be debilitating and expensive, and are likely to be much more common than previously realized. But with major advances in genetics and the exponential growth of knowledge about the immune system, scientists are within reach of discovering new ways to not only treat immune disorders, but also predict susceptibility to these diseases and possibly prevent them.

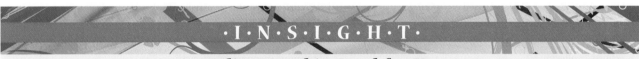

·I·N·S·I·G·H·T·
Feeling Good is Good for You

Researchers are discovering convincing evidence to support the age-old claim that simple pleasures such as laughter are beneficial to the immune system.

Researchers are finding that the mind—the keeper of thoughts, memories, emotions, and personality—is related to the activity of high-level neurons that make descending connections to other neurons lower in the brain, then in the spinal cord, and ultimately to the rest of the body. According to Nobel Prize-winner Sir Francis Crick in his book, *The Astonishing Hypothesis*, these neurons can influence all aspects of the immune system, from B and T cells to lymph organs such as the spleen and thymus.

Although the lay person can "believe" in a mind-body connection to good health, researchers are looking for the exact mechanisms by which specific brain-immunity effects are achieved. A team from Carnegie Mellon University in Pittsburgh found that people who had a positive emotional attitude were not infected as often and experienced fewer symptoms of the common cold than people with a negative emotional outlook. The researchers interviewed 334 healthy volunteers three evenings a week for two weeks to assess their emotional states. After their assessment, each volunteer received a squirt in the nose of a rhinovirus—a germ that causes colds. The researchers kept the subjects under observation for five days to see whether or not they became infected and how they manifested symptoms. Tests showed that although positive people were just as likely to be infected with the virus, infection seemed to produce fewer signs and symptoms of illness.

Although traditional medicine focuses on the body to cure disease, research on the mind-body connection continues to advance, enabling scientists to establish absolutely that far from functioning independently from the rest of the body, the immune system interacts intimately and extensively with the nervous system, which governs all of the body's thoughts and psychological processes. Research in such fields as "behavioral medicine" and "psychoneuroimmunology" continues to focus on the role the mind plays in influencing the body to promote good health and protect itself against disease.

Common Soundalike Words

Word	Word Pronunciation	Soundalike	Soundalike Pronunciation
thymus: A gland that produces mature T cells, found in the thorax under the breastbone.	thī′mŭs	**thyroid**: A butterfly-shaped gland located in the neck, just below the larynx.	thī′royd
complement: A collective term for a system of serum proteins designed to destroy foreign cells and help remove foreign materials.	kom′plĕ-ment	**compliment**: A remark (or act) of praise or admiration.	kom′pli-ment
flare: An acute period of increased disease activity, such as in lupus.	flār	**flair**: A distinctive and stylish elegance; or a natural talent.	flār
allergen: Any substance that can cause an allergy.	al′er-jen	**antigen**: Any substance that initiates a state of immune responsiveness by the body.	an′ti-jen
pheresis: A procedure in which blood is removed from a donor, separated, and a portion retained, with the remainder returned to the donor.	fe-rē′sis	**-phoresis**: A suffix meaning "transmission," such as in *electrophoresis*, which is the migration of electrically charged molecules through a fluid or gel under the influence of an electric field.	fŏr′ē-sis
lymph: A clear fluid that circulates through the lymphatic vessels.	limf	**lymphs**: An abbreviated form for *lymphocytes*.	limfs
occlusion: The act of closing or being closed.	ŏ-klū′zhŭn	**exclusion**: A shutting out or disconnection from the main portion.	eks-klū′zhŭn

Combining Forms

Combining Form	Meaning	Combining Form	Meaning
aden/o	gland	mon/o	one; single
angi/o	blood vessel; lymphatic vessel	myel/o	bone marrow
blast/o (-blast, also a suffix)	germ or bud	opportun/o	well timed; taking advantage of
cyt/o	cell		
defici/o	lacking, inadequate	path/o	disease; suffering
immun/o	immune system	phag/o	eating, swallowing
inhibit/o	block; hold back	splen/o	spleen
leuk/o	white	suppress/o	press down
lymph/o, lymphat/o	lymph or lymphatic system	thromb/o	thrombus (blood clot)
lymphaden/o	lymph nodes	thym/o	thymus
macr/o, meg/a, megal/o	large	tonsill/o	palatine tonsil (a lymph node)
micr/o	small		

Add Your Own Combining Forms Here:

_____

_____

_____

_____

ABBREVIATIONS

Abbreviation	Meaning
ABVD	Adriamycin, bleomycin, vinblastine, and dacarbazine (drug combination)
aCL	anticardiolipin
AIDS	acquired immunodeficiency syndrome
ANA	antinuclear antibody
APL	antiphospholipid antibody
APS	antiphospholipid syndrome
BMT	bone marrow transplant
BRM	biological response modifier
CBC	complete blood count
CMP	comprehensive metabolic panel
COPP	cyclophosphamide, prednisone, procarbazine, and vincristine
CT	computed tomography (scan)
DMARD	disease-modifying antirheumatic drug
DVT	deep venous thrombosis
EBV	Epstein-Barr virus
ESR	erythrocyte sedimentation rate
FNA	fine-needle aspiration
GCA	giant cell arteritis
HAART	highly active antiretroviral therapy
HIV	human immunodeficiency virus
IgA	immunoglobulin A

Abbreviation	Meaning
IgD	immunoglobulin D
IgE	immunoglobulin E
IgG	immunoglobulin G
IgM	immunoglobulin M
IVIG	intravenous immunoglobulin
KS	Kaposi sarcoma
LA	lupus anticoagulant
MOPP	mechlorethamine, vincristine, prednisone, and procarbazine
MRI/MRA	magnetic resonance imaging/magnetic resonance angiography
NSAID	nonsteroidal anti-inflammatory drug
PET	positron emission tomography
RA	rheumatoid arthritis
RF	rheumatoid factor
SCID	severe combined immunodeficiency disease
SLE	systemic lupus erythematosus
SLEDAI	SLE disease activity index
TNF	tumor necrosis factor
TSH	thyroid stimulating hormone
VDRL	Venereal Disease Research Laboratory (test)

Add Your Own Abbreviations Here:

_____

_____

_____

_____

_____

_____

TERMINOLOGY

Term	Meaning
active immunity	The body's response and defense against pathogens it has encountered before.
acquired immunodeficiency syndrome (AIDS)	An often fatal disease of the immune system caused by the human immunodeficiency virus (HIV), which damages the immune system to the extent that opportunistic infections and cancers can attack the body.
adaptive immune system	A system of highly specialized systemic cells that can recognize what belongs in the body and what does not, and remember specific pathogens in order to mount stronger attacks each time the pathogen is encountered.
adenoids	Clumps of lymphoid tissue located in the back of the nasal passages.
allergen	A specific environmental antigen that initiates an allergic response.
allergic salute	The upward motion of the hand against the nose to relieve nasal itching.
allergic shiner	A bluish circle resembling a black eye seen frequently in children with an allergy affecting the sinuses.
allergy	An abnormal reaction to a specific environmental antigen.
allogeneic bone marrow transplant	A bone marrow transplant that uses marrow taken from another person and that is later infused back into the patient.
anemia	Abnormally low levels of red blood cells in the blood.
aneurysm	The weakening of a blood vessel wall, causing it to stretch and bulge.
angioplasty	A procedure in which a balloon-type catheter is threaded into a blood vessel in order to widen narrow arteries.
antibodies	Proteins that are secreted into the body's fluids to destroy bacteria, viruses, or other harmful toxins.
anticardiolipin (aCL)	An antiphospholipid antibody that causes damage to blood vessels and acts against proteins in the blood promoting clotting problems.
anti-double-stranded DNA	A test that tags antibodies which bind to DNA.
antigen	Any substance that initiates an immune response by the body.
anti-La	A specific type of autoantibody that helps to narrow down the diagnosis of a particular autoimmune disorder.
antinuclear antibody (ANA)	An antibody that reacts with a cell's nucleus, or command center.
antiphospholipid antibodies (APLs)	Antibodies that cause damage to blood vessels and act against proteins in the blood to promote clotting problems.
antiphospholipid syndrome (APS)	A disorder in which autoantibodies promote blood clots that can cause unrelated problems such as miscarriages and strokes.
anti-Ro	A specific type of autoantibody that helps to narrow down the diagnosis of a particular autoimmune disorder.
anti-Sm	Dictated as *anti-Smith*, a specific type of autoantibody that helps to narrow down the diagnosis of a particular autoimmune disorder.
apheresis	A procedure whereby whole blood is removed from the body and a desired component is retained, whereas the remainder of the blood is returned to the donor.
appendix	A small pouch of tissue that extends from the large intestine containing lymphoid tissue that scientists believe may be useful in fighting infection.
arthralgia	Pain in the joints.

Term	Meaning
arthrocentesis, syn. joint aspiration	A type of biopsy in which a thin, hollow needle is used to remove synovial fluid from a joint for examination under a microscope.
arthroplasty, syn. joint replacement	A surgical procedure in which a diseased joint is replaced with long-lasting artificial parts affixed with cement.
articular	Referring to a joint (in RA, the disease affecting only the joints).
autoantibodies	Abnormal antibodies produced against the body's own tissues.
autoimmunity	An abnormal condition in which the immune system confuses normal body tissue (self) and attacks the tissues of the body, causing pain and loss of function.
autologous bone marrow transplant	A bone marrow transplant that uses marrow taken directly from the donor patient.
B cells	A type of lymphocyte that matures in the bone marrow and makes antibodies that destroy bacteria, viruses, and other foreign substances that enter the body.
biopsy	A procedure whereby a small sample of tissue is removed from the body for examination under a microscope.
bone marrow	The soft tissue in the hollow shafts of long bones where blood cells are produced.
bone marrow transplant (BMT)	A procedure in which marrow is taken from the bones of a patient before chemotherapy treatment and then put back into the patient later to replace the marrow that was destroyed by chemotherapy.
collagen	The substance that makes skin elastic and supports other connective tissues inside the body.
collateral vessels	Pre-existing blood vessels that help restore blood flow by bypassing areas of narrowing in other blood vessels.
complement	A collective term for a system of serum proteins designed to destroy foreign cells and help remove foreign materials.
cytokines	Chemical messengers used by the cells of the immune system to communicate with one another to coordinate an appropriate immune response.
deep venous thrombosis (DVT)	Blood clots in leg veins.
disease-modifying antirheumatic drug (DMARD)	Any drug that actually reverses the disease process of an autoimmune disorder, as opposed to just treating symptoms.
ecchymoses (singular, ecchymosis)	Larger blotches of discoloration caused by bleeding from the blood vessels under the skin.
Epstein-Barr virus (EBV)	A herpeslike virus that causes one of the two kinds of mononucleosis.
erythrocyte sedimentation rate (ESR), syn. sed rate	A test that determines the rate of speed at which red blood cells settle in a glass tube containing a specimen of unclotted blood.
excisional biopsy	A surgical procedure in which an entire node or part of a node is removed for examination under a microscope.
exophthalmos	A condition in which the eyes bulge in appearance as a result of water retention.
extra-articular	Outside the joints (in RA, affecting not only the joints but tissues, muscles, and organs outside of the joints).
fibrosis	The formation of scar tissue.
fine needle aspiration (FNA)	A type of biopsy in which a thin, hollow needle is used to withdraw fluid or tissue from the body for examination under a microscope.
flare	An acute period of increased disease activity, such as in lupus.
free thyroxine (T4)	A hormone produced by the thyroid gland that helps to regulate the body's metabolism.

Term	*Meaning*
fusion inhibitors	A class of drugs to treat HIV, which work by interfering with HIV's ability to enter the body's healthy immune system cells by blocking the merging of the virus with the cell membranes.
giant cell arteritis (GCA), syn. temporal arteritis	A form of vasculitis; an inflammation of the arteries that primarily supply the head.
goiter	A mass on the neck that is actually an enlarged, inflamed thyroid gland.
Graves disease	An autoimmune thyroid disease caused by an overactivity of the thyroid gland.
Hashimoto thyroiditis, syn. thyroiditis	An autoimmune condition that occurs when antibodies attack the thyroid gland directly, leading to insufficient production of thyroid hormone.
helper T cells	T cells that communicate with other cells to organize and destroy foreign substances.
high-dose chemotherapy with stem cell rescue	A procedure that involves harvesting of healthy stem cells, purifying and freezing them, and then infusing them back into the patient after high-dose chemotherapy has destroyed his/her immune system.
highly active antiretroviral therapy (HAART)	The name given to multiple drugs used in combination to help suppress the HIV virus.
histamine	A chemical that is released during an allergic reaction, causing symptoms in the eyes, nose, throat, lungs, skin, or gastrointestinal tract.
Hodgkin lymphoma, Hodgkin disease	A cancer that starts in the lymphatic tissue and is characterized microscopically by the presence of Reed-Sternberg cells.
human immunodeficiency virus (HIV)	The virus that infects and destroys T cells, paving the way for other infections and cancers to enter the body.
hypercalcemia	An abnormally high level of calcium in blood.
hyperthyroidism	An overactivity of the thyroid gland, producing too much thyroid hormone.
hypothyroidism	An underactivity of the thyroid gland, producing too little thyroid hormone.
immune response	The coordinated effort between the blood and lymphatic system to destroy invading microorganisms.
immune system	A complex network of specialized cells and organs that defends the body against attack by infections and foreign substances.
immunodeficiency	A condition that is caused when the immune system fails to respond effectively to foreign substances that enter the body.
immunoelectrophoresis	A test that identifies immunoglobins in a blood sample.
immunoglobulins	A class of proteins produced and secreted by B cells in response to stimulation by antigens.
immunologist	A clinician who specializes in the field of immunology.
immunology	The study of the human immune system and the treatment of diseases involving that system.
immunotherapy	A type of biological therapy used to treat autoimmune disorders.
infarction	An area of tissue necrosis resulting from a sudden insufficiency of arterial or venous blood supply.
innate immune system	The body's system of cells and mechanisms that provide an immediate defense against infection by other organisms.
intravenous immunoglobulin (IVIG)	A pooled solution of antibodies compiled from the blood of many people, sterilized, and then administered to a patient with an autoimmune disorder.
ischemia	A condition in which blood flow is restricted to a part of the body.

Term	Meaning
killer T cells	T cells that engulf and destroy all types of pathogens.
leukopenia	Abnormally low levels of white blood cells in the blood.
localized scleroderma	A form of scleroderma that usually affects only the skin, causing hard patches to form on the skin or streaks of thickened skin to form on various areas of the body.
lupus anticoagulant (LA)	An antiphospholipid antibody that causes damage to blood vessels and acts against proteins in the blood to promote clotting problems.
lupus flare	A period of acute lupus disease activity.
lymph	A clear fluid containing immune cells that bathes tissues and organs throughout the body.
lymph nodes	Small, bean-shaped structures in the lymph vessels, which act as filters, collecting bacteria or cancer cells that may travel through the lymphatic system.
lymphatic system	A body system consisting of lymphatic vessels and nodes, along with a few specialized structures that serve to function as the immune system.
lymphatic vessels	A circulating system of vessels that transport lymph to the immune organs and into the bloodstream.
lymphocytes	A type of white blood cell that helps the body fight infection.
lymphoid organs	The name given to the organs of the immune system.
lymphoma	A general term for a group of cancers that originate in the lymphocytes.
lymphoma cells	Lymphocytes that become cancerous.
macrophage	A type of specialized cell produced by the bone marrow, which quickly appears at the site of infection to ingest and destroy foreign particles.
memory T cells	T cells that are created when they are exposed to a pathogen, remaining inactive until the same pathogen re-enters the body, at which time they remember the pathogen and reactivate to destroy it.
metabolism	The rate at which the body converts food into energy.
monoclonal antibodies	Antibodies produced in the laboratory to target specific antigens.
neutropenia	A condition of abnormally low levels of neutrophils in the blood.
neutrophil	A type of specialized blood cell produced by the bone marrow, which quickly appears at the site of infection to ingest and destroy foreign particles.
nodules	Bumps under the skin that are found close to the joints.
non-Hodgkin lymphoma	All lymphomas that originate in the lymphatic system that are not Hodgkin lymphoma.
nucleoside reverse transcriptase inhibitors	A group of drugs to treat HIV, which involves interruption of the ability of the virus to make copies of itself in early stages of infection.
occlusion	The state of closing or being closed; in vasculitis, a blood vessel that is closed off entirely, causing a blockage of blood flow altogether.
passive immunity	The immunity provided when a person is given antibodies to a disease rather than producing them through his or her own immune system.
pathogen	Microorganisms that cause disease.
peripheral blood stem cell transplant	A method of collecting and freezing stem cells from the circulating blood-stream before chemotherapy, allowing the patient to receive higher-than-conventional doses of chemotherapy and/or radiation to destroy cancer cells. After completing high-dose chemotherapy or radiotherapy, the frozen stem cells are thawed and reintroduced to the patient via an intravenous infusion.

Term	Meaning
petechiae (singular, petechia)	Tiny localized hemorrhages of the blood vessels just beneath the surface of the skin.
Peyer patches	A clump of lymphoid tissue located in the mucosa of the small intestine.
photosensitivity	Sensitivity to light.
polyarthritis	Inflammation and soft tissue swelling of many joints at the same time.
protease inhibitors	A group of drugs to treat HIV, which involves interrupting the ability of the virus to make copies of itself in later stages of infection.
purpura	Red or purple discolorations caused by bleeding from blood vessels under the skin.
Raynaud phenomenon	A symptom of scleroderma in which blood vessels in the fingers become narrow, diminishing blood supply and causing fingers to become pale, waxy-white, or purple in cold temperatures.
receptor	A molecule on the surface of a T cell that receives signals from antigens.
Reed-Sternberg cells	A kind of cell specific to Hodgkin lymphoma.
rheumatic fever	An acute inflammatory disease involving the heart (as well as the skin, joints, and other tissues) caused by the body's immune reaction to a preceding streptococcal infection.
rheumatoid arthritis (RA)	An autoimmune disorder in which the immune system attacks and causes inflammation of the joints and surrounding tissues of the body.
rheumatoid factor (RF)	An antibody found in the blood of most patients with rheumatoid arthritis.
SCL-70	A blood test that isolates the scleroderma antibody.
sclerodactyly	A symptom of scleroderma in which the skin becomes thickened and tight from loss of subcutaneous tissue.
scleroderma	A chronic autoimmune disorder that affects the blood and connective tissue of the body, causing skin to harden and scar.
self and nonself	A concept that describes the ability of cells to recognize what belongs in the body and what does not.
severe combined immuno-deficiency disease (SCID)	A rare congenital disorder in infants resulting in a lack of all major immune defenses.
Sjögren syndrome	An autoimmune disorder in which the immune system attacks and destroys cells in the excretory glands, resulting in lack of saliva and tears.
SLE disease activity index (SLEDAI)	A score derived from the level of activity of a lupus flare.
spleen	The largest organ of the lymphatic system, which stores lymphocytes that assist the body in fighting infections.
stem cells	Immature cells that grow into different types of cells.
synovectomy	The removal of inflamed synovial tissue from the joints.
systemic lupus erythematosus (SLE), syn. lupus	A multisystem autoimmune disease characterized by achy joints; inflammation of the fibrous tissue surrounding the heart; unexplained rashes on the face, neck, or scalp; and other disorders.
systemic scleroderma	A more widespread form of scleroderma, initially affecting the skin and then gradually involving the esophagus, lungs, intestines or other organs, causing them to function abnormally.
T cells	A type of lymphocyte that matures in the thymus, which detects invading bacteria or viruses and stimulates B cells to produce antibodies against them.
Takayasu arteritis	A form of vasculitis that affects the aorta and its branches.

Term	Meaning
tendon reconstruction	A procedure in which an intact tendon is attached to a damaged one.
thrombocytopenia	Abnormally low levels of platelets in the blood.
thymus	A gland that produces mature T cells, found in the thorax under the breastbone.
thyroglobulin	A protein produced by normal thyroid tissue.
thyroid	A butterfly-shaped gland located in the neck, just below the larynx.
thyroid-stimulating hormone (TSH)	A hormone produced by the pituitary gland that enables the thyroid gland to produce thyroid hormone.
thyroxine (T4)	A hormone produced by the thyroid gland which helps to regulate the body's metabolism.
titer	The concentration or strength of a substance in a particular solution.
tonsils	A clump of lymphoid tissue located in the back of the throat.
triiodothyronine (T3)	A hormone produced by the thyroid gland that helps regulate the body's metabolism.
vasculitis	An inflammation of the blood vessels and the different disorders that can result therefrom.
vasodilators	Drugs that improve blood flow to vessels by dilating them.
Venereal Disease Research Laboratory (VDRL) test	A test used to diagnose syphilis but which is also used to diagnose the presence of the anticardiolipin antibody in lupus.
Wegener granulomatosis	A form of vasculitis that affects primarily the lungs, kidneys, and upper respiratory tract.

Add Your Own Terms and Definitions Here:

_____

_____

_____

_____

_____

_____

_____

_____

REVIEW QUESTIONS

1. Describe the components of the immune system's defense layers.
2. What are lymphatic vessels and what is their function?
3. What is the difference between active and passive immunity?
4. What is the SLEDAI scoring system?
5. Name one theory proposed by researchers as to why the body's immune system may attack itself.
6. What is the difference between immunodeficiency and autoimmunity?
7. How do vasodilators improve the symptoms of some autoimmune diseases?
8. What types of cells engulf and destroy all types of pathogens?
9. Name four places in the body where clumps of lymphoid tissue may be found.
10. How do monoclonal antibodies work to fight autoimmune disease?

CHAPTER ACTIVITIES

Soundalike Word Choice

Circle the correct word in the following sentences.

1. Ms. Sanders is a 54-year-old African American female with a history of systemic lupus (erythrocytosis, erythematosus).
2. During his most recent hospitalization, Mr. Smith was found to have a small axillary (lymph, limp) node.
3. Her laboratory results showed that anti-double-stranded (DNA, DMA) was borderline positive at 30.
4. Imaging studies revealed the patient to have a right upper extremity (inclusion, occlusion) of the brachial and cephalic veins that was repaired in the operating room.
5. Joint examination was without evidence of (syringitis, synovitis) and with full range of motion in all of the joints.
6. Quantitative (myoglobulins, immunoglobulins) revealed an elevated IgA at 763, with the upper limit of normal being 474.
7. Because of further relapses in her disease, she was given (Remicade, Remeron) infusions every 2 months in addition to the (cyclobenzaprine, cyclosporine).
8. The patient is on Coumadin for his antiphospholipid (antigen, antibody) syndrome and history of pulmonary (embolism, embolization).
9. This 35-year-old female with (SLE, SBE) is known to have (anticardiolyte, anticardiolipin).
10. On questioning, it seems that the patient has noticed some improvement in his symptoms, with only occasional aches and pains and (flares, flairs) of his disease.

Immune Disorder Match

Match the immune disorder with the following descriptive characteristics (some disorders may be used more than once).

Clue

1. _____ exophthalmos
2. _____ bone marrow transplant
3. _____ petechiae
4. _____ dry eyes
5. _____ hyperthyroidism
6. _____ cancer of lymphocytes
7. _____ weakened blood vessel walls
8. _____ nodules on hands
9. _____ hypothyroidism
10. _____ SLEDAI
11. _____ histamine
12. _____ Reed-Sternberg cells
13. _____ deviated fingers
14. _____ "like a wolf"
15. _____ Raynaud phenomenon
16. _____ HIV
17. _____ hard, scarred skin
18. _____ tendon reconstruction
19. _____ goiter
20. _____ giant cell arteritis

Disorder

A. rheumatoid arthritis
B. lupus
C. Sjögren syndrome
D. allergies
E. Graves disease
F. Hashimoto thyroiditis
G. Hodgkin disease
H. vasculitis
I. scleroderma
J. lymphoma
K. AIDS

Choose the Correct Abbreviation

Circle the correct abbreviation in the following sentences. Then write out the meaning of the abbreviation.

1. A pooled solution of antibodies administered intravenously is called (ILIG/IVIG).

   _____

2. In an (ESE/ESR) test, the speed at which red blood cells settle in a glass tube containing a specimen of unclotted blood is measured.

   _____

3. A common manifestation of (RP/RA) is inflammation and swelling of the joints and tissues of the hands.

   _____

4. A (BMT/BMP) is used to treat patients whose bone marrow is destroyed by high doses of chemotherapy.

   _____

5. The (ADA/ANA) test looks for antibodies that react against the nuclear material of cells.

   _____

6. Abnormally low levels of red blood cells can be detected in a (CBC/CDC) test.

   _____

7. (LA/LC) is an antibody test used to check for antiphospholipid syndrome.

   _____

8. A (TTF/TNF) inhibitor is a drug that bolsters a person's immune responses.

   _____

9. Physicians use the (SLEDAK/SLEDAI) test to measure the degree of a patient's lupus activity.

   _____

10. A positive response to a (VDDL/VDRL) test does not mean a patient has syphilis.

   _____

Medicine Match

How well do you remember the medications you have learned about so far? Match the names of the following medications with their corresponding descriptions.

Description

1. _____ An anticonvulsant medication used to treat epilepsy.

2. _____ An immune system suppressor used to treat, among other diseases, some gastrointestinal (GI) disorders.

3. _____ An angiotensin-converting enzyme (ACE) inhibitor used to prevent the formation of angiotensin II that constricts the blood vessels; this drug causes blood vessels to dilate and blood pressure to decrease.

4. _____ A drug used to stimulate ovulation.

5. _____ A calcium channel blocker used to treat hypertension.

6. _____ A medication used to remedy dizziness.

7. _____ Used as an antispasmodic for an overactive bladder.

8. _____ A proton pump inhibitor (PPI) used to treat gastroesophageal reflux disease (GERD).

9. _____ A bronchodilator used in reversible airway obstruction due to asthma or chronic obstructive pulmonary disease (COPD).

10. _____ A drug given with levodopa to treat Parkinson disease.

Name

A. Procardia

B. Albuterol

C. Nexium

D. Ditropan

E. Carbidopa

F. Clomid

G. Depakote

H. Lisinopril

I. 6-MP

J. Antiver

Converting Nouns to Adjectives

Convert each of the following nouns into its adjectival form.

1. immunology _____

2. nodule _____

3. spleen _____

4. vasculitis _____

5. cell _____

6. allergy _____

7. petechia _____

8. vein _____

9. lymph _____

10. arthritis _____

Proofreading for Context

Read the following note and circle the inappropriate words in the clinic report that would not fit in context (there are no errors in punctuation or formatting, only words). Then write the correct word in the numbered space below the report. There are 17 errors in total. The first one has been identified for you.

REASON FOR VISIT: Systemic lupus erythema.

INTERVAL HISTORY: This 32-year-old Caucasian female comes in for routine file-up of her lupus. She has had SBE for 10 years now. She mentions some morning stillness in her joints that is not any worse from previous visits. She also has had 2 episodes of either lower back pain or hip pain in the last 7 months. Most recently was 2 weeks ago and it lasted about 2 weeks. This is slowly resulting. She did actually have a bilateral hip MTI scan which was completely negative.

PHYSICAL EXAMINATION: On physical exam, the weight is 160 pints, temperature 99.1 degrees, blood pressure 121/65, height 5 feet 5 feet. On physical examination of the skin, there is no rash present. She does have some acne present and will be following up with a dermatologist. On HENNT, there are no nasal ulcers and no aural thrush in the buccal mucosa present. On chest exam, she is clear to auscultation bilaterally. Cardiac exam reveals regular right and rhythm without murmurs, rubs, or gallops. Abdominal exam shows she is soft and nontender with positive bowl sounds. On extremity exam, there is no clubbing, cyanosis, or edema. On comprehensive muscular-skeletal exam, she does have some arthralgias of her MVPs of the hands and knees. There is no synovitis present. Neurologically she is nonfocal.

ASSESSMENT AND PLAN:

1. SLE with arthralgias. On the SLEDOG, there are no descriptors circled.
2. She does have some facial acne. She will follow up with a dermatologist. I do not think that it is in relation to any of her current medications.
3. We do recommend a DEKA scan as she has never had one done and she was on chronic prednisone use in childhood.
4. She has had these episodes of lower back pain and questionable hop pain. At the next occurrence, we asked her to contact the office and we would consider medication such as Flexeril as a muscle relaxant to see if some of this is due to muscle spasm.

CORRECT TERMS:

1. _____erythematosus_____
2. _____
3. _____
4. _____
5. _____
6. _____
7. _____
8. _____
9. _____
10. _____
11. _____
12. _____
13. _____
14. _____
15. _____
16. _____
17. _____

TRANSCRIPTION PRACTICE

Open your word-processing software. Insert the student CD-ROM and locate the dictation for this chapter. For each of the words in the "listen for these terms" list for each report, use a medical dictionary or other resources to identify and write down a brief definition of the term on a separate sheet of paper to attach with your work. Then listen to the dictation and transcribe each report. Use the current date for each report where a date is indicated. Insert a heading into the document if the text falls to a second page.

At the end of each report, indicate the name of the dictating physician under the signature line and insert reference initials. For date dictated and transcribed and date of admission, use the current date. Proofread your work, print one copy for your instructor along with your term definitions, and save the completed report to your student disk.

Report T19.1: Clinic Note
Patient Name: Jodie Kleinfeld
Medical Record No.: 168903
Attending Physician: Kamraan George, MD

Listen for these terms:
CREST syndrome
metformin
calcinosis cutis
telangiectasia

Report T19.2: Consultation Letter
Patient Name: Sandy Barber
Medical Record No.: 35-43922
Attending Physician: Lena Kushner, MD
Letter addressed to: Stefanie Warner, MD, Medical Pavilion, 500 South Commerce Street, Suite 203, St. Louis, MO 63109

Listen for these terms:
follicular small cleaved cell lymphoma
intrapulmonary parenchymal mass
hypoproteinemia
hypogammaglobulinemia
CHOP
Rituxan
nephrotic syndrome
perineoplastic
hematopathologists

Report T19.3: Clinic Note
Patient Name: Nicole Burgess
Medical Record No.: 463711
Attending Physician: Andrea Biggs, MD

Listen for these terms:
serositis
retropubic lymph nodes
serpiginous
speckled pattern
RVVT
beta-2 glycoprotein

20

ONCOLOGY

OBJECTIVES

After completing this chapter, you will be able to:

- Discuss the concept of cancer and cell structure.
- Explain the genetic development of cancer.
- Describe risk factors related to the development of cancer.
- Discuss the systems used to grade and classify cancers according to their severity or metastasis.
- Describe common laboratory tests and diagnostic procedures used to analyze, detect, and diagnose cancer.
- Describe common treatment modalities used to treat cancer.

INTRODUCTION

The word *cancer* scares most people, and with good reason. Although typically cancer develops over a long period before producing symptoms, the disease often makes its presence known without warning, altering one's course of life and causing anxiety and uncertainty about the future. Despite regular media reports of potential cures, this disease continues to be one of the leading causes of death in the United States, exceeded only by heart disease.

Oncology is the branch of medicine that deals with the study of the development, diagnosis, treatment, and prevention of cancer. The term derives from the combining form, *onc/o*, meaning mass or bulk, referring to tumors. An **oncologist** is a physician who specializes in the treatment of cancer. Because cancer can occur in any body system, the field of oncology is broad. Many oncologists specialize in a particular branch of the disease, such as organ cancer or blood diseases. Some oncologists concentrate their practices on cancer treatments, such as chemotherapy, radiation, or surgery, whereas others serve in areas of research and clinical studies.

Because cancer is a complex and serious illness, medical management of the disease consists of care from a variety of professionals who comprise a patient's oncology healthcare team. A medical transcriptionist working in the field of oncology might transcribe reports from social workers, rehabilitation specialists, nutritionists, specialists in several areas of oncology, and other healthcare providers. These professionals work together to help patients maintain their quality of life while providing the best possible medical treatment and support through the entire process. This chapter provides a basic explanation of the process by which cancer develops from a single cell, the methods used to diagnose cancer, and various treatment options for management of the disease.

The term **cancer** is the name given to a group of related diseases that all have to do with the abnormal transformation, or **carcinogenesis**, of normal cells in the body into cancer. Carcinogenesis involves normal cells that enlarge and divide more rapidly than normal and serve no useful purpose. The word *cancer* is derived from the Latin word for *crab*, so named for the invasive extensions that emanate from the main body of a tumor mass. It is estimated that 90% of all cancers develop because of complex interactions among the cells in the body, lifestyle, genetic makeup, and environment. In all, there are around 200 different types of cancer that can affect the human body. Some types of cancer are more serious than others, and some can be treated more easily than others.

CELL STRUCTURE

Cells are called the *building blocks of life*. All living things, whether plants, animals, people, or tiny microscopic organisms, are made up of cells. A **cell** is the smallest living unit of the structure that makes up all living organ-

isms. Cells are organized into tissues, which are then organized into organs. Cells carry out metabolism, the sum of all of the physical and chemical activities that occur in the body in order for it to survive, as well as the various signals used by cells to communicate with each other. Although these fundamental processes seem relatively straightforward, many of them require complicated cascades of biochemical reactions. All body functions derive from the activities of trillions of cells.

Figure 20.1 illustrates a diagram of a typical animal cell. Cells are surrounded by a **cell membrane**, which is the permeable barrier that envelopes the cell and protects its contents. The cell membrane allows water and nutrients to enter the cell and waste products to leave the cell. The cell is filled with a gel-like substance called **cytoplasm**. The cytoplasm contains different structural units called **organelles**, which are responsible for different functions of cell development, including the production of proteins, the generation of energy, and the process of cell division. Think of organelles as being similar to the organs in the body; your heart, liver, and brain are all organs performing specific functions to make the body work.

In the center of each cell is the **nucleus**, which contains the cell's control center. The nucleus of each cell

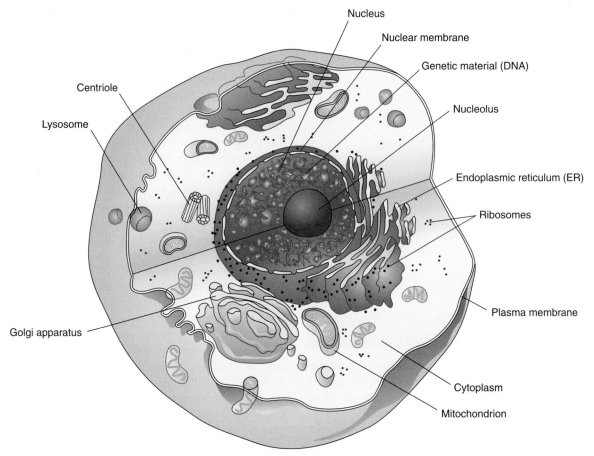

FIGURE 20.1. The Cell. This diagram shows a typical animal cell containing the main organelles. Reprinted with permission from Cohen BJ, Wood DL. *Memmler's The Human Body in Health and Disease.* 9th ed. Philadelphia: Lippincott Williams & Wilkins, 2000.

Strand 1   Strand 2

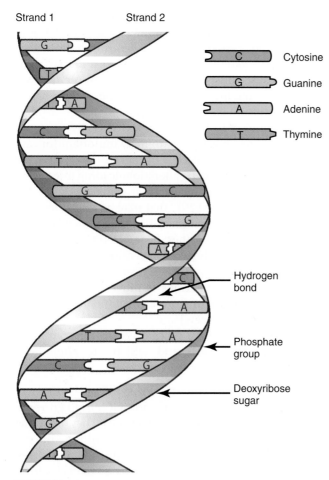

C   Cytosine

G   Guanine

A   Adenine

T   Thymine

Hydrogen
bond

Phosphate
group

Deoxyribose
sugar

FIGURE 20.2. **The Structure of DNA**. The four main chemical bases of DNA can be arranged in countless ways. Reprinted with permission from Premkumar K. *The Massage Connection Anatomy and Physiology*. Baltimore: Lippincott Williams & Wilkins, 2004.

contains 46 **chromosomes**, which carry genetic information. Chromosomes are composed of long strands of a complex organic substance called **deoxyribonucleic acid** (DNA). DNA is a vast chemical information database that carries the complete set of instructions for making all the proteins a cell will ever need. DNA appears as two long, paired strands spiraled into a double helix, as shown in Figure 20.2. Each strand is made up of millions of chemical building blocks called bases. There are only four different chemical bases in DNA, but they can be arranged and rearranged in countless ways. The order in which the bases occur determines the messages to be conveyed, much as specific letters of the alphabet combine to form words and sentences. Each cell has 46 molecules of DNA. Each DNA molecule is made up of 50 to 250 million bases housed in a single chromosome.

DNA is organized into separate functional units of heredity called **genes**. Genes occupy specific places on the chromosomes of cells and control the formation of enzymes needed for metabolic reactions. Within each chromosome, there are many hundreds to thousands of genes. Genes tell the cell to do a specific task, usually to make a particular protein. **Proteins** are large, complex molecules that perform a wide variety of activities in a cell. Some genes direct the formation of structural proteins that eventually determine physical features such as brown eyes or curly hair; other genes provide instructions for the body to produce proteins that help direct and control the chemical reactions that occur in the body. For example, certain proteins help one cell divide into two, whereas other proteins prevent the cell from dividing too often. Each human cell has about 30,000 genes; each one makes a protein with a unique function. A healthy body depends on the continuous interplay of thousands of proteins acting together in just the right amounts and in just the right places—and each properly functioning protein is the product of an intact gene. Sometimes, depending on the codes of a specific gene, an error within the DNA structure can produce serious problems that affect the entire body, resulting in significant physical disability or a shortened lifespan.

Cells undergo a process of **mitosis**, or cell division, which keeps the body supplied with healthy cells. In mitosis, a cell's chromosomes are doubled and then equally divided between two daughter cells. The process goes on continuously in an orderly fashion in response to a particular need by the body. For example, skin cells are constantly being shed from the surface of the body and must be replaced. When cell division runs out of control and the daughter cells invade other tissues, a cancer results.

HOW CANCER DEVELOPS

Like all of nature, the cells of the human body conduct their life cycles in a predictable biological pattern of growth, reproduction, and death. The body is composed of trillions of cells, which all behave in accordance with natural laws that have evolved to follow a prearranged routine unless disrupted by a disease or abnormality that causes that cycle to go awry.

Every cell in the body is programmed to perform a certain job. With the exception of the brain and nerve cells, the rest continually develop, divide, die, and are replaced with new cells. Just as in any society, some individuals choose to ignore the societal norms and march to the tune of their own drummers. In the body, some rogue cells deviate from the laws regulating their growth and function. Cancer is a biological process of these rogue cells, which aim to reproduce not for the good of the host, but to kill it.

Cancer begins when genes that control the orderly replication of cells become damaged, allowing the cells to reproduce without restraint. No one knows what causes the genetic machinery that directs a cell's division to go awry, but when it happens, the cell may continue growing at a faster-than-normal rate or may keep dividing indefinitely, rather than dying. These aberrant cells create dysfunctional masses of tissue that compress other organs and commandeer nutrients the body needs to survive. They grow and spread rapidly, uncontrollably, and independently, and may spread from the primary site of growth to other tissues.

The body has the ability to protect itself against a cell that contains flawed genetic messages to overproduce. For instance, killer T cells, discussed in Chapter 19, *Immunology*, can detect and eliminate a mutated cell. However, sometimes the body's search-and-destroy immune system fails, and a malformed cell can continue on its present course of generating more and more copies of itself. These cells can escape their normal habitats and move to other parts of the body, like rampant marauders, to invade and conquer every tissue group they encounter. Eventually this invasion causes our bodies to fall into ruin.

Despite the complexities and varieties of cancer, it all begins in the genes of just one cell. The cell's progress from normal to malignant appears to involve a series of distinct changes in the tumor and its immediate environment, and each is influenced by different sets of genes. Under a microscope, cancer cells appear to be different from normal cells in that they lose a number of their vital control systems. This change is referred to as a **mutation**. A gene mutation is a permanent change in the DNA sequence that makes up a gene, which causes changes in the way a cell behaves. Mutations range in size from a single DNA building block to a large segment of a chromosome. There are two ways in which DNA can become mutated:

- Mutations can be inherited. If a parent has a mutation in his or her DNA, then the mutation is passed on to his or her children. This occurrence, however, is actually small and comprises perhaps only 5% to 10% of all cancer cases.
- Mutations can be acquired. Most cancers derive from random mutations that develop in body cells during one's lifetime, either as a mistake when cells are going through cell division or in response to injuries from environmental agents such as radiation or chemicals. Cells often self-destruct if they carry a mutation, or they may be recognized by the immune system as abnormal and be destroyed. Some mutations, however, escape these safeguards to turn into a cancer. It can also occur as a result of a viral infection, a chronic inflammation, or from a chemical, such as those found in tobacco smoke.

Genes can be mutated in several different ways. The simplest type of mutation involves a change in a single base along the base sequence of a particular gene—much like a typographical error in a word that has been misspelled. In other cases, one or more bases may be added or deleted. And sometimes large segments of a DNA molecule are accidentally repeated, deleted, or moved. If the mutation occurs in a gene that helps control how often a cell divides or one that checks for errors in cell division, it may contribute to a person developing cancer, or cancer may occur because the mutation happens in a gene that normally causes a defective cell to die. Most scientists today believe that cancer develops in a process that involves more than one, and likely several, mutation.

The discovery of certain types of genes that contribute to cancer has been extremely important for cancer research. More than 90% of cancers are observed to have some type of genetic alteration, leading researchers to think that most cancers have genetic origins. For example, a gene called *PTC* that may be linked to basal cell carcinoma has been identified on a particular chromosome, whereas another gene, *HNPCC*, has been identified by researchers as increasing an individual's chance of getting colon cancer. A small percentage (5% to 10%) of these alterations is inherited, whereas the rest occur by chance or from environmental exposures (usually over many years).

There are two main types of genes that can affect cancerous cell growth and which are altered, or mutated, in certain types of cancers:

- **Oncogenes** are mutated forms of genes that activate cell division, causing normal cells to grow out of control and become cancer cells. They are mutations of genes that normally control how often a cell divides and the degree to which it specializes. For example, cells multiply to repair damage after a wound or operation. When these genes mutate into oncogenes, they alter the cells' DNA to signal cells to grow uncontrollably. To use a simple comparison, an oncogene is like the gas pedal of an automobile. The effect of a damaged oncogene is similar to that of a gas pedal that becomes stuck to the floorboard, causing the automobile to move faster and faster. When this occurs, the cell continually grows and divides, which can lead to cancer.
- **Tumor suppressor genes** are typically found in normal human cells. These genes can recognize abnormal growth and reproduction of damaged cells, or cancer cells, and can halt cell division and prevent the cell from multiplying or doubling until the defect is corrected. They slow down cell division, repair DNA mistakes, and tell cells when to die. If the tumor suppressor genes are mutated, however, the cells will carry on multiplying. For example, *p53* is a well-known tumor suppressor gene. This gene normally stops cells with other damaged genes from reproducing, but certain kinds of mutations transform these cells and they cannot perform properly. This gene is damaged or missing in most human cancers.

In order for cancer to develop and grow, there must be a change in the gene that affects cell growth and exposure to something that promotes such growth, called a

carcinogen. A carcinogen is something that causes cells with DNA mutations to multiply and become tumors. This explains why not all women who inherit a breast cancer gene actually develop the disease and why not all smokers get lung cancer. A carcinogen speeds up the pace of cell division, which can create more genetic mutations and eventually lead to cancer. It can be a hormone, such as estrogen, or a toxic substance, such as a chemical in tobacco smoke. The abnormal cell then progresses to out-of-control growth, which forms the basis for all cancers. Cells accumulate to form a tumor, and the tumor keeps growing, sometimes extending into adjacent tissues. In addition to all the molecular changes that occur within a cancer cell, the environment around the tumor changes dramatically as well. The cancer cell loses receptors that would normally respond to neighboring cells that call for growth to stop. Instead, tumors amplify their own supply of growth signals.

In addition, the cells may metastasize to other parts of the body, forming clusters there. How quickly this progression takes place is determined in part by genetic programming, but also is influenced by conditions in the body, such as the presence of hormones that may encourage the growth of cancer cells. However, even during this process, the immune system may still destroy cancer cells, significantly affecting how quickly the disease progresses. Theoretically, the body develops cancer cells continuously, but the immune system recognizes them as foreign cells and destroys them. Because of this action on the part of the immune system, cancer growth may be so slow that the malignant cells never cause a problem. In fact, it is estimated that cancer is present in the organs of 10% to 15% of people who die from other causes.

A **lesion** is a general term that refers to any area of altered tissue. A dense mass of abnormal cells is called a **tumor**. A tumor mass, inflammation, scar tissue, or dead tissue are all examples of lesions that may be found in the body. Determining the nature of a tumor is the work of a pathologist. Cells that grow beyond their normally defined limits are called **neoplastic cells**. The word **neoplasia** literally means *new growth*, and this term is used to describe an abnormal, disorganized growth in a tissue or organ, usually forming a distinct mass. Such a growth is called a **neoplasm**, also known as a *tumor*. The terms *neoplasia* and *cancer* are often incorrectly used interchangeably. *Neoplasia* refers to both benign and malignant growths, whereas the term *cancer* refers specifically to malignant neoplasia. Therefore, neoplastic cells that invade and destroy tissue, or spread to other parts of the body, are cancerous. Although all cancers are neoplasias, not all neoplasias are cancerous. For example, common warts are neoplastic but not cancerous. Most problems associated with aging arise from neoplasias. Cataracts, arthritis, and even arthrosclerosis result from the unchecked proliferation of normal tissue cells. Cancer occurs when cells that are not normal begin to grow and divide uncontrollably and do not die.

Not all cancers behave in the same way. The progression from a tiny, unnoticeable cluster of abnormal cells to a detectable tumor may take years, or the growth can be so swift as to be almost immediately detectable. For example, one man may have prostate cancer that grows extremely slowly, produces no symptoms, and never spreads beyond the prostate; eventually he dies from some other cause. Another man may learn that he has advanced metastatic prostate cancer less than a year after a normal screening test.

Cancers can originate almost anywhere in the body and are classified by their histologic origin:

- **Carcinomas**, the most common types of cancer, arise from the epithelial tissues, or cells that cover external and internal body surfaces, such as the lungs, breasts, or colon.
- **Adenocarcinomas** arise from epithelial and glandular tissues.
- **Sarcomas** arise from connective or supporting tissues such as bone, cartilage, or muscle.
- **Gliomas** arise from glial cells.
- **Melanomas** arise from pigmented skin cells.
- **Myelomas** arise from plasma cells.
- **Lymphomas** arise from lymphatic tissues of the body's immune system, as discussed previously in Chapter 19, *Immunology*.

Leukemias are cancers of the blood derived from the overabundance of very immature white blood cells called **leukocytes**. The term derives from the Greek words for *white* and *blood*, and is often considered a disease of children, yet it actually affects far more adults. Every day, hundreds of billions of new blood cells are produced in the bone marrow, most of them red cells called **erythrocytes**. In people with leukemia, however, the body starts producing more white leukocytes than it needs. Many of these extra white cells do not mature normally, yet they live well beyond their normal life span and continue to replicate uncontrollably. These immature cells are unable to fight infection the way normal white blood cells do, and as they accumulate, they crowd out other vital cell production in the bone marrow that are needed for vital body function. As a result, the body does not have enough erythrocytes to supply oxygen to organs and tissues, enough **platelets** (clotting cells, also called *thrombocytes*) to ensure proper blood clotting, or enough normal, mature white blood cells to fight infection, making people susceptible to bruising, bleeding, and infection. Leukemias are classified according to the type of blood cell involved and whether the onset of symptoms is acute (of rapid onset) or chronic (occurring more slowly).

- **Acute myelogenous leukemia** (AML), caused by too many myeloblasts and myelocytes.

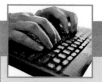

TRANSCRIPTION TIP:

You may hear a physician use a term that sounds like "b-c-r, able." This refers to a genetic abnormality common to CML patients. These patients have what is called the **Philadelphia chromosome**, a defective chromosome in a cell's genetic makeup. This chromosome is caused when a piece of one chromosome (22) breaks off and attaches to the end of another chromosome (9), and a piece of chromosome 9 also breaks off and attaches to the end of chromosome 22. The break on chromosome 9 involves a gene called *Abl*. The break on chromosome 22 involves a gene called *Bcr*. The *Bcr* and *Abl* genes combine to make the CML-causing gene called the **bcr/abl gene**, which is transcribed in all lowercase letters.

- **Chronic myelogenous leukemia** (CML), a result of too many myeloblasts and myelocytes as well as mature neutrophils, eosinophils, and basophils.
- **Acute lymphocytic leukemia** (ALL), a result of too many lymphoblasts.
- **Chronic lymphocytic leukemia** (CLL), caused by too many mature lymphocytes.

Tumors can be either benign or malignant. **Benign** tumors are not cancerous; in fact, the word *benign* means *harmless*. A benign tumor consists of a cluster of cells that grows very slowly. The tumor has a distinct border and rarely spreads to other parts of the body. Benign tumors are almost never life-threatening in and of themselves; however, they are usually removed surgically when their growth begins to interfere with the ability of healthy tissues to grow and thrive. If allowed to grow unchecked, they can displace soft tissue (such as that found in the brain) or apply pressure to vital body organs, resulting in organ dysfunction or death. A benign tumor may also be removed surgically when it becomes unsightly. For example, a brain tumor composed of benign cells, but located in a vital area, could be considered life-threatening even though the tumor and its cells would not be classified as malignant. Once removed, a benign tumor usually does not return.

Malignant tumors, on the other hand, are dangerous. A malignant tumor is characterized by progressive and uncontrolled growth. The mass does not have distinct borders, is fast growing, invasive, and can spread throughout the body. By definition, the term *cancer* applies only to malignant tumors.

Malignant tumors spread throughout the body by two mechanisms: invasion and metastasis. **Invasion** refers to the direct migration and penetration by cancer cells into neighboring tissues. **Metastasis** refers to the migration of cancer cells from the original tumor site to produce cancers in other parts of the body. Cancerous cells can metastasize to healthy tissue and organs in other sites in a variety of ways, as shown in Figure 20.3. A cancer that is growing at the site in which it originated in the body is called the **primary cancer**, or sometimes dictated simply as *the primary*. The place to which a cancer spreads and starts growing is called the **secondary cancer**, or *the metastasis*.

Regardless of where a cancer may spread, cancerous tumors are usually named after the part of the body where the cancer first began. The name does not change even if the cancer spreads to another part of the body. For example, if a breast cancer (the primary) spreads, or metastasizes, to the lung (the secondary), it is still termed a breast cancer primary but with lung metastasis. This fact is important with regard to treatment. In the preceding example, if chemotherapy is indicated as the best treatment, breast cancer drugs would be used to treat the lung tumor.

CANCER RISK FACTORS

A **risk factor** is something that may increase the chance of developing a disease. Examples of risk factors for cancer include age, a family history of certain cancers, use of tobacco products, diet and obesity, exposure to radiation or other cancer-causing agents, and certain genetic changes. Some cancers, particularly in adults, have been associated with certain risk factors. A risk factor does not necessarily cause the disease, but it may make the body less resistant to it. Common cancer risk factors discussed by physicians in medical reports include:

- Diet. Food additives such as nitrates and food preparation methods like charbroiling may introduce carcinogens into the body. Diets high in fat have been linked to increased risk of cancer as well. Obesity is the second biggest risk factor for some types of cancer.
- Genetic factors. Scientists believe that family history, or **heredity**, may play an important role in some adult and childhood cancers. By definition, heredity is the genetic inheritance passed on from the DNA of the mother and father to child. Although some gene alterations are inherited, this does not necessarily mean that the person will develop cancer, but rather indicates that the chance of developing cancer increases. About 50 types of cancer have a tendency to run in families.
- Virus exposure. Exposures to certain viruses, such as the human papillomavirus (HPV), human immunodeficiency virus (HIV), and the herpes virus, have been linked to an increased risk of developing certain types of cancers. Researchers believe the virus may alter a cell in some way, causing

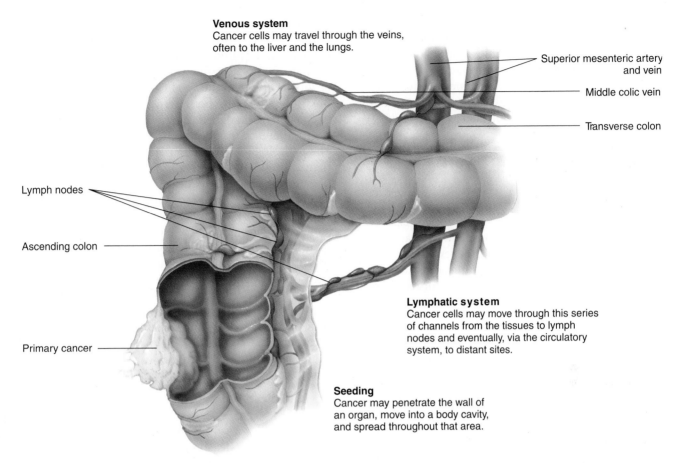

Venous system
Cancer cells may travel through the veins, often to the liver and the lungs.

Superior mesenteric artery and vein

Middle colic vein

Transverse colon

Lymph nodes

Ascending colon

Lymphatic system
Cancer cells may move through this series of channels from the tissues to lymph nodes and eventually, via the circulatory system, to distant sites.

Primary cancer

Seeding
Cancer may penetrate the wall of an organ, move into a body cavity, and spread throughout that area.

FIGURE 20.3. **How Cancer Spreads.** Cancer cells may invade nearby tissues or spread to other organs. Cancer cells may move to other tissues by any or all of three routes: venous system, lymphatic system, seeding. Asset provided by Anatomical Chart Co.

it to become a cancer cell that reproduces more cancer cells.

- Environmental exposures. Many substances commonly found in the environment may induce carcinogenesis by damaging cellular DNA. Some proven carcinogens in humans include asbestos, vinyl chloride, airborne hydrocarbons, pesticides, and tobacco smoke.
- Ineffective immune response. Theoretically, the body develops cancer cells continuously but the

immune system recognizes them as foreign cells and destroys them. Tumor growth is enhanced when the immune system is weakened or destroyed as a result of other factors, such as infection, acquired immunodeficiency syndrome (AIDS), or cytoxic drugs, as discussed in Chapter 19, *Immunology*.

Unfortunately, it is common for cancer to return months or years after the primary tumor has been removed. This occurs because by the time the primary tumor was discovered, cancer cells had already broken

QUICK CHECK 20.1

Fill in the blanks with the correct answers.

1. The formal name given to cell division is _____.

2. Cancers that arise from cells found in the connective tissues of the body are called _____.

3. A dense mass of abnormal tissue is called a _____.

4. A change in a cell's genes is referred to as a _____.

5. The word *benign* means _____.

away and lodged in distant locations in the body but had not yet formed tumors large enough to be detected. Cancer that recurs after all visible tumor had been eradicated is referred to as **recurrent disease**. Disease that recurs in the area of the primary tumor is referred to as a **local recurrence**, and disease that recurs as metastases is referred to as a **distant recurrence**.

CANCER CLASSIFICATION SYSTEMS

When analyzing tumor cells, pathologists classify a tumor's appearance by stage and grade to establish the severity and amount of spread of the lesion. This information helps to facilitate communication among a patient's various medical providers in order to plan treatment and to predict the outcome of treatment.

Grade

A tumor's **grade** indicates its degree of intensity or severity in relation to what normal cells in the area look like. Whereas normal cells tend to have an orderly and mature structure, cancer cells appear immature and incompletely developed. To determine the grade of a tumor, a sample of tissue (or, on occasion, the entire tumor) is removed during a biopsy for microscopic examination by a pathologist. Based on the microscopic appearance of cancer cells, the pathologist describes tumor grade by four degrees of severity, transcribed in arabic numbers 1 through 4, as follows:

- Grade 1: Cells differ slightly from normal cells.
- Grade 2: Cells are more abnormal than grade 1 cells.
- Grade 3: Cells are very abnormal and hard to differentiate.
- Grade 4: Cells are immature, primitive, and undifferentiated. It is difficult to decide the origin of the cells.

The cells of a grade 1 tumor nearly resemble normal cells and tend to grow and multiply slowly, whereas the cells of a grade 3 or 4 tumor that appear immature and not normally developed tend to grow rapidly and spread faster than tumors with a lower grade. A tumor's grade is transcribed with the word "grade" in lowercase letters, followed by the arabic number 1, 2, 3, or 4.

> Example:　grade 1
> 　　　　　grade 2

In addition, other classifications are used for specific types of cancer. For example, pathologists use the **Gleason system** to describe the degree of differentiation of prostate cancer cells. The Gleason system uses scores ranging from 1 to 5 to indicate each dominant pattern

and secondary pattern, with the two numbers then totaled for the score. Lower total Gleason scores describe well-differentiated, less aggressive tumors. Higher scores describe poorly differentiated, more aggressive tumors. The final Gleason score is the combination of two numbers, derived from adding the two highest grades assigned to two tissue samples extracted from different areas of the prostate during the biopsy. The pathologist will assign patterns to each section of tissue samples, the most common pattern in one sample and the second most common pattern in another specimen. Assigning a combined grade to the two most common patterns allows for a better prediction about the prognosis. The lowest possible Gleason score is 2 (1 + 1), where both the primary and secondary patterns have a Gleason score of 1. A typical Gleason score might be 5 (2 + 3), where the primary pattern has a Gleason grade of 2 and the secondary pattern has a grade of 3. In dictation, a Gleason score is typically heard as a formula, such as "The patient had a Gleason score of 4 plus 3 equals 7." This sentence would be transcribed with the word "grade" or "score" in lowercase letters, followed by arabic numbers.

> Example:　The patient had a Gleason score of 4 + 3 = 7.
> 　　　　　The patient was diagnosed with a Gleason grade 3 + 3 = 6 carcinoma of the prostate.

Stage

A cancer's **stage** indicates whether a tumor has spread, or metastasized, beyond the site of its origin. Staging a tumor helps physicians evaluate its aggressiveness and prognosis, and the tumor is evaluated by physical examinations, imaging studies, laboratory tests, and pathology reports. The stage is indicated using zero and then roman numerals. The more a tumor has spread throughout the body, the higher the stage of the tumor, as follows:

- Stage 0: The cancer is located only in a precise tumor and is not invading the organ.
- Stage I: Cancer cells are breaking through to normal tissue but no lymph nodes are involved.
- Stage II: There is a limited, local spread of cancer to the lymph nodes but the disease has not yet advanced to stage III.
- Stage III: There is an extensive local and regional spread of cancer cells.
- Stage IV: The cancer has spread (metastasized) to a distant part of the body.

In transcription, the word "stage" is not capitalized, followed by a roman numeral of I through IV. For many cancers, the overall staging is further divided within subdivisions using capital letters and arabic numbers, and without internal commas, spaces, or hyphens.

TABLE 20.1   Staging Cancer by the TNM System

Letter	Meaning	Description	Structure
T	Tumor	The anatomic extent of the primary tumor is based on size, depth of invasion, and surface spread.	TX: Primary tumor cannot be assessed T0: No evidence of primary tumor T1: Tumor invades submucosa T2: Tumor invades muscular coating of a structure T3: Tumor invades through muscle layer to connective tissue T4: Tumor directly invades organs or structures
N	Nodes	Nodal involvement reflects tumor's spread to the lymph nodes.	NX: Regional lymph nodes cannot be assessed N0: No evidence of regional lymph node metastasis N1: Metastasis in 1 to 3 regional lymph nodes N2: Metastasis in 4 or more regional lymph nodes
M	Metastasis	The extent or spread of disease from the original site.	MX: Distant metastasis cannot be assessed M0: No evidence of distant metastasis M1: Distant metastasis present

Example: stage III
                 stage IIIA
                 stage IIB3

The **TNM system** is a staging system for primary malignant tumors developed by the American Joint Committee on Cancer. This system uses the letters T, N, and M, and numbers 1 through 4 to help describe the size of a primary tumor (T), whether there are lymph nodes with cancer cells in them (N), and whether the cancer has spread to a different part of the body, as in metastasis (M). As the size of the primary tumor increases, the T number increases. Likewise, the amount of lymph nodes involved determines the N number, and whether metastases exist determines the M number. The staging is transcribed with no spaces between the letter and the number, and no space between each letter designation. An uppercase "X" next to the letter indicates that a parameter could not be assessed. See Table 20.1 for a description of the structure of this system. For example, breast cancer T3N2M0 refers to a large tumor that has spread outside the breast to nearby lymph nodes, but not to other parts of the body.

Example: T2N1M0
                 T1aN1MX
                 T1NXMX

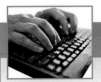

TRANSCRIPTION TIP:

Do not use an apostrophe with the word *Dukes*. The term is *Dukes*, not *Duke's* or *Duke*.

Other classification systems are also used for specific types of cancers. For example, colon carcinoma is staged by the **Dukes classification system**. This system is used to classify cancers relating to the colon or rectum. It is transcribed using the word *Dukes* followed by a capital letter, and subdivided by arabic numbers with no spaces in between.

Example: Dukes A
                 Dukes C3

The **Clark level system** is used to describe the level of malignant melanoma of the skin from the epidermis. It is transcribed using roman numerals and the word "level" in lowercase.

Example: Clark level I
                 Clark level IV

FIGO staging is used to measure gynecologic malignancy, particularly involving the ovary. FIGO is an acronym for the *Federation Internationale de Gynecologie et Obstetrique*, the originators of the system. FIGO grades are transcribed with the word "stage" in lowercase letters, followed by a roman numeral and lowercase letters to indicate subdivisions within the stage. In dictation, this acronym sounds like one word, *FI-go*.

Example: FIGO stage II
                 FIGO stage IIIc

The **Jewett classification** is used to classify bladder carcinomas using the letters O, A, B, C, or D. It is indicated by typing the name Jewett followed by the letter classification.

Example: Jewett class B
                 Jewett class O

Performance Status

The term **performance status** relates to quantification of a cancer patient's general well-being. Physicians use this measure to determine whether a patient can receive chemotherapy, whether a dose adjustment is necessary, and as a measure of the patient's quality of life when used in oncological controlled trials of new medications and treatments.

The **Karnofsky Performance Status** (KPS) is a scale used to rate a cancer patient's general well-being and ability to perform ordinary tasks. The total score ranges from 0 to 100 using intervals of 10, where 100 is "perfect" health and 0 is death. A higher score means the patient is better able to carry out daily activities. KPS may be used to determine a patient's prognosis, to measure changes in a patient's ability to function, or to decide if a patient could be included in a clinical trial. This value is indicated with the word *Karnofsky* and arabic numbers.

Example: 10, 20, 30, 40, 50, 60, 70, 80, 90, 100
Karnofsky 10

A second system used to rate a cancer patient's performance is the **ECOG scale**. ECOG stands for the *Eastern Cooperative Oncology Group* and uses a rating scale from 0 to 5, with 0 indicating the patient is fully active and able to carry on all pre-disease performance without restriction, and 5 indicating the patient is deceased. In dictation, this acronym sounds like one word: *E-cog*.

Example: The patient's status is ECOG 3.
The patient's status is currently ECOG 2.

DIAGNOSTIC STUDIES AND PROCEDURES

In general, the sooner a cancer is diagnosed, the better the chance of treating it successfully; most cancers, if left alone, are fatal. Physicians use laboratory tests and imaging studies not only to detect and assess malignant disease and monitor the effects of treatment, but also to increase the chance of early detection of a new or metastasized cancer.

Laboratory Studies

Laboratory tests serve an important function in identifying and measuring particular substances characteristic of various tumors. Some of the tests commonly performed to look for evidence of disease include the following:

Blood Tests

Blood tests are routinely performed to check the levels of substances in the blood that indicate how healthy the body is, whether an infection is present, and how well a patient's body is responding to therapy. For example, a comprehensive metabolic panel (CMP) can indicate an elevated level of waste products such as creatinine or blood urea nitrogen (BUN) in the body, which may indicate that the kidneys are not working efficiently to filter toxic substances. Electrolytes, such as sodium and potassium, can be checked to ensure they are at adequate levels for the body's healthy functioning.

A complete blood count (CBC) provides information about the white blood cells (WBCs), red blood cells (RBCs), and platelets present in a sample of blood, including the number, type, size, shape, and some of the characteristics of the cells. If there are abnormalities in the counts in one or more of these cell populations, it may be an indication that additional tests are necessary. For example, WBCs that are found in low numbers in a normal sample may appear elevated in a person with an abnormal proliferation of cells, such as in leukemia. A blood sample may also show large numbers of more primitive blood cells called myeloblasts (commonly dictated as, simply, *blasts*). A depletion of RBCs in a blood sample may indicate the presence of **anemia**, which is a condition in which blood does not carry enough oxygen to the rest of the body due to a deficiency in red blood cells. A drop in platelet count may indicate a problem with **coagulation**, or how quickly blood clots.

Tumor Markers

A **tumor marker** is a substance produced by tumor cells or other cells in the body in response to cancer. They are either released into the blood, urine, tumor tissue, or in other tissues. Different tumor markers are found in different types of cancer, and although their presence does not confirm the presence of cancer by themselves, a tumor marker can signal cancer that affects many parts of the body. To date, researchers have identified more than a dozen substances that increase to abnormal levels when some types of cancer are present; therefore, they can help to detect tumors, evaluate the extent of disease, monitor response to treatment, and check for tumor recurrence. Some of the more common tumor markers include the following:

- **Prostate-specific antigen** (PSA). PSA, as discussed in Chapter 15, *Urology*, is a substance made only by the prostate. An elevated PSA level may help detect prostate cancer in its early stages, before a tumor is large enough to be felt by the physician during a rectal examination. Because other factors elevate PSA, such as an enlarged prostate or infection of the prostate, this test is often used in conjunction with other blood tests to make a definitive diagnosis.
- **CA125** (which sounds like *C-A one twenty-five* when dictated). This protein is often found on the surface of ovarian cancer cells, although cancers of the uterus, cervix, pancreas, liver, colon, breast,

QUICK CHECK 20.2 ✓

Circle the letter corresponding to the best answer to the following questions.

1. The Gleason system is used to describe cancer cells related to the
   A. bladder.
   B. urethra.
   C. prostate.
   D. scrotum.

2. Something that may increase the chance of developing a disease is called a(n)
   A. risk factor.
   B. primary recurrence.
   C. tumor grade.
   D. performance status.

3. Cancer that returns after all visible tumor had been eradicated is called
   A. a primary tumor.
   B. recurrent disease.
   C. a distant metastasis.
   D. secondary cancer.

4. The "N" in the TNM staging system stands for
   A. necrosis.
   B. lymph node.
   C. metastasis.
   D tumor.

5. The quantification of a patient's general well-being is called the
   A. risk factor.
   B. stage.
   C. Jewett classification scale.
   D. performance status.

lung, and digestive tract can also raise CA125 levels. CA125 is mainly used to evaluate and monitor cancers of the reproductive system, including the uterus, fallopian tubes, and ovaries.

- **Carcinoembryonic antigen** (CEA). This tumor marker can signal cancer that affects the large bowel, stomach, pancreas, lungs, or breasts as well as some sarcomas, such as leukemias and lymphomas.
- **Alpha-fetoprotein** (AFP). This substance is normally elevated in pregnant women, since it is produced by the fetus. However, in men and in women who are not pregnant, an elevation of AFP can suggest testicular, ovarian, gastric, pancreatic, or primary lung cancers.
- **Human chorionic gonadotropin** (hCG). hCG, another substance that appears normally in pregnancy, is produced by the placenta. In men and in women who are not pregnant, however, elevated hCG levels may indicate cancer in the testis, ovary, liver, stomach, pancreas, or lung.
- **CA19-9** (which sounds like *C A nineteen dash nine* when dictated). This marker is a protein that exists on the surface of certain cells, making it useful as a tumor marker commonly associated with cancers in the colon, stomach, and biliary tract.
- **CA27.29** (which sounds like *C A twenty-seven twenty-nine* when dictated). This marker is used to

follow the course of treatment for women with advanced breast cancer, although cancers of the colon, stomach, kidney, lung, ovary, pancreas, uterus, and liver may also raise CA27.29 levels. Note this tumor marker is transcribed using a period instead of a hyphen.

- **HER2/neu** (which sounds like *HER-two-NEW* in dictation). HER2/neu is a protein found on the surface of breast cells, which sends messages to the cells from growth factors outside the cell, instructing them to grow. Although everyone has the HER2/neu protein, in some breast cancers, the cells produce many more HER2/neu proteins than normal. These breast cancers are called **HER2/neu-positive** cancers. Breast cancers that have very few HER2/neu proteins, or none at all, are called **HER2/neu-negative** cancers. HER2/neu-positive breast cancers grow faster than HER2/neu-negative breast cancers, tend to resist conventional treatment therapies, and have an overall poorer prognosis than HER2/neu negative cancers.

Fecal Occult Blood Test

A fecal occult blood test, also called a stool guaiac test (pronounced like *GWI*-yac in dictation), evaluates stool samples for traces of hidden, or *occult*, blood that cannot be seen with the naked eye. This test is used as a screening test to detect colorectal cancer, especially when the cancer is in its early stages and is not causing any symptoms. Sometimes physicians refer to the test using the name of the commercially produced slide kit that is given to patients to use in order to obtain the stool sample for testing. A positive finding usually leads to further tests, such as a colonoscopy or sigmoidoscopy, to detect polyps or tumors.

Genetic Testing

New technology in genetic testing has revolutionized the ability of researchers to detect cancer remotely and to ensure the correct form of treatment for a particular cancer. These techniques involve the direct examination of the DNA molecule itself, which has enabled scientists to understand how the genes within the human chromosomes determine how the body will be built in the womb and control its further growth and development. Researchers now understand the relationship of genes to cancer; that is, that cancer is a disease of the genes, which manifests when the normal genetic control mechanisms overtake cell function.

Genetic testing involves analysis of a patient's DNA to assess that individual's risk of a particular disease. The test determines whether the DNA contains a genetic mutation that has also been found in many other people with that disease. For example, it is estimated that about 10% of breast cancer cases are hereditary. In many of these cases, a person has inherited a gene from his or her parents that has mutated. This mutated gene makes it easier for a person to get cancer.

For example, the test for the BRCA1 and BRCA2 genes assesses the risk of developing breast or ovarian cancer associated with inheriting the genetic abnormalities in *BRCA1* or *BRCA2*, the genes linked with these cancers. Everyone has two genes called BRCA1 and BRCA2. Normally, these genes help to prevent cancerous tumors from growing. But sometimes a person inherits an abnormal form of BRCA1 or BRCA2 from his or her family. The mutation of these genes provides a significantly elevated risk for developing primarily breast cancer and ovarian cancer. BRCA mutations are inherited and are passed from generation to generation.

Women from Ashkenazi Jewish families are more likely than other women to carry abnormal BRCA1 and BRCA2 genes, and this ethnic group is often mentioned by physicians in dictation when discussing genetic testing for breast cancer.

Genetic testing enables physicians to take several approaches to manage cancer risk in those individuals who have been found to have a genetic mutation or predisposition for a certain cancer. These include:

- Surveillance by careful monitoring of symptoms and signs for the onset of cancer, with screening tests that include regular physical examinations and measurement of blood tumor markers.
- Prophylactic surgery, which entails the removal of as much of the at-risk tissue as possible in order to reduce the chances of developing cancer. The term **prophylaxis** means the prevention of disease or of a process that can lead to disease. For example, preventive mastectomy, or the removal of healthy breasts, or oophorectomy, the removal of healthy ovaries, may be performed to help lessen the risk of a woman developing cancer.
- Chemoprevention in the form of medications, such as tamoxifen, or nutritional supplements, like vitamin E or selenium, can be used to help prevent new cancers from developing when the existence of certain genetic mutations is known.
- Gene therapy which, in the future, can be used to repair or manipulate the genes or sets of genes that cause or increase one's risk for cancer and other illnesses.

Biopsy

A **biopsy** is also referred to as *diagnostic surgery*. Diagnostic surgery can remove a small tissue sample or the entire tumor so that it can be examined under a microscope and identified. Common types of diagnostic surgeries include the following:

- **Excisional biopsy**, in which the entire tumor is removed for microscopic examination.
- **Incisional biopsy**, in which a small piece of the tumor is removed for analysis under the microscope.
- **Fine-needle biopsy**, in which a fine needle is used to withdraw a small tissue sample or fluid from the tumor.
- **Core biopsy**, in which a large needle is used to withdraw samples of tissue.
- **Endoscopy**, in which a flexible tube with a camera or viewing lens, called an endoscope, is passed through a very small incision made in the body (or through a natural body opening) to view and remove a sample of suspicious tissue located in the thorax or gastrointestinal system. Specific types of endoscopies include **laparoscopy**, **thoracoscopy**,

TRANSCRIPTION TIP:

Hemoccult is the brand name of the fecal occult blood test kit used by physicians for this test. Therefore, this term is capitalized when used in dictation.

Example: "The patient's Hemoccult test was negative for blood in the stool."

and **mediastinoscopy**, in which a tube with a lighted lens is passed through a very small incision into the abdomen, thorax, or mediastinum, respectively, to view suspicious areas and to remove a sample of tissue.

Imaging Studies

Imaging studies alone cannot treat cancer, but they do help physicians make better decisions about treatments. Imaging techniques produce pictures of what is going on inside the body, using different types of energy such as x-rays, sound waves, radioactive particles, and magnetic fields. The changes in energy patterns caused by different body tissues are detected by special imaging devices, which convert the changes into images. These images enable a physician to find a cancer, evaluate how far it has spread, determine the type of treatment needed, or find out if a specific treatment is working. In addition, imaging studies can be used to see if a previously treated cancer has returned.

The most familiar type of imaging, x-rays (or radiographs), produce shadowlike images of certain organs and tissues that may reveal tumors or other diseases in the body. In dictation, the image or series of images produced by the x-ray machine are sometimes referred to collectively as **radiographic studies**. For example, a chest x-ray is used to detect lung disorders such as cancer. A **mammogram** is a special type of x-ray that allows doctors to visualize breast tissue to look for tumors or suspicious lumps in the breasts. Pictures are taken of each breast from top to bottom and from side to side to detect any abnormality more precisely.

A **digital mammogram** also uses x-rays, but the data are collected on a computer instead of film. These computer-enhanced images are sharper in detail and can also be magnified, theoretically detecting suspicious areas that the human eye might miss. **Computer-aided detection** (CAD) technology is an important component of digital mammography. It increases the sensitivity for detecting small lesions and calcifications in the breast. Once breast images have been taken, CAD technology acts like a second pair of eyes, reviewing the images after the radiologist has made an initial interpretation—similar to the way a spell-checker program might alert a writer to a misspelled word in a document—without altering the original films. Using sophisticated pattern recognition computer software, CAD technology can mark patterns of bright spots that suggest **microcalcifications**, which are tiny calcium deposits that may indicate cancer. In addition, it can detect dense regions in the breast that may suggest a mass or distortion.

To use CAD technology, the original mammogram films are first loaded into a special processing unit that digitizes the mammogram images. The CAD unit then analyzes the digitized images of the films and highlights any detected breast abnormalities using special pattern recognition computer software. The digitized mammogram files are then transmitted to a computer monitor so the radiologist can compare the original films to the digitized mammogram image. The radiologist can magnify that portion of the image indicated by computer as potentially abnormal and further study these areas to determine whether any areas are suspicious and might require further evaluation. Based on the results of the CAD marker information, the radiologist may choose to reexamine the original mammogram films and modify his or her interpretation, when appropriate.

Studies show that CAD analysis can improve the detection of early cancers by as much as 20% by reviewing a patient's mammogram films after the radiologist has already made an initial interpretation. Some radiologists cite the high cost of CAD technology and the tendency of the software to sometimes mark a fairly high number of "normal" areas on mammograms as abnormalities that may lead to additional unnecessary and costly breast imaging and/or biopsies. However, many physicians believe that CAD will become more widespread in the coming years as more mammography facilities acquire digital mammography and CAD technology.

Computed tomography (CT) scanning uses computer-controlled x-rays to create three-dimensional images of the body that are more vivid than standard x-rays. Unlike a standard x-ray machine, which produces only single-view, flat-type images, the CT scanner creates hundreds of images from several different angles via a rotating device, which are then assembled on a computer. The detailed pictures show the body in cross-sectional views, or slices, from head to toe (as if looking down through the head or up through the feet). The images can be enlarged, making them easier to read and interpret. With CT scans, not only can physicians determine if a tumor is present, but also the approximate depth of the tumor in the body. The images can show a tumor's shape, size, volume, and location, and can even reveal the blood vessels that feed the tumor. Physicians often use these sharp, three-dimensional images to help precisely guide a needle into the tumor to remove a tissue sample, called a **CT-guided biopsy**, or to guide a needle into a tumor to facilitate certain cancer treatments, such as to obtain a biopsy or completely excising the tumor.

A **spiral CT scanner** is faster type of CT machine. In this procedure, the scanner part of the machine rotates around the body continuously, allowing images to be collected more quickly than with a standard CT scanner and lowering the chance of blurred images occurring as a result of the patient moving or breathing while the images are being taken. The spiral CT yields even more detailed three-dimensional images, and by placing the images on top of each other, doctors can create an image on a computer screen that can be rotated to allow for different views.

The use of highly advanced computers to aid in locating and creating a three-dimensional image of a tumor in the body is called **stereotaxy**. When used during surgery, the technique is called **stereotactic surgery**. When used to obtain a biopsy of a sample of tissue, the term is **stereotactic biopsy**. Stereotactic surgery may be used during a biopsy or for tumor removal, while implanting radiation wafers or pellets, or to provide a system of navigation during surgery. This technique is especially useful in locating and removing tumors deep in the brain. Sometimes a frame to position and steady the skull is used for the procedure. In this case, a lightweight frame is attached to the skull at four points and an image is produced by CT or magnetic resonance imaging (MRI). Because the scan shows both the tumor and the frame, the exact location of the tumor in three dimensions in relation to the head frame is displayed. The neurosurgeon is then able to insert a probe through a small incision in the skull to perform the biopsy or other procedure more precisely.

Like CT scans, MRI displays a cross-section of the body, but it uses powerful magnetic fields instead of radiation to create the images. The MRI measures the electromagnetic signals given off naturally by the body and can create images of soft tissue parts of the body that would sometimes be hard to see using other imaging techniques.

An MRI scanner houses a very strong magnet weighing several tons. As the patient lies on a table within the scanner, the device surrounds him or her with a powerful magnetic field. The magnetic force causes the hydrogen atoms in the body to line up in one direction. Once the atoms are lined up, the machine emits a burst of radiofrequency waves, causing the atoms to change their alignment. When they return to their original positions, the atoms emit certain signals that the scanner detects. A computer interprets the signals from these changes and converts them into two-dimentional and three-dimensional images. The MRI is especially helpful in detecting tumors in the brain, spinal cord, head, neck, bones, and muscles.

Positron emission tomography (PET) produces computerized images of chemical changes, such as sugar metabolism, that take place in cells. Physicians track how much glucose is metabolized in different areas of the body by injecting a radioactive tracer to map the body's use of the fuel. The PET scanner and computer work together to create images of the cells at work. Because cancer cells are dividing rapidly, they break down glucose at a much higher rate than do normal cells. This activity will show up on the scan as a *hot spot*, or glow, on the PET image. Unlike CT, the PET scan is able to detect microscopic amounts of cancer cells that remain after treatment and to verify that a suspicious mass is truly cancer. Because they can actually see the metabolism of the tumor, physicians can determine whether it is benign or malignant, if it has spread, and whether treatment has been successful.

Ultrasound is a diagnostic test that uses sound waves with frequencies above those which humans can hear to create images of internal organs. A transducer sends sound waves traveling into the body. These waves are then reflected back from organs and tissues, allowing images to be made of those anatomic structures. Ultrasound can show tumors and, like CT, can also guide physicians in the placement of a needle into a tumor to remove a tissue sample for biopsy; this procedure is called an **ultrasound-guided biopsy**.

In addition to the diagnostic and imaging tests described in this chapter, regular medical checkups along with regular laboratory studies and imaging of organs increase the chance of early detection of a new or metastasized cancer. These regularly scheduled tests, called **screening tests**, enable physicians to find hidden cancers before they reach advanced stages or to detect abnormalities before they become full-fledged cancers. These tests are referred to as screening tests because they are performed on healthy people who have no symptoms

QUICK CHECK 20.3 ✓

Fill in the blanks with the correct answers.

1. The lab test that checks for blood in stool is called a _____ test.

2. A procedure in which a large needle is used to withdraw samples of tissue is called a _____.

3. A substance produced by cells in response to cancer are called _____.

4. Regular medical checkups and imaging of organs to detect new or metastasized cancer are called _____.

5. The two genes linked to an increased risk of inheriting breast or ovarian cancer are _____ and _____.

for the sole purpose of looking for a condition that could lead to cancer or on patients with an existing cancer to look for any evidence of recurrence. For example, a Pap smear is a screening test that detects not only cervical cancer but changes in cervical cells that suggest cancer may develop in the future. The detection of cellular and tissue changes early with the use of screening tests is the first step in halting the possible development of cancer later.

CANCER TREATMENTS

The effectiveness of any kind of cancer treatment depends on a number of factors: the type of cancer, the location of the disease, and the extent to which the cancer has spread to other parts of the body. Treatment for cancer is focused mainly on removing the cancer cells or destroying them in the body with medicines or other agents. This treatment is usually a combination approach, which may include surgery to remove the cancerous cells, chemotherapy and radiation therapy, as well as methods of chemoprevention to keep the cancer from recurring.

Surgery

When a person has cancer, surgical intervention is often indicated. Surgery can be a simple procedure, such as removal of a small skin cancer or lump, or it can become complex, involving nearby organs, tissues, and lymph nodes.

Often more than one surgical procedure is required. The surgical biopsy is used first to remove a sample of tissue or, using a fine needle, to obtain a fluid sample. The specimen is examined by a pathologist to provide grading and staging information about its size, spread, and type of cancer. Another surgery may then follow to remove as much of the affected tissue as possible.

Surgical excision of a tumor in its early stage, along with some healthy tissue around it, may completely cure the cancer. Such curative surgery requires that the tumor be confined to a particular area, such as an organ, so that it can be safely removed in its entirety. Some special curative surgeries commonly used include:

- Laser surgery, which uses high-intensity light to shrink or destroy tumors on the surface of the body or the linings of internal organs.
- Cryosurgery, which destroys abnormal tissues with the use of extreme cold produced by liquid nitrogen. This type of surgery is often used to treat external tumors, such as skin cancers. If used internally, the liquid nitrogen is applied to the tumor with the use of a hollow tube called a cryoprobe.
- Mohs surgery is commonly used to treat skin cancers by shaving the tumor off the skin, one layer at a time. Each layer is inspected under the micro-

scope, and the shaving is stopped when all the cells of the shaved tissue look normal.
- Laparoscopic surgery is performed by passing a small lighted tube through a small incision in the body. The laparoscope can than be used to both remove the tumor and examine the tissues and organs surrounding the tumor for any additional suspicious areas.
- Electrosurgery uses high-frequency electrical current to destroy cancer cells and is used mostly for cancers of the skin and mouth.

When it is not possible to completely remove a tumor, **debulking surgery** is used to excise as much of the cancerous tissue as possible to reduce its size. The remaining tumor cells are then treated with chemotherapy or radiation. In some cases, surgery is used to only relieve the symptoms caused by a cancerous tumor. This procedure, called **palliative surgery**, can relieve pain or other symptoms to give a person more comfort and an improved quality of life, even though the surgery is not likely to cure the cancer or even prolong a person's life. For example, some cancers in the abdomen may grow large enough to affect bowel function, thereby warranting the use of surgery to provide effective relief. Surgery to remove an organ that has a high chance of developing cancer is called prophylactic, or preventive, surgery. For example, polyps in the colon may be considered precancerous and, therefore, preventive surgery is used to remove the tissue to prevent transformation to colon cancer. Finally, **reconstructive surgery** is a followup to other surgeries in order to help return the function and appearance of the area of the body where the tumor was located.

Chemotherapy

Chemotherapy is any regimen of therapy that makes use of **cytotoxic** chemicals, or drugs poisonous or destructive to cells, to treat cancer. Chemotherapy works by impairing the ability of cancer cells to duplicate themselves or by artificially starting the normal process of cell death, called **apoptosis**. Normally apoptosis, or programmed cell death, occurs when a cell detects that it has become infected or damaged. Apoptosis controls the numbers of cells in the body at a given time and provides signals to the body when new cells are needed. Cancerous cells resist apoptosis and continue to reproduce more rapidly than the number of cells dying, leading to overall tumor growth. Chemotherapy drugs are used to stop this process by altering the behavior of tumor cells or by killing the tumor cells entirely. As a palliative treatment, chemotherapy can improve a patient's quality of life by relieving pain and other symptoms.

The drugs used in chemotherapy often vary with the type of cancer being treated and how much the tumor has spread to other parts of the body. Chemotherapy regimens are typically administered in regular intervals and doses according to the number of days that make up a cell's reproductive process in order to stop cancer cells from completing the duplication process. Some chemotherapy drugs act during specific parts of the cell cycle. This type of drug includes etoposide (VP-16), hydroxyurea (Hydrea), methotrexate (MTX), procarbazine (Matulane), and temozolomide (Temodar). Other drugs are given any time during the cell cycle. Common non-cell-cycle-specific drugs include cisplatin (CDDP), carmustine (BCNU), lomustine (CCNU), irinotecan (CPT-11), sirolimus (Rapamune), and vincristine (Vincasor PFS).

Chemotherapy, whether given orally or via an injection or infusion, travels through the body via the blood to enter tumor cells. **Interstitial chemotherapy** is the term used to describe the placement of chemotherapy drugs directly into a tumor, as shown in Figure 20.4. With some tumors, such as those involving the brain or spine, chemotherapy can be delivered directly into the cerebrospinal fluid (CSF) of the brain and spinal cord, a method called **intrathecal chemotherapy**.

The most common system used in intrathecal chemotherapy is an **Ommaya reservoir**, which is a small channel-type device through which medications or fluids can be given directly into the brain or spinal cord. It consists of a dome-shaped container that is placed under the scalp and a tube that leads off the dome. The end of the tube may be directed into a cyst or tumor in the brain or spinal cord, or in one of the four ventricles of the brain where CSF is produced. Chemotherapy medications are injected via a syringe into the reservoir and then the reservoir is pumped by pressing the dome up and down to push the medication through the tube into the target space and to prevent it from becoming blocked.

Another method of delivering chemotherapy directly to a tumor is the implantation of a **polymer implant wafer** directly into the tumor site. The implantable, biodegradable wafer, which is saturated with a chemotherapy drug, is commonly referenced in reports pertaining to patients with high-grade malignant brain tumors. After resection of as much of the tumor as possible, several wafers are inserted into the tumor cavity and are left there to dissolve over a two- to

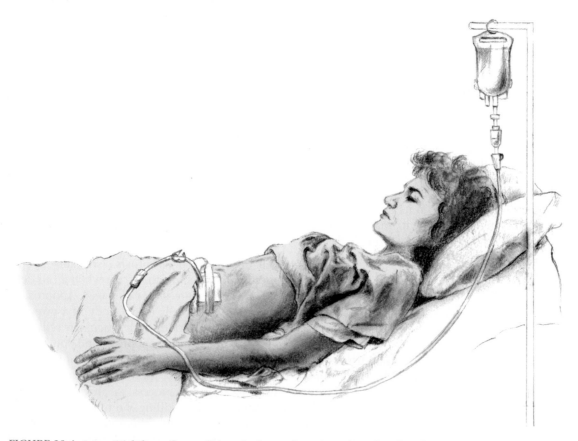

FIGURE 20.4. Interstitial Chemotherapy. This method passes drugs via a catheter directly to the tumor area, exposing cancer cells to high concentrations of chemotherapy—up to 1,000 times the amount that can be safely given by other methods. Reprinted with permission from *Nursing Procedures*, 4th ed. Ambler: Lippincott Williams & Wilkins, 2004.

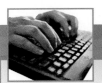

three-week period. In this way, concentrated doses of the drug (approximately 100 times higher than can be infused intravenously) are delivered directly to the tumor site. In dictation, physicians most often refer to the wafers by their brand name, **Gliadel**, with the phrase, "Gliadel wafers."

In some instances, higher doses of chemotherapy drugs are more effective than lower drug doses spread over a longer period. **High-dose chemotherapy** is a procedure that involves the administration of massive doses of a chemotherapy drug, followed by an antidote, which reverses the effect of the drug on healthy cells. For example, methotrexate is often used for high-dose chemotherapy with another drug, Leucovorin, as the most common antidote. In this instance, a physician may dictate, "The patient was given high-dose methotrexate with Leucovorin rescue."

Chemotherapy is often associated with debilitating side effects, but many types of chemotherapy used today cause only mild problems. Physicians are constantly trying out new chemotherapy combinations and regimens to improve treatment. Therefore, transcription of reports detailing chemotherapy sessions frequently involves learning new regimens and the new terminology used to describe them.

Radiation Therapy

Radiation therapy, also called *radiotherapy*, consists of using high-energy radioactive waves to destroy or disable cancerous cells. Radiation treatment is designed to destroy the rapidly dividing cancer cells by targeting and destroying the cell's DNA while, at the same time, damaging the surrounding normal cells as little as possible. A **radiation oncologist** is a physician who coordinates and manages a patient's radiation treatment.

Radiation therapy is a local treatment in that it affects cancer cells only in the treated area. It may be used with other forms of treatment such as chemotherapy and surgery. In fact, it is often used to shrink the size of a tumor, which is then removed during surgery. It can also be used to treat a malignancy not accessible through surgery.

The machinery used in radiotherapy is similar to x-ray equipment except that it contains a source of high-

energy radiation, such as radium or a radioactive isotope of cobalt. There are two types of radiation treatments. **External beam radiation**, as shown in Figure 20.5, is delivered externally to the specific part of the body affected by the tumor. This type of radiation targets only the tumor and a small percentage of surrounding healthy tissue. **Internal radiation treatment** is administered through ingestion, injection, or by catheter.

Chemoprevention

Chemoprevention involves the use of a natural or synthetic substance, such as a nutrient or a drug, to keep cancer at bay or to derail the disease process before the cancer becomes invasive. The basic principle behind chemoprevention is to change the way in which cells behave. Some chemopreventatives interfere with whatever is stimulating cellular reproduction, whereas others improve the body's ability to detoxify a harmful substance or to repair genetic damage caused by a virus.

Today scientists are studying several hundred compounds for possible chemopreventive actions through clinical trials. In breast cancer, tamoxifen and raloxifene are drugs that have been found to dramatically reduce the chances of breast cancer in women at high risk for the disease. These drugs belong to a class of drugs called **selective estrogen receptor modulators** (SERMs). Throughout the body, these drugs block the function of estrogen by binding to cell receptors that would otherwise bind to estrogen. Drugs like tamoxifen and raloxifene bind to the receptors in place of estrogen, thereby blocking the effects of estrogen. They are used to treat estrogen-receptor-positive advanced breast cancer and, for women whose estrogen-receptor breast cancer is early stage, to keep the cancer from recurring after treatment.

Aromatase inhibitors are a group of drugs designed to reduce estrogen levels in a woman's body by preventing an enzyme called **aromatase** from converting other hormones (such as testosterone) to estrogens. By reducing the amount of estrogen in the body, breast cancer cells are deprived of the fuel they need to grow and thrive. Three aromatase inhibitors commonly encountered in medical reports are anastrozole (Arimidex), exemestane (Aromasin), and letrozole (Femara).

Clinical Trials

A **clinical trial** is a research study that tests how well a new medical treatment works in people. There are many clinical trials in progress at any one time, and each one seeks to answer specific questions about how to prevent, detect, diagnose, or treat a disease, including cancer.

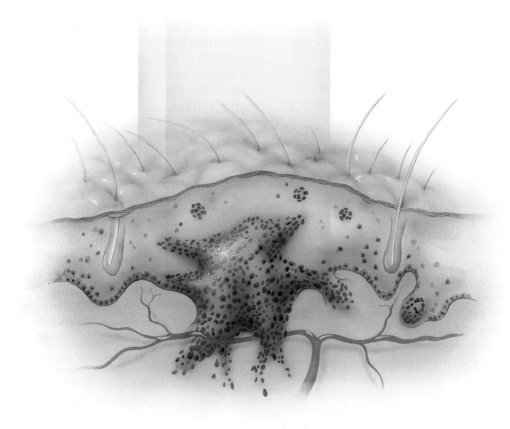

FIGURE 20.5. Radiation Chemotherapy. External beam radiation consists of using high-energy radioactive waves (in yellow) delivered externally to a specific part of the body to destroy or disable cancerous cells (in purple). Asset provided by Anatomical Chart Co.

Patients who take part in these studies are called **participants**.

Clinical trials help to move the setting for basic scientific research about a drug or condition from the laboratory into the patient's treatment room. They are the final step in a long research process required to make a new drug or treatment modality available to the public.

TRANSCRIPTION TIP:

The amount of radiation energy absorbed by irradiated tissue is measured in centigray (cGy) and should always be transcribed using the abbreviated form.

For example:

Dictated:	"The patient was given radiation at a dose of six thousand centigray."
Transcribed:	"The patient was given radiation at a dose of 6000 cGy."

Government agencies, such as the National Cancer Institute (NCI) or National Institutes of Health (NIH), sponsor and conduct clinical trials. In addition, medical organizations such as hospitals, foundations, and pharmaceutical companies also sponsor clinical trials. The name of the trial may have a simple title (such as the STAR trial, an actual NIH-sponsored study comparing breast cancer treatment drugs) or use a combination of letters and numbers indicating a particular name or property of the drug being studied, such as RTOG-0522.

Every clinical trial has a plan, called a **protocol**, which acts as a blueprint for the physicians and research centers conducting the trial. The protocol describes what will be done in the study, how it will be conducted, and why each part of the study is necessary. The protocol also contains guidelines about who can or cannot participate in the study. These guidelines, called **eligibility criteria**, describe characteristics that must be shared by all participants in the study. For example, treatment studies may require that the patients have the same age, gender, or medical history. They often require that patients have a particular type and stage of cancer in order to participate. The enrollment of

QUICK CHECK 20.4 ✓

Indicate whether the following sentences are true (T) or false (F).

1. Clinical trials are open only to women.   T   F

2. Interstitial chemotherapy refers to the delivery of radioactive waves to the tumor.   T   F

3. A Gliadel wafer is biodegradable and will dissolve in the body on its own.   T   F

4. Aromatase inhibitors are designed to aid in providing better images of a tumor on x-ray.   T   F

5. A clinical trial typically consists of four phases.   T   F

---

participants with similar characteristics ensures that the results of the trial can be accurately attributed to what is being studied and not other factors related to the participants.

A clinical trial typically takes place in four phases, each designed to answer different research questions:

- Phase I looks at the safety of a new cancer agent or treatment in patients. This part of the trial studies the best way to give patients the new agent (for example, by pill or injection), how often it should be given, what the safest dose is, and whether the new agent is of benefit.

- Phase II continues to test the safety of the new agent and begins to evaluate how well it works against a specific type of cancer. Participation in phase II trials is often restricted based on the previous treatment received; that is, participants in these trials have been treated with chemotherapy or other treatment modalities, but the treatment has not been effective.

- Phase III compares a new treatment to the standard, or most widely accepted treatment, for a disease. Researchers investigate whether the new treatment is better than, the same as, or worse than the standard treatment. These studies are called **randomized clinical trials**, as participants are randomly (i.e., by chance) assigned to one of two or more treatment groups in the trial. Most randomized trials have at least two groups, called **arms**, but

some have three or more, depending on the treatments being compared. The participants are placed into one of the arms of the study at random, via a computer program or table of random numbers. Randomization ensures that unknown factors, such as human choices, beliefs about which treatment they think is best, or other factors, do not influence the trial results. Participants have an equal chance of being assigned to a group of patients who are receiving the standard treatment or to the group that is getting the new treatment.

- Phase IV continues to further evaluate the long-term safety and effectiveness of the new treatment. These trials usually take place after the new treatment has been approved by the U.S. Food and Drug Administration (FDA) for standard use.

After the clinical trial is completed, researchers analyze all of the collected data, interpret the results, and make decisions about further testing. The researchers then inform the medical community and the public of the trial results. Once a new drug or intervention is proven safe and effective in a clinical trial, it may become the new standard of practice for physicians.

CHAPTER SUMMARY

Despite years of research and millions of dollars in funding, scientists have yet to discover a cure for cancer. Although early detection, prevention, and new, aggressive treatments have led to improved success rates and longer life expectancies for cancer patients, a definitive cure for the disease continues to elude medical experts. But research continues, and a medical transcriptionist working in this field will be among the first to learn of the advancements and discoveries researchers make as they work toward eradicating this disease.

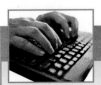

TRANSCRIPTION TIP:

Physicians often will revert to acronyms when dictating about cancer trials. For example, physicians may pronounce the S-W-O-G trial as *swog* and the E-C-O-G trial as *E-cog*.

· I · N · S · I · G · H · T ·

"Nanospheres" Can Diagnose and Treat Cancer

Scientists have been working on novel ways to target and destroy tumor cells without affecting healthy tissue. Recently researchers have developed polymer-coated gold "nanospheres" that can target tumors using a photothermal technique to ablate cancer tissue. These particles are designed to be injected intravenously. They then locate the tumor site, breach the cancerous cell membrane, and are drawn directly into the cells. Once in the tumor, the nanospheres can be precisely heated with noninvasive, nearly-infrared light to destroy the cancerous cells. In preliminary tests, scientists found that the cells with targeted nanospheres died and the rest were severely damaged, all while sparing surrounding tissue. This method would enable doctors to better target therapy to tumors with few side effects or damage to healthy tissue.

Despite the promising results, there are obstacles to overcome as research continues. The most important biological obstacle to using nanospheres is their effect on the liver and spleen. The body naturally tends to route foreign particles (such as the nanospheres) toward these organs for destructive processing. Researchers found that while most of the nanospheres injected into mice collected within a target tumor, a small amount gathered in the liver and spleen. Thus, more research into the effect of this technique on these organs from this technique is needed, as well as additional work in selective targeting of the nanospheres. In addition, more focused study is needed on the excretion and clearance of the nanospheres from the body, as well as on safety concerns (including toxicity from introducing gold into the body) and on the overall efficacy of the technique.

Although more research is needed, researchers envision a time when a doctor might inject millions of the tiny nanospheres into a patient to detect and treat cancer using the body's complex chemical composition instead of chemotherapy and radiation.

Common Soundalike Words

Word	Word Pronunciation	Soundalike	Pronunciation
necrosis: Pathologic death of one or more cells, or of a portion of tissue or organ, resulting from irreversible damage.	ně-krō′sis	**narcosis**: Unconsciousness induced by narcotics or anesthesia.	nar-kō′sis
mitosis: The process of cell division.	mī-tō′sis	**mycosis**: Any disease caused by a fungus.	mī-kō′sis
cytoplasmic: Relating to the cytoplasm, or substance of a cell.	sī-tō-plaz′mik	**cytotoxic**: Detrimental or destructive to cells.	sī-tō-tok′sik
estramustine: A drug used to treat prostate cancer.	es tră mus′ těn	**exemestane**: A drug used to treat breast cancer.	eks e mes′-tān
neoplasm: An abnormal tissue that grows by cellular proliferation more rapidly than normal.	ně′ōplazm	**neoprene (sleeve)**: A sheath of synthetic rubber used to provide warmth and minor support to an upper or lower limb.	ně′ōprēn
palliative: Reducing the severity of; denoting the alleviation of symptoms without curing the underlying disease.	pal′ē-ă-tiv	**palatal**: Relating to the palate or palate bone.	pal′ă-tăl
thalidomide: A drug that prevents the growth of new blood vessels into a tumor.	thal li′ dō mīd	**flutamide**: An antiandrogen drug used to treat prostate cancer.	flū′tă mīd

Combining Forms

Name	Definition	Name	Definition
cancer/o, carcin/o	cancer	lapar/o	abdomen
chem/o	chemical or drug	lymph/o	lymph; lymphatic system
cry/o	cold	malign/o	intentionally causing harm
cyt/o	cell	mamm/o	breast
gen/o	arising from; produced by	mutat/o	to change
gene/o	gene	onc/o	tumor; mass
gonad/o	gonads (ovaries and testes)	plas/o	growth, formation
hered/o	genetic inheritance	radi/o	radiation
incis/o	incise or cut	recept/o	receive
interstiti/o	spaces within tissue	sarc/o	connective tissue
invas/o	to go into; invade	surg/o	operative procedure

Add Your Own Combining Forms Here:

_____

_____

_____

_____

_____

_____

ABBREVIATIONS

Abbreviation	Meaning
AFP	alpha-fetoprotein
ALL	acute lymphocytic leukemia
AML	acute myelogenous leukemia
CAD	computer-aided detection
CBC	complete blood count
CEA	carcinoembryonic antigen
CLL	chronic lymphocytic leukemia
CML	chronic myelogenous leukemia
CMP	comprehensive metabolic panel
CSF	cerebrospinal fluid
CT	computed tomography (scan)
DNA	deoxyribonucleic acid
ECOG	Eastern Cooperative Oncology Group
FDA	U.S. Food and Drug Administration

Abbreviation	Meaning
FIGO	Federal Internationale de Gynecologie et Obstetrique
hCG	human chorionic gonadotropin
KPS	Karnofsky performance status
MRI	magnetic resonance imaging
NCI	National Cancer Institute
NIH	National Institutes of Health
PET	positron emission tomography
PSA	prostate-specific antigen
RBC	red blood cell
SERM	selective estrogen receptor modulator
TNM	tumor, nodes, metastasis
WBC	white blood cell

Add Your Own Abbreviations Here:

_____

_____

_____

_____

_____

_____

TERMINOLOGY

Term	Meaning
acute myelogenous leukemia	A fast-growing cancer that develops in the myelocytes of the blood and bone marrow.
adenocarcinomas	Cancers that arise from epithelial and glandular tissues of the body.
alpha-fetoprotein (AFP)	A tumor marker evaluated in liver, ovarian, or testicular cancers.
anemia	A condition in which blood does not carry enough oxygen to the rest of the body due to a deficiency in red blood cells, leading to damage of the heart, brain and other organs.
apoptosis	The normal process of cell death.
arm	A branch or part of a clinical study.
aromatase	An enzyme that converts other hormones (such as testosterone) to estrogens.
aromatase inhibitors	A group of drugs designed to reduce estrogen levels in a woman's body by preventing aromatase from converting other hormones to estrogen.
benign	Another word for *harmless*.
biopsy, syn. diagnostic surgery	A procedure in which a small tissue sample or the entire tumor is removed so that it can be examined under a microscope and identified.
BRCA1 and BRCA2	The name given to the two genes that with mutations are linked with breast cancer.
CA125	A protein and tumor marker evaluated in cancers of the reproductive system.
CA19-9	A protein and tumor marker evaluated in cancers of the colon, stomach, and biliary tract.
CA27.29	A tumor marker evaluated in advanced breast cancer as well as other cancers.
cancer	The name given to a group of many related diseases that all have to do with the abnormal division of cells in the body.
carcinoembryonic antigen (CEA)	A tumor marker evaluated in colorectal cancer and other cancers.
carcinogen	Something that promotes the abnormal growth of cells.
carcinogenesis	The abnormal transformation of normal cells in the body into cancer.
carcinoma	Cancer that arises from the epithelial tissues, or cells that cover external and internal body surfaces.
cell	The smallest living unit of structure that make up all living organisms.
cell membrane	The permeable barrier that surrounds the cell and protects its contents.
chemoprevention	The use of natural or synthetic products to keep cancer at bay or to derail the disease process before it becomes invasive.
chemotherapy	A regimen of therapy that uses chemicals to treat cancer.
chromosomes	The containers in the nucleus of cells that hold the cell's genetic material.
Clark level system	A staging classification system used for malignant melanoma of the skin.
clinical trial	A formal research study that tests how well a new medical treatment works in people.
computer-aided detection (CAD)	The use of a computer to more accurately analyze x-ray films for areas suspicious for cancer.
core biopsy	A biopsy in which a large needle is used to withdraw samples of tissue.
CT-guided biopsy	A procedure whereby a CT scanner is used to help guide a needle into a tumor more precisely to obtain a sample of tissue.

Term	Meaning
cytoplasm	The gel-like substance that fills a cell.
cytotoxic	A term meaning poisonous or destructive to cells.
debulking surgery	Surgery used to excise as much of cancerous tissue as possible to reduce the size of the tumor.
deoxyribonucleic acid (DNA)	A spiral-shaped molecule found inside the chromosomes of each body cell.
digital mammogram	An imaging study that allows doctors to visualize breast tissue for tumor or suspicious lumps in the breasts and uses a computer instead of x-ray film to collect the images.
distant recurrence	Disease that recurs at a location distant from that of the primary tumor.
Dukes classification system	A staging classification system used for colon carcinoma.
ECOG scale	A performance status scale used to rate a cancer patient's general well-being and ability to perform ordinary tasks.
eligibility criteria	The guidelines that describe the details that must be shared by all participants enrolled in a clinical trial.
endoscopy	A procedure in which a flexible tube with a viewing or camera lens (endoscope) is used to view and remove a sample of suspicious tissue located in the thorax or gastrointestinal system.
erythrocytes	A mature red blood cell.
excisional biopsy	A biopsy in which the entire tumor is removed for microscopic examination.
external beam radiation	A type of radiation treatment that is delivered externally to a specific part of the body affected by the tumor.
FIGO staging	A staging classification system used for gynecologic malignancies.
fine-needle biopsy	A biopsy in which a fine needle is used to withdraw a small tissue sample or fluid from the tumor.
genes	Functional unit of heredity that occupies a specific place on a chromosome of a cell.
Gleason system	A cancer classification system used for prostate tumors.
Gliadel	The brand name of the polymer implant wafer used in patients with high-grade malignant brain tumors.
gliomas	Cancers that arise from the glial cells of the body.
grade	The name given to a tumor's degree of malignancy.
Hemoccult	The brand name of the test kit used in colorectal cancer screening.
HER2/neu	A protein and tumor marker used to evaluate breast cancer.
HER2/neu negative	The classification of a breast cancer that has very few HER2/neu proteins, or none at all.
HER2/neu positive	The classification of a breast cancer that contain many more HER2/neu proteins than normal.
heredity	The genetic inheritance passed on from the DNA of the mother and father to the child.
high-dose chemotherapy	A procedure that involves administration of massive doses of a chemotherapy drug, followed by an antidote which reverses the effect of the drug on healthy cells.
human chorionic gonadotropin (hCG)	A tumor marker evaluated in testicular, ovarian, liver, stomach, pancreatic, or lung cancer.

Term	Meaning
incisional biopsy	A biopsy in which a small piece of tumor is removed for analysis.
internal radiation therapy	A type of radiation treatment administered through ingestion, injection, or by catheter.
interstitial chemotherapy	The method of placing chemotherapy drugs directly into a tumor.
intrathecal chemotherapy	The procedure of delivering chemotherapy drugs into the spinal canal.
invasion	Direct migration and penetration of cancer cells into neighboring tissues.
Jewett classification	A staging classification system used for bladder carcinomas.
Karnofsky performance status (KPS)	A scale used to rate a cancer patient's general well-being and ability to perform ordinary tasks.
laparoscopy	A procedure in which a flexible tube with a viewing or camera lens (laparoscope) is used to view and remove a sample of suspicious tissue located in the abdomen.
lesion	A general term that refers to any change in tissue.
leukemia	Cancer of the blood derived from the overabundance of very immature lympho-cytes that cannot prevent anemia, infection, or bleeding.
leukocytes	White blood cells.
local recurrence	Cancer that returns in the area of the primary tumor after all the visible tumor had been eradicated previously.
lymphoma	Cancer that arises in the lymph nodes and tissues of the body's immune system.
malignant	A descriptive word for something characterized by progressive and uncontrolled growth capable of causing harm, such as a tumor.
mammogram	A special type of x-ray that allows doctors to visualize breast tissue for tumor or suspicious lumps in the breasts.
mediastinoscopy	A procedure in which a flexible tube with a viewing or camera lens (endoscope) is used to view and remove a sample of suspicious tissue located in the chest cavity.
melanomas	Cancers that arise from pigmented skin cells of the body.
metastasis	The migration of cancer cells from the original tumor site through the blood and lymph vessels to produce cancers in other tissues.
microcalcifications	Tiny calcium deposits that may indicate cancer.
mitosis	The process of cell division.
mutations	A growth change triggered in a cell's genes.
myelomas	Cancers which arise from plasma cells in the body.
neoplasia	A condition of abnormal and uncontrolled cell growth.
neoplasm, syn. tumor	An abnormal, disorganized growth in a tissue or organ
neoplastic cells	Cells that grow beyond their normally defined limits.
nucleus	The center of a cell that contains the cell's control mechanisms.
Ommaya reservoir	A container system for delivering chemotherapy drugs to tumors in the brain and spinal cord.
oncogenes	Genes that regulate the normal growth of cells.
oncologist	A physician who specializes in the treatment of cancer.
oncology	The branch of medicine that deals with the study of the development, diagnosis, treatment, and prevention of cancer.
organelles	Structural units in a cell which are responsible for different functions of cell development.

Term	Meaning
palliative surgery	Surgery used to relieve pain or other symptoms of cancer but not to cure it.
participants	The name given to those patients who participate in clinical trials.
performance status	A method of quantifying a patient's general well-being.
Philadelphia chromosome	A defective chromosome in a cell's genetic makeup that is common in patients with chronic myelogenous leukemia.
platelets, syn. thrombocytes	A type of blood cell that prevents bleeding by forming clots.
polymer implant wafer	A biodegradable wafer saturated with chemotherapy drug and inserted into a tumor site; commonly used in patients with brain tumors.
primary cancer	A cancer that is growing in the body at its site of origin.
prophylaxis	The prevention of disease or of a process that can lead to disease.
prostate-specific antigen (PSA)	A substance made by the prostate gland that, at elevated levels, may indicate the existence of prostate cancer.
proteins	Large complex molecules that perform a wide variety of activities in a cell.
protocol	The blueprint or plan for the physicians and research centers that conduct a clinical trial.
radiation oncologist	A physician who coordinates and manages a patient's radiation treatment.
radiographic studies	An image, or series of images, produced by an x-ray machine.
radiation therapy, syn. radiotherapy	A procedure of using high-energy radioactive waves to destroy or disable cancerous cells.
randomized clinical trials	A clinical trial in which participants are placed in one of the parts (arms) of the study at random, determined by computer or table of random numbers.
reconstructive surgery	Surgery used to return the function and appearance of the area of the body where a tumor was located.
recurrent disease	Cancer that returns after all remnants of visible tumor has been eradicated.
risk factor	Something that may increase the chance of the development of disease.
sarcomas	Cancers that arise from connective or supporting tissues of the body such as bone, cartilage, or muscle.
screening tests	A collection of medical checkups and diagnostic studies obtained on a regular basis to increase the chance of early detection of a new or metastasized cancer.
secondary cancer	The place to which a cancer spreads and begins to grow.
selective estrogen receptor modulator (SERM)	A type of drug that block the effects of estrogen, thereby preventing cancer from returning after treatment. It is primarily used in advanced breast cancer.
spiral CT scan	A faster type of CT scan in which images are collected more quickly, allowing for more detailed three-dimensional images.
stage	Refers to whether a tumor has spread beyond the site of its origin.
stereotactic biopsy	A sample of tissue obtained from the body using the aid of highly advanced computers.
stereotactic surgery	A surgery that is performed using highly advanced computers to aid in the surgical removal of a tumor.
stereotaxy	Refers to the use of highly advanced computers to create a three-dimensional image of a tumor.
thoracoscopy	A procedure in which a flexible tube with a viewing or camera lens is used to view and remove a sample of suspicious tissue located in the thorax.
TNM system	A type of staging system used for primary malignant tumors.

Term	Meaning
tumor marker	A substance produced by cells in the body in response to cancer.
tumor suppressor genes	Genes able to recognize abnormal growth and reproduction of damaged cells and which can interrupt their reproduction until the defect is corrected.
ultrasound-guided biopsy	A procedure whereby an ultrasound machine is used to help guide a needle into a tumor more precisely to obtain a sample of tissue.

Add Your Own Terms and Definitions Here:

_____

_____

_____

_____

_____

_____

_____

_____

REVIEW QUESTIONS

1. What is mitosis and why is it important?
2. Why is a spiral CT scan better than a conventional CT in some instances?
3. Describe the function of oncogenes.
4. Why is assessing a patient's performance status useful?
5. What are neoplastic cells?
6. What is the purpose of a clinical trial's protocol?
7. What is the difference between external beam radiation and internal radiation treatment?
8. Explain apoptosis and how this process affects body function.
9. What is the advantage of implementing polymer wafers into a tumor site?
10. How does a drug like tamoxifen work to keep cancer at bay?

CHAPTER ACTIVITIES

Soundalike Word Choice

Circle the correct word in the following sentences.

1. The biopsy was taken from the right (areolar, aural) area of the breast using a #24 blade.
2. Mr. Hilliard is a gentleman who was recently diagnosed (stage, state) IIIB non-small-cell lung cancer.
3. The patient will continue to be monitored by Dr. Smith for the possibility of (metatarsal, metastatic) disease.
4. She received a total of 5940 (cGy, cGi) of radiation to her tumor site.
5. The recent CT scan revealed that the patient had no new pulmonary (nodules, modules) identified and had generally stable disease.
6. Ms. Braden's CT scan was read by the radiologist and was stated to have shown a reduction in the size of the left upper lobe (lesson, lesion).
7. The patient is a 52-year-old female who came to the clinic for evaluation after a finding of a right breast mass found on routine (microgram, mammogram).
8. This is a pleasant female with recently diagnosed (colon, collum) cancer who recently underwent a subtotal colectomy.
9. The patient had a cervical biopsy with the finding of carcinoma (incited, in situ).
10. Admission labs were remarkable for (hyperkalemia, hypokalemia), with a potassium level noted to be 7.3.

Abbreviations

Provide the meaning for each of these abbreviations.

Abbreviation	*Definition*
1. NCI	_____
2. SERM	_____
3. ECOG	_____
4. AFP	_____
5. PET	_____
6. KPS	_____
7. DNA	_____
8. CEA	_____
9. AML	_____
10. NIH	_____

True or False

Read each statement and indicate whether it is true or false. If false, rewrite the sentence in the Correction column to make the statement true.

Statement	True (T) or False (F)	Correction, if False
1. Aromatase inhibitors are a group of drugs designed to deliver chemotherapy to a tumor.	_____	_____
2. Sarcomas are cancers that arise in the lymph nodes.	_____	_____
3. Laser surgery uses a high intensity light to shrink or destroy tumors.	_____	_____
4. Chemotherapy makes use of high energy radioactive waves to treat cancer.	_____	_____
5. The ECOG scale is used to assess a cancer patient's performance.	_____	_____
6. A tumor's grade indicates its degree of malignancy.	_____	_____
7. A Hemoccult test assesses blood in the stool.	_____	_____
8. External beam radiation is delivered by injection.	_____	_____
9. Malignant tumors are harmless.	_____	_____
10. The word *benign* means *harmless*.	_____	_____
11. A promoter is a change in a gene that suppresses cancer growth.	_____	_____
12. The *N* in the TNM system stands for the amount of tumor necrosis.	_____	_____
13. An incisional biopsy is a procedure in which the entire tumor is removed for microscopic analysis.	_____	_____
14. Patients who take part in clinical trials are called participants.	_____	_____
15. Mitosis is the depletion of red blood cells.	_____	_____

Fill in the Blanks

Fill in the blanks with the correct answers.

1. Normal cells undergo a process of cell death called _____.

2. A substance produced by cells in response to cancer is called a _____.

3. Something that may increase the chance of developing cancer is called _____.

4. A cancer that grows in the site where it originated is called a _____.

5. The classification indicating whether a tumor has spread beyond the site of its origin is called _____.

6. The protective barrier that surrounds a cell is called the _____.

7. Changes in a cell's genes that trigger the development of cancer are called _____.

8. A treatment group in a clinical trial is none as a(an) _____.

9. A container system that delivers chemotherapy drugs to tumors in the brain and spinal cord is called a(n) _____.

10. The system used to classify cancers relating to the colon or rectum is called the _____ classification system.

Creating Medical Words

1. Using the root word *lapar*/o, write a word for each of the following definitions.

   An instrument used to examine the abdominal cavity.   _____

   Incision into the abdomen.   _____

   A swelling or hernia in the abdomen.   _____

2. Using the root word *carcin*/o, write a word for each of the following definitions.

   A cancer-producing substance or organism.   _____

   A cancerous tumor or neoplasm.   _____

   Widespread dissemination of carcinoma in various organs or tissues of
   the body.   _____

3. Using the root word *lymph*/o, write a word for each of the following definitions.

   A white blood cell.   _____

   Resembling lymph or lymphatic tissue.   _____

   A neoplasm of lymphoid tissue.   _____

4. Using the root word *radi*/o, write a word for each of the following definitions.

   A negative image on photographic film made by exposure to x-rays that
   have passed through matter or tissue.   _____

   The science of high-energy radiation and of the sources and the
   chemical, physical, and biologic effects of such radiation.   _____

   Necrosis due to radiation.   _____

5. Using the root word *onc*/o, write a word for each of the following definitions.

   Origin and growth of a neoplasm.   _____

   A specialist in the study or science dealing with the physical,
   chemical, and biologic properties and features of neoplasms,
   including causation, pathogenesis, and treatment.   _____

   Destruction of a neoplasm.   _____

Punctuation Practice

Fill in and circle the correct punctuation and capitalization omissions in the following paragraph. Then retype the paragraph to include the correct punctuation. Proofread your work, print one copy for your instructor, and save the completed report to your student disk. There are 15 missing punctuation marks and capitalization errors.

INTERVAL HISTORY The patient has been doing relatively well since her last appointment last seen by me in October. She has intermittent bony pain swelling and tenderness secondary to her bone metastasis but has been continuing to take her Arimidex and Zometa as prescribed she complains of right femur pain and left sided rib pain both in the areas of known metastasis. This she states has improved somewhat since originally being diagnosed and has not worsened in intensity. She denies any fevers no shortness of breath no cough no constipation and no diarrhea she denies any dysuria. She does have some frequency in urination at night possibly secondary to her hydrochlorothiazide.

TRANSCRIPTION PRACTICE

Open your word-processing software. Insert the student CD-ROM and locate the dictation for this chapter. For each of the words in the "listen for these terms" list for each report, use a medical dictionary or other resources to identify and write down a brief definition of the term on a separate sheet of paper to attach with your work. Then listen to the dictation and transcribe each report. Use the current date for each report where a date is indicated. Insert a heading into the document if the text falls to a second page.

At the end of each report, indicate the name of the dictating physician under the signature line and insert reference initials. For date dictated and transcribed and date of admission, use the current date. Proofread your work, print one copy for your instructor along with your term definitions, and save the completed report to your student disk.

Report T20.1: Clinic Note
Patient Name: Myra Jackson
Medical Record No.: 681112
Attending Physician: Lena Kushner, MD

Listen for these terms:
glioblastoma
Temodar
craniotomy
gliacyte
necrosis

Report T20.2: Clinic Note
Patient Name: Samuel Goldberg
Medical Record No.: 880–35200
Attending Physician: Michael Josephs, MD

Listen for these terms:
apical
hilar adenopathy
AP window
FTG
Taxol
cGy (centigray)
myelolipoma

Report T20.3: Discharge Summary
Patient Name: Uma Hayes
Medical Record No.: 7990
Attending Physician: Andrea Biggs, MD

Listen for these terms:
meningeal
carcinomatosis
parenchymal
cytology

21

ENDOCRINOLOGY

OBJECTIVES

After completing this chapter, you will be able to:

- Identify the glands that make up the endocrine system, their locations in the body, and the hormones secreted by each.
- Describe common diseases and disorders affecting the endocrine system.
- Describe common laboratory tests and procedures used to analyze, detect, and diagnose endocrinologic disorders.

INTRODUCTION

The endocrine system plays a vital role in its communication, control, and coordination of the work accomplished by the other body systems, especially the work pertaining to metabolism and internal balance, called **homeostasis**. The word *endocrine* comes from the prefix *endo-*, meaning *within*, and the Greek word *krino*, which means *to separate or secrete*.

Endocrinology is a subspecialty within the field of internal medicine and is the scientific study of the function and pathology of the endocrine glands. **Endocrinologists** are specially trained physicians who diagnose

and treat hormone problems by helping to restore the normal balance of hormones in the body. Included in their field of expertise are diseases of the pancreas, thyroid, adrenal, and pituitary glands, and gonads. This chapter reviews the anatomy of the major glands of the endocrine system and the different types of hormones produced by each; common abnormalities that affect endocrine function; and the studies and tests utilized to detect and diagnose endocrine disorders.

ANATOMY OF THE ENDOCRINE SYSTEM

The endocrine system is different from other body systems in that its specialized organs, called **endocrine glands**, are located in different parts of the body but not connected to each other, as shown in Figure 21.1. These glands control very important body functions by releasing chemical transmitters and **hormones**, which are chemical substances secreted by the glands in response to stimulation from the nervous system and other sites in the body. Hormones are chemical messengers that regulate bodily processes such as growth, reproduction, metabolism, digestion, mineral and fluid balance, and the functioning of various organs. Hormones are secreted by organs, tissues, and glands of the endocrine system directly into the blood and are carried in the

and the endocrine system. Recall from Chapter 18, *Neurology*, that the hypothalamus serves as part of the nervous system by regulating autonomic functions such as body temperature control and appetite. As part of the endocrine system, this gland secretes **neurohormones**, which in turn control the secretion of hormones from the adjacent anterior pituitary gland. The hypothalamus also produces two hormones, antidiuretic hormone (ADH) and oxytocin (described in subsequent text), that are stored in the posterior pituitary gland, and which are released when the hypothalamus sends nerve impulses to the posterior pituitary gland.

Pituitary Gland

The **pituitary gland**, also called the **hypophysis**, is a small, teardrop-shaped gland lying immediately below the hypothalamus of the brain (see Figure 21.2). It is attached to the underside of the brain by a stalk of tissue called the **infundibulum**. The **circle of Willis**, which is a connection of arteries in the brain, surrounds the pituitary gland and provides it with blood exchange. The pituitary gland is sometimes called the "master gland" of the endocrine system because it controls the functions of the other endocrine glands. The release of hormones from the pituitary gland is controlled by the hypothalamus.

The pituitary is divided into two basic parts, called **lobes**, each of which actually functions independently of the other. The **anterior pituitary gland** regulates many body functions that are in turn regulated by releasing hormones from the hypothalamus. As the releasing hormones are absorbed by the anterior pituitary gland, they stimulate the secretion of several hormones, including the following:

- **Prolactin (PRL).** This hormone is responsible for the initiation of milk production in the mammary

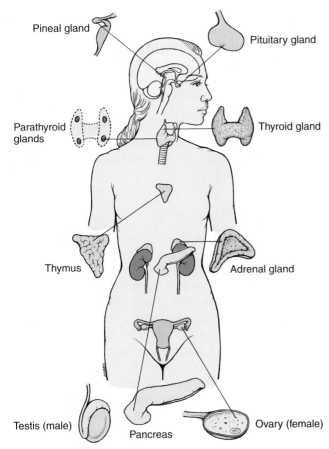

FIGURE 21.1. The Endocrine System. Reprinted with permission from *Stedman's Medical Dictionary*, 27th ed. Baltimore: Lippincott Williams & Wilkins, 2000.

bloodstream to target organs. Once there, the hormones alter the activities of the organ or regulate the production of other hormones.

Hormones are secreted by the endocrine glands as needed. The cells of the endocrine glands respond to changes in the blood, or perhaps to other hormones in the blood, by increasing or decreasing secretion of their respective hormones. When a hormone brings about the intended effects, secretion of that hormone decreases until the stimulus recurs. For example, insulin, a hormone secreted by the pancreas (discussed later), is secreted when the level of glucose (blood sugar) is high. Insulin enables cells to remove the glucose from the blood and use it for energy production. As a result of the action of insulin, blood glucose level decreases. Insulin secretion then decreases until the blood glucose level increases again.

The glands of the endocrine system include the hypothalamus, pituitary, pineal, thyroid, parathyroid, thymus, adrenals, pancreas, and the gonads.

Hypothalamus

The hypothalamus is a small structure at the base of the brain that functions as part of both the nervous system

Pituitary gland

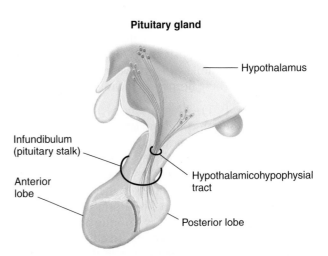

FIGURE 21.2. The Pituitary Gland. Also called the hypophysis, or master gland, the pituitary connects with the hypothalamus via the infundibulum, through which it receives chemical and neural stimuli. Asset provided by Anatomical Chart Co.

glands after childbirth and can affect sex hormone levels from the ovaries in women and the testes in men.

- **Growth hormone (GH).** Also known as **somatotropin**, this chemical controls linear growth in children and adolescents. Growth hormone releasing hormone (GHRH) from the hypothalamus increases the secretion of GH, whereas **somatostatin**, a growth hormone-inhibiting hormone also secreted by the hypothalamus, causes a decrease in the production of GH.
- **Adrenocorticotropic hormone (ACTH).** ACTH, also called **corticotropin**, stimulates the secretion of cortisol and other hormones by the adrenal glands, which helps to maintain blood pressure and blood glucose levels.
- **Thyroid-stimulating hormone (TSH).** This hormone, also called **thyrotropin**, stimulates the normal growth of the thyroid gland and the secretion of thyroid hormones **triiodothyronine** (T3) and **thyroxine** (T4), as discussed later, which regulate the body's metabolism. The secretion of TSH is stimulated by the secretion of thyrotropin-releasing hormone (TRH) from the hypothalamus. When metabolic rate, or energy production, decreases, TRH is produced.
- **Gonadotropins.** Gonadotropins is a collective term for **follicle-stimulating hormone** (FSH) and **luteinizing hormone** (LH), which stimulate production of various hormones in the gonads. In women, FSH is responsible for the release of an ovum from an ovarian follicle, as discussed in Chapter 16, *Obstetrics and Gynecology.* LH then stimulates that follicle to develop into the corpus luteum, which secretes progesterone. In men, where LH had also been called **interstitial cell stimulating hormone** (ICSH), LH stimulates production of testosterone.

The two hormones secreted by the **posterior pituitary gland** are actually produced by the hypothalamus and simply stored in the posterior pituitary until needed. Their release is stimulated by nerve impulses from the hypothalamus. These hormones include:

- **Oxytocin (OT)**—This hormone stimulates contractions during childbirth and the production of milk in nursing mothers. As labor begins, the cervix of the uterus begins to stretch, generating sensory impulses to the hypothalamus. The hypothalamus, in turn, stimulates the posterior pituitary to release oxytocin. This hormone then causes contractions of the uterus to bring about delivery of the baby and the placenta. In addition, when a baby is breast-fed, the sucking of the baby stimulates sensory impulses from the mother's nipple to the hypothalamus, which, in turn, stimulates the posterior pituitary gland to release oxytocin, which contributes to the contraction of the smooth muscle cells around the mammary ducts.
- **Antidiuretic hormone (ADH).** ADH, also called **vasopressin**, is a hormone that reduces the production of urine in the kidneys and, therefore, prevents water loss from the body. Any type of dehydration stimulates the secretion of ADH to conserve water balance. In addition, the release of ADH also causes constriction of blood vessels, which contribute to the maintenance of normal blood pressure.

Pineal Gland

The **pineal gland** is a tiny, cone-shaped structure located at the back of the third ventricle of the brain. It produces the hormone **melatonin**, which regulates a person's internal clock and sleep-wake pattern (called the **circadian rhythm**) and plays a role in mood regulation. The pineal gland's production of melatonin varies both with the time of day and with age; production of melatonin increases during the nighttime hours and falls off during the day, and melatonin levels are much higher in children younger than age seven than in adolescents, and these levels are lower still in adults.

Melatonin also seems to play an important role in regulating sleep cycles; test subjects injected with the hormone become sleepy, suggesting that the increased production of melatonin coincident with nightfall acts as a fundamental mechanism for making people sleepy. With dawn the pineal gland stops producing melatonin, and wakefulness and alertness ensue. The high level of melatonin production in young children may explain their tendency to sleep longer than adults.

In addition, in mammals other than humans, melatonin may act as a breeding and mating cue, since it is produced in greater amounts in response to the longer nights of winter and less so during summer. Animals who time their mating or breeding to coincide with favorable seasons (such as spring) may depend on melatonin production as a kind of biological clock that regulates their reproductive cycles on the basis of the length of the solar day.

Thyroid Gland

The **thyroid gland** is a butterfly-shaped gland with two lateral sides, called lobes, which wrap around the trachea. The lobes are connected by a thin bridge of tissue called the **isthmus**. The thyroid gland regulates the body's metabolism, which permits growth, development, reproduction, physical movement, and constant body temperature. Essentially all the cells in the body are target cells of thyroid hormones, which regulate metabolism by promoting normal cardiac function, normal growth of muscles and bones, and normal neurologic function.

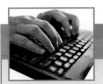

The hormones produced by the thyroid include T3 and T4, collectively called **thyroid hormone**, and **calcitonin** (CT). Thyroid hormone is released from the thyroid follicles when stimulated by TSH from the anterior pituitary gland. When the body's metabolism, or rate of energy production, decreases, this change is detected by the hypothalamus; the hypothalamus stimulates the anterior pituitary gland to secrete TSH, which signals the thyroid to release T3, thereby raising the metabolic rate and increasing energy production. Although the thyroid secretes more T4 than T3, it is the T3 that does most of the work of regulating metabolism. When the optimum metabolic rate is achieved, secretion of T3 then stops until the metabolic rate decreases again. Hypothyroidism is a condition caused by low levels of thyroid hormone in the body. The thyroid gland responds by becoming abnormally large (**thyromegaly**) and forming a goiter, as discussed in Chapter 19, *Immunology*.

Calcitonin regulates the balance of calcium and phosphate in the blood by decreasing the absorption of these minerals from the bones to the blood, thereby lowering blood levels of these minerals. Calcitonin is secreted when blood calcium levels are too high, which ensures that no more will be removed from the bones until there is a real need for more calcium in the blood.

Parathyroid Glands

The **parathyroid glands** are four tiny (pea-sized) endocrine glands, two located on the back of each lobe of the thyroid gland. The purpose of the parathyroid glands is to produce **parathyroid hormone** (PTH), which, as an antagonist to calcitonin, helps maintain the level of calcium as well as phosphate concentrations in the blood. The overall effect of PTH is to raise the blood calcium level and lower the blood phosphate level.

A reduction in the level of calcium in the blood stimulates the parathyroid gland to release PTH. This hormone, in turn, stimulates the release of calcium from the bones by increasing the activity of cells called **osteoclasts**, which break down the mineral part of the bone. In doing so, parathyroids also control how much calcium is in the bones, and therefore, the strength and density of the bones. PTH has an action opposite from that of calcitonin, which is secreted by the thyroid gland; the levels of PTH are decreased when levels of blood

calcium are too high, as discussed previously. If the parathyroid gland is too active (**hyperparathyroidism**), excess PTH causes a decreased concentration of phosphate and increased level of calcium in the blood. Conversely, reduced parathyroid activity (**hypoparathyroidism**) causes an increase in blood phosphate and decreases in the level of blood calcium.

Thymus

The **thymus** is a small gland located in the thoracic cavity behind the sternum. The thymus reaches its maximum weight during childhood and puberty, and then slowly decreases in size during adulthood as it is gradually replaced by fat tissue. The thymus gland functions as part of both the body's immune system, as discussed in Chapter 19, *Immunology*, and the endocrine system. As part of the endocrine system, the thymus gland secretes **thymosin**, which causes immature T cells in the thymus to develop and mature.

Adrenal Glands

The two **adrenal glands**, also called **suprarenal glands**, are cone-shaped structures that lie one on top of each kidney at the back of the abdomen. Each adrenal gland has an outer region, called the **adrenal cortex**, and a core, called the **medulla**. Both parts of the gland secrete hormones, but the hormones released by each have very different functions and, in a sense, the adrenal cortex and adrenal medulla function as two separate endocrine glands.

The adrenal cortex secretes the following hormones, which have an effect on the body's metabolism, on chemicals in the blood, and on certain body characteristics:

- **Cortisol**. This hormone controls the body's use of fats, proteins, and carbohydrates. It increases the use of fats and excess amino acids for energy and decreases the use of glucose. Cortisol is secreted in response to a stress situation by the body, such as disease, injury, fear or anger, exercise, or hunger.
- **Corticosterone**. This hormone, together with cortisol, suppresses inflammatory reactions in the body.
- **Aldosterone**. This hormone regulates the balance of electrolytes, such as sodium and potassium, in the body, and helps maintain blood volume and pressure. The secretion of aldosterone is stimulated by a deficiency of sodium, loss of blood, or dehydration that lowers blood pressure, or an elevated level of potassium.

The cells of the adrenal medulla, the inner part of the adrenal gland, secrete hormones, collectively called **catecholamines**, which help control the effects of physically and emotionally stressful situations and help prepare the body for a "fight or flight" response, as follows:

- **Epinephrine** (also called **adrenaline**). This hormone allows for the body's "fight or flight" reaction to stressful situations by increasing the heart rate and force of heart contractions, facilitating blood flow to the muscles and brain, and increasing respirations in the lungs, in addition to controlling other activities regulated by the sympathetic nervous system.

- **Norepinephrine** (also called **noradrenaline**). This hormone, secreted in smaller amounts than epinephrine, causes blood vessels and skeletal muscles to constrict, which raises blood pressure.

Pancreas

The **pancreas** is an elongated gland located near the stomach in the left upper quadrant of the abdomen. The pancreas plays a role in both the digestive system and the endocrine system. Most of its cells secrete enzymes that assist in the digestive function of the body, as discussed in Chapter 14, *Gastroenterology*. However, other cells, called **islets of Langerhans**, produce the hormones that are essential to metabolizing carbohydrates and regulating blood sugar, both after meals and during periods of fasting, as a function of the endocrine system. The islets of Langerhans are tiny clusters of cells scattered throughout the pancreas. These spherical clumps of pancreatic tissue secrete hormones directly into the bloodstream in response to abnormal levels of **glucose**, a simple sugar that is the main source of energy for the body.

Insulin is a hormone made by the pancreas, the production of which is stimulated by rising levels of glucose in the blood (called **hyperglycemia**). The pancreas secretes insulin in response to the increase in blood sugar, stimulating cells to absorb glucose from the bloodstream and move it into the cells for energy. Without insulin, the cells in the body would not be able to process the glucose and, therefore, would have no energy for movement, growth, repair, or other functions. Insulin increases the permeability of cell membranes in order to allow the glucose to be transferred from the bloodstream into the cell. Ordinarily, when glucose enters the blood, the pancreas automatically produces the right amount of insulin to move glucose into cells. **Glucagon**, like insulin, is a hormone produced by the islets of Langerhans in the pancreas, but it is secreted in response to low blood glucose levels in the blood (called **hypoglycemia**). These hormones then stimulate release of glucose, fats, and other substances from body stores to provide energy to cells.

Gonads

The **gonads** are the body's sex glands—the ovaries in the female and the testes in the male. Hormones found in the gonads control sexual development and reproductive processes.

The **ovaries** are small, egg-producing glands located in the pelvic cavity, one on each side of the uterus. The

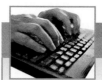

ovaries function as part of the female reproductive system, as discussed in Chapter 16, *Obstetrics and Gynecology*, as well as the endocrine system. As part of the endocrine system, the ovaries secrete two hormones:

- **Estrogen**. This hormone, commonly called **estradiol**, is secreted by the follicle cells of the ovary when stimulated by FSH from the anterior pituitary gland. The ovaries control the development and maintenance of female sex-related traits, regulate the menstrual cycle, and maintain the uterus for pregnancy. Along with other hormones, they also prepare the mammary glands for lactation.
- **Progesterone**. When a mature ovarian follicle releases an ovum, the follicle becomes the corpus luteum and begins to secrete progesterone, stimulated by LH from the anterior pituitary gland.

In males, the **testes** (singular, **testis**), or **testicles**, are egg-shaped glands located in the scrotum between the upper thighs. The testes function as a part of both the male genitourinary system, discussed in Chapter 15, *Urology*, and the endocrine system. The testes secrete two hormones when stimulated by LH from the pituitary gland:

- **Testosterone**. The most abundant and biologically active of all the **androgens** (male hormones), testosterone stimulates and maintains male sex-related traits. These include growth of all the reproductive organs, growth of facial and body hair, growth of the larynx and deepening of the voice, and growth of the skeletal muscles.
- **Inhibin**. This hormone is secreted by the cells of the testes when there is increased testosterone. The function of inhibin is to decrease the level of FSH by the anterior pituitary gland. Together, inhibin, testosterone, and the pituitary hormones maintain the process of producing sperm at a constant rate.

COMMON ENDOCRINE DISEASES AND TREATMENTS

An endocrine disorder is defined as the production of too much or too little of a specific hormone. There could be a problem with the system regulating the hormones in the bloodstream, or the body may have

QUICK CHECK 21.1 ✓

Match the hormone with the endocrine gland for which it is associated (some glands may be used more than once).

Hormone

1. _____ thymosin
2. _____ prolactin
3. _____ melatonin
4. _____ aldosterone
5. _____ calcitonin
6. _____ PTH
7. _____ oxytocin
8. _____ estrogen
9. _____ ADH
10. _____ insulin

Gland

A. thyroid

B. gonads

C. adrenals

D. pituitary

E. parathyroid

F. pancreas

G. thymus

H. pineal

difficulty controlling hormone levels because of problems clearing hormones from the blood. Endocrine disorders can be grouped into many different areas depending on what part of the system is affected.

Generally, endocrine disorders marked by hormone deficiency are managed by hormone replacement therapy, whereas disorders that result from overproduction of a particular hormone may be treated by surgery, radiation, or a drug therapy to reduce the activity of the endocrine gland. Drugs that contain hormones as their active ingredients come from natural or synthetic sources that mimic the actions of hormones in the body. The chemical structures of these medications are modified or improved upon to make the hormone more potent or to adapt it for use in a specific form (such as a pill to be swallowed as opposed to an injection). The most common endocrine disorders and their treatments are described later.

Pituitary Disorders

The most frequent cause of pituitary disorders is benign tumors called **pituitary adenomas**, which result in abnormalities in the function of the pituitary gland. There are no known environmental causes for pituitary tumors. Very rarely they can run in families and may be associated with some other diseases such as high blood-calcium level and a certain type of abdominal tumors. Although the tumor is benign, it can cause the normal pituitary gland to become underactive or to produce excess hormones.

Growth hormone (GH or *somatropin*) is a hormone produced by the anterior pituitary gland. As its name implies, growth hormone stimulates the growth of cells in the body. It acts not on a specific group of cells or organs but rather on all the cells of the body to promote their growth and proliferation. Abnormal output of growth hormone from the pituitary gland early in life can result in one of two disorders—**dwarfism** if there is too little growth hormone excreted during childhood or **gigantism** if there is too much, as illustrated in Figure 21.3.

Overproduction of growth hormone in middle-aged adults can cause **acromegaly**, a serious disorder in which bones, cartilage, and other organs become severely oversized. Acromegaly is most often caused by a tumor in the pituitary gland. The term acromegaly comes from the Greek words for *extremities* and *enlargement* and reflects one of its most common symptoms—the abnormal growth of the hands and feet. Gradually bony changes occur, which affect a person's facial features, such as brow and jaw protrusion, nasal bone enlargement, and increased spacing between the teeth. In addition, enlargement of body organs, including the liver, spleen, kidneys, and heart, may occur.

Surgery is the treatment of choice for acromegaly. The tumor is removed by means of a **transsphenoidal adenectomy**, which is a procedure whereby the surgery is performed through the sphenoid sinuses behind the nose, which obviates the need for drilling a hole or cutting through the skull. Removal or reduction of the size of the pituitary tumor reduces the growth hormone levels and relieves the pressure caused by the tumor mass.

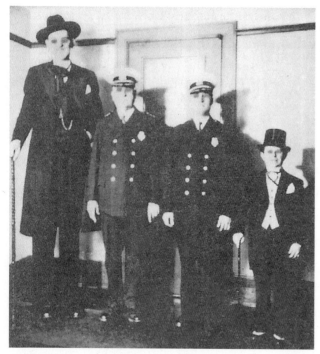

FIGURE 21.3. Pituitary Gland Disorders. The effects of abnormal output of growth hormone from the pituitary gland result in gigantism (far left) if there is too much or dwarfism (far right) if there is too little. Two men of normal stature appear in between. Reprinted with permission from Thibodeau GA and Patton KT. *Anatomy and Physiology*. 3rd ed. St. Louis: Mosby-Year Book, 1996.

If there is still residual tumor or hormone levels do not return to normal, medical therapy in the form of a drug called octreotide is given, which controls the overproduction of growth hormone.

Hypopituitarism is a complex syndrome that affects the function of the anterior lobe of the pituitary gland, usually resulting in a partial or complete loss of hormone secretion of that lobe. The resulting symptoms depend on which hormones are no longer being produced by the gland and include metabolic dysfunction, sexual immaturity, and growth retardation in childhood. If all the hormones produced by the pituitary are affected, this condition is known as **panhypopituitarism** (the word *pan* means *all*). Hypopituitarism is most often caused by a benign adenoma in the pituitary gland. Pituitary underactivity may be caused by the direct pressure of the tumor mass on the normal pituitary or by the effects of surgery or radiation used to treat the tumor. Sometimes hypopituitarism can be caused by an infection in or around the brain, such as meningitis, or by a head injury.

The goal of treatment is to restore the pituitary gland to normal function, where it produces normal levels of hormones. Replacement of hormones normally secreted by the target glands is the most effective treatment for hypopituitarism and panhypopituitarism. If the cause of the disorder is a tumor or lesion, radiation or surgical removal is a treatment option. Success-

ful removal of the tumor may reverse the hypopituitarism. However, even after removal of the mass, hormone replacement therapy may still be necessary.

Hyperparathyroidism

Hyperparathyroidism is a disorder of the parathyroid glands. Most people with this disorder have one or more enlarged, overactive parathyroid glands that secrete too much PTH. This hormone is secreted by the parathyroid glands and helps maintain the correct balance of calcium and phosphorus in the body. PTH regulates release of calcium from bone, absorption of calcium in the intestine, and excretion of calcium in the urine. If too much PTH is secreted, blood calcium levels rise, called **hypercalcemia**. The bones may lose calcium, and too much calcium may be absorbed from food. The levels of calcium may increase in the urine, causing kidney stones. PTH also acts to lower blood phosphorus levels by increasing excretion of phosphorus in the urine.

In many cases, hyperparathyroidism is caused by a benign adenoma that has formed on one of the parathyroid glands, causing it to become overactive. The excess hormone may be due to the abnormal enlargement of the parathyroid glands, a condition called **hyperplasia**, or in rare cases can be caused by cancer of a parathyroid gland. Hyperparathyroidism is diagnosed when tests show that blood levels of calcium as well as parathyroid hormone are too high. Surgery to remove the parathyroid gland (or glands), called **parathyroidectomy**, is the only treatment for the disorder and is effective in most cases.

Adrenal Disorders

Cushing syndrome, also called **hypercortisolism**, is a hormonal disorder caused by prolonged exposure of the body's tissues to abnormally high levels of the hormone cortisol. Cortisol helps maintain blood pressure and cardiovascular function, reduces the immune system's inflammatory response, balances the effects of insulin in breaking down sugar for energy, and regulates the metabolism of proteins, carbohydrates, and fats. In addition, cortisol helps the body respond to stress. People with depression, alcoholism, malnutrition, and panic disorders typically have increased cortisol levels. Symptoms include, among other things, upper body obesity, facial puffiness (a moon-shaped appearance), **hirsutism** (excessive hair growth), hyperglycemia, thin and easily bruised skin with **striae** (stretch marks), and hypertension, as illustrated in Figure 21.4.

Cortisol resembles the cortisone found in some medicines, and Cushing's may also be caused by taking too much cortisonelike medication over a long period. Prednisone is the most common medicine in this category and is routinely prescribed for patients with

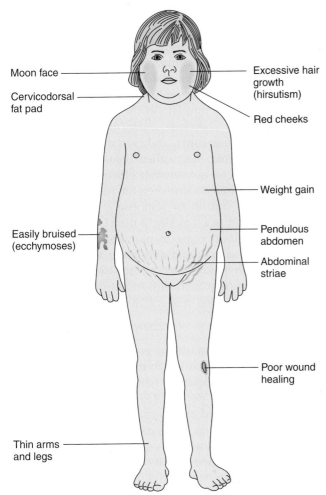

Moon face

Cervicodorsal fat pad

Easily bruised (ecchymoses)

Thin arms and legs

Excessive hair growth (hirsutism)

Red cheeks

Weight gain

Pendulous abdomen

Abdominal striae

Poor wound healing

FIGURE 21.4. Cushing Syndrome. Signs and symptoms of Cushing syndrome affect various parts of the body. Reprinted with permission from Pillitteri, A. *Maternal and Child Nursing*, 4th ed. Philadelphia: Lippincott Williams & Wilkins, 2003.

asthma, rheumatoid arthritis, lupus, or other inflammatory diseases. In addition, an adrenal gland tumor can cause excessive secretion of corticosteroids.

Others develop Cushing's because of overproduction of cortisol by the body due to an abnormality in the pituitary gland. **Cushing disease** is the name physicians use when Cushing syndrome is caused by a tumor in the pituitary gland. A pituitary adenoma can cause the adrenal glands, which are near the kidneys, to make too much cortisol.

Treatment depends on the specific reason for cortisol excess and may include surgery, radiation, chemotherapy, or the use of cortisol-inhibiting drugs. Medications used alone or in combination to control the production of excess cortisol include bromocriptine (Parlodel), cyproheptadine (Periactin), octreotide (Sandostatin), and ketoconazole (Nizoral). If the cause is long-term use of cortisone-type medications to treat another disorder, the medication is gradually reduced to the lowest dose adequate for control of that disorder.

Tumors on the adrenal glands are removed by surgery. If there is a tumor on just one adrenal gland, the other gland usually shrinks and ceases normal productivity. Hormone supplements are usually given before surgery and must be taken for weeks and sometimes months after surgery, until the second gland recovers normal function. Pituitary adenomas are removed or reduced through the use of transsphenoidal surgery, as described previously. Finally, for patients in whom surgery has failed or for patients who are not suitable candidates for surgery, another possible course of treatment is radiotherapy to weaken and lower the pituitary's production of ACTH, which stimulates the production of cortisol by the adrenal gland.

Addison disease, also referred to as **adrenal insufficiency**, is the name given to the hyposecretion of cortisol. This hormonal disorder occurs when the adrenal glands do not produce enough of the hormone cortisol and, in some cases, the hormone aldosterone. This leads to weight loss, muscle weakness, fatigue, low blood pressure, and sometimes darkening of the skin in both exposed and nonexposed parts of the body. Most cases are caused by the gradual destruction of the adrenal cortex by the body's immune system, in which the immune system makes antibodies that attack the adrenal cortex and slowly destroy it. As a result, often both cortisol and aldosterone hormones are lacking.

Treatment of Addison's involves replacing, or substituting, the hormones that the adrenal glands are not making. Cortisol is replaced orally with hydrocortisone tablets taken once or twice a day. If aldosterone is also deficient, it is replaced with oral doses of fludrocortisone acetate (Florinef), taken once a day. The doses of each of these medications are adjusted to meet the needs of individual patients.

A **pheochromocytoma** is a benign tumor of the adrenal medulla characterized by hypersecretion of the hormones epinephrine and norepinephrine. These catecholamines are responsible for regulating heart rate and blood pressure, among other functions, and the hypersecretion of these hormones causes the gland to produce too much adrenaline, resulting in symptoms such as pounding headaches, very high blood pressure, and flushing of the face. Most pheochromocytomas start in the cells of the adrenal glands, called **chromaffin cells**, which store and secrete catecholamines (they are called *chromaffin* because of the ability of chromium salts to stain them when viewing under a microscope). These tumors rarely spread to other parts of the body.

A definitive cause of pheochromocytoma is not known, but researchers have found that certain families have an increased risk of the disease. The most common familial condition is called **multiple endocrine neoplasia** (MEN). Two types of MEN—MEN2A and MEN2B—are associated with pheochromocytoma. Both are genetic syndromes that run in families and are transmitted from parent to child.

Surgical removal of a pheochromocytoma is the treatment of choice. If surgery is not possible, medications such as phenoxybenzamine (Dibenzyline) and propranolol (Inderal) are beneficial in controlling the adverse effects of catecholamine hypersecretion.

Diabetes Mellitus

Diabetes mellitus (DM) literally means *passing through honey sweet*. It is a chronic disease characterized by the body's failure to manufacture or properly use insulin, resulting in sugar in the blood rising to dangerously high levels. As discussed previously, insulin is a hormone produced by the pancreas that regulates the level of glucose which provides energy for the proper functioning of body cells. Insulin is a key player in the control of metabolism. Abnormalities in insulin secretion have widespread and devastating effects on many organs and tissues.

Although the exact cause of diabetes is unknown, the disease displays certain symptoms that are often heard in medical reports, including frequent urination (**polyuria**), excessive thirst (**polydipsia**), extreme hunger (**polyphagia**), unusual weight loss, and blurred vision.

The human body requires a steady amount of glucose throughout the day to function, and that glucose comes from food. When the stomach digests food, glucose is liberated from the digested food within the small intestine and then is absorbed into the blood where it is carried to all the cells in the body to be used for energy. However, glucose cannot enter the cells alone and needs insulin to aid in its transport into the cells. Without insulin, the cells become starved of glucose energy despite the presence of abundant glucose in the bloodstream. This unused glucose is excreted in the urine.

Elevated concentrations of glucose in the blood stimulate release of insulin, and insulin acts on cells throughout the body to stimulate uptake, utilization, and storage of glucose. Some of the glucose absorbed from the small intestine is immediately taken up by the liver, which converts the glucose to **glycogen**. When the supply of glucose is abundant, insulin *tells* the liver to bank as much of it as possible for later use.

In addition to helping glucose enter cells, insulin also regulates the level of glucose in the blood. After a meal, the blood glucose level rises. In response to this, the pancreas releases more insulin into the bloodstream, which helps glucose enter the cells and lower blood glucose levels after a meal. When blood glucose levels are lowered, the insulin release from the pancreas is lowered. In diabetes, the insulin is either absent, insufficient for the body's needs, or not used properly by the body, all of which cause elevated levels of blood glucose.

Diabetes can have acute and chronic complications. Acute complications include:

- **Diabetic ketoacidosis (DKA)**, a serious condition that develops when insulin levels are insufficient to transport glucose to cells to use for energy. Without insulin, the body cannot use sugar for energy and begins to break down fat and muscle instead. This results in byproducts of fat breakdown, called ketones, to accumulate in the blood and urine. If the condition becomes severe, difficulty breathing, brain swelling, coma, and even death can result.
- **Hypoglycemia**, also called insulin shock, results when there is not enough glucose in the blood. Hypoglycemia occurs when the pancreas sends out too much insulin in response to a rapid rise in blood sugar (such as after a meal), causing the glucose, or blood sugar, to plummet below the level necessary to maintain well-being. Common symptoms of hypoglycemia include sweating, tremor, anxiety, vertigo, and diplopia, followed by delirium, convulsions, and collapse.

Chronic complications of diabetes include:

- **Diabetic retinopathy**, a progressive degeneration of retinal blood vessels in the eyes.
- **Diabetic neuropathy**, which is a condition of damage to the nerves of the body. This problem can be classified as peripheral, autonomic, proximal, or focal. Each affects different parts of the body in various ways:
  - **Peripheral neuropathy**, the most common type of diabetic neuropathy. In medicine, the word *peripheral* means *away from the center* and refers to the areas away from the center of the body or a body part. This type of neuropathy affects the feeling in the toes, feet, legs, hands, and arms.
  - **Autonomic neuropathy** causes changes in digestion, bowel and bladder function, sexual response, and perspiration as well as the nerves that serve the heart, lungs, and eyes.
  - **Proximal neuropathy** causes pain in the thighs, hips, or buttocks and leads to weakness in the legs.
  - **Focal neuropathy** affects one nerve or specific group of nerves, causing muscle weakness or pain. Any nerve in the body can be affected.
- **Diabetic nephropathy**, which is a progressive deteriorating disease of the kidneys. Diabetic nephropathy can lead to chronic renal failure, eventually requiring dialysis.
- **Macrovascular disease**, a condition in which fat builds up in the large (*macro-*) blood vessels and sticks to the vessel walls.
- Coronary artery disease, leading to heart complications such as angina or myocardial infarction (see Chapter 13, *Cardiology*).
- Cerebrovascular disease, leading to stroke.
- **Peripheral vascular disease (PVD)**, which is the narrowing and damage to the vessels distant from the heart, specifically the peripheral arteries and

veins that carry blood to the legs, arms, stomach, and kidneys.

There are two major types of diabetes: type 1 and type 2. In **type 1 diabetes**, also called **insulin-dependent diabetes mellitus** (IDDM), the body's immune system incorrectly identifies the precise cells in the pancreas responsible for insulin production, resulting in destruction of the cells in the islets of Langerhans and rendering the pancreas useless for making insulin. Without insulin, the body's blood sugar refinery is effectively shut down. Thus, individuals with type 1 diabetes must rely on lifelong insulin medication for survival.

In **type 2 diabetes**, also referred to **non-insulin-dependent diabetes mellitus** (NIDDM) or **adult-onset diabetes**, the pancreas can still produce insulin—sometimes even at high levels—but the level of insulin production can be too low or other tissues in the body are resistant to it, impairing the absorption and conversion of blood sugar. This condition is called **insulin resistance**. Over time, insulin production decreases to the point where glucose builds up in the blood and the body cannot make efficient use of its main source of fuel. The main problem with type 2 diabetes is that the cells do not respond adequately to the insulin and, therefore, do not absorb glucose properly. This makes blood sugar levels higher than they should be. When the body can no longer get the energy from the glucose into the cells, it stores the extra energy in fat cells, which explains why diabetics tend to gain weight easily and find it difficult to lose it. This leads to even less efficient use of glucose and eventually requires insulin therapy.

A third category, **gestational diabetes**, occurs only in pregnancy and usually resolves once the pregnancy is delivered. It can lead to a condition in the newborn called **macrosomia**, which means an abnormally large size of the body and is used to describe a newborn with an excessive birth weight. Unfortunately, a diagnosis of fetal macrosomia can be made only by measuring birth weight after delivery. Therefore, the condition is confirmed only retrospectively. Fetal macrosomia is encountered in up to 10% of deliveries.

Finally, **secondary diabetes** refers to elevated blood sugar levels as a result of another body condition. This form of the disease may develop when the pancreas is destroyed by disease, such as chronic pancreatitis or trauma, or from surgical removal of the pancreas. It can also develop from hormonal disturbances, such as in the case of acromegaly or Cushing syndrome. In addition, certain medications may bring on secondary diabetes, which is commonly seen where steroid medications such as prednisone are taken in combination with medications used in the treatment of human immunodeficiency virus (HIV) infection and acquired immunodeficiency syndrome (AIDS).

Treatment for diabetes is focused on controlling the levels of blood glucose, which is essential for overall body health, and for avoiding long-term complications. Physicians typically prescribe a program of diet, exercise, and lifestyle changes to keep blood sugar levels under control. Other patients, however, may need to use insulin or other medications to supplement these lifestyle changes.

Patients with diabetes often test their levels of blood sugar to see whether glucose levels are in the target range recommended by their physicians. These values are transcribed as milligrams per deciliter, or mg/dL. A typical target range might be 80 to 120 mg/dL before meals, and less than 180 mg/dL after eating. Uncontrolled blood sugar can increase in the range of 300 and over, and life-threatening blood sugar values can reach even as high as 1000 mg/dL.

When diet, exercise, and maintenance of a healthy weight are not enough, physicians may prescribe medication to help control diabetes by helping the body process insulin more effectively. A variety of oral medications can be prescribed for patients with diabetes. Each type of pill helps lower blood glucose in a different way. As a transcriptionist, you should listen very carefully to the type and name of drug being dictated, as many of the medications sound alike. The following are some of the common groups of diabetic medications encountered in medical transcription:

- **Sulfonylureas.** These medications work by stimulating insulin secretion in the pancreas and by helping the body better use the insulin it makes. These medications include glipizide (Glucotrol, Glucotrol XL), glyburide (DiaBeta, Micronase), and glimepiride (Amaryl).
- **Biguanides.** These drugs inhibit the production and release of glucose from the liver, resulting in less insulin being required to transport glucose to the cells of the body. Currently, metformin (Glucophage, Glucophage XR) is the only drug in this class available in the United States.
- **Alpha-glucosidase inhibitors.** These drugs block the action of enzymes in the digestive tract that break down carbohydrates, resulting in glucose being absorbed into the bloodstream more slowly. Drugs in this class include acarbose (Precose) and miglitol (Glyset).
- **Thiazolidinediones.** These drugs make the body tissues more sensitive to insulin, which helps to lower blood glucose levels. Common drugs in this category include rosiglitazone (Avandia) and pioglitazone hydrochloride (Actos).
- **Drug combinations.** Combination medications put together different types of drugs into a single pill, enabling blood sugar to be controlled in several different ways. Most physicians prescribe two drugs in combination, with the combination of glyburide and metformin hydrochloride (Glucovance) being the most common.

If these medications fail to control blood sugar levels, physicians may prescribe insulin, injected directly into the bloodstream, to replace what the pancreas is unable to produce. Insulin cannot be taken in pill form because enzymes in the stomach break it down so that it becomes ineffective. For that reason, many people inject themselves with insulin using a syringe or penlike device. Others may use an insulin pump, which provides a continuous supply of insulin, eliminating the need for daily shots. The most widely used form of insulin is synthetic human insulin, which is chemically identical to human insulin but manufactured in a laboratory.

There are six types of insulin used to control diabetes:

- Rapid-acting (Humalog and NovoLog), which starts working in 5 to 20 minutes and lasts up to 5 hours.
- Short-acting (called regular, or R insulin), which starts working in 30 minutes and lasts up to 8 hours.
- Intermediate-acting (NPH or N insulin), which starts working in 1 to 3 hours and lasts up to 24 hours.
- Long-acting (Ultralente or U insulin), which starts working in 4 to 6 hours and lasts up to 28 hours.
- Very long-acting (Lantus), which starts working in 1 hour and lasts up to 24 hours.
- Premixed (NPH and regular insulin), which are two types of insulin mixed together in one bottle. This medication starts working in 30 minutes and lasts up to 24 hours.

In recent years, researchers have focused increasing attention on transplantation for people with type 1 diabetes. Current procedures include a pancreatic transplant, which is usually carried out in conjunction with a kidney transplant. Kidney failure is one of the most common complications of diabetes, and receipt of a new pancreas along with a new kidney may improve kidney survival. In addition, many people do not require injectable insulin after a successful transplantation. However, the body may reject the new organ days or even years after the transplantation, requiring a person to take immunosuppressive drugs for life.

A less invasive treatment option includes pancreatic islet transplantation, in which pancreatic islet cells are taken from a donor pancreas and transferred to a recipient. Once implanted, the beta cells in these islets begin to make and release insulin. Researchers hope that islet transplantation will help people with type 1 diabetes live without daily injections of insulin. In this procedure, pancreatic islets are removed from the pancreas of a deceased donor. Because the islets are fragile, transplantation occurs soon after they are removed. During the transplantation procedure, the surgeon uses ultrasound to guide placement of a small plastic catheter through the upper abdomen and into the liver. The islets are then injected through the catheter into the liver. Over time, the transplanted cells attach to new blood vessels and begin releasing insulin. Blood glucose levels are monitored after the procedure, and insulin may be needed until control is achieved.

Diabetes Insipidus

Diabetes insipidus is a water metabolism disorder caused by deficiency of the hormone ADH, also called vasopressin. ADH is a hormone released by the pituitary gland, which controls the body's ability to retain water. The absence of ADH allows water to be excreted in the urine instead of being reabsorbed by the cells of the body where it is needed. This results in excessive urination and excessive thirst and fluid intake. Diabetes insipidus is not the same as diabetes mellitus. Diabetes insipidus resembles diabetes mellitus because the symptoms of both diseases are increased urination and thirst. However, in every other respect, including the causes and treatment of the disorders, the diseases are completely unrelated. Sometimes diabetes insipidus is referred to as *water* diabetes to distinguish it from the more common diabetes mellitus or *sugar* diabetes.

Possible causes of diabetes insipidus include a pituitary or hypothalamic tumor, a cranial injury, use of certain medications such as lithium and Dilantin, or even excessive alcohol intake. This disorder is treated with the administration of antidiuretic medications, given orally or intravenously, to control fluid balance and prevent dehydration. Oral medications such as desmopressin acetate (DDAVP) are given in the form of tablets

QUICK CHECK 21.2

Fill in the blanks with the correct answers.

1. Another name for hypercortisolism is _____.
2. The hormone _____ is secreted when blood sugars are low.
3. The familial condition, MEN, is associated with _____.
4. _____ forms a class of drugs that stimulate the pancreas to produce more insulin.
5. A disease in which too much growth hormone is secreted by the pituitary gland is called _____.

or a nasal spray to increase urine concentration and decrease urine production.

DIAGNOSTIC STUDIES AND PROCEDURES

Physicians use a variety of tests to diagnose possible endocrine abnormalities. These tests are also often used on an ongoing basis in a patient's followup care and serve as a foundation for ongoing treatment of disease. As with other disorders, endocrine function is tested through laboratory testing and imaging studies.

Laboratory Tests

When a person exhibits signs and symptoms of an endocrine disorder, laboratory studies provide valuable clues as to the possible cause. The typical method used is the measurement of hormone levels in the blood or urine, which can suggest, confirm, or rule out an endocrine disorder. The following list includes the most common of these tests:

- Calcium. This test is used to measure the level of calcium in the blood to detect bone and parathyroid disorders, such as hyperparathyroidism.
- Catecholamines. This test is used to assess adrenal medulla function to help diagnose pheochromocytoma.
- Cortisol. This test is used to evaluate the status of adrenal function; above-normal values can indicate Cushing syndrome or disease.
- **Glucose tolerance test** (GTT). This test is used to detect abnormally high or low blood sugar levels such as that found in diabetes mellitus at the time the test is taken.
- **Glycosylated hemoglobin**, also called **hemoglobin A1c**. This is a measure of the degree of glucose control in diabetes mellitus over a three-month period. Above-normal hormone levels may indicate uncontrolled diabetes.

- Follicle-stimulating hormone (FSH) and luteinizing hormone (LH). These gonadotropins are measured to distinguish between a gonadal abnormality and pituitary gland insufficiency.
- Growth hormone (GH). This test is used to diagnose acromegaly by measuring oversecretion of growth hormone. This test also helps diagnose dwarfism as well as hypothalamic or pituitary tumors.
- Parathyroid hormone (PTH). This test is used to evaluate parathyroid gland function and can confirm a diagnosis of hyperparathyroidism or hypoparathyroidism.
- Thyroid-stimulating hormone (TSH), thyroxine (T4), and triiodothyronine (T3). These tests are used to evaluate thyroid function (hypothyroidism or hyperthyroidism) and also to monitor the effects of iodine or antithyroid medication therapy.
- The **rapid ACTH stimulation test**. This test is used to measure the integrity of the adrenal glands. In this test, blood cortisol, urine cortisol, or both, are measured before and after a synthetic form of ACTH is given by injection. Measurement of cortisol in blood is repeated 30 to 60 minutes after an intravenous ACTH injection. The normal response after an injection of ACTH is a rise in blood and urine cortisol levels. Patients with either form of adrenal insufficiency respond poorly or do not respond at all.
- Serum aldosterone. This test measures serum aldosterone levels. Above-normal levels may indicate hyperaldosteronism, manifested by high blood pressure, muscle cramps and weakness, numbness or tingling in the hands, and low levels of potassium in the blood. Low aldosterone levels may indicate hypoaldosteronism (also called Addison disease), or may occur in people who have diabetes.

Imaging Studies

Imaging studies play a vital role in the evaluation of endocrine diseases. They are performed either alone or in conjunction with other tests. Routine x-rays are used to evaluate how endocrine dysfunction affects bones and

---

QUICK CHECK 21.3 ✓

Indicate whether the following sentences are true (T) or false (F).

1. A hot spot is an area of little or no radionuclide uptake.   T   F

2. The rapid ACTH stimulation test is used to measure the integrity of the adrenal glands.   T   F

3. A gamma camera is used to obtain images of insulin in a blood sample.   T   F

4. Another name for the glycosylated hemoglobin test is hemoglobin A1c.   T   F

5. Obtaining a calcium level measurement in a blood sample is useful in diagnosing a gonadal disorder.   T   F

body tissues, even though they do not reveal endocrine glands. For example, a bone x-ray, routinely ordered for a suspected parathyroid disorder, can show the effects of calcium imbalance on bones. CT scan and MRI are used to assess the various glands of the endocrine system by providing high-resolution images of the gland's structure and may be used to identify tumors or other structural abnormalities causing endocrine dysfunction.

Nuclear medicine studies are also used in endocrinologic diagnostic studies. A **radioactive iodine uptake** (RAIU) test is an imaging study performed to evaluate thyroid function and to distinguish between different types of thyroid disorders. In this procedure, the patient ingests an oral dose of radioactive iodine. The thyroid is then scanned at two hours, six hours, and 24 hours with a special counting probe. The amount of radioactivity detected by the probe is compared with the amount of radioactivity contained in the original dose to determine the percentage of radioactive iodine retained by the thyroid. Below-normal levels of iodine may indicate hypothyroidism, whereas above-normal uptake may indicate hyperthyroidism, or Graves disease.

Another iodine uptake test, called **radionuclide thyroid imaging**, is performed to evaluate the size, structure, and position of the thyroid gland itself. It is usually ordered after a palpable mass, enlarged gland, or goiter is found. In this procedure, a radioactive material is administered to the patient, either orally or intra-venously. The radionuclide scanner, also called a **gamma camera**, is positioned above the thyroid area as it obtains images of the distribution of the radioactive substance in and around the thyroid gland. Nodules with areas of increased radionuclide uptake appear as black regions, or **hot spots**, on the scan, whereas areas of little or no radionuclide uptake appear as white regions, or **cold spots**. These images can determine whether the enlargement is caused by a diffuse increase in the total amount of thyroid tissue or by a nodule or nodules that may need to be biopsied to rule out malignancy.

CHAPTER SUMMARY

Endocrinology is a diverse specialty that incorporates an enormous range of clinical conditions. The work performed by endocrinologists spans a continuum from basic science through clinical investigation to new drug trials. As the incidence of endocrine disorders such as type 2 diabetes continues to climb throughout the developed world, the ability of physicians to modify disease progression steadily improves with new technology and groundbreaking research in cellular biology and genetics. Many medical transcriptionists who have experience in transcribing reports in this field appreciate learning about the fascinating impact of hormonal imbalance on the body, both in physical and emotional terms.

·I·N·S·I·G·H·T·

Only the Lonely

A new study shows that when adults go to bed lonely, sad, or overwhelmed, they have elevated levels of cortisol shortly after waking the next morning. Elevated levels of cortisol—a stress hormone linked to depression, obesity, and other health problems when chronic—actually provide a boost in the morning that cues the body that it is time to rev up to deal with loneliness and other negative experiences, according to Northwestern University's Emma K. Adam, the lead investigator of the study. This study reached across several social and biomedical disciplines to demonstrate that it is not just that people who have more negative emotions have higher levels of cortisol. Rather, with its detailed and intricate methodology, the study shows a complex day-to-day relationship between experience and cortisol levels.

In this study, the cortisol levels of 156 older adults across a range of socioeconomic classes living in the Chicago area were measured three times a day for three consecutive days. Study participants reported their feelings each night in a diary, and researchers looked at whether cortisol levels on a particular day were predicted by experiences the day before or were predictive of experiences that same day.

In addition to noting that loneliness the night before predicted higher cortisol the next morning, Adam and colleagues found that people who experienced anger throughout the day have higher bedtime levels of cortisol and more uniform overall levels of the stress hormone, like the biological signature of a bad day. The study also proved that, in addition to simply being at the mercy of one's daily experiences, cortisol also plays a role in influencing them. Individuals with lower levels of cortisol in the morning experienced greater fatigue during the day, a result with potential implications for understanding chronic fatigue.

Hormonal studies of this type help researchers understand how people's changing social environments influence their biology and health. Hormonal systems are designed to translate social experience into biological action. The bigger question for researchers is whether overuse of these systems plays a role in disease outcomes.

Common Soundalike Words

Word	Word Pronunciation	Soundalike	Pronunciation
endocrine: General term that describes the glands and organs that release hormones directly into the blood.	en'dō-krin	**exocrine**: General term that describes glands that release substances through ducts and not directly into the blood.	ek'sō-krin
gland: An organized aggregation of cells functioning as a secretory or excretory organ.	gland	**glans**: A conic, acorn-shaped structure.	glanz
adrenal: The suprarenal gland.	ă-drē'năl	**aline**: A catecholamine that is the chief hormone of the adrenal medulla.	ă-dren'ă-lin
pineal: Relating to the pineal body.	pin'ē-ăl	**penile**: Relating to the penis.	pē'nīl
thyroid: A gland located in the larynx.	thī'royd	**thymus**: A gland located in the superior mediastinum and lower part of the neck.	thī'mŭs
melatonin: Hormone secreted by the pineal gland.	mel-ă-tōn'in	**melanin**: Dark brown or black pigment produced by melanocytes in the skin.	mel'ă-nin
gonadotropin: A hormone capable of promoting gonadal growth and function.	gō'nad-ō-trō'pin	**goniotomy**: Surgical opening of the trabecular meshwork in congenital glaucoma.	gō-nē-ot'ŏ-mē
adren/o: Combining form meaning the *adrenal gland*.	ă-drē'-nō	**aden/o**: Combining form meaning a *gland*.	ad'ĕ-nō
GTT: Abbreviation for *glucose tolerance test*.	GTT	**gtt**: Abbreviation for *drops* (used in pharmacology).	gtt
inhibin: A substance secreted by the testes and ovaries that regulates FSH levels.	in-hib'in	**inhibit**: To curb or restrain.	in-hib'it

Combining Forms

Combining Form	Definition	Combining Form	Definition
aden/o, glandul/o	gland	medull/o	inner region
adren/o, adrenal/o	adrenal gland	melan/o	black
andr/o	male	ovari/o	ovary
calc/i	calcium	ox/y	oxygen
cortic/o	cortex	pancreat/o	pancreas
crin/o	to secrete	parathyr/o, parathyroid/o	parathyroid gland
dips/o	thirst	somat/o	body
endocrin/o	endocrine	stimul/o	strengthening
gluc/o, glyc/o	sugar	testicul/o	testicle
gonad/o	gonads (ovaries and testes)	thalam/o	thalamus
hormon/o	hormone	thym/o	thymus gland
hypophys/o, pituit/o	pituitary gland	thyr/o, thyroid/o	thyroid gland
insul/o	island	toc/o	labor and childbirth
iod/o	iodine		
lact/o	milk		

Add Your Own Combining Forms Here:

_____

_____

_____

_____

_____

_____

ABBREVIATIONS

Abbreviation	Meaning	Abbreviation	Meaning
ACTH	adrenocorticotropic hormone	LH	luteinizing hormone
ADH	antidiuretic hormone	MEN	multiple endocrine neoplasia
BG	blood glucose	NIDDM	non-insulin-dependent diabetes mellitus
CBG	capillary blood glucose		
CT	calcitonin	NPH	intermediate-acting (insulin)
DDAVP	desmopressin acetate	OT	oxytocin
DKA	diabetic ketoacidosis	PRL	prolactin
DM	diabetes mellitus	PTH	parathyroid hormone
FSH	follicle-stimulating hormone	PVD	peripheral vascular disease
GH	growth hormone	RAIU	radioactive iodine uptake (test)
GHRH	growth hormone-releasing hormone	T3	triiodothyronine
GTT	glucose tolerance test	T4	thyroxine
ICSH	interstitial cell-stimulating hormone	TSH	thyroid-stimulating hormone
IDDM	insulin-dependent diabetes mellitus		

Add Your Own Abbreviations Here:

_____

_____

_____

_____

_____

_____

TERMINOLOGY

Term	Meaning
acromegaly	Overproduction of growth hormone from the pituitary gland that affects middle-aged adults.
Addison disease, syn. adrenal insufficiency	A hormonal disorder of the adrenal glands caused by the hyposecretion of cortisol.
adrenal cortex	The upper region of the adrenal gland.

Term	Meaning
adrenal glands, syn. suprarenal glands	Two cone-shaped structures that lie on top of each kidney.
adrenocorticotropic hormone (ACTH), syn. corticotropin	A hormone that stimulates the secretion of cortisol in the adrenal glands.
aldosterone	A hormone secreted by the adrenal cortex that helps regulate the balance of electrolytes in the body and helps maintain blood volume and pressure.
alpha-glucosidase inhibitors	A class of drugs which block the action of enzymes in the digestive tract, enabling glucose to be absorbed into the bloodstream more slowly.
androgens	The name given to male hormones.
anterior pituitary gland	The anterior, or front, part of the pituitary gland.
antidiuretic hormone (ADH), syn. vasopressin	A hormone produced by the pituitary gland that reduces the production of urine in the kidneys, and, therefore, prevents water loss from the body.
autonomic neuropathy	A type of neuropathy that causes changed in digestion, bowel and bladder function, sexual response, and perspiration as well as the to the nerves of the heart, lungs and eyes, as a complication of diabetes mellitus.
biguanides	A class of drugs which inhibit the production and release of glucose from the liver, resulting in less insulin being required to transport glucose to the cells of the body.
blood glucose (BG), syn. capillary blood glucose (CBG)	The principal sugar of the blood.
calcitonin	A hormone secreted by the thyroid gland that regulates the balance of calcium and phosphorus in the blood.
catecholamines	The collective term for *epinephrine and norepinephrine.*
chromaffin cells	The cells of the adrenal glands.
circadian rhythm	The body's biological internal clock and sleep-wake pattern.
circle of Willis	A connection of arteries in the brain that provides the pituitary gland with blood exchange.
cold spots	White or gray regions that appear in the image of a radionuclide thyroid imaging study.
corticosterone	A hormone secreted by the adrenal cortex that helps suppress inflammatory reactions in the body.
cortisol	A hormone secreted by the adrenal cortex that controls the body's use of fats, proteins, and carbohydrates.
Cushing disease	The name used when Cushing syndrome is caused by an abnormality (such as a tumor) in the pituitary gland.
Cushing syndrome, syn. hypercoritsolism	A hormonal disorder of the adrenal glands caused by prolonged exposure of the body's tissue to abnormally high levels of cortisol.
diabetes insipidus	A water metabolism disorder caused by deficiency of ADH.
diabetic ketoacidosis (DKA)	A serious condition that develops when insulin levels are insufficient to transport glucose to cells to use for energy, leading the body to break down fat and muscle for energy use instead.
diabetes mellitus (DM)	A chronic disease characterized by the body's failure to manufacture or properly use insulin.
diabetic nephropathy	A progress deteriorating disease of the kidneys as a result of long-term complications of diabetes mellitus.

Term	Meaning
diabetic neuropathy	A condition of damage to the nerves of the body as a result of long-term complications of diabetes mellitus.
diabetic retinopathy	A progressive degeneration of retinal blood vessels in the eyes as a result of long-term complications of diabetes mellitus.
dwarfism	A disorder caused by too little growth hormone secreted by the pituitary gland in childhood.
endocrine glands	The specialized organs that make up the endocrine system.
endocrinologist	A specially trained physician who diagnoses and treats hormone problems.
endocrinology	The scientific study of the function and pathology of the endocrine glands.
epinephrine, syn. adrenaline	A hormone secreted by the adrenal medulla that increases heart rate and facilitates blood flow to muscles and the brain, as well as other activities regulated by the sympathetic nervous system. This hormone allows for the body's "fight or flight" reaction to stressful situations.
estradiol	The most common type of estrogen secreted by the follicles of the ovary.
estrogen	A hormone secreted by the follicles of the ovary when stimulated by FSH from the anterior pituitary gland.
focal neuropathy	A type of diabetic neuropathy that affects one nerve or a specific group of nerves, causing muscle weakness or pain.
follicle-stimulating hormone (FSH)	A gonadotropic hormone that promotes sperm production in men and ovulation in women.
gamma camera	A special scanner used to obtain images during a radionuclide thyroid imaging study.
gestational diabetes	Diabetes that occurs only in pregnancy.
gigantism	A disorder caused by too much growth hormone excreted by the pituitary gland in childhood.
glucagon	A hormone produced by the pancreas in response to low blood glucose levels.
glucose	A simple sugar that is the main source of energy for the body.
glucose tolerance test (GGT)	A test to detect abnormally high or low blood sugar levels at a given moment.
glycogen	The storage form of glucose found in the liver and muscles.
glycosylated hemoglobin, syn. hemoglobin A1c	Also called *hemoglobin A1c,* the blood sugar levels measured over a three-month period.
gonadotropins	A group of hormones that stimulate the production of various hormones in the gonads.
gonads	The sex glands of the body, namely the ovaries in females and testes in males.
growth hormone (GH), syn. somatotropin	A hormone that controls linear growth in children and adolescents.
hirsutism	Excessive hair growth.
homeostasis	The maintenance of the body's metabolic activities and internal balance.
hormones	Chemical substances secreted by the endocrine glands in response to stimulation from the nervous system and other sites in the body.
hot spots	Black regions that appear in the image of a radionuclide thyroid imaging study.
hypercalcemia	The condition of elevated levels of calcium in the blood.
hyperglycemia	A condition of elevated levels of blood glucose.

Term	Meaning
hypoglycemia, syn. insulin shock	A condition that results when there is not enough glucose in the blood due to the pancreas secreting too much insulin in response to a rapid rise in blood sugar.
hyperparathyroidism	A disorder of the parathyroid glands resulting in the secretion of too much parathyroid hormone (PTH), resulting in decreased phosphorus and increased calcium in the blood.
hyperplasia	An abnormal increase in the elements composing a part, such as abnormal enlargement of the thyroid gland.
hypoglycemia	A condition of low levels of blood glucose.
hypoparathyroidism	A disorder of the parathyroid glands resulting in the secretion of too little parathyroid hormone (PTH), resulting in increased phosphorus and decreased calcium in the blood.
hypopituitarism	A condition resulting in complete loss of function and hormone secretion of the anterior lobe of the pituitary gland.
infundibulum	A stalk of tissue that connects the pituitary gland to the hypothalamus.
inhibin	A hormone secreted by the testes in response to increased testosterone.
insulin	A hormone made by the pancreas in response to rising levels of glucose in the blood.
insulin resistance	The suboptimal or defective production of insulin by the pancreas.
interstitial cell-stimulating hormone (ICSH)	A gonadotropic hormone that stimulates production of various hormones in the gonads.
islets of Langerhans	Cells located in the pancreas that produce insulin.
isthmus	The thin bridge of tissue that connects the lobes of the thyroid gland.
lobe	Each of two divisions of the pituitary gland; also the name given to each lateral side of the thyroid gland.
luteinizing hormone (LH)	A gonadotropic hormone that stimulates an ovarian follicle to develop into the corpus luteum.
macrosomia	A term that means an abnormally large size of the body and is often used to describe a newborn with an excessive birth weight.
macrovascular disease	A condition in which fat builds up in the large blood vessels of the body and sticks to vessel walls, as a result of long-term complications of diabetes mellitus.
medulla	The inner or core region of the adrenal gland.
melatonin	A hormone secreted by the pineal gland that regulates the body's internal clock and plays a role in mood regulation.
multiple endocrine neoplasia (MEN)	A familial genetic condition that leads to an increased risk of acquiring pheochromocytoma.
neurohormones	Hormones that control the secretion of hormones from the adjacent anterior pituitary gland in the brain.
norepinephrine, syn. noradrenaline	A hormone secreted by the adrenal medulla that causes blood vessels and skeletal muscles to constrict, which raises blood pressure.
osteoclasts	Cells located in the bones, which break down the mineral part of the bone and release calcium into the blood.
ovaries	Small, egg-producing glands located in the pelvic cavity in women.
oxytocin	A hormone secreted by the pituitary gland that stimulates the production of prolactin in nursing mothers and contractions during childbirth.

Term	Meaning
pancreas	An elongated gland located near the stomach in the left upper quadrant of the abdomen.
panhypopituitarism	A condition resulting in complete loss of function and hormone secretion of the entire pituitary gland.
parathyroid glands	Four small glands located on the back of each lobe of the thyroid gland.
parathyroid hormone (PTH)	A hormone secreted by the parathyroid glands that helps conserve levels of calcium in the blood.
parathyroidectomy	The surgical removal of the parathyroid gland(s).
peripheral neuropathy	A type of diabetic neuropathy that causes pain in the toes, feet, legs, hands, and arms.
peripheral vascular disease (PVD)	Damaged to the vessels distant from the heart, specifically the peripheral arteries and veins that carry blood to the legs, arms, stomach or kidneys, resulting from long-term complications of diabetes mellitus.
pheochromocytoma	A benign tumor of the adrenal medulla characterized by hypersecretion of hormones epinephrine and norepinephrine.
pineal gland	A tiny, cone-shaped structure located in the third ventricle of the brain.
pituitary adenoma	A tumor located in the pituitary gland.
pituitary gland, syn. hypophysis	A small, teardrop-shaped gland lying below the hypothalamus of the brain.
polydipsia	Excessive thirst.
polyphagia	Extreme hunger.
polyuria	Frequent urination.
posterior pituitary gland	The posterior, or rear, part of the pituitary gland.
progesterone	A hormone secreted by the corpus luteum in response to LH from the pituitary gland.
prolactin (PRL)	A hormone responsible for lactation in the breasts after childbirth.
proximal neuropathy	A type of diabetic neuropathy that causes pain in the thighs, hips, and buttocks and leads to weakness in the legs.
radioactive iodine uptake (RAIU) test	An imaging study performed to evaluate thyroid function.
radionuclide thyroid imaging	An imaging study performed to evaluate the size, structure, and position of the thyroid gland itself.
rapid ACTH stimulation test, syn. rapid corticotropin test	A test used to measure the integrity of the adrenal glands.
secondary diabetes	The condition of elevated blood sugar levels as a result of another body condition or illness.
somatostatin	A hormone produced by the pancreas, which inhibits the release of growth hormone from the pituitary gland.
striae	Stretch marks.
sulfonylureas	A class of drugs which stimulate the pancreas to produce and release more insulin.
testes (singular, testis)	Egg-shaped glands located in the scrotum of males.
testicles	Another name for *testes*.
testosterone	A hormone secreted by the testes that maintains male sex-related traits.
thiazolidinediones	A class of drugs which make the body tissues more sensitive to insulin.

Term	Meaning
thymosin	A hormone secreted by the thymus gland that causes immature T cells to develop and mature.
thymus	A small gland located in the thoracic cavity behind the sternum.
thyroid gland	A butterfly-shaped gland that wraps around the trachea.
thyroid hormone	The collective hormones T3 and thyroxine (T4).
thyroid-stimulating hormone (TSH), syn. thyrotropin	A hormone that stimulates the normal growth of the thyroid and the secretion of thyroid hormones.
thyromegaly	Enlargement of the thyroid gland.
thyroxine (T4)	A hormone secreted by the thyroid gland that helps regulate body metabolism.
transsphenoidal adenectomy	The surgical removal of a pituitary adenoma through the sphenoid sinuses behind the nose.
triiodothyronine (T3)	A hormone secreted by the thyroid gland that helps regulate body metabolism.
type 1 diabetes, syn. insulin-dependent diabetes (IDDM)	A condition whereby the pancreas undergoes an autoimmune attack by the body itself, rendering it useless for making insulin.
type 2 diabetes, syn. non-insulin-dependent diabetes (NDDM) or adult-onset diabetes	A condition whereby the pancreas can produce insulin, but this production is insufficient or suboptimal.

Add Your Own Terms and Definitions Here:

_____

_____

_____

_____

_____

_____

_____

_____

REVIEW QUESTIONS

1. Name and describe the procedure used to remove a pituitary tumor.
2. Where in the pancreas is insulin produced?
3. Name the hormones stored in the posterior pituitary gland and describe the function of each.
4. What is the purpose of the parathyroid glands?
5. What is the function of insulin?
6. Describe Cushing syndrome.
7. What is the difference between a glucose tolerance test and a glycosylated hemoglobin test?
8. List the hormones secreted by the adrenal cortex and adrenal medulla, respectively.
9. What type of imaging study evaluates the size and structure of the thyroid gland?
10. What is diabetes mellitus?

CHAPTER ACTIVITIES

Soundalike Word Choice

Circle the correct word in the following sentences.

1. After the induction of general endotracheal anesthesia, the low collar incision was injected with 8 mL of Naropin without (ephedrine, epinephrine).
2. During her hospital stay, she was able to tolerate oral foods and obtain relief of her nausea with (parenteral, parental) medications.
3. On examination, tympanic membranes are intact and mobile bilaterally. There are no (infusions, effusions) present.
4. As you recall, this is a 26-year-old female with a history of left thyroid (nodule, nodosum).
5. As part of his workup, Danny received a radioactive (iodide, iodine) uptake test to evaluate the thyroid.
6. During the operation, the right superior (parathyroid, paratyphoid) was identified and preserved.
7. The patient previously underwent removal of her left thyroid and (isthmus, island).
8. Working in the subcapsular (plane, plain) along the lateral border of the thyroid, the right (thymus, thyroid) lobe was elevated up out of the tracheoesophageal groove.
9. The patient was eventually diagnosed with type 1 diabetes (melotia, mellitus).
10. I believe she will probably need continued monitoring while taking calcium to ensure that she does not become (hypercalcemic, hyperkalemic).

Multiple Choice

Circle the letter corresponding to the best answers to the following questions.

1. Hormones are
    A. another name for brain waves.
    B. neurons on which messages travel.
    C. chemicals that respond to stimulation from the nervous system and other sites in the body.
    D. substances containing tumor markers.

2. Which of the following are mismatched?
    A. thyroxine—pituitary gland
    B. insulin—pancreas
    C. glucagon—pancreas
    D. oxytocin—hypothalamus

3. Which gland is part of both the digestive system and the endocrine system?
    A. the thyroid
    B. the pineal
    C. the pituitary
    D. the pancreas

4. The posterior lobe of the pituitary gland
   A. secretes hormones that stimulate the anterior pituitary gland.
   B. stores hormones produced by the hypothalamus.
   C. is responsible for all hormone secretion.
   D. sends nerve signals to other parts of the brain.

5. Type 1 diabetes is also called
   A. non-insulin-dependent diabetes mellitus.
   B. secondary diabetes.
   C. insulin-dependent diabetes mellitus.
   D. adult-onset diabetes.

6. The hormones T3 and T4 are collectively called
   A. calcitonin.
   B. thyroid hormone.
   C. aldosterone.
   D. pituitary hormone.

7. All of the following are produced by the pituitary gland except
   A. growth hormone.
   B. prolactin.
   C. oxytocin.
   D. insulin.

8. A person's internal clock and sleep-wake cycle is referred to as the
   A. regular routine.
   B. sleep routine.
   C. biological clock.
   D. circadian rhythm.

9. When the level of calcium drops,
   A. one should immediately eat a bowl of vanilla ice cream.
   B. the thyroid gland releases calcium into the blood.
   C. the parathyroid glands secrete a hormone the causes the release of calcium from bone into the blood.
   D. the thyroid gland releases iodine into the blood.

10. Low levels of thyroid hormones cause the disease known as
    A. hypothyroidism.
    B. diabetes mellitus.
    C. gigantism.
    D. hyperthyroidism.

11. What hormone is secreted by the adrenal medulla?
    A. epinephrine
    B. cortisol
    C. PTH
    D. oxytocin

12. The part of the endocrine system called the "master gland" is the
    A. thymus.
    B. hypothalamus.
    C. adrenals.
    D. pituitary.

13. A decrease in blood glucose stimulates the release of the hormone
    A. oxytocin.
    B. insulin.
    C. TSH.
    D. glucagon.

14. Which category of diabetes occurs only during pregnancy?
    A. type 2 diabetes
    B. type 1 diabetes
    C. secondary diabetes
    D. gestational diabetes

15. Cortisol is a hormone produced by the
    A. adrenal medulla.
    B. adrenal cortex.
    C. pancreas.
    D. thymus.

16. A high concentration of calcium in the blood suggests a disorder of the
    A. adrenals.
    B. thyroid.
    C. parathyroid glands.
    D. liver.

17. Which gland produces progesterone?
    A. the ovaries
    B. the testes
    C. the adrenals
    D. the parathyroid glands

18. The procedure whereby surgery is performed through the sphenoid sinuses behind the nose to remove a pituitary tumor is called
    A. transsphenoidal adenectomy.
    B. transdermal pituitectomy.
    C. transmaxillary adenectomy.
    D. transsphenoidal ethmoidectomy.

19. If the amount of blood glucose is high, the islets of Langerhans will secrete
    A. glucagon.
    B. insulin.
    C. testosterone.
    D. ADH.

20. Cushing syndrome is characterized by
    A. a moon-face appearance.
    B. upper body obesity.
    C. hyperglycemia.
    D. All of the above.

Medical Terminology Review

Circle the correct word in the following sentences.

1. If you ate four sugar-glazed doughnuts, (insulin/insudate) would be secreted at higher levels.
2. (Vasosporin/vasopressin) is the same hormone as ADH.
3. (THS/TSH) causes activation of thyroid follicular cells.
4. Oxytocin is a hormone actually produced by the (hypothalamus/hypopotamus).
5. The thymus gland produces (thymosin/thyroxine).
6. The adrenal (medusa/medulla) is an endocrine gland.
7. The pineal gland secretes a hormone called (melanin/melatonin).
8. (ACTH/ACH) is also called corticotropin.
9. The hypothalamus produces the hormone (oxycontin/oxytocin).
10. The hormone (cortisol/cortisone) helps control the body's use of fats, proteins, and carbohydrates.

Understanding Medical Documents

Read the following excerpt from a clinic note and using resource materials or the Internet to locate terms you do not know, answer the questions that follow.

This is a 60-year-old white female who is status post total thyroidectomy for thyroid cancer. She is complaining of pain and the swelling in her left neck. She states that she has had reflux symptoms and shortness of breath for the last 6 months. She was recently started on 125 mcg of Synthroid daily but she says this has only helped slightly. Palpation of the neck reveals no masses. Indirect laryngoscopy was performed. No masses or lesions were noted. True vocal cords were mobile bilaterally.

Questions:

1. Did the patient undergo thyroid surgery in the past or is this a future event? How did you know?
2. For which of the patient's symptoms would the physician have prescribed Synthroid?
3. What does "palpation" mean?
4. Why do you think the physician would perform an indirect laryngoscopy as part of the physical examination?
5. Which of the following disorders do you think the patient likely has—hypothyroidism or hyperthyroidism—and on which symptom(s) do you base your conclusion?

Matching

Match the disorder or symptom on the left with the gland affected on the right (some glands may be used more than once).

Disorder/Symptom

1. _____ acromegaly
2. _____ Addison disease
3. _____ panhypopituitarism
4. _____ polyuria
5. _____ Cushing syndrome
6. _____ dwarfism
7. _____ hyperglycemia
8. _____ circadian rhythm disruption
9. _____ hypercalcemia
10. _____ moon-shaped appearance
11. _____ pheochromocytoma
12. _____ gigantism
13. _____ diabetes mellitus
14. _____ thyromegaly
15. _____ hyperparathyroidism

Gland Affected

A. pituitary

B. pineal

C. thyroid

D. parathyroid

E. thymus

F. adrenals

G. pancreas

H. gonads

Hormone Function and Abbreviations

Write the function and abbreviation for each of the hormones on the left in the space at the right. The first one is done for you.

Hormone	*Function*	*Abbreviation*
1. somatotropin	stimulates growth	GH
2. corticotropin		
3. interstitial cell-stimulating hormone		
4. prolactin		
5. calcitonin		
6. luteinizing hormone		
7. follicle-stimulating hormone		
8. antidiuretic hormone		
9. parathyroid hormone		
10. triiodothyronine		

TRANSCRIPTION PRACTICE

Open your word-processing software. Insert the student CD-ROM and locate the dictation for this chapter. For each of the words in the "listen for these terms" list for each report, use a medical dictionary or other resources to identify and write down a brief definition of the term on a separate sheet of paper to attach with your work. Then listen to the dictation and transcribe each report. Use the current date for each report where a date is indicated. Insert a heading into the document if the text falls to a second page.

At the end of each report, indicate the name of the dictating physician under the signature line and insert reference initials. For date dictated and transcribed and date of admission, use the current date. Proofread your work, print one copy for your instructor along with your term definitions, and save the completed report to your student disk.

Report T21.1: Clinic Note
Patient Name: Brittany Randolph
Medical Record No.: 060355
Attending Physician (dictator): Sabrina Scott, MD

Listen for these terms:
thyroidectomy
central compartment dissection
papillary thyroid cancer
deltoid
clavicular

Report T21.2: Consultation Letter
Patient Name: Kristen Webb
Medical Record No.: WE-2119
Attending Physician: Kamraan George, MD

Listen for these terms:
hyperplasia
hypocalcemia
vascularized
calcitriol

Report T21.3: Clinic Note
Patient Name: Alma Tucker
Medical Record No.: 245
Attending Physician: Andrea Biggs, MD

Listen for these terms:
petechial
Skelaxin
cushingoid
adrenalectomy

PART III

Your New Career

22

CAREER MANAGEMENT

OBJECTIVES

After completing this chapter, you will be able to:

- Develop clear job search strategies.
- Create a resumé and application letter.
- Describe methods and strategies for taking online application tests.
- Demonstrate effective interview techniques.
- Identify personal and professional strategies in order to work optimally as a medical transcriptionist.
- Understand the key concepts and procedures involved in owning a medical transcription business.

INTRODUCTION

Congratulations! You have successfully completed your medical transcription training and are ready to start a new and exciting career as a medical transcriptionist.

Medical transcription companies are referred to as **medical transcription service organizations** (MTSOs), and they are always looking for qualified individuals to transcribe reports for medical facilities. Although it is true that MTSOs always need experienced medical transcriptionists, you can still obtain a meaningful position in the workforce even if you have little or no work experience. Experience, including qualities in those important areas of emotional intelligence, communications, creativity, responsibility, determination, integrity, compassion, and problem-solving—the qualities all employers value—accumulates from everything we do. As a new graduate, you can demonstrate that you have the qualities that employers will recognize and desire.

JOB SEARCH STRATEGIES

The primary obstacle to launching a career in the medical transcription industry is overcoming the "experience" requirement. You may hear from prospective employers that you do not have enough experience, or worse, that you have no experience at all. This hurdle is not impossible to overcome, however. You have selected a field where job openings far outnumber the candidates qualified to fill them. It is a fact that most students will not have a job by the time they graduate, but do not feel discouraged. If you are persistent and use the following tools to find an employer willing to give you your first job, a wide range of opportunities for acquiring experience and work will open up before you.

Professional Associations

Joining a professional organization is one of the most important first steps in building a career as a medical transcriptionist. The Association for Healthcare Documentation Integrity (**AHDI**)—formerly the American Association for Medical Transcription—is the organization that represents the interests of medical transcriptionists and other healthcare documentation providers. The AHDI works to set and uphold standards of practice in the field of medical documentation that ensure the highest level of quality, privacy, and security of health information. The association has a variety of membership categories, some at reduced rates, to help you get started. Although the membership rate may be somewhat costly at first for a graduating medical transcriptionist, you can learn a tremendous amount about the medical transcription industry by attending the organization's meetings and reading its newsletter or journal. Armed with this knowledge, you will be much more informed about the field you have chosen and better prepared for upcoming interviews. Joining your trade association is a great way to meet other medical transcriptionists. Members of organizations such as the AHDI are impassioned about their work and enjoy the company of other medical transcriptionists.

AHDI national, state/regional, and local chapters will help you meet other medical transcriptionists and make new friends as well as to keep you up to date on the latest trends in the field. Most organizations have regularly scheduled meetings that offer programs featuring speakers who not only teach you about the latest happenings in the industry, but also who may know of job openings in your local area. In addition to monthly meetings, state/regional and local chapters have member lists, education symposia, and other events where members can network and exchange information about job opportunities. Association work and industry-wide networking go hand in hand. When you serve on a committee or as an officer of your local, state, or regional organization, you have an opportunity to meet your counterparts in chapters in other regions, expanding your networking contacts in multiple directions. Then when it comes time to look for a new job, you will be able to explore a broader range of opportunities.

Network Opportunities

The term **networking** refers to the process of connecting particular people or objects. For example, a computer network is a series of computers hooked together so that information can be transmitted and shared between members of the same network. A social network is a group of people who are connected or affiliated through a common interest or need. The objective of social networks can be either personal or related to business. Statistics show that more than 70% of jobs are found through networking, and medical transcription is no different. Networking, therefore, should be a key component of your job-search program.

The important byproduct of all networks is the relationships that develop among the group members. There is a certain level of personal allegiance and responsiveness that evolves naturally as a result of the group's common interest and the relationships fostered through personal affiliation with the group. The members of your professional network (either directly or indirectly through their contacts) are often in a position to provide valuable job leads. Each member of your immediate network is probably connected to several other people connected to other networks; the opportunities to make contacts that can help you with your job search are significant.

Networking is so powerful because it gives you access to a hidden job market. The word "hidden" in this instance refers to employment opportunities that either are not known by the public or job openings that are never advertised. These job openings are usually known to only a small handful of internal employees (such as human resource managers). These jobs are reserved for word-of-mouth referrals from others in the field; so even if a recruiter received your resumé, you would likely receive a polite rejection to your query despite the fact that an opportunity for which you were qualified actually existed. This is because managers prefer to hire a known quantity, rather than fish through a mountain of resumés and applications to find just the right person. When a candidate is introduced through another company employee, a hiring manager has a tendency to feel more comfortable with that candidate than with someone who is "just off the street." In addition, when another employee takes the time to make a candidate referral, the hiring manager may feel a sense of obligation to devote some extra time to evaluating that person's candidacy. Such personal referrals are to the candidate's advantage and greatly enhance the probability of success.

To use networking effectively, begin by identifying those individuals who are closely related to the field, such as your school instructors, trade association members and officers, or even your personal medical providers. To keep track of calls made to your contacts and results, you might want to create a simple call log (or e-mail log) that indicates the person contacted (including title, location, and phone number), the result of the call, and a potential follow-up date on which to call the person back, a sample of which is shown in Figure 22.1.

One of the secrets of networking is to know what you want—or at least to appear to know what you want. When you talk to people about a potential job opportunity, you will appear more intelligent, professional, and even more of an industry insider if you are knowledgeable about your field. Try to keep up to date in any

Network Contact Sheet

Date of Contact	Name	Company	E-mail and/or Phone Number	Source of Contact (Internet, Friend, etc.)	Summary of Conversation and Notes	Date to Call Again

FIGURE 22.1. **Network Contact Sheet.** Use a call log to keep track of calls made to your networking contacts.

way you can. Read trade publications and browse Internet web sites that are particular to medical transcription. Program your browser settings to alert you of newspaper or magazine articles written about the field. For example, Yahoo and Google both send alerts by e-mail when articles from reliable news sources that match the topics you specify appear online. In the news alert section of these search engines, you can request as many types of alerts as you want, and you can request that they be sent once a day or as news happens. Enter subject words such as *medical transcription* or *health care documentation* to stay alert to articles wherever the word or phrase appears in a headline, in the text of an article, or even in a byline. The service is free.

INDUSTRY TERMINOLOGY

It is helpful to know some of the common terms used in the medical transcription industry. Companies for which you will eventually work use these terms to describe the nature of their work and the reports submitted by medical transcriptionists:

- **Turnaround time** (TAT). This term refers to the measurement of time between the point at which a dictated report is submitted for transcription and time the report is typed by the medical transcriptionist and returned to the facility. A medical transcription company pays close attention to the turnaround time of documents because they have promised the facility specific turnaround times for certain documents. For example, some reports require a 12-hour TAT, while others require a faster TAT. Should a typed report exceed the promised turnaround time, any number of events at the facility might be delayed as people await the return of the document. Delays can not only be costly, but can even affect patient care. For example, perhaps a patient is in the operating room, awaiting surgery. The surgery cannot commence because the physicians are waiting for the report from a CT scan of the patient's lungs before beginning. Or, a patient's surgery might have to be stopped should the pathology report on a specimen arrive late. Turnaround time, then, is not just a matter of money when it could conceivably mean the life or death of a patient.
- **Work type** (WT). Reports are categorized by the type of document dictated, and there are many different document types. The report may be a history and physical, a consultation, an operative report, or a progress note. Often times the first thing a company wants to know when you apply for a job is what kind of documents you do best. Work types typically have a number or abbreviation assigned to them to make it easier to direct certain report types to a particular transcriptionist. For example, a consultation note might be designated as a work type 4, or CN, in the company computer system. The medical transcriptionist who is unskilled at consultations will not be sent this work type— thus, division of reports by work type makes it easier for the company to disburse work to the most qualified employee. It also allows the facility to quickly locate the particular reports they might need. Some work types are notoriously more difficult to type than others. For example, many transcriptionists with years of experience still find operative reports a challenge.
- **Outsourcing**. This term refers to the process by which a healthcare organization contracts with a medical transcription company to handle the production of their dictated medical records. Currently in the field of medical transcription, the term *outsourcing* refers to contracting with companies located overseas to perform medical transcription services.
- **Overflow**. This term is used by MTSOs to refer to the work that a facility's in-house staff cannot complete within the required TAT.
- **Line counts**. Line counts are measurements of lines typed by a medical transcriptionist. Your value as a medical transcriptionist has a lot to do with your line count; a higher line count indicates that you can produce more typed lines, and, hence, more reports. Be ready to answer when a company asks, "What is your typical daily line count?" Line counts are based on certain criteria, which might include:
  - Character. A character is any letter, number, symbol, or function key necessary for the final appearance and content of a document, including the spacebar, return key, underscore, bold, and any character contained within a macro, header, or footer.
  - Word. A word consists of a set number of characters. Total words in a document are determined by dividing the total character count by the specified number of characters in a word, for example 5.
  - Line. A line of text consists of a certain number of characters. A typical typed line consists of sixty-five (65) characters. Some companies measure line counts with a seventy (70) character line. The total number of lines for reporting purposes is determined by dividing the total characters by the specified number of characters in a line (such as 65).

Volunteer Prospects

Perhaps the biggest problem graduating students face is lack of experience, but this can be overcome. Your school may have internship programs designed to give students exposure to the medical transcription field, as well as the opportunity to make valuable contacts. Check out your school's career services department to see what internships are available. If your school does not have a formal internship program, or if no internships appeal to you, try contacting local businesses, such as doctor's offices and local hospitals, to offer your services. Many businesses are more than willing to have an extra pair of hands (especially for free!) for a day or two each week. Call your local hospital to check for volunteering opportunities in the facility. Volunteering your time in your field demonstrates dedication—qualities that most MTSOs look for in employees. It looks good on your resumé as well. In addition, volunteering can introduce you to more contacts you can call upon for possible work opportunities in the future.

Internet Strategies

The Internet is probably the most effective source for leads on medical transcription jobs, and most medical transcription jobs landed are the result of Internet listings. Most MTSOs have web sites and use them to invite job applications. Because most medical transcriptionists work at home, MTSOs use the Internet not only to communicate with their employees but also to load their software platforms and to work with their clients. When you explore an MTSO's web site, the company can see that you are proficient with online communications and that you can effectively navigate application windows and other features of the web site. This is very important for performing research for potential employers as well. Proficiency in using Internet research to find information, for job seeking now and later, and for actual research purposes on the job is essential.

Company Web Sites

Company web sites are probably the most effective source of hiring for MTSOs. However, from a job seeker's perspective, locating these web sites may be the most time-consuming process. How can you find the thousands of MTSOs?

The fastest way to locate MTSOs is by means of a search engine such as Google, Yahoo, or Ask. Simply type the words "medical transcription companies" into the search box and click on the search button. In most cases, you should receive thousands of hits of companies located all over the country, if not all over the world. Review the search results to target the companies to which you would like to apply. As most transcriptionists work at home, geographic area is not as important a consideration as the type of work in which the company specializes. For example, if you love radiology and pathology, you might want to focus your job search on companies that specialize in radiology. Then click on

those MTSOs in which you have an interest and follow the online instructions on the company's web site for completing the application process. Many new graduates are often discouraged when they go to a company's web site and see "experienced only." As mentioned previously, many companies will make an exception if you have a winning resumé and cover letter and demonstrate your abilities.

Forums

Forums are specific Internet message boards whose posts focus on a particular subject or industry. Medical transcription forums are a wonderful place to find information not only about job opportunities but also about companies and the work of a medical transcriptionist in general. These sites have career boards as a convenience for medical transcriptionists seeking employment, but many employers either sponsor such boards or participate in them in order to reach a more narrowly targeted audience of qualified professionals than they might through generalized job-seeking boards.

Because medical transcriptionists and MTSOs tend to post on these boards, you should check focused boards and forums regularly as part of your job search strategy. Your instructor or networking sources may know of the popular forum sites, or you may search for them using an Internet search engine. Type in the search box a term such as *www.mt* or *www.medicaltranscription*, or *www.transcription* and evaluate the search results. Visit each site and look for a job or classified board where you can learn more about the field and the jobs available. Look at each job opportunity listed and apply for each one for which you feel qualified. Again, if the site calls for experience, but you feel that you possess other required qualifications, apply anyway.

Employment Web Sites

An **employment web site**, as the name implies, is a web site that deals specifically with employment. These sites are designed to allow employers to post classified ads for a position to be filled, and for prospective employees to seek out job listings, fill out applications, and submit resumés for advertised positions over the Internet. In addition, many employment web sites offer articles and tips on preparing resumés and cover letters, as well as interview techniques.

Employment web sites provide job positions in real time all over the world. This means that when jobs are posted, applicants can find that opening and submit an application and/or resumé within minutes instead of hours or days. Job seekers can search, browse, and apply for jobs anytime they wish. The search engines that are a part of these web sites can match the skills of a job seeker not only to a particular company or type of work, but also to preferred locales. Job seekers can use a single search engine to search a multitude of job listings from thousands of job listing sources across the Internet, all at the same time.

Currently the two largest employment web sites on the Internet are Monster (www.monster.com) and Career Builder (www.careerbuilder.com). Once you have registered for a free account on the site with a user name and password, you have access to all of the site's search capabilities. When you click on a job posting, a full description of the position is displayed. From here, you can either e-mail the employer directly or click on a button that enables you to submit a pre-stored resumé and cover letter for use in completing the application. You can create and store several versions of your resumé for future use, choosing the version most appropriate for the job you seek. In addition, you can choose and send one of several versions of a cover letter to an employer without having to open your word-processing software on your computer to retrieve, copy, and paste the information into your browser.

You can register with several job search agents at a time, enabling the employment site search engine to search for new job postings as employers list them on the web site. When these new listings match your search criteria, an e-mail is automatically sent to you, alerting you to the new listing. This eliminates the need to manually search the site's new listings, thereby saving you considerable time and effort. Some employment web sites contain a salary calculator, which allows you to get salary information for the type of position you are seeking as well as for the location of a given job listing. A helpful cost-of-living calculator also displays the cost of living in a specific location.

Newspapers and Publications

Although the use of advertising in newspapers and magazines for jobs has declined in recent years in favor of Internet job boards, print advertising still accounts for many job hires in medical transcription. To use print advertising effectively in your job search, browse the classified ads later in the evening while using daylight and early evening hours principally for networking and making personal contacts with those who can help you with job referrals.

Many of the nation's largest newspapers have a circulation well beyond the major cities in which they are published, and most post their classified ad sections online. In addition, many newspaper online classified ad sites contain links to helpful articles about resumé writing, interview tips, salary comparisons, and other job-hunting tools. Because the larger newspapers cover a large geographic area, many national MTSOs post vacancies in these media as opposed to smaller community newspapers to take advantage of the large pool of potential candidates reading these ads. The following are some of the major national newspapers, along with their Internet addresses, that you can consult for job listings:

New York Times: jobmarket.nytimes.com/pages/jobs
Baltimore Sun: www.baltimoresun.com/classified/jobs
Washington Post: www.washingtonpost.com/wl/jobs/home
Atlanta Journal-Constitution: www.ajcjobs.com
Chicago Tribune: www.chicagotribune.com/classified/jobs
Los Angeles Times: www.latimes.com/classified/jobs
Miami Herald: www.miamiherald.com/classifieds

Career Fairs

Career fairs are another great, often overlooked job-hunting resource. A career fair is an event that gathers representatives and hiring managers from various companies in the medical transcription field in one place to give you the opportunity to introduce yourself and often to interview on the spot. Putting a face and personality to a resumé helps recruiters remember you and gives you the opportunity to make a good impression that will help get your foot in the door.

QUICK CHECK 22.1

Fill in the blanks with the correct answers.

1. A _____ consists of a set number of characters.

2. Specific message boards that focus on a particular industry are called _____.

3. The objective of _____ is to connect people with a common interest or need.

4. Web sites that deal specifically with helping people find jobs are called _____.

5. The measurement of lines typed by a medical transcription is called the _____.

Check with local community colleges and medical transcription schools, as well as the local chamber of commerce, hospitals, local newspapers, trade associations, and other medical organizations that host career fairs. Information on upcoming career fairs is often advertised in the *Community* or *Business* sections of your local newspaper and can also be obtained online through employment web sites as well as web sites dedicated solely to providing career fair information. Attend conventions and symposia hosted by your state and local chapters of the AHDI to meet potential employers. Once you locate a career fair in your area, find out which companies are participating in the career fair and do some research in advance so that when you speak to the recruiter, you appear knowledgeable about the field and interested in working for that company.

At the career fair event, you can exhibit your skills and enthusiasm to many different companies, some of which have specific openings to fill, all in one day at one location. Be sure to dress as you would for a formal interview and have lots of resumés to pass out to potential employers.

Word of Mouth

Finally, do not underestimate the power of nonindustry contacts all around you. People in all walks of life can help you in your job search. Although such relationships are not readily apparent, you might be surprised to learn that the least likely contact has some powerful industry connection you never would have imagined. Some of these nonindustry people you may know would include relatives, friends, neighbors, church members, social club members, and school alumni contacts.

EFFECTIVE RESUMÉS AND APPLICATION LETTERS

Imagine working as a recruiter for a large MTSO. You sit down at your desk to find more than 50 e-mails with attachments of resumés of individuals who believe they are qualified for a position as a medical transcriptionist for the company.

The recruiter's job is to review the resumés, scanning each one to see if the applicant might be a good prospect for the company. On average, a recruiter spends 30 seconds reviewing an incoming employment request. Those that do not capture his/her interest immediately are deleted. Therefore, your employment future depends on your making a favorable first impression on a recruiter who receives a sea of e-mails every single day.

It is critical to have a powerful message that grabs a reader's attention quickly, or you may not be considered for the position—even if you have the experience required for success. To create a powerful message—one that will warrant a second look from a recruiter—tailor your resumé and cover letter to each medical transcription company. Although all MTSOs function the same way in providing typed medical reports for facilities, each company (its infrastructure) is different in subtle ways. Tailor your message with that thought in mind. Use your cover letter and resumé as an advertisement of who you are and what services you can provide that particular company. Include information and terminology in your message that is appropriate for the medical transcription field. For example, you will want to include industry phrases such as *turnaround time*, *work types*, and *line counts*. The use of specific terms shows a recruiter that you have knowledge of the industry and might integrate easily into the company's operation.

Resumé

What exactly is a resumé? A **resumé** is a document containing a summary or listing of relevant job experience, education, and achievement for the purpose of seeking employment. A resumé is also called a *curriculum vita (CV)*, which is a Latin term meaning *course of life*. Having a powerful resumé is crucial to any successful job hunt. When creating a resumé, the most challenging task is to determine what details to include and how to organize that information on the page. Two types of resumés used most often are the **chronological resumé** and the **functional resumé**.

A chronological resumé is organized according to dates during which you were employed by each company for which you have worked, with the most recent job listed first, as shown in Figure 22.2. This format is constructed by listing the date, job history, and accomplishments in reverse chronological order.

For people with a strong and consistent employment history, this format is the most beneficial. However, if you have large lapses of time between jobs, or do not have a lot of job-related experience, the functional resumé format is recommended. Also called a *skills-based resumé*, the functional resumé lists accomplishments by job description or job function instead of by date. Rather than listing each job by date, list your experience by category. A functional resumé contains the same required information; however, your skills and expertise are emphasized over chronological work history. Functional resumés are the most useful for individuals who are changing careers or whose work skills have been acquired through nontraditional work venues, such as volunteering or educational pursuits. Graduating students often use this type of resumé. Medical transcription recruiters prefer the functional resumé because it quickly highlights everything they need to know about an applicant's skills and experience. Figure 22.3 illustrates an example of a functional resumé of a graduating medical transcription student who was once in the

Kira Johnson
350 Spring Hill Road
Chicago, IL 60610
Telephone: (708) 555-5833
E-mail: kjjohnson99@lww.com

Profile

Highly organized and accomplished medical transcriptionist with a proven track record of achieving production objectives by surpassing required line counts with greater than 99% accuracy on all accounts.

Professional Experience

A Transcription Company   Jan. 20xx – Present

- Consistently scored above 99% on in-house audits
- Never called in sick
- Named "MT Manager's Award" three times in one year for exceeding production quotas

B Transcription Company   Aug. 19xx – Jan. 20xx

- Met and exceeded line counts each pay period
- Lead computer technology training program for company employees
- Assisted in updating text and exhibits for employee handbook

Other Experiences

Volunteer Coordinator for Valley Hill Hospital's annual Breast Cancer Walk-A-Thon
Writer and Newsletter Editor for "Pulse," local trade association membership newsletter

Skills and Expertise

MS Word ◆ MS Excel ◆ MS POWERPoint ◆ MS Access ◆ Various Windows-Integrated Transcription Software Programs ◆ Document Preparation Skills ◆ ESL Dictator Styles ◆ Digital Transmission of Files

Education

Medical Transcription Certification   Graduated in June 19xx
American Community College
Graduated with Honors

Associate of Arts, Computer Technology   Graduated in June 19xx
University of West Indiana
Member of Phi Delta Beta Academic Sorority

FIGURE 22.2. **Chronological Resumé**. Professional experience is placed first, followed by skills and other experiences relevant to the job.

Jennifer A. Smith
JAS@lww.com

100 Northeast First Street
Miami, FL 33004

Phone: (555) 826-2447
Cell Phone: (555) 866-8661

SUMMARY OF QUALIFICATIONS

Industrious medical transcription student graduate with top grades and references. Over 5 years' experience in legal clerical and computer skills as well as excellent communication and organizational skills. Active member of national and local chapter of AHDI.

SKILLS PROFILE

5+ years transcription experience in legal field.
Consistently exceed 1,400 lines per day in acute care; familiar with all work types.
Very experienced with ESL dictators.
Routinely score over 98.5% accuracy in medical transcription audits in school.
Head organizer for city-wide breast cancer awareness walk-a-thon for past 2 years.
Proficient with MS Word, Excel, Lanier, and various dictation systems.

PROFESSIONAL ACHIEVEMENTS

Recipient of City Local Hero Award (4 years) for organizing city-wide fundraising charity events.

PROFESSIONAL ACTIVITIES

President and newsletter editor of local chapter of AHDI.
Obtain medical education speakers for local chapter meetings.
Coordinated school advertising campaign for Medical Transcription Week.
Organized school field trip to State Capitol for Lobby Day.

PROFESSIONAL EXPERIENCE

2000 to Present
Phone: (555) 393-5000

Waldon's Legal Transcription Service
Miami, FL 33130

Legal transcription of all pleadings, depositions, and trial proceedings for city's largest law firm. Organized filing of appellate briefs, hearings, and assembly of parties and witnesses for court events. Designed office network and calendaring computer system, resulting in 52% increase in work efficiency.

EDUCATION

Medical Transcription Degree (2-year)
Gator County Community College
Graduated with Top Honors
Wilson Academic Award Recipient (2 years)
Chaired Student Advisory Committee

FIGURE 22.3. **Functional Resume**. This resumé style stresses the skills and achievements of an applicant rather than specific jobs held.

legal field and changed careers. Note that this resumé highlights skills derived primarily from clerical and volunteer activities as well as an employment history that stresses work in a field requiring a strong background in English and grammar.

Generally, your resumé should be a concise summary of your qualifications—not something verbose or full of subjective opinions. Make your points short and concise; the fewer words the better, and stick with the objective facts. Instead of saying, "I was the best typist the company (or school) had ever seen," you might say something like, "Consistently exceeded the quota of typed reports required by 65 percent." This shows a quantifiable result and evidence that you are a fast, accurate typist.

Make your resumé easy to read. Most recruiters will spend only about 30 seconds to initially scan your resumé. If they cannot find the information they are looking for immediately, they will most likely discard your resumé. Recruiters want to know what you can bring to the job and the company, and what skills you have that set you apart from other candidates. Therefore, keep the information relevant to the position. Do not include personal items that have no relevance to the reader, such as hobbies, political ideology, or even religious beliefs.

Every resumé should contain a summary, list of accomplishments, overview of expertise or skills, education, and work experience.

Summary or Profile

The first lines of a resumé are a one- or two-sentence description that provides an overview of your personality and experience. The summary must capture the recruiter's attention right away and show him/her that you are the most qualified candidate for the position—or, at least, that you are someone on whom the company can successfully take a chance. Use powerful words and visual cues. For example, an opening statement such as, "Bright, enthusiastic individual who is impassioned about the field of medicine and is known for consistently exceeding expectations . . ." is a much stronger opening to a resumé than "I am interested in a position that will help me become a better medical transcriptionist."

Accomplishments

The next part of your resumé includes highlights of pertinent accomplishments and results. This section shows your capabilities up-front and gives a recruiter a general idea of who you are and what you can do. For example, bulleted items, such as "In charge of organizing all of the PTA fundraising drives for the last five years" or "Regularly scored over 98% accuracy in audits of my reports," will grab attention. In addition, if you are a student, you can highlight your educational accomplishments here.

Bullet points such as "Scored greater than 95% on all chapter exams and finished course in the top 5% of the class" or "Completed all dictation activities with a typing speed of 120 words per minute and accuracy of greater than 98%" would make a recruiter take a second look, even if you have no work experience.

Expertise or Skills

The next section of your resumé should be a summary of your skills and expertise. You may want to further break it down into subcategories, such as "Medical Transcription Expertise," "Technical Skills" or "Organizational Skills."

In this section, think about what criteria would be important to the company to which you are applying. Study the classified ad or the job description for clues about what the job entails. For example, an ad may specify that applicants be proficient in Microsoft Word or have expertise in certain fields of medicine, such as radiology. Edit your skills list to highlight those items.

Education

Include all education relevant to the job for which you are applying. If you have prior medical experience (i.e., if you are changing specific careers within the medical field), limit this section to what is important. However, if you lack significant work-related experience (i.e., if you are a student), expand on this section. In this case, you can include not just the names of courses you have taken but grades achieved and other information about your education. Did you attend an educational seminar or program? Include that. Did a speaker come to your class and give a presentation about a particular medical topic? That could be added as well.

Work Experience

The last component of your resumé details your work experience. List the various jobs you have held and provide objective details about your duties while in these positions. Relevant information includes the names of the employers for which you have worked, the period of time you worked for each employer, and the responsibilities you had that demonstrate your ability to succeed in the job for which you are applying.

Application Letter

A powerful resumé opens the door to many interview opportunities. However, a resume is only one component of the job application. A cover letter is an essential part of your correspondence with employers. Figure 22.4 illustrates a conventional cover letter that should be included with your resumé. Although the resumé provides an overview of your background, the cover letter

ANDREW J. HILL
1230 South First Street
West Moreland, Texas 77001

March 31, 20xx

Christine LaGrange, CMT, AHDI-F
Hiring Manager
LWW Medical Transcription Service
2330 Union Avenue
Los Angeles, CA 90211

Dear Ms. LaGrange:

Please consider my application for a position as a medical transcriptionist with LWW Medical Transcription Service. Your company has an excellent reputation for customer satisfaction, and I know that my education, background, and motivation to excel will make me an asset to the company.

As a medical transcription major at Valley College, I have taken classes in anatomy and physiology, medical terminology, and computer technology, among others. While taking a full load of courses and volunteering in patient care at our local medical facility 30 hours per week, I consistently surpassed my class line count requirements with 99.5% accuracy and maintained a 3.8 grade point average. In addition, I am an active member of the Association for Healthcare Documentation Integrity (AHDI) and currently serve as student liaison and membership chairperson, which has given me additional experience dealing with individuals and groups in the medical community. I was also recently recognized as the Student Medical Transcriptionist of the Year by my chapter.

My resumé is attached for your review, and I look forward to speaking with you further about a possibility of an interview. I can be reached via telephone at (281) 555-4392 or e-mail at ajhill@lww.com. Thank you for your consideration.

Sincerely,

Andrew J. Hill

FIGURE 22.4. Application Letter. This letter highlights the applicant's academic and relevant extracurricular activities because he has no work experience. He does not draw attention to the fact he has no experience; he simply outlines his strong points.

shows your personality and invites a reader to look further at your resume. It not only interprets and humanizes your resume, but also reveals your ability to write and convey your thoughts effectively. An effective cover letter gives a prospective employer insight into your abilities that cannot be obtained from the resumé alone. The cover letter also allows you to highlight your skills and selling points and enables you to request an interview.

It is important to keep the intended recipient in mind when drafting the cover letter. The letter must relate to the reader even though it is describing the writer. The choice of words and level of formality in addressing the reader reflects the writer's attitude toward that person as well as the situation that occasions the letter.

In addition, the spirit in which the writer conveys the message to the reader is important. This attitude, called tone, sends a strong message about who you are—positive or negative—to the reader. A letter that is overly formal in tone may appear unfriendly or impersonal and create an impression of a cold and disinterested applicant. An employer, to some degree, is as concerned about the personality of an applicant as about his or her skills. After all, most people can be trained to perform a job, but if they do not get along with their co-workers, everyone will suffer. A thoughtful, sincere letter demonstrates an attitude of consideration and respect for its reader. In addition, the message being conveyed, involving work skills and experience, needs to be conveyed clearly and courteously. The key to choosing the appropriate words and tone of a letter is to focus on the recipient. Ask yourself, "How would I respond if I were the recipient of this letter?" A letter tailored to meet the needs of the recipient stands a better chance of being understood and receiving a positive response. The key to a good application letter is a pleasant, enthusiastic, but professional, tone that will make the reader want to meet you.

Most MTSOs require application by e-mail as opposed to regular mail. E-mail cover letters can be submitted as a general distribution e-mail or in response to a single classified advertisement.

General Distribution Letter

A cover letter should be submitted when you want to send your resume to a number of MTSOs to be considered for present or future positions as opportunities arise. This letter is short, concise, and contains the basic information every recruiter initially looks for in a potential candidate for employment.

Even though the cover letter is distributed to a wide variety of recipients at once, each letter should be addressed to an individual, preferably a hiring manager or recruiter, if possible. Names of persons to contact may be obtained by checking the company's web site under the company's contact information. However, in many cases, the e-mail address for the recruiter is simply listed as "HR" or "Recruiter," followed by the company's network address. In that instance, a generic greeting in the cover letter is appropriate.

The letter begins with a sentence or two about your qualifications and general interest. The second part of the letter lists a series of qualifications and accomplishments that a recruiter would find of interest for the job you are seeking. A single sentence reference to your resume that accompanies the e-mail cover letter is sufficient to direct the recruiter to open the attachment. The next part of the letter includes a sentence or two requesting action on the part of the reader and expressing a desire to talk with the recruiter about your qualifications. Be sure to provide contact information, such as an e-mail address or a phone number where you can be reached during business hours. The letter closes with a thank you to the reader, followed by a traditional letter closing (such as "Sincerely" or "Respectfully submitted") and your signature. Despite the brevity of this letter, it is concise, powerful, and effective in conveying your qualifications, writing ability, and personality—the very things that entice a recruiter with little time to spare to take notice.

Ad Response Letter

When a cover letter is used to respond to a specific ad placed by an employer, the first paragraph of your letter should reference the employer's job listing, affirm confidence in your ability to perform the job, and direct the reader's attention to your qualifications. The next part of the letter, as in the letter described previously, should be used to highlight your skills and accomplishments as they relate to your potential successful performance of the job. The rest of the letter, similar to a general distribution letter, should make a brief statement drawing the recruiter's attention to the fact that a resumé is attached to the e-mail, as well as to include basic contact information. This letter, too, should end with a "thank you" and traditional closing.

Many applicants use the Internet to mass-mail their resumé to a number of employers. However, many MTSOs have set their spam filters to block out resumés that have been mass-mailed to prevent junk e-mail or spam from filling up the company's network mail server. A large number of recipients in the address line of your e-mail may cause it to be flagged as "spam" by an MTSO's mail filter. If your e-mail is classified as spam, it will be deleted or stored in a temporary file for an unspecified amount of time and then discarded. In addition, the company's network provider may "remember" your e-mail address incorrectly as spam and prevent any e-mail you send to that company from ever reaching anyone.

To prevent this from happening, it is best to send your e-mail cover letter and resume to only one individual e-mail address per e-mail submission so that your message will not be flagged as spam and your e-mail will be delivered as you had intended. In addition, when a recruiter sees only one addressee on the e-mail received, the recruiter believes that she or he was singled out for the query.

Written communications, whether on paper or by e-mail, tell a lot about the sender. Therefore, the importance of both clear, accurate content and neat appearance cannot be overemphasized. Mastering the essential skills of writing and producing an effective resumé and

QUICK CHECK 22.2 ✓

Match the detail item on the left with the section of a resumé with which it is associated on the right (some resumé section entries may be used more than once).

Item

1. _____ prior background in radiology
2. _____ knowledge of Excel
3. _____ "bright and enthusiastic"
4. _____ dates of prior employment
5. _____ names of courses completed
6. _____ attendance award at school
7. _____ typing speed
8. _____ surpassed 98% accuracy on weekly audits
9. _____ responsibilities of current job
10. _____ student of the month

Resumé Section

A. Summary or profile

B. Accomplishments

C. Expertise or skills

D. Education

E. Work experience

---

cover letter convey an image of professionalism and competence to a prospective employer.

Whether you send your letter to one person or many, keep the following tips in mind when creating and sending a cover letter with your resumé:

- Remember that one size does not fit all. Each letter, although structured in a similar manner, should be tailored to the particular position and company to which you are applying. Your letter should show that you have researched the company and the positions it has open, and that you are a good fit with its culture and mission.
- The cover letter should not merely review highlights of your resumé, it should also create a picture of your personality.
- Keep your letter simple and keep it short. One page consisting of paragraphs that address why you are an ideal candidate for the job and providing a few details about your qualifications will get to the point for recruiters who do not have the time to read lengthy letters.
- Focus your letter on the specific skills and interests you possess that you can offer to an employer. Stress what you can do for the company, not what the company can do for you. Sound upbeat and confident. Sell yourself!
- Make sure that the letter is *perfect* in terms of spelling, punctuation, and grammar. Have someone proofread the letter before you send it.

ONLINE TESTING

You have done your research, created a winning resumé, and found an MTSO interested in hiring you. The next step in the hiring process is taking the company's online test. An **online test** is an examination conducted by an MTSO via the Internet to gain an objective measure of a potential employee's skills and to help the company match the transcriptionist's skills with account requirements. Most online tests are located on an MTSO's web site, and many recruiters consider them invaluable assessment tools when used in conjunction with direct interviews. Some are used for the initial screening of an applicant, some midway through the interview process, and others as the last evaluation before making a final decision about a candidate. Sometimes these same tools are used for internal promotion.

A pre-employment test not only evaluates your skills as a medical transcriptionist, but also helps the potential employer learn more about you and can help you learn more about yourself, too. Companies want to see how you deal with new experiences and information and how you resolve problems you may encounter on the job. Are you a self-starter, seeking to solve problems on your own? Do you have a natural curiosity to verify the meaning of a phrase or term you have not heard before, which was used during the dictation portion of the exam? Or do you give up, abandoning a project (such as a test) as soon as you encounter a difficulty? A pre-employment test can be viewed as an indication of how you would function in similar circumstances on the job.

Taking online tests can be a nerve-wracking experience, even for the most seasoned medical transcriptionist. You may be apprehensive about the testing process, but do not let that intimidate you. Your scores are only one factor among many that an employer will consider in judging your job qualifications.

Medical transcriptionist pre-employment tests typically cover topics that are crucial to the creation of accurate medical reports—spelling, grammar, proofreading skills, medical abbreviations and terminology, and actual transcription of sample reports. Some companies emphasize the written portion of the examination but provide only a few excerpts of dictation for transcription. Other companies focus their examinations on transcription with only a few written questions about medical language and usage. Questions might be multiple-choice, true/false, or fill-in-the-blank. They typically test one's ability to identify commonly misspelled words, differentiate between soundalike words, and choose the correct word for a given sentence. Proofreading questions may involve correcting errors in grammar, spelling, punctuation, and context in a given sentence or paragraph. You may also be tested on commonly used abbreviations, covering areas of dosage frequency (such as the difference between b.i.d. and t.i.d.), or the correct transcription of case-specific abbreviations (such as pH or mEq). The transcription portion of the examination may involve typing two or three actual medical reports in the space provided on the computer screen. This portion of the examination is probably the most important to a potential employer as it evaluates your ability to listen carefully and to promptly and accurately transcribe what was dictated. Excellent transcription skills may actually help compensate for lack of formal work experience.

No matter what the purpose of an examination, an online test can be a challenge and cause anxiety. The following tips will help you prepare for and successfully complete a medical transcription pre-employment test.

First, keep a positive attitude when taking the test. A negative or anxious approach to the test will make you doubt your skills, which may subconsciously show up in the exam as a wrong answer to a simple question. Companies test applicants not to see how stupid they are, but to fill available positions with the right people. You do not want to set yourself up to fail on the job, and companies do not want to waste time hiring someone who is not suited for the position they need to fill. If your skills do not match the needs of a company's accounts, types of work, or operating style, that is not a mark against you.

Carefully read and follow all test instructions. Recruiters seek candidates who pay attention to details and complete the test on time. An applicant who cannot follow simple instructions or who takes days to complete the test sends a red flag about how she or he will perform on the job. Select a time to take the test when you can complete it in one sitting without distractions.

Before beginning the examination, make note of how to seek technical support in case a problem arises during testing. Sometimes problems with the testing software, the computer network, or even your own computer, will cause the test to "freeze up" or to perform improperly. If you encounter a technical difficulty during the examination process, contact the company's technical support personnel for assistance. In addition, let the recruiter know that you have encountered a technical problem while taking the test and that you will complete the examination as soon as the problem is resolved. A recruiter will appreciate your providing the status update rather than haven given up because of a technical snafu.

Pay attention to time management when taking the test. Although most online tests do not indicate a specific time-period for completion of the examination, the MTSO's computer network may make a note of how long you took to answer the questions. Then, as you progress through the examination, watch your time per question. Obviously, some questions will consume more time, others less; but be aware of the average.

Be sure you understand the question being asked. Some medical transcriptionist tests ask you to select an *incorrect* word in a sentence, whereas others ask for the *correct* word. Although this sounds obvious, all too often we assume things that are not actually mentioned in examination questions. Just because you see a keyword or phrase that triggers an idea in your mind does not mean that the question is about that idea or that you need to answer the question immediately. The trigger could simply be a distraction and cause you to select the wrong answer. Read each question thoroughly and completely, and pause for a moment or two to collect your thoughts before selecting your answer.

For examinations that allow you to return to previous questions, you can use a technique that enables you to flag the difficult questions and go back to them after answering the easy questions. First, on a piece of paper, create two columns called *hard* and *guess* so you can create columns of question numbers below them. As you work through the examinations, answer those questions for which you know the answer immediately after reading the question. If you have to read a question more than twice to figure out what is being asked or to begin pondering the correct answer, write the question number in the *hard* column and move on. After you have gone through the entire examination once, go back and answer the *hard* questions. If you answer the question, mark it off from the *hard* column. If you cannot answer the question, move it to the *guess* column.

For multiple-choice-type questions, once you are sure you know what is being asked, choose an answer from the listed selections. Then, re-read the question to make sure your selection makes sense and that it is relevant to the question being asked. If you do not immediately know the correct answer, seek to eliminate all incorrect answers. If you can identify and eliminate the obviously wrong answers, then the correct answer will become clearer.

The transcription portion of most online tests includes actual medical reports that must be transcribed, proofread, and edited. The reports (usually about three or four) consist of dictation that is representative of reports encountered during actual working conditions, including operative notes, discharge summaries, and history and physical exams. The transcription tests are designed to test your knowledge, skill, and ability to transcribe medical reports effectively. Before beginning the transcription portion of the test, make sure your foot pedal and headset are working properly so you can hear and transcribe the report correctly. If you encounter a problem, contact your recruiter or the company's technical support personnel so that you will be able to complete the transcription portion of the examination.

Once you have completed the test, notify the recruiter so the test can be scored and the results evaluated. Do not dwell on it or think about how you could have done better. Use each online test you encounter as a learning experience and a way to display your talent. Eventually your skills will be a perfect match for a particular company, and you will have your first job as a medical transcriptionist.

INTERVIEW SUCCESS

Although the most stressful part of the job-search process for some, the interview is one of the most exciting parts of the job-hunting process, as it shines the spotlight on you.

When preparing for a job interview, try to put yourself in the employer's shoes. What are the skills and knowledge that the employer is looking for to fill this position, and what skills and knowledge (such as terminology and computer skills) do you possess? What other "soft skills," or personal traits and qualities, do you possess that would be beneficial to the company? Are you friendly, well organized, and a good communicator? Can you adapt easily to new situations or multitask several jobs at once? If you can determine the technical skills and personal qualities required by the job, you will have a much better chance of having a successful interview.

Whether in person or by phone, be prepared to talk about yourself. If you are not prepared to answer a soft opening question, like "tell me about yourself," you have missed a valuable opportunity to introduce the qualities that make you a good fit for that position. To avoid an awkward response, prepare. Write down five

words that describe you. Write down your strengths and weaknesses. Collect a few anecdotes that illustrate your accomplishments. Then practice your answers.

Because most medical transcription employees work from home, many interviews are conducted by phone. Here your voice must be the main selling point. Make an effort to sound pleasant and friendly. When you talk to a stranger on the phone, what impressions do you get from the tone and quality of that person's voice? Do you create a mental picture of that person while you are talking to him or her? A telephone interview works the same way. The interviewer's first impression of you is the mental picture created by the sound of your voice. Behavioral observations made during the interview will help an interviewer predict how you might get along with co-workers or management in the position and, therefore, help predict success on the job. Before the phone interview, close your eyes and visualize the outcome you want. Imagine the interviewer saying to you, "You are just the type of person we are looking for!" Believing in yourself is an attitude that is contagious: If your voice sounds confident and enthusiastic, your interviewer will pick up on that enthusiasm and believe in you, too. When an interviewer leaves an interview jazzed up, it is very difficult for him or her to forget that candidate.

Prepare for a phone interview just as you would for a regular interview. Compile a list of your strengths and weaknesses, as well as a list of answers to typical interview questions regarding your work history and accomplishments and answers to questions about your place in the new job and company. In addition, be prepared for a discussion about your background and skills. Rehearse your answers to some of the typical interview questions you may be asked, such as:

"Tell me about yourself."
"Why do you want to work here?"
"Why did you leave your last job?"
"How do you handle pressure?"
"What do you consider to be your greatest strengths? Your shortcomings?"

An interviewer will also ask you about the computer capabilities in your home, the types of software and hardware equipment you are familiar with, and the type of Internet connection you currently have (DSL, cable, satellite, broadband, or dial-up). Depending on the type of equipment you already have, you may be required to purchase a foot pedal for a nominal fee that would be compatible with the company's software platform you will be using. In addition, your type of Internet connection is important in terms of compatibility with the transmission of work through the company's network system. For example, some MTSOs find that satellite service is not compatible with their network servers. Dial-up service may not be fast enough to transmit information. Be sure you are familiar with the equipment and service you use currently and be prepared to elaborate on these topics during the interview.

Keep your resumé in view so that you can reach it easily if needed to help you answer a question. Have a pen and paper handy to jot down information that the interviewer may provide you; and on the same sheet of paper, make a little *cheat sheet* list of your accomplishments so you do not forget them. Turn your phone's call waiting feature off so that the call is not interrupted. Make sure the room is quiet for the interview—no kids, pets, or music.

Interviewing by phone is not as easy as a face-to-face conversation. During the interview, it might be helpful to focus on an object, such as the telephone or a calendar on your desk, to substitute for a person's face. Do not eat or drink during the interview, but do keep a glass of water handy in case you need it. Often the interview will begin, after some small talk, with the interviewer telling you about the company and the position. Even if you have already done your research before the interview and find this information repetitive, do not interrupt the interviewer by saying you are already familiar with it. Simply listen to the background information, interjecting words or phrases as appropriate to indicate you are listening. This will help build rapport with the interviewer and show your interest in what he or she has to say.

Some interviewers chat informally between questions to help you feel more relaxed; do not interrupt the interviewer, and answer only when you are sure the interviewer has finished speaking. Speak slowly and enunciate your words clearly. Do not give long, elaborate answers. And smile, even if it is only at the telephone or desk calendar. Smiling will project a cheerful, confident tone to your voice and convey a positive image to the listener.

As a new graduate, you probably have little or no work history in the medical field. It is a daunting dilemma: It is difficult to get a job without experience, but it is equally difficult to get experience without a job. However, you can get around this problem during an interview by emphasizing your strengths and educational achievements. For example, put a positive spin on your answers about your school activities, emphasizing the extra effort you made to learn about the field, your volunteer work, or your class projects (rather than the grades you received). Talk about your favorite class and your desire to learn more about a particular field of medicine. Describe your extracurricular activities in such a way that an interviewer can see how the experience you gained might benefit the company. For example, you can say that you participated in certain activities (organizing school functions or joining outside clubs) to broaden your experience and meet new people. Talk about the great relationship you had with your prior employers and how much you enjoyed working with people and learning new ideas.

Watch for informational questions. These questions are designed to learn as much as possible about you as a person and to identify your level of honesty, integrity, and dedication to the field. Be ready to answer questions like:

"What made you choose the medical profession as a
    career?"
"What do you think are the qualities of a successful
    employee in this field?"
"Do you think it is okay to take office supplies home?"
"What are your long-term goals?"

Some recruiters may ask a "trick" or "loaded" question, called a **zinger**, knowing you are probably not prepared for it or cannot answer it, to judge how you might respond to pressure or tension on the job. If you are asked a question you cannot answer, such as, "What would you do if an irate client called you because you put a formatting code in your report that short-circuited their printer at the moment it starting printing your reports?" Think about it for a few seconds. If you cannot think of an answer immediately, then, with a confident tone to your voice and without apology, simply say, "I don't know," or "I can't answer that question right now."

At the conclusion of the interview, thank the interviewer for his or her time and indicate that you look forward to hearing from the company in the future. Follow up with a thank you note, sent by regular mail or e-mail, to the interviewer, thanking him or her again for the opportunity to interview and reiterating your interest in the job.

Preparing for an on-site interview is similar to preparing for a phone interview except that the first impression you make on an interviewer derives not from your tone of voice, but from your appearance. In face-to-face interviews, more than 90% of all initial impressions are nonverbal. Therefore, you want to look good because it has a major impact on your chances of getting a job. Dress professionally—a professional suit for men; and a skirt suit or fashionable pant suit for women. Bring extra copies of your resumé to the interview and arrive a few minutes early. Greet the interviewer with a firm but professional handshake. Establish eye contact during the interview; it shows you are listening and communicating and that you mean what you say. Most important, leave your cell phone in the car or turn it off before entering the interview. Nothing is more annoying or disrupting than a ringing cell phone. The interruption ruins the flow of conversation; and if you commit the grievous error of making the interviewer wait while you take the call, it conveys the impression that your call is more important than the interview.

One advantage of a face-to-face interview is the opportunity to bring a professional **portfolio**, a collection of documents outlining your achievements, the scope and quality of your experience and training, and your abilities. To organize your portfolio, choose items that will show a potential employer how your skills relate to the company's needs. Enclose your documents in plastic covers to help protect them and make the arranging of your portfolio easier. Place the covered items in a small notebook or report folder. Label the different sections for ease in finding information in the portfolio. Make several sets of the portfolio so that you can leave a copy for the interviewer to look at later.

Items to include in your medical transcription portfolio might include:

- A copy of your resumé.
- An official copy of your school transcript.
- Certificates of awards and honors, degrees, diplomas, or special certifications for special training you received.
- A list of educational programs or workshops you have attended outside of school and a description of each.
- Samples of reports you have completed in class showing knowledge of medical terminology and formatting of documents.
- Documentation of technical or computer skills; for example, a PowerPoint slide show you created for a class project or samples of newsletters or flyers you may have designed.

As an alternative to a traditional portfolio, you might want to create an electronic portfolio as a supplement to your resumé. It can be organized on a CD-ROM, with each document as a separate file, or you can even set it up as a PowerPoint slideshow that can be transmitted as an attachment via e-mail for the employer to view either before or after your interview. Electronic portfolios on a CD-ROM brought to the interview or included in an e-mail attachment may be more convenient for potential employers to access and view than a bulky paper notebook. Inclusion of an e-mail hyperlink in your electronic portfolio will allow employers to contact you easily simply by clicking on the link and typing in a message for you. Electronic portfolios also show employers that you are familiar with various types of computer technology and programs and have the ability to use them creatively.

At the conclusion of the interview, remain positive, self-assured, and enthusiastic. Offer a handshake and thank the interviewer for his or her time. As with a telephone interview, write a follow-up thank you note and mail it immediately, while the interview is still fresh in the interviewer's mind. The thank you note may be handwritten or typed and sent by e-mail or regular mail. Handwritten notes are more personal, but e-mail is appropriate when that has been your previous contact with the person you want to thank. A thank you note is a courteous gesture and helps maintain good relations with people you may want to contact again. This advice may seem obvious; but in fact, the majority of people interviewed for a job do not take the time to send a thank you note. This simple gesture can make a big difference in separating you from your competition.

Figure 22.5 illustrates a typical post-interview thank you note. The three main components are:

- A thank you to the interviewer for his or her time during the interview. You may also mention something learned during the interview about the company, especially those things relevant to your qualifications.
- A review of your qualifications relevant to the job opportunity to serve as a reminder to the interviewer about why you are the best person for the position.
- A courteous closing paragraph, inviting the employer to contact you for more information if necessary and indicating that you are looking forward to the employer's positive decision.

Be sure you spell the name of the interviewer and the company correctly. If you are unsure of the spelling, call the company and ask the receptionist. Make sure the note is delivered as quickly as possible, preferably by the end of the following day, because the sooner your letter arrives, the greater the likelihood of its having a positive impact.

Do not be discouraged if you do not receive an immediate response from an employer. Companies often interview many candidates before making a final decision. In the meantime, contact other companies with job openings and schedule more interviews, so that if you do not get hired for the first job, you have other options. If you do get rejected for the job, send a note to the interviewer, which makes a positive statement. Thank the interviewer for considering your qualifications and emphasize your ongoing interest in being considered for other medical transcription openings in the future. Be sure to use an upbeat tone. Although you may be disappointed at not getting the job, you do not want to imply to the interviewer that you do not respect his or her decision. This small but gracious gesture may help the interviewer remember you when a new opening arises.

PERSONAL AND PROFESSIONAL DEVELOPMENT

Becoming an experienced, professional medical transcriptionist requires more than just fast typing speed and good listening skills. Invest in yourself by integrating your interests, abilities, and preferences more fully into your work as a medical transcriptionist. These strategies will enable you to plan, develop, and advance toward a more challenging and rewarding career.

Personal Development

In the world of medical transcription, personal development means optimizing your work environment and

September 5, 20xx

Maryann Spivak, CMT
Director of Human Resources
LWW Medical Transcription Service
9000 Church Avenue
St. Louis, MO 63101

Dear Ms. Spivak:

Thank you for the opportunity to discuss your opening for a medical transcriptionist by telephone today. I enjoyed learning more about LWW Medical Transcription Service's operations and business goals for the next five years.

I believe that my experience as a working medical transcriptionist as well as my outside activities involving my volunteer work at my neighborhood hospital and activities in my professional association qualify me for the position. In addition, my extensive knowledge of computers and medical transcription software platforms would also be especially valuable to me as a medical transcriptionist with the company.

I look forward to having the opportunity to be a part of your winning team. If there is any further information I can provide as you consider my qualifications, please feel free to contact me at (615) 555-3771 or myname@lww.com. Again, thank you for your time and consideration.

Jane Smith

FIGURE 22.5. **Post-Interview Thank You Note**. This small gesture can leave a positive and lasting impression on an interviewer.

mastering medical transcription tools that allow you to work more efficiently and make more money.

Optimize Your Work Environment

Most medical transcription jobs involve working from home. This can have definite advantages in terms of flexible hours and of money saved on a work wardrobe, day-care expenses, gasoline, and commute time. However, working from home entails a whole set of distractions, which will require discipline and the ability to effectively manage your work time.

If you are working from home, strive to create a work space that is conducive to transcribing. If possible, separate your work area from the rest of your family's living space and set the ground rules for the family's sharing of *your office*, both for professional purposes and to comply with HIPAA regulations. Avoid distractions that can affect your overall production. For instance, turn the ringer off on your personal telephone or let the answering machine take calls during work hours. Turn the television and radio off if they interfere with getting your

work done. Discourage neighbors from stopping by *because you are home*, or family from hanging around in your office when you are at work. You can easily save one to two hours or more by controlling distractions that can have a detrimental effect on your line count.

Ergonomics is the science of designing and arranging objects, systems, and environments in such a way as to maximize productivity by reducing operator fatigue and discomfort. The word derives from two Greek words: *ergon*, meaning *work*, and *nomos* meaning *laws*, and this concept involves arranging the environment to fit the person in it. When ergonomics is applied correctly in your work environment, visual and musculoskeletal discomfort and fatigue are reduced significantly.

Good work habits are effective in preventing injury on the job. To create an ergonomically friendly space that will enhance efficiency and safety, consider the following when setting up your home office:

- Space. Ideally, your office space should be a separate room in the house, with good lighting and plenty of electrical outlets. It should have a comfortable temperature and plenty of ventilation. It should be situated out of the family traffic pattern. The office should be sufficiently spacious to contain a desk large enough to hold your computer and shelves within arm's reach to hold the reference books you use most often.

- Lighting. Both natural and artificial lighting should be considered when setting up your home office. Natural lighting comes in from outside and will change with the time of day. Does the window in your office present a glare? Is it pleasant or distracting? Is the artificial light in the room bright enough to work but not to cast a shadow over your desk?
- Workstation. The design of your workstation can have a big impact on your overall health and well-being. Discomfort and musculoskeletal disorders can result from ergonomically incorrect computer workstation setups. For example, the wrong chair and/or bad posture can cause lower back strain; a chair that is too high can cause loss of circulation in legs and feet. Both desk and chair should be properly adjusted to avoid placing stress on the wrists or back. Your feet should be flat on the floor; and when your hands are placed on the keyboard, the forearms should be straight and shoulders relaxed. When sitting at the computer in an upright position, your head should be over your shoulders and your shoulders over your hips.
- Computer System. Analyze the placement of your computer on the desktop. For example, positioning the monitor lower and farther away may cause less strain on your neck. Make sure your computer is set up so that it is centered in front of you, an arm's length away. The top of the document screen should be at eye level, about two to three inches below the top of the monitor, and positioned to reduce glare. An ergonomic keyboard is a split keyboard that makes it easier for your hands to rest in a curved position above the keys, avoiding stress on the hands, arms, and tendons. Use an ergonomic mouse. Reaching for a mouse is one of the primary causes of shoulder and elbow pain. An ergonomically designed mouse incorporated into the keyboard increases productivity and reduces upper extremity pain by as much as 85%.
- Body position. Arrange your surroundings to promote a comfortable and relaxed body position. Awkward reaches or angles will create problems. The chair and keyboard should be set high so that your thighs and forearms are level or sloping slightly downward away from the body. Your wrists should remain level, not bent far down or way back. Two sponges or a smaller towel rolled flatly can be used for simple wrist rests and cost virtually nothing. Sit straight, do not slouch, and do not stretch forward to reach the keys or see the computer screen. Sit back

in the seat so that your lower back is supported firmly by the chair or a lumbar support cushion. If necessary, roll a towel to a three-inch diameter and place it behind your lower back to relieve pressure and provide support. Place your feet on a foot rest so that your knees are not lower than your hips. This will relieve "pull" on your lower back. Finally, taking frequent breaks to get up and stretch will help prevent repetitive stress injuries.

By practicing ergonomics, you can avoid the aches and pains caused by muscle stress and fatigue that can plague medical transcriptionists. As you work, pay attention to the signals your body gives you. If you have pain in the wrists or hands after a long day of typing, examine your work area and work practices to see if they may be causing the problems and make adjustments accordingly. Raise or lower chairs to avoid typing with your wrists at an odd angle. Adjust computer monitors to avoid glare. Take frequent breaks from repetitive tasks to give your body a rest. Sometimes small modifications in work procedures, posture, habits, and/or work station design can make a big difference in the way you feel at the end of a day.

Master Your Resources

There are many "tools of the trade," or resources, that medical transcriptionists use to maximize productivity.

Text-Expansion Software

Also referred to as **macros** (not to be confused with Microsoft Word's macro feature), these abbreviations increase productivity and reduce mistakes. Text-expansion software is not only for medical words, but also can be used to program commonly used words and phrases. For example, a little phrase like *as mentioned above* can be entered as *ama* in your text expander. The phrase *left greater than right* can be abbreviated as *lgr* in a text expander.

You can even use the word expander to create shortcuts for various forms of words. For example:

eso=esophagus; esot=esophagitis; esol=esophageal; esov=esophageal varices
gen=general; genl=generally
th=the; oth=of the; ath=at the; fth=for the; wth=with the; toth=to the

You can make shortcuts for numbers that indicate dosage or time:

1p=1+; e34=every 3-4 hours; 1v=1-0 Vicryl; 2w=2 weeks; 3tw=3 times per week

In addition, you can use word expanders to enter entire paragraphs of text commonly dictated by a physician. If a doctor always dictates the same text in certain parts of a specific type of report, you can enter that text into the text expander, along with a code to instruct the expander to go back and find a particular character (such as * or ??) to pause while you enter the information. For example, in a physical examination report, you can program the expander to include the standard language with pauses for you to enter vital signs of one individual patient:

> *Blood pressure ??, pulse ??, weight ?? pounds. General: Patient alert and cooperative with exam. No apparent distress. HEENT: Sclerae are anicteric. Conjunctivae are normal. Nares patent. No lymphadenopathy. Cardiovascular: Regular rate and rhythm. No murmurs, gallops, or rubs. Lungs: Clear to auscultation. Extremities: No clubbing, cyanosis, or edema.*

Parts of reports that physicians dictate using the same language all the time are referred to as **normals** by MTSOs. Many companies have sets of normals available on their web sites for medical transcriptionists to use when transcribing reports for certain physicians. The medical transcriptionist obtains the text and creates a macro in the text-expansion software for use when needed. With a few keystrokes, the text appears in the document and the medical transcriptionist is paid for all of the lines generated, even though they were not typed manually.

The possibilities are endless. Make a text expander your friend and challenge yourself to find as many words in your routine transcription as possible to enter as text-expander entries to increase your production and your pay. Before you know it, you will have upwards of 10,000 entries at your fingertips to maximize your daily line counts. Your goal should be to manually type as few words as possible into a report. As you are typing, take a moment or two to enter a new macro or phrase into your word expander immediately, or make a written list of abbreviations to add later. *Saving Keystrokes*, by Diana Rolland (Lippincott Williams & Wilkins) is a comprehensive guide to creating a logical, organized text-expander file that you may find helpful.

Medical References

Get to know which word books and references will provide you with the information you need right away and where they are located. Keep your most often-used word books on the same shelves and always return them to the same place on the shelf so you can find them easily. Keep a binder for each of your transcription accounts, containing all the information about that specific account. The binder might contain the site's document and formatting rules, the list of physicians who practice at that facility, a printout of any templates and boilerplate-type information used regularly on that account, sample reports, and any other instructions pertinent to that account. Place icons for the programs you use most often at work (such as *The Book of Style for Medical Transcription*, electronic medical dictionary, and specific programs related to the company for which you work) on your computer desktop for easy accessibility.

The Internet

The ability to navigate the Internet to find credible information is crucial to your productivity. The Internet is an invaluable tool for locating information that is not readily available in reference books. New medical words, such as names of the latest surgical equipment or treatment protocols, can be found on the Internet years before they appear in print in a reference book. A medical transcriptionist can locate hundreds of resources on the Internet, web sites that list physicians' names by state, geographic locations not spelled by the dictator, and healthcare facilities, to name a few. Use the "My Favorites" list on the computer to organize the web sites you use most frequently. You can create separate folders in the "My Favorites" list to organize your preferred sites by account or geographic location.

Professional Development

Professional development means mastering the knowledge and skills of your profession so that you grow and learn in your day-to-day work life.

Trade-association membership activities and networking are as important after you are working as a medical transcriptionist as they were during your job search. The AHDI is a national organization of medical transcriptionists and other healthcare documentation workers. Membership in the AHDI demonstrates a professional attitude toward your career and also provides a wealth of benefits that can help you grow professionally if you take advantage of the opportunities afforded: continuing education opportunities, opportunities to develop leadership skills, networking opportunities at regularly scheduled meetings, and educational symposia.

The Internet also provides avenues for professional development. Interaction with other medical transcriptionists through online web sites and forums, as well as newsgroups, allows transcriptionists to exchange information and ideas about the newest technologies, terminology, and business conditions in the field, as well as to keep up with professional association news. The Internet is also a useful source for keeping abreast of the standards required by **The Joint Commission** (formerly the Joint Commission on Accreditation of Healthcare Organizations, JCAHO) for institutional accreditation. As discussed in earlier chapters, these standards relate to such medical transcriptionist interests as confidentiality of patient information, records reviews to audit for completeness, timeliness of data collection, and other requirements relevant to the practice of medical transcription. Familiarity with the standards outlined by The Joint Commission will help a new transcriptionist understand the legalities and regulations that govern the healthcare industry as well as the importance of accurate and timely transcription of medical information.

The AHDI awards the certification designations of **Registered Medical Transcriptionist** (RMT) and **Certified Medical Transcriptionist** (CMT) to those who earn passing scores on certification examinations. As in many other fields, credentialing is recognized as a sign of competence. The RMT credential was developed for new medical transcription program graduates and for MTs who do not have the years or variety of experience to be eligible for the CMT exam. Like the CMT examination, the RMT examination consists of both medical transcription-related knowledge items and transcription performance items. The transcription performance section of the examination requires that you transcribe dictation, edit, and proofread.

As a newcomer to the field, you should strive to attain RMT, and later, CMT credentialing. Although you are not currently required to become credentialed in order to work as a medical transcriptionist, earning the credential can be very helpful in advancing your career because it demonstrates to your employers and peers that you are a professional and committed to being the best you can be. Credentialing also serves the public interest by assuring that those who become credentialed meet accepted standards of practice. Credentialing elevates the profession as well as the individual and is a great addition to your resumé of achievements in the field of medical transcription.

Finally, AHDI also enables an MT to become a **Fellow of the Association for Healthcare Documentation Integrity** (AHDI-F), a designation that recognizes a transcriptionist's involvement in both work-related and community activities. As discussed in Chapter 1, *A Career Profile*, the AHDI-F designation requires an MT to get involved in other activities, such as community and association events, by earning a specific number of points for activities performed in different service categories in the five years preceding the application. The designation does not expire as long as the transcriptionist remains a member in good standing with AHDI.

Once you are on the job, there are many ways to build and maintain a professional image, even if you are working from home:

- Always strive to learn more about medical transcription. Speak with your supervisor about taking on more challenging work; learn new accounts and new work specialties. Be someone that the company can depend on to be flexible, to adapt to new situations, and to learn new skills. Strive to learn more about the computer skills you may need. If your company sends out data-type documents using Microsoft Excel, learn how to use Excel. Familiarity with the software used by your employer will help you advance your skills, build your resumé, and flag you as a candidate to work on projects requiring these skills.
- Communicate in a professional way with your peers. Take care to make sure your phone calls and e-mails portray an appropriate image. Be sure the message on your phone answering machine is professional and appropriate, not in questionable taste ("I ain't here, so leave a message"), and be sure that the machine is functioning properly. Adopt a professional e-mail address for your work contacts, preferably simply your name or a variation of it. An e-mail address like wildncrazy@ISP.com does not conjure up a professional image. Keep e-mails simple and to the point, without fancy fonts, garish colors, or goofy clip-art images.
- Dress professionally at association meetings and other functions. Remember: The world of medical transcription is really quite small, and dressing and acting inappropriately in front of your fellow medical transcriptionists does not create an impression of you as someone who could be called upon to assist with projects or leadership opportunities.

QUICK CHECK 22.3 ✓

Indicate whether the following sentences are true (T) or false (F).

1. A portfolio documents your skills and abilities.   T   F

2. Macros are used to place your signature on documents.   T   F

3. You do not have to continue learning about medical transcription once you get a job.   T   F

4. A post-interview thank you note helps maintain good relations with potential employers.   T   F

5. Ideally your office space at home should be in the middle of the living room so you can work and watch television with the family at the same time.   T   F

OWNING YOUR OWN BUSINESS

Working for an MTSO can be a satisfying experience, but the time may come when you want to consider operating a home-based medical transcription business of your own. An **entrepreneur**, also called a **freelancer**, is someone who undertakes and operates a business and assumes all responsibility for its inherent risks as well as its rewards. Medical transcriptionist entrepreneurs have the best of both worlds: the ability to earn money at a job they love while, at the same time, being the person who makes all the decisions.

The startup of any small business obviously requires sound financial planning, but there are other aspects of operating a business that need to be considered carefully before you make the decision to work for yourself. You may discover that your personality and temperament are not compatible with the constant demands of owning a business. You may lose the business if you do not have strong record-keeping, personnel management, or communication skills. Owning a business is an individual choice that should be made only after serious study of a variety of factors. Individual preparation, both personal and professional, is the key to successfully starting and maintaining any business.

Personality and Work Preferences

As much as everyone likes to fantasize about it, not everyone is well suited to owning and operating a business. Think about your personality and work preferences. A chief trait of a successful entrepreneur is determination and the drive to put plans into action. In addition to determination, you need discipline and a strong desire to succeed even when the hours get long and the decisions are difficult. You also need to be flexible and adaptable to change, as each day will bring new challenges you may or may not have anticipated.

Do you think you have the personality to own your own medical transcription business? Answer the questions in Table 22.1 to see how you measure up. Although not every successful medical transcription freelancer starts with an affirmative answer to all of the questions, three or four "negative" or "undecided" answers should be sufficient reason for you to stop and give a second thought to going it alone. Many potential proprietors seek extra training or counseling from small business advisors such as accountants and lawyers.

Equipment

The advantage of a home-based medical transcription business is that you probably already have much of the equipment needed to start on a basic level, such as a desk, computer, modem, Internet service, printer, and telephone answering machine. You also will need a filing cabinet, fax machine, and a copier; the price ranges for these items can be well within a start-up budget.

Of course, transcription equipment is a must, and costs vary by technology. Smaller clinics and offices may still use desktop machines and dictate reports onto a cassette tape or use a dedicated telephone line for incoming dictation, which is more convenient and speeds up turnaround time.

Many larger offices and facilities today use a production and workflow document management system. A **document management system** is a computer software

TABLE 22.1 Am I an Entrepreneur?		
	Yes	*No*
Do I have a strong desire to be my own boss?		
Can I take responsibility for my own financial destiny?		
Can I use power in a constructive way?		
Can I effectively allocate my time between personal and business matters?		
Do I have excellent medical transcription skills based on my education and experience?		
Do I have a broad view of business procedures and how each individual part relates to other parts?		
Do I have the courage to pursue new ideas and technology, even if I do not succeed?		
Am I a risk-taker?		
Am I self-disciplined and responsible for the work that I do?		
Do I have the willingness to persevere, even in hard times?		
Can I accept criticism about my work and learn from my mistakes in order to perform better?		
Can I meet the deadlines required of me?		
Do I have a high level of energy?		
Do I have the flexibility to work long and variable hours to make a business successful?		

program accessible to dictating physicians as well as home-based medical transcriptionists through an online network server connected to the facility's internal phone and medical record-keeping systems. The Internet is used to send and receive files through secure encrypted pathways. This type of software platform, however, is expensive and requires constant maintenance and supervision by qualified technical staff. You should investigate this technology thoroughly before making the investment for your own home-based business.

In addition, you may be required to install a dedicated phone line for business purposes. And you need to be available to your customers when you are not at home working, so a cell phone is required. You can restrict the use of your cell phone to business calls by giving out the number to your clients only.

Because most facilities rely on the Internet to send and receive files, a high-speed Internet connection is a must. Consider investing in the fastest connection you can get where you live in order to avoid signal drops or slow transmission speeds. A fast connection is far more amenable to transmitting a high volume of work anywhere, and the prompt turnaround time is preferable to the agony of any dial-up connection no matter how reliable. You can move more work faster, saving time that can be spent working on other aspects of your business as opposed to dealing with connection delays and inopportune line disconnections. If cable Internet service is not available in your area, consider a **digital subscriber line** (DSL), which is a method of providing digital data transmission over the wires of a local telephone network. If your area is limited to dial-up service, look into a satellite connection. Fast modem connections can be expensive, but are well worth the cost in the digital age of medical transcription.

Financing

One of the most appealing aspects of owning a medical transcription business is the relatively low start-up costs. Most freelance medical transcriptionists use their own personal savings and the equipment they already own to start their businesses and concentrate initially on building a small local client base with which to expand. Many freelancers start their businesses on the side while working full-time jobs. If you plan to plunge into your new business from the start, however, be sure you have enough cash on hand to cover your expenses until the revenue starts coming in. At a minimum, you should have the equivalent of six months' expenses in a savings account to tap into if you need it.

Because start-up costs are relatively low, you may find traditional financing difficult to obtain—banks and lenders would rather lend amounts much larger than you will need or likely qualify for. Yet reserve capital is critical for a successful business. Investigate other areas of financing for your business, such as using personal savings or investments from family and friends, certificates of deposits, or loans against insurance policies. You can also check out low-interest loans from the Small Business Administration (SBA), a branch of the U.S. Government designed to aid, counsel, and assist small businesses. Loan application guidelines can be found on the SBA's website located at www.sba.gov.

Insurance

Insurance is essential for protecting a home-based business against unforeseen losses or financial burdens. You should consider calling your insurance agent for help in properly insuring all aspects of your business operations. Typical requirements include fire, liability, and vehicle insurance. You will also need workers' compensation insurance if you later choose to hire employees for your business.

Type of Business

There are also legal requirements for starting a business. You may need a business license, and you must operate your business according to the laws of your city and state with regard to location and other local ordinances as well as HIPAA regulations. In addition, check to see that your business complies with local zoning requirements. Many communities forbid, through zoning ordinances, the establishment of some types of home-based businesses. Check local restrictions prior to investing time and money.

You also will have to consider the laws concerning state and federal taxes with regard to the income generated by your business. There are different types of business organizations, each of which offers distinct advantages and disadvantages.

Sole Proprietorship

A **sole proprietorship** is owned and operated by an individual, and many home-based freelance medical transcriptionists fall into this category. Advantages of this form of organization include ease of formation and freedom from government controls and restrictions. You can keep simple, unaudited accounts of your income and expenses; and if you form a corporation or other business entity later, you can transfer your sole proprietorship business dealings to it. The disadvantage to this type of business ownership is that you are entitled to fewer employment security benefits. For example, if you cannot work or lose your business, you cannot claim unemployment benefits from the government. The main disadvantage of this form of organization; however, is that it provides less protection with regard to personal liability. This means that in the event of losses incurred by the business or litigation brought against you concerning work you have performed, you may be required to sell personal property such as a car, house, or other assets to satisfy debts owed.

Partnership

Generally, a **partnership** is defined as a business comprised of two or more individuals who carry on an association as co-owners of a business for profit. This type of business is entered into using a partnership agreement prepared by an attorney. The agreement defines how much each owner must contribute in equity, the extent to which each partner will work in the company, and the share of the profits or losses to be assigned to each of them. Although the advantages to a partnership include more working capital and a chance to test the old adage, "two heads being better than one," a general partnership exposes all of the owners to personal liability in the event of business losses, even if only one partner caused the debt to occur. If the business is not successful and the partnership cannot pay all of its debts, the general partners may be required to do so using their personal assets.

Corporation

A **corporation** is a distinct legal entity that conducts business and is given many of the same legal rights as an actual person. It is the most complex, but most protective, form of business organization. A corporation may sell shares of stock, which are certificates indicating ownership in the company, to as many people as needed to obtain working capital. A board of directors elected by the shareholders runs the company on a day-to-day basis. The distinct advantage of a corporation is the limited liability of the corporation's shareholders for debts owed by the company. This concept is called the **corporate veil**, a legal term referring to the separation between a shareholder and a corporation and the fact that a shareholder is not liable for the debts of the corporation. However, doing business through a corporation carries several tax disadvantages. Because a corporation has its own existence, it pays taxes on its own income. However, if a corporation has losses, only the corporation, and not the shareholders, can claim those losses as a tax deduction.

A **C corporation** is the most common type of corporation in the United States. It allows for theoretically unlimited amounts of stock to be issued for a company to obtain capital, and it usually has a small board of directors that makes decisions. A C corporation pays taxes on its income at the corporate level, and shareholders also pay taxes on the income they receive from the corporation. An **S corporation** is another form of corporate entity and is nearly identical to a C corporation, except that an S corporation does not pay a tax on its income. The income and expenses of the corporation are divided among its shareholders, who then report the income on their own income tax returns. To qualify for S corporation status, a corporation must meet several requirements, one of which limits the number of shareholders who can participate in the business.

Taxes

Taxation for a small business can be simple or complex, depending on the size and type of the company. Of course, every company making a profit must pay a tax based on net income. A sole proprietor must pay individual income taxes on earnings from the business. In a partnership, each partner must pay taxes on the distributive share of the partnership income, whereas a corporation must pay corporate income tax.

The IRS estimates that up to 80% of home-based workers report income and expenses as either a sole proprietorship, partnership, or S corporation. Maintaining a home office for generating income offers many tax benefits or "write-offs" that can be credited against a person's tax liability, as the expenses are prorated between personal and business use. These expenses include interest on a home mortgage, utilities, major home maintenance costs, and other legitimate business expenses. Seek the advice of a professional who is well versed in federal and state tax laws to get accurate advice about what is and is not tax deductible for your home office.

Developing a Client Base

For the first time ever, the Internet allows you to participate in a global economy without leaving your living room, making the world a freelancer's oyster. As an entrepreneur, you have the potential to market your services not only to healthcare providers in your neighborhood, but to those all over the country and perhaps, one day, the world.

Advertising is the primary way to obtain new business. Newspaper and journal ads, a directory yellow page listing, and direct mailings to area clinics and hospitals are some methods of advertising. Target your own direct-mail campaign using the telephone directory and trade journals as a resource. A presence on online networking communities such as Facebook and Twitter can generate long-term responses.

Join your local chapter of the AHDI to develop networking opportunities for your business. Your local chamber of commerce is another potential avenue for client contacts. Joining and actively participating in professional organization activities and programs will help you make friends with your peers and give you an opportunity for business leads and advice from other business professionals.

Try door-to-door introductions by visiting facilities to introduce yourself and to leave a business card and flyer. You might want to invest in small promotional items such as pens, emery boards, desk calendars, or other products to leave a lasting impression of your name and services. Stress the advantages for the company that uses your services. Stress your knowledge and dependability to get the job done quickly, the prompt turnaround time of the work, reliability, and flexibility in meeting the facility's transcription needs.

You can also put your best foot forward on personal visits by showing the same portfolio you used when you were looking for a job with a medical transcription company. If your work and credentials are excellent, show them off by leaving a small portfolio of samples (with identifying information obliterated, of course) and other documented achievements with potential clients you visit. If you are presenting the portfolio in a one-on-one setting with an office manager or physician, show enthusiasm for the work you did and the experience you had with that particular part of the portfolio. The presentation will be more interesting if you relay stories and details about your experiences while presenting your items and giving a potential client a sense of who you are and of your work ethic.

Another key element in advertising your services is a professional-appearing web site. Today a web site has become a requirement for almost every business. Among other things, an effective web site can improve the image of your business, save time in presenting your services to prospective clients, and can help you reach more people who may want to use your services. You can invest in a professional designer to create your web site, or you can create your own using web site design software. Either way, be sure to include a comprehensive description of your services, the equipment used, and your contact information. Be sure to update your web site frequently to keep it current and inviting.

Billing Considerations

The inevitable question facing freelance medical transcriptionists is what to charge for services rendered. As an entrepreneur, you decide what your services are worth based on your knowledge and experience and what you want to earn. Do not price yourself out of the market, but do not charge a rate that is not commensurate with your skills.

Some freelance medical transcriptionists charge their customers by the hour, whereas others charge a flat fee per page, with more than one-half of the page completed constituting a full page. Most MTSOs charge their customers for services rendered by the line. The rate may vary by location, so you could try to contact local competitors to obtain information on rates charged to their corporate customers per line. However, since you will be a potential competitor to them, it would be unrealistic

---

QUICK CHECK 22.4 ✓

Circle the letter corresponding to the best answer to the following questions.

1. The advantage of a sole proprietorship is

    A. the ease of formation of the business.
    B. the freedom from government controls and restrictions.
    C. the simple accounting of income and expenses.
    D. all of the above.

2. A standard unit of measure for the line-rate billing by most MTSOs is called

    A. the visible line rate.
    B. the virtual black character.
    C. the visible black character.
    D. the document management system.

3. A method of providing digital data transmission over telephone wires is called a

    A. satellite transmission service.
    B. digital subscriber line.
    C. dial-up server.
    D. digital transmission line.

4. The legal term referring to a separation between a shareholder and the corporation is called the

    A. shareholder agreement.
    B. corporate veil.
    C. S corporation status.
    D. dividend.

5. In a general partnership, the liabilities are

    A. shared equally by both partners.
    B. incurred only by the partner who created them.
    C. shared by neither partner.
    D. erased at the end of each year.

to assume they would be forthcoming with such proprietary information. The U.S. Government offers informational bulletins about wages and prices for small businesses at the U.S. Department of Labor Bureau of Labor Statistics' web site located at www.bls.gov.

When working out a line rate or hourly fee, remember to include any state or local taxes, federal income tax, social security, or other extraneous expenses that may be taken from your gross pay for the job. Some freelance medical transcriptionists charge a line rate that is double the going medical transcription employee rate in order to cover expenses. For example, if an employee typically makes 10 cents per line through an MTSO, a freelancer may charge 20 to 25 cents per line. Or you might determine a percentage markup from a base rate for services rendered, for example, a base line rate plus 25%.

Recently the **visible black character** (VBC) has become the standard unit of measure for the line-rate billing by many MTSOs. This standard, endorsed by the Clinical Documentation Industry Association (CDIA, formerly the Medical Transcription Industry Association, MTIA) and the American Health Information Management Association (AHIMA), is defined as "a character that can be seen with the naked eye in which spaces, carriage returns, and hidden formatting instructions (such as bolding, underline, text boxes, printer configurations, and spell checking) are not counted in the total character count." The standard unit of measure is intended to resolve the confusion surrounding the vast number of billing methods used by different MTSOs for lines billed to their customers. This standard unit of measure can be applied to all types of medical reports and various technologies. It is hoped that this uniformity in billing will create understandable billing

practices and improve customer relations. The entire position statement with regard to the VBC and how it applies to the invoicing of customers and compensation of medical transcription employees can be viewed on the AHDI web site at www.ahdionline.org.

Despite the comfort of playing it safe by working for someone else, the pleasure of owning your own business, if done correctly, can far outweigh the potential risks associated with it. If you know the basics of business ownership and operation, you can achieve your entrepreneurial dream of working for yourself. A business based on a solid foundation of professionalism and trust will guarantee your success as a business owner for years to come.

CHAPTER SUMMARY

Congratulations! You have finished this book as part of your learning curriculum and have laid the foundation you need to be a successful medical transcriptionist. It is hoped that this has been a fun and rewarding experience for you and that you are ready to begin your new career armed with knowledge, tips, and techniques to help you achieve success.

The greater your desire to learn and explore your profession, the greater will be your opportunities for advancement and success on the job. There are many paths you can take to advance your career in medical transcription, including owning your own medical transcription service, and each step contributes to growth and learning. Take one step at a time, look forward, and take in everything you can as you go. And most important, have fun. Welcome to the world of medical transcription!

·I·N·S·I·G·H·T·

The Benefits of Ergonomics

Tingling fingers, aching forearms, or painful wrists are all early warning signs of repetitive stress disorders such as carpal tunnel syndrome or tendonitis. Once a rare occurrence in business environments, the U.S. Department of Labor's Occupational Safety & Health Administration (OSHA) indicates that more than two million U.S. workers now have this type of musculoskeletal disorders caused primarily by repetitive motion such as typing.

Carpal tunnel syndrome was rare during the era of manual typewriters because typewriter tables were a standard 26 inches above the floor. In addition, typists were constantly moving in different ways, hitting the return bar, pulling paper out, putting paper in, and standing or walking to filing cabinets or to get more paper. Today, computers enable employees to sit in one place without moving. A poorly designed workstation, combined with poor work habits and postures, can result in carpal tunnel syndrome and tendonitis. Files are now stored on hard drives, eliminating the standing and walking. Printers and refill paper are usually near workstations. Keyboards often sit at a height of 29 to 30 inches from the floor and often the mouse is not within easy reach, creating awkward stress on the forearms. Sitting in a static position at a workstation throughout the day requires muscles to flex and remain taut to hold the body in position—an unnatural activity. These workplace automations cause back injuries and stress injuries such as carpal tunnel syndrome, resulting in lost work days, workers' compensation claims, and repetitive trauma disorders that require costly medical care.

In the past, individual complaints were looked upon as individual problems, not human problems. Attention to the workplace was focused on the interaction of machines and environments with little attention paid to the role of employees. The concept of ergonomics was born when researchers began to consider how humans functioned in a workplace environment dominated by machines.

Today the science of ergonomics is used to design the workplace to accommodate the worker. Companies now strive to identify potential problems and supply their workers with ergonomically designed work tools, furniture and supplies, and effective training programs to help them derive maximum benefit from those items.

For employees and employers alike, good ergonomics equal good economics. Aggressive application of the principals of ergonomics on the job has resulted in the reduction of crippling repetitive strain injuries and increased productivity on the job. Employees feel happier and better about their workplaces, which means less absenteeism and more productivity on the job.

ABBREVIATIONS

Abbreviation	Meaning	Abbreviation	Meaning
AHDI	Association for Healthcare Documentation Integrity	JCAHO	The Joint Commission on Accreditation of Healthcare Organizations, now known as The Joint Commission
AHDI-F	Fellow of the Association for Healthcare Documentation Integrity	MTSO	medical transcription service organization
AHIMA	American Health Information Management Association	RMT	registered medical transcriptionist
CDIA	Clinical Documentation Industry Association	SBA	Small Business Administration
CMT	certified medical transcriptionist	TAT	turnaround time
CV	curriculum vitae		
DSL	digital subscriber line		

Add Your Own Abbreviations Here:

_____

_____

_____

_____

_____

_____

TERMINOLOGY

Term	Meaning
AHDI	The professional organization representing the interests of medical transcriptionists and other healthcare documentation providers.
AHDI-F	A designation awarded by the AHDI that signifies a balance of successful activities in the medical transcription profession in a variety of core areas involving practice duties, professional experience, leadership, and community involvement.
C corporation	A type of corporation that pays taxes on its income at the corporate level, and shareholders also pay taxes on the income (dividends) they receive from the corporation.
career fair	An event that brings together representatives and hiring manager from various companies in one place.

Term	*Meaning*
certified medical transcriptionist (CMT)	A credential awarded by the AHDI to those with greater than two years of experience in the field who earn a passing score on a certification examination.
chronological resumé	A resumé in which experiences and achievements are listed in reverse chronological order by dates.
corporate veil	A legal term referring to the separation between a shareholder and a corporation and the fact that a shareholder is not liable for the debts of the corporation.
corporation	A distinct legal entity that conducts business and is given many of the same legal rights as an actual person.
digital subscriber line (DSL)	A method of providing digital data transmission over the wires of a local telephone network.
document management system	A computer software program accessible to dictating physicians as well as home-based medical transcriptionists through an online network server connected to the facility's internal phone and medical record keeping systems.
employment web site	A web site that deals specifically with employment.
entrepreneur, syn. freelancer	Someone who undertakes and operates a business and assumes all responsibility for its inherent risks as well as rewards.
ergonomics	The science of designing and arranging objects, systems, and environments in such a way as to maximize productivity by reducing operator fatigue and discomfort.
forums	Specific Internet message boards whose posts focus on a particular subject or industry.
functional resumé, syn. skills-based resume	A resumé in which skills and expertise are highlighted, not a chronological work history or timeline.
Joint Commission (The)	Formerly called JCAHO, a nonprofit organization with a mission to maintain and elevate standards of healthcare delivery through evaluation and accreditation of healthcare organizations by sending surveyors to healthcare organizations to evaluate their operational practices and facilities.
line count	The measurement of lines type by a medical transcriptionist.
macros	The name given to abbreviations entered into text-expansion software to increase productivity and reduce mistakes (not to be confused with macros in word-processing software such as *Microsoft Word*).
medical transcription service organization (MTSO)	A medical transcription company or provider.
networking	The process of connecting particular people or objects.
normal	A part of a report that contains a dictator's standard language.
online test	An examination conducted by an MTSO via the Internet to gain an objective measure of a potential employee's skills as well as to help match the transcriptionist's skills with account requirements.
outsourcing	The process by which a healthcare organization contracts with a medical transcription company to handle the production of their dictated medical records.
overflow	A term referring to the work that the in-house staff cannot complete within the required turnaround time.
partnership	A business comprised of two or more individuals who carry on an association as co-owners of a business for profit.
portfolio	A collection of documents outlining one's achievements, the scope and quality of experience and training, and abilities.

Term	*Meaning*
resumé	A document containing a summary or listing of relevant job experience, education, and achievement for the purpose of seeking employment.
S corporation	A type of corporation that is nearly identical to a C corporation, except that the income and expenses of the corporation are divided among its shareholders, who then report the income on their own income tax returns.
sole proprietorship	A business owned and operated by an individual.
turnaround time (TAT)	The measurement of time between the point at which a dictated report is submitted for transcription and the time the report is typed by the medical transcriptionist and returned to the facility.
visible black character (VBC)	A standard unit of billing measure where a character can be seen with the naked eye. Carriage returns and hidden formatting instructions (such as bolding, underline, text boxes, printer configurations, and spell checking) are not counted in the total character count.
work type (WT)	Reports categorized by the type of document dictated.
zinger	A question asked by an interviewer that is difficult, if not impossible to answer, to judge how a candidate might respond to pressure or tension on the job.

Add Your Own Terms and Definitions Here:

_____

_____

_____

_____

_____

_____

_____

_____

REVIEW QUESTIONS

1. Name three sources of job leads.
2. What is the purpose of text-expansion software?
3. What is a general-distribution cover letter?
4. When is a chronological resumé more effective than a functional one? When is a functional resumé more effective?
5. What is the benefit of volunteering?
6. Why should a medical transcriptionist be familiar with and practice ergonomics?
7. What is the purpose of an online test?
8. Name three functions of an effective cover letter.
9. Where can information about career fairs be found?
10. What is the RMT and why is it beneficial to a student graduate?

CHAPTER ACTIVITIES

Strengths and Skills Evaluation

Complete the following worksheet listing the strengths and skills you possess that would be useful to a potential medical transcription employer. Consider not only school-related activities and achievements, but also those in which you engage in your spare time that have given you skills and experience that would be helpful on the job.

Strengths and Skills
Worksheet

Personality Traits:
(outgoing, social, quiet, inquisitive, studious, motivated, etc.)
1. _____
2. _____
3. _____

Work-Related Personality Traits:
(team-oriented, can multitask, easy to get along with, organized, prompt, reliable, etc.)
1. _____
2. _____
3. _____

Personal Achievements:
(PTA chairman, youth league coach, community service, charity activities, etc.)
1. _____
2. _____
3. _____

Functional Skills:
(computer skills, typing speed, test scores, etc.)
1. _____
2. _____
3. _____

Professional Activities:
(Association activities, school honors and awards, certifications, medical education events, etc.)

1. _____

2. _____

3. _____

Other Marketable Skills:

1. _____

2. _____

3. _____

Revise Resumé Descriptions

Revise the following unimpressive descriptions from resumés. Recast the sentences into phrases, removing personal pronouns.

1. "When the company needed a manual on the new Windows platform program, I helped to organize and write it."
2. "I was always passing my line count quotas every single week."
3. "I was the most accurate medical transcriptionist in my company. I always received at least 99% in all my audits all the time."
4. "I was able to train all newbie MTs during the first week they are hired the right way."
5. "I was instructed to draw, using my own creativity, first in pencil tracings and then in final form, all of the illustrations used in the wants ads used by the company in magazines and newspapers."

Create a Resumé

Create a functional resumé using the tips and information provided in this chapter. First write down a list of the different items that should be included in the resumé that contain the five key areas: summary, accomplishments, skills, education, and work experience. Design the layout of your resumé on a separate piece of paper to make it as aesthetically appealing as possible, or you may refer to one of the resumé templates in Microsoft Word to help list the information you need to include on your resumé. Review sample resumés online or in job-search books to help you incorporate your resumé template information into an appropriate format. Use the resumé template to generate a list of information to include on your resumé; then compile the details from the resumé template to format your resumé into a customized resumé to send to employers.

Create an Application Cover Letter

Create a cover letter to accompany your resumé. Think of a fictitious company and name of a recruiter to address your cover letter to. In your cover letter, creatively state the following:

1. The title of the position for which you are applying and where you learned of the position (you may indicate the newspaper, through networking, online forum, etc.).
2. Your interest in that particular company.
3. Your most relevant skills and experiences.
4. How your abilities relate or can be used for the position.
5. Your interest in the field as well as your motivation and strengths.
6. Your outside achievements.
7. How you will follow up on your submission of your resumé and cover letter.

Appendix 1

ISMP'S LIST OF ERROR-PRONE ABBREVIATIONS, SYMBOLS, AND DOSE DESIGNATIONS

The abbreviations, symbols, and dose designations found in this table have been reported to ISMP through the ISMP Medication Error Reporting Program (MERP) as being frequently misinterpreted and involved in harmful medication errors. They should NEVER be used when communicating medical information. This includes internal communications, telephone/verbal prescriptions, computer-generated labels, labels for drug storage bins, medication administration records, as well as pharmacy and prescriber computer order entry screens.

The Joint Commission has established a National Patient Safety Goal that specifies that certain abbreviations must appear on an accredited organization's "do-not-use" list; we have highlighted these items with a double asterisk (**). However, we hope that you will consider others beyond the minimum Joint Commission requirements. By using and promoting safe practices and by educating one another about hazards, we can better protect our patients.

Abbreviations	Intended Meaning	Misinterpretation	Correction
μg	Microgram	Mistaken as "mg"	Use "mcg"
AD, AS, AU	Right ear, left ear, each ear	Mistaken as OD, OS, OU (right eye, left eye, each eye)	Use "right ear," "left ear," or "each ear"
OD, OS, OU	Right eye, left eye, each eye	Mistaken as AD, AS, AU (right ear, left ear, each ear)	Use "right eye," "left eye," or "each eye"
BT	Bedtime	Mistaken as "BID" (twice daily)	Use "bedtime"
cc	Cubic centimeters	Mistaken as "u" (units)	Use "mL"
D/C	Discharge or discontinue	Premature discontinuation of medications if D/C (intended to mean "discharge") has been misinterpreted as "discontinued" when followed by a list of discharge medications	Use "discharge" and "discontinue"

(Continued)

Abbreviations	Intended Meaning	Misinterpretation	Correction
IJ	Injection	Mistaken as "IV" or "intrajugular"	Use "injection"
IN	Intranasal	Mistaken as "IM" or "IV"	Use "intranasal" or "NAS"
HS hs	Half-strength At bedtime, hours of sleep	Mistaken as bedtime Mistaken as half-strength	Use "half-strength" or "bedtime"
IU**	International unit	Mistaken as IV (intravenous) or 10 (ten)	Use "units"
o.d. or OD	Once daily	Mistaken as "right eye" (OD-oculus dexter), leading to oral liquid medications administered in the eye	Use "daily"
OJ	Orange juice	Mistaken as OD or OS (right or left eye); drugs meant to be diluted in orange juice may be given in the eye	Use "orange juice"
Per os	By mouth, orally	The "os" can be mistaken as "left eye" (OS-oculus sinister)	Use "PO," "by mouth," or "orally"
q.d. or QD**	Every day	Mistaken as q.i.d., especially if the period after the "q" or the tail of the "q" is misunderstood as an "i"	Use "daily"
qhs	Nightly at bedtime	Mistaken as "qhr" or every hour	Use "nightly"
qn q.o.d. or QOD**	Nightly or at bedtime Every other day	Mistaken as "qh" (every hour) Mistaken as "q.d." (daily) or "q.i.d." (four times daily) if the "o" is poorly written	Use "nightly" or "at bedtime" Use "every other day"
q1d	Daily	Mistaken as q.i.d. (four times daily)	Use "daily"
q6PM, etc.	Every evening at 6 PM	Mistaken as every 6 hours	Use "daily at 6 PM" or "6 PM daily"
SC, SQ, sub q	Subcutaneous	SC mistaken as SL (sublingual); SQ mistaken as "5 every;" the "q" in "sub q" has been mistaken as "every" (e.g., a heparin dose ordered "sub q 2 hours before surgery" misunderstood as every 2 hours before surgery)	Use "subcut" or "subcutaneously"
ss SSRI SSI	Sliding scale (insulin) or ½ (apothecary) Sliding scale regular insulin Sliding scale insulin	Mistaken as "55" Mistaken as selective-serotonin reuptake inhibitor Mistaken as Strong Solution of Iodine (Lugol's)	Spell out "sliding scale;" use "one-half" or "½" Spell out "sliding scale (insulin)"
i/d	One daily	Mistaken as "tid"	Use "1 daily"
TIW or tiw (also BIW or biw)	TIW: 3 times a week BIW: 2 times a week	TIW mistaken as "3 times a day" or "twice in a week" BIW mistaken ad "2 times a day"	Use "3 times weekly" Use "2 times weekly"
U or u**	Unit	Mistaken as the number 0 or 4, causing a 10-fold overdose or greater (e.g., 4U seen as "40" or 4u seen as "44"); mistaken as "cc" so dose given in volume instead of units (e.g., 4u seen as 4cc)	Use "unit"
UD	As directed ("ut dictum")	Mistaken as unit dose (e.g., diltiazem 125 mg IV infusion "UD" misinterpreted as meaning to give the entire infusion as a unit [bolus] dose)	Use "as directed"

Dose Designations and Other Information	Intended Meaning	Misinterpretation	Correction
Trailing zero after decimal point (e.g. 1.0 mg)**	1 mg	Mistaken as 10 mg if the decimal point is not seen	Do not use trailing zeros for doses expressed in whole numbers
No leading zero before a decimal point (e.g., .5 mg)**	0.5 mg	Mistaken as 5 mg if the decimal point is not seen	Use zero before a decimal point when the dose is less than a whole unit
Drug name and dose run together (especially problematic for drug names that end in "l" such as Inderal40 mg; Tegretol300 mg)	Inderal 40 mg Tegretol 300 mg	Mistaken as Inderal 140 mg Mistaken as Tegretol 1300 mg	Place adequate space between the drug name, dose, and unit of measure
Numerical dose and unit of measure run together (e.g., 10mg, 100mL)	10 mg 100 mL	The "m" is sometimes mistaken as a zero or two zeros, risking a 10- to 100-fold overdose	Place adequate space between the dose and unit of measure
Abbreviations such as mg. or mL. with a period following the abbreviation	mg mL	The period is unnecessary and could be mistaken as the number 1 if written poorly	Use mg, mL, etc. without a terminal period
Large doses without properly placed commas (e.g., 100000 units; 1000000 units)	100,000 units 1,000,000 units	100000 has been mistaken as 10,000 or 1,000,000; 1000000 has been mistaken as 100,000	Use commas for dosing units at or above 1,000, or use words such as 100 "thousand" or 1 "million" to improve readability

Drug Name Abbreviations	Intended Meaning	Misinterpretation	Correction
ARA A	vidarabine	Mistaken as cytarabine (ARA C)	Use complete drug name
AZT	zidovudine (Retrovir)	Mistaken as azathioprine or aztreonam	Use complete drug name
CPZ	Compazine (prochlorperazine)	Mistaken as chlorpromazine	Use complete drug name
DPT	Demerol-Phenergan-Thorazine	Mistaken as diphtheria-pertussis-tetanus (vaccine)	Use complete drug name
DTO	Diluted tincture of opium, or deodorized tincture of opium (Paregoric)	Mistaken as tincture of opium	Use complete drug name
HCl	hydrochloric acid or hydrochloride	Mistaken as potassium chloride (The "H" is misinterpreted as "K")	Use complete drug name unless expressed as a salt of a drug
HCT	hydrocortisone	Mistaken as hydrochlorothiazide	Use complete drug name
HCTZ	hydrochlorothiazide	Mistaken as hydrocortisone (seen as HCT250 mg)	Use complete drug name
MgSO4**	magnesium sulfate	Mistaken as morphine sulfate	Use complete drug name
MS, MSO4**	morphine sulfate	Mistaken as magnesium sulfate	Use complete drug name
MTX	methotrexate	Mistaken as mitoxantrone	Use complete drug name

(Continued)

Drug Name Abbreviations	Intended Meaning	Misinterpretation	Correction
PCA	procainamide	Mistaken as patient controlled analgesia	Use complete drug name
PTU	propylthiouracil	Mistaken as mercaptopurine	Use complete drug name
T3	Tylenol with codeine No. 3	Mistaken as liothyronine	Use complete drug name
TAC	triamcinolone	Mistaken as tetracaine, Adrenalin, cocaine	Use complete drug name
TNK	TNKase	Mistaken as "TPA"	Use complete drug name
ZnSO4	zinc sulfate	Mistaken as morphine sulfate	Use complete drug name

Stemmed Drug Names	Intended Meaning	Misinterpretation	Correction
"Nitro" drip	nitroglycerin infusion	Mistaken as sodium nitroprusside infusion	Use complete drug name
"Norflox"	norfloxacin	Mistaken as Norflex	Use complete drug name
"IV Vanc"	intravenous vancomycin	Mistaken as Invanz	Use complete drug name

Symbols	Intended Meaning	Misinterpretation	Correction
℥ ℳ	Dram Minim	Symbol for dram mistaken as "3" Symbol for minim mistaken as "mL"	Use the metric system
x3d	For three days	Mistaken as "3 doses"	Use "for three days"
>and<	Greater than and less than	Mistaken as opposite of intended; mistakenly use incorrect symbol; "<10" mistaken as "40"	Use "greater than" or "less than"
/ (slash mark)	Separates two doses or indicates "per"	Mistaken as the number 1 (e.g., "25 units/10 units" misread as "25 units and 110" units)	Use "per" rather than a slash mark to separate doses
@	At	Mistaken as "2"	Use "at"
&	And	Mistaken as "2"	Use "and"
+	Plus or and	Mistaken as "4"	Use "and"
°	Hour	Mistaken as a zero (e.g., q2° seen as q 20)	Use "hr," "h," or "hour"
Ø	zero, null sign	Mistaken as the numerals 4, 6, or 9	Use the number "0" or the word "zero"

**These abbreviations are included on The Joint Commission's "minimum list" of dangerous abbreviations, acronyms, and symbols that must be included on an organization's "Do Not Use" list, effective January 1, 2004. Visit www.jcaho.org for more information about this Joint Commission requirement.

Report medication errors or near misses to the ISMP Medication Errors Reporting Program (MERP) at 1-800-FAIL-SAF(E) or online at www.ismp.org. Reprinted with permission from the Institute for Safe Medication Practices, www.ismp.org

Appendix 2

SELECTED NORMAL LABORATORY VALUES

Test	Conventional Units	SI Units
Acetaminophen, serum or plasma (Hep or EDTA)		
Therapeutic	10–30 mcg/mL	66–199 mcmol/L
Toxic	>200 mcg/mL	>1324 mcmol/L
*Alanine aminotransferase, serum	6–37 U/L	1–62 × 10⁻⁷ kat/L
Albumin		
Serum		
Adult	3.5–5.2 g/dL	35–52 g/L
>60 y	3.2–4.6 g/dL	32–46 g/L
	Avg. of 0.3 g/dL higher in patients in upright position	Avg. of 3 g/L higher in patients in upright position
Urine		
Qualitative	Negative	Negative
Quantitative	50–80 mg/24 h	50–80 mg/24 h
CSF	10–30 mg/dL	100–300 mg/L
*Aldolase, serum	1.0–7.5 U/L (30°C)	0.02–0.13 mckat/L (30°C)
Aldosterone		
Serum		
Supine	3–16 ng/dL	80–444 pmol/L
Standing	7–30 ng/dL	190–832 pmol/L
Urine	3–19 mcg/24 h	8–51 nmol/24 h
Alkaline phosphatase, serum	30–90 U/L	30–95 U/L (Bowers and McComb)
Alpha₁ antitrypsin, serum	110–200 mg/dL	1.10–2.0 g/L

(Continued)

623

Test	Conventional Units	SI Units
Ammonia (EDTA)	<50–ng/dL	<36 nmol/L
Ammonia		
Plasma (Hep)	7–27 mcmol/L	7–27 mcmol/L
*Amylase		
Serum	27–131 U/L	0.46–2.23 mckat/L
Urine	1–17 U/h	0.017–0.29 mckat/h
Amylase:creatinine clearance ratio	<3%	<.03
Androstenedione, serum		
Male	75–205 ng/dL	2.6–7.2 nmol/L
Female	85–275 ng/dL	3.0–9.6 nmol/L
Anion gap		
($[Na + K] - [Cl + HCO_3]$)	10–20 mEq/L	10–20 mmol/L
α_1-Antitrypsin, serum	78–200 mg/dL	0.78–2.00 g/L
Apolipoprotein A-1		
Male	94–178 mg/dL	0.94–1.78 g/L
Female	101–199 mg/dL	1.01–1.99 g/L
Apolipoprotein B		
Male	63–133 mg/dL	0.63–1.33 g/L
Female	60–126 mg/dL	0.60–1.26 g/L
*Aspartate aminotransferase (SGOT) serum	5–30 U/L	$8.3–50 \times 10^{-8}$ kat/L
Base excess, blood (Hep)	22 to +3 mEq/L	22 to +3 mmol/L
Bicarbonate,		
serum (venous)	22–29 mEq/L	22–29 mmol/L
plasma (arterial)	22–25 mEq/L	22–25 mmol/L
††Bilirubin		
Bilirubin, direct		
Birth–death	0.0–0.4 mg/dL	
Bilirubin, total		
Birth–1 day	1.0–6.0 mg/dL	
1–2 days	6.0–7.5 mg/dL	
2–5 days	4.0–13.5 mg/dL	
5 days–death	0.2–1.2 mg/dL	
Total bilirubin, neonatal (full term infant)		
Birth–1 day	1.0–6.0 mg/dL	
1–2 days	6.0–7.5 mg/dL	
2–5 days	4.0–6.0 mg/dL	
5 days–1 month	0.0–1.8 mg/dL	
1 month–death	0.0–1.8 mg/dL	
Bone marrow, differential cell count		
Adult		
Undifferentiated cells	0–1%	0–0.01
Myeloblast	0–2%	0–0.02
Promyelocyte	0–4%	0–0.04

*Test values depend on laboratory methods.
*Test values depend on laboratory methods.
†Bilirubin data—Source: http://labs-sec.uhs-sa.com/clinical_ext/dols/soprefrange.asp

Test	Conventional Units	SI Units
Myelocytes		
Neutrophilic	5–20%	0.05–0.20
Eosinophilic	0–3%	0–0.03
Basophilic	0–1%	0–0.01
Metamyeolocytes and bands		
Neutrophilic	5–35%	0.05–0.35
Eosinophilic	0–5%	0–0.05
Basophilic	0–1%	0–0.01
Segmented neutrophils	5–15%	0.05–0.15
Pronormoblast	0–1.5%	0–0.015
Basophilic normoblast	0–5%	0–0.05
Polychromatophilic normoblast	5–30%	0.05–0.30
Orthochromatic normoblast	5–10%	0.05–0.10
Lymphocytes	10–20%	0.10–0.20
Plasma cells	0–2%	0–0.02
Monocytes	0–5%	0–0.05
CA-125, serum	<35 U/mL	<35 kU/L
CA 15-3, serum	<25 U/mL	<30 kU/L
CA 19-9, serum	<37 U/mL	<37 kU/L
Calcitonin, serum or plasma		
Male	≤100 pg/mL	≤100 ng/L
Female	≤30 pg/mL	≤30 ng/L
Calcium, serum	8.6–10.0 mg/dL	2.15–2.50 mmol/L
Child	8.6–10.6 mg/dL	2.5–2.65 mmol/L
Calcium, ionized, serum	4.64–5.28 mg/dL	1.16–1.32 mmol/L
Calcium, neonate, serum	4.8–5.9 mg/dL	1.20–1.48 mmol/L
Calcium, urine		
Low calcium diet	50–150 mg/24 h	1.25–3.75 mmol/24 h
Usual diet; trough	100–300 mg/24 h	2.50–7.50 mmol/24 h
Carbon dioxide, total, serum/plasma	(Hep) 22–28 mmol/L	22–28 mmol/L
Carbon dioxide (PCO_2), blood, arterial	Male 35–48 mmHg	4.66–6.38 kPa
	Female 32–45 mmHg	4.26–5.99 kPa
Catecholamines, plasma (EDTA)		
Dopamine	<30 pg/mL	<196 pmol/L
Epinephrine	<110 pg/mL	<680 pmol/L
Norepinephrine	<1700 pg/mL	<10,047 pmol/L
Catecholamines, urine		
Dopamine	65–400 mcg/24 h	425–2610 nmol/24 h
Epinephrine	0–20 mcg/24 h	0–109 nmol/24 h
Norepinephrine	15–80 mcg/24 h	89–473 nmol/24 h
CEA, serum		
Nonsmokers	<5.0 ng/mL	<5.0 mcg/L
Cell counts, adult		
Erythrocytes		
Male	4.5–5.5 × 10^6/mcL	4.5–5.5 × 10^{12}/L
Female	4.0–5.0 × 10^6/mcL	4.2–5.0 × 10^{12}/L

(Continued)

Test	Conventional Units		SI Units
Leukocytes			
Total	4.5–11.0 × 10³/mcL		4.5–11.0 × 10⁹/L
Leukocyte differential	Percentage Absolute		Absolute (SI)
Myelocytes	0 0/mcL		0/L
Neutrophils			
Band	3–5%	0.0–0.7 × 10³/mcL	0.0–0.7 × 10⁹/L
Segmented	40–80%	1.8–7.0 × 10³/mcL	1.8–7.0 × 10⁹/L
Lymphocytes	25–35%	1.0–4.8 × 10³/mcL	1.0–4.8 × 10⁹/L
Monocytes	2–10%	0.0–0.8 × 10³/mcL	0.0–0.8 × 10⁹/L
Granulocytes	42.2–75.2%	1.4–6.5 × 10³/mcL	1.4–6.5 × 10⁹/L
Eosinophils	0–5%	0.0–0.4 × 10³/mcL	0.0–0.4 × 10⁹/L
Basophils	0–0.2%	0.0–0.2 × 10³/mcL	0.0–0.2 × 10⁹/L
Platelets	150–450 × 10³/mcL		150–450 × 10⁹/L
Reticulocytes	0.5–2.5% RBCs		0.005–0.015 of RBCs
	18,000–158,000/mcL		18–158 × 10⁹/L
Cells, CSF	<5 lymphocytes/mm³		<5 lymphocytes/mm³
	0 RBC/mm³		0 RBC/mm³
Ceruloplasmin, serum	20–60 mg/dL		0.2–0.6 g/L
Chloride			
Serum or plasma (Hep)	98–107 mmol/L		98–107 mmol/L
Sweat			
Normal	5–35 mmol/L		5–35 mmol/L
Cystic fibrosis	60–200 mmol/L		60–200 mmol/L
Urine, 24 h (vary greatly with Cl intake)			
Infant	2–10 mmol/24 h		2–10 mmol/24h
Child	15–40 mmol/24 h		15–40 mmol/24h
Adult	110–250 mmol/24 h		110–250 mmol/24 h
CSF	118–132 mmol/L (20 mmol/L higher than serum)		118–132 mmol/L (20 mmol/L higher than serum)
Cholesterol, serum			
Adult desirable	<200 mg/dL		<5.2 mmol/L
borderline	200–239 mg/dL		5.2–6.2 mmol/L
high-risk	>240 mg/dL		≥6.2 mmol/L
*Chorionic gonadotropin, intact			
Serum or plasma (EDTA)			
Male and nonpregnant female	<5.0 mIU/mL		<5.0 IU/L
Pregnant female	Varies with gestational age		
Urine, qualitative			
Male and nonpregnant female	Negative		Negative
Pregnant female	Positive		Positive
Coagulation tests			
Activated partial thromboplastin time (APTT)	21–35 sec		
Activated protein C resistance	>2.1		
Antithrombin (AT)			
Activity	80–120%		
Antigen	22–40 mg/dL		

*Test values depend on laboratory methods.

Test	Conventional Units	SI Units
Bleeding time, template	3.0–10.0 min	
D-dimer	<250 ng/L	<1.37 nmol/L
Dilute Russell viper venom test (dRVVT)	<40 sec	
Euglobin lysis time	No lysis of plasma clot at 37°C in 60–120 min	
Factor II	80–120%	
Factor V	50–150%	
Factor VII	65–140%	
Factor VIII	55–145%	
Factor IX	60–140%	
Factor X	45–155%	
Factor XI	65–135%	
Factor XII	50–150%	
Fibrin degradation products (FDP)	Negative at 1:4 dilution or <10 mg/L	
Fibrinogen	200–400 mg/dL	2.0–4.0 G/L
International normalized ratio (INR)	2.0–3.0, varies by specific disorder	
Lupus anticoagulant	Negative	
Plasminogen activity		
Females	65–153%	
Males	76–124%	
Plasminogen activator inhibitor-1 (PAI-1)		
Activity	78–142%	
Antigen	4–43 mcg/mL	
Protein C		
Activity	70–140%	
Antigen	65–150%	
Protein S		
Activity	70–140%	
Antigen, free & total	70–160%	
Prothrombin time (PT)	11.0–13.0 sec	
Reptilase time	18–22 sec	
Thrombin time	7.0–12.0 sec	
von Willebrand factor		
Activity	42–139%	
Antigen	60–150%	
Complement components		
Total hemolytic complement activity, plasma (EDTA)	40–90 U/mL	0.4–0.9 kU/L
Total complement decay rate (functional), plasma (EDTA)	10–20%	Fraction decay rate: 0.10–0.20
	Deficiency: >50%	>0.50
C1q, serum	14.9–22.1 mg/dL	149–221 mg/L
C1r, serum	2.5–10.0 mg/dL	25–100 mg/L
C1s (C1 esterase), serum	5.0–10.0 mg/dL	50–100 mg/L
C2, serum	1.6–3.6 mg/dL	16–36 mg/L
C3, serum	90–180 mg/dL	0.9–1.8 g/L

(Continued)

Test	Conventional Units	SI Units
C4, serum	10–40 mg/dL	0.1–0.4 g/L
C5, serum	5.5–11.3 mg/dL	55–113 mg/L
C6, serum	17.9–23.9 mg/dL	179–239 mg/L
C7, serum	2.7–7.4 mg/dL	27–74 mg/L
C8, serum	4.9–10.6 mg/dL	49–106 mg/L
C9, serum	3.3–9.5 mg/dL	33–95 mg/L
Coombs test		
Direct	Negative	Negative
Indirect	Negative	Negative
Corpuscular values of erythrocytes		
Erythrocyte indices		
MCV	86–94 fL	
MCH	28–34 pg	
MCHC	32–36 g/dL	
Cortisol, serum		
Plasma (Hep, EDTA, Ox)		
8 AM	9–35 mcg/dL	250–650 nmol/L
4 PM	3–12 mcg/dL	80–330 nmol/L
10 PM	<50% of 8 AM value	<0.5 of 8 AM value
Free, urine	<50 mcg/24 h	<138 mmol/24 h
*C-Peptide, serum	0.78–1.89 ng/mL	0.26–0.62 nmol/L
C-Reactive protein, serum	<0.5 mg/dL	<5 mg/L
*†Creatine kinase, serum		
Male	15–105 U/L (30°C)	0.26–1.79 mckat/L (30°C)
Female	10–80 U/L (30°C)	0.17–1.36 mckat/L (30°C)
Note: Strenuous exercise or intramuscular injections may elevate transient levels of creatine kinase.		
*Creatine kinase MB isoenzyme, serum	0–7 ng/mL	0–7 mcg/L
*Creatinine		
Serum or plasma, adult		
Male	0.7–1.3 mg/dL	62–115 mcmol/L
Female	0.6–1.1 mg/dL	53–97 mcmol/L
Urine		
Male	14–26 mg/kg body weight/24 h	124–230 mcmol/kg body weight/24 h
Female	11–20 mg/kg body weight/24 h	97–177 mcmol/kg body weight/24 h
*Creatinine clearance, serum or plasma and urine		
Male	94–140 mL/min/1.73 m²	0.91–1.35 mL/s/m²
Female	72–110 mL/min/1.73 m²	0.69–1.06 mL/s/m²
Cryoglobulins, serum	Negative	Negative
*Estradiol, serum		
Adult		
Male	10–50 pg/mL	37–184 pmol/L
Female	Varies with menstrual cycle	

*Test values depend on laboratory methods.
†Actual therapeutic range should be adjusted for individual patient.

Test	Conventional Units	SI Units
Ethanol (alcohol), whole blood (Ox) or serum		
Depression of CNS	>100 mg/dL	>21.7 mmol/L
Fatalities reported	>400 mg/dL	>86.8 mmol/L
†Fat, fecal, F, 72 h		
Infant, breast-fed	<1 g/d	
Pediatrics (0–6 y)	<2 g/d	
Adult	<7 g/d	
Adult (fat-free diet)	<4 g/d	
Ferritin, serum		
Male	20–300 ng/mL	20–300 mcg/L
Female	20–120 ng/mL	20–120 mcg/L
Ferritin values of <20 ng/mL (20 mcg/L) have been reported to be generally associated with depleted iron stores.		
*Follicle-stimulating hormone serum and plasma (Hep)		
Male	5–20 mIU/mL	5–20 IU/L
Female	5–20 mIU/mL	5–20 IU/L
Follicular phase	1–10 mIU/mL	1–10 IU/L
Midcycle	5–20 mIU/mL	5–20 IU/L
Luteal phase	5–15 mIU/mL	5–15 IU/L
Postmenopausal	5–100 mIU/mL	5–100 IU/L
*Free thyroxine index (FTI), serum	4.2–13	4.2–13
Free thyroxine, serum	0.9–2.3 ng/dL	10–30 nmol/L
Free triiodothyronin, serum	0.2–0.6 ng/dL	0.003–0.009 nmol/L
Gastrin, serum	50–150 pg/mL	50–150 ng/L
Glucose (fasting)		
Blood	70–110 mg/dL	3.9–6.0 mmol/L
Plasma or serum	74–106 mg/dL	4.1–5.9 mmol/L
Glucose, 2 h postprandial, serum	<140 mg/dL	<7.8 mmol/L
Glucose, urine		
Quantitative	<500 mg/24 h	<2.8 mmol/24 h
Qualitative	Negative	Negative
Glucose, CSF	50–80 mg/dL	2.8–4.4 mmol/L
*Glucose-6-phosphate dehydrogenase in erythrocytes, whole blood (ACD, EDTA, or Hep)	12.1 ± 2.1 U/g Hb (SD)	0.78 ± 0.13 mU/mol Hb
	351 ± 60.6 U/10^{12} RBC	0.35 ± 0.06 nU/RBC
	4.11 ± 0.71 U/mL RBC	4.11 ± 0.71 kU/L RBC
Glycated hemoglobin (Hemoglobin A1c), whole blood (EDTA)	4.2% – 5.9%	0.042–0.059
Growth hormone, serum		
Male	<0–4 ng/mL	0–4 mcg/L
Female	<0.8–18 ng/mL	0–18 mcg/L
Haptoglobin, serum	40–180 mg/dL	0.4–1.8 g/L

*Test values depend on laboratory methods.
†Reference values vary from laboratory to laboratory, but are generally found within the range of 5–7 g/d. It should be noted that children, especially infants, cannot ingest the 100 g/d of fat that is suggested for the test. Therefore, a fat retention coefficient is determined by measuring the difference between ingested fat and fecal fat, and expressing that difference as a percentage. The figure, called the fat retention coefficient, is 95% or greater in healthy children and adults. A low value indicates steatorrhea.
http://www.labcorp.com/datasets/labcorp/html/chapter/mono/sc008000.htm

(Continued)

Test	Conventional Units	SI Units
HDL-lipid panel		
Cholesterol, HDL	>40 mg/dL	
Cholesterol, LDL (calculated)		
optimal	<100 mg/dL	
near optimal	100–129 mg/dL	
borderline high	130–159 mg/dL	
high	>160 mg/dL	
very high	>190 mg/dL	
Cholesterol, total		
0–1 year	50–120 mg/dL	
1–2 years	70–190 mg/dL	
2–16 years	120–220 mg/dL	
>16 years	0–199 mg/dL	
desirable	<200 mg/dL	
borderline	200–239 mg/dL	
high	>240 mg/dL	
*Tryglycerides		
desirable	<250 mg/dL	
borderline high	250–500 mg/dL	
high	>500 mg/dL	
Hematocrit		
Males	42–52%	0.42–0.52 L/L
Females	36–46%	0.36–0.46 L/L
Hemoglobin (Hb)		
Males	14.0–17.4 g/dL	140–170 g/L
Females	12.0–16.0 g/dL	120–160 g/L
Immunoglobulins, serum		
IgG	800–1200 mg/dL	8–12 g/L
IgA	80–312 mg/dL	0.7–3.12 g/L
IgM	50–280 mg/dL	0.5–2.8 g/L
IgD	0.5–2.8 mg/dL	0.005–0.2 mg/L
IgE	0.01–0.06 mg/dL	0.1–0.6 mg/L
Immunoglobulin G (IgC), CSF	0.5–6.1 mg/dL	0.5–6.1 g/L
†Iron, serum		
Males	65–175 mcg/dL	11.6–31.3 mcmol/L
Females	50–170 mcg/dL	9.0–30.4 mcmol/L
Iron binding capacity, serum, total	300–310 mcg/dL	54–64 mcmol/L
Iron saturation, serum		
Male	20–50%	0.2–0.5
Female	15–50%	0.15–0.5
Iron total binding capacity (serum)	300–360 ng/dL	54–64 nmol/K
17-Ketogenic steroids, urine		
Males	4–14 mg/24 h	13–49 mcmol/24 h
Females	2–12 mg/24 h	7–42 mcmol/24 h
	(decreases with age)	(decreases with age)

*If the triglyceride value is >400 mg/dL, the LDL calculation is invalid. http://webserver01.bjc.org/slch/pro/Professional.htm?
http://webserver01.bjc.org/labtestguide/Lab%20Test%20Guidebook/slchlabsiteoneline.htm
†Test values depend on laboratory methods.

Test	Conventional Units	SI Units
LDL-cholesterol, serum or plasma (EDTA)		
Adult desirable	<130 mg/dL	<3.36 mmol/L
borderline	130–159 mg/dL	3.37–4.11 mmol/L
high risk	≥160 mg/dL	≥4.13 mmol/L
Lead		
Whole blood (Hep)	<25 mcg/dL	<0.48 mcmol/L
Urine, 24 h	<80 mcg/d	<0.39 mcmol/d
Lecithin: sphingomyelin	2.0–5.0 indicates probable fetal lung	2.0–5.0 indicates probable fetal lung
ratio, amniotic fluid	maturity; >3.5 in diabetic patients	maturity; >3.5 in diabetic patients
*Lipase, serum	<160 U/L	<2.72 nkat/L (37°C)
*Luteinizing hormone, serum or		
plasma (Hep)		
Male	5–20 mIU/mL	5–20 IU/L
Female		
Follicular phase	5–15.0 mIU/mL	5–15.0 IU/L
Mid-cycle peak	30–60 mIU/mL	30–60 IU/L
Luteal phase	5–15 mIU/mL	5–15 IU/L
Postmenopausal	5–100 mIU/mL	5–100 IU/L
Magnesium		
Serum	1.3–2.1 mEq/L	0.65–1.07 mmol/L
Urine	6.0–10.0 mEq/24 h	3.0–5.0 mmol/24 h
Myoglobin, serum	30–70 ng/mL	30–70 mcg/mL
Occult blood, feces, random	Negative (<2 mL blood/150 g stool/d)	Negative (<13.3 mL blood/kg stool/d)
Qualitative, urine, random	Negative	Negative
Oxygen, blood		
Capacity	16–24 vol% (varies with hemoglobin)	7.14–10.7 mmol/L (varies with hemoglobin)
Content		
Arterial	15–23 vol%	0.15–0.25 mmol/L
Venous	10–16 vol%	4.46–7.14 mmol/L
Saturation		
Arterial and capillary	95–98% of capacity	0.95–0.98 of capacity
Venous	60–85% of capacity	0.60–0.85 of capacity
Tension		
pO$_2$ arterial and capillary	83–108 mmHg	11.1–14.4 kPa
Venous	35–45 mmHg	4.6–6.0 kPa
Partial thromboplastin time activated	<35 sec	<35 sec
*Phosphatase, alkaline, total, serum	30–90 U/L (30°C)	30–90 U/L (Bowers and McComb)
Phosphate, inorganic, serum		
Adults	2.7–4.5 mg/dL	0.87–1.45 mmol/L
Children	4.5–5.5 mg/dL	1.45–1.78 mmol/L
Phospholipids, serum	150–250 mg/dL	1.5–2.55 g/L
Phosphorus, urine	0.4–1.3 g/24 h	12.9–42 mmol/24 h
Potassium, plasma (Hep)		
Males	3.5–4.5 mEq/L	3.5–4.5 mmol/L
Females	3.4–4.4 mEq/L	3.4–4.4 mmol/L

*Test values depend on laboratory methods.

(Continued)

Test	Conventional Units	SI Units
Potassium		
Serum		
Premature		
Cord	5.0–10.2 mEq/L	5.0–10.2 mmol/L
48 h	3.0–6.0 mEq/L	3.0–6.0 mmol/L
Newborn, cord	5.6–12.0 mEq/L	5.6–12.0 mmol/L
Newborn	3.7–5.9 mEq/L	3.7–5.9 mmol/L
Infant	4.1–5.3 mEq/L	4.1–5.3 mmol/L
Child	3.4–4.7 mEq/L	3.4–4.7 mmol/L
Adult	3.5–5.1 mEq/L	3.5–5.1 mmol/L
Urine, 24 h	25–125 mEq/d, varies with diet	25–125 mmol/d; varies with diet
CSF	70% of plasma level or 2.5–3.2 mEq/L; rises with plasma hyperosmolality	0.70 of plasma level or 2.5–3.2 mmol/L; rises with plasma hyperosmolality
Prealbumin (transthyretin), serum	10–40 mg/dL	100–400 mg/L
*Progesterone, plasma		
Adult		
Male	13–97 ng/dL	0.4–3.1 nmol/L
Female		
Follicular phase	<150 ng/dL	<5 nmol/L
Luteal phase	300–1200 ng/dL	10–40 nmol/L
Pregnancy	Varies with gestational week	
1st Trimester	15000–5000 ng/dL	50–160 nmol/L
2nd and 3rd Trimesters	8000–20,000 ng/dL	250–650 nmol/L
*Prolactin, serum		
Males	Undetectable to 23 ng/mL	Undetectable to 23 mcg/L
Females	2.5–19.0 ng/mL	2.5–19.0 mcg/L
*Prostate-specific antigen, serum		
Male <60 years	<4.0 ng/mL	<4.0 mcg/L
Male >60 years	<7.5 ng/mL	<7.5 mcg/L
*Protein, serum		
Total		
Albumin	6.5–8.3 g/dL	65–83 g/L
Globulin	3.5–5.5 g/dL	35–55 g/L
α_1	0.2–0.4 g/dL	2–4 g/L
α_2	0.4–0.8 g/dL	4–8 g/L
β	0.5–1.0 g/dL	5–10 g/L
γ	0.6–1.3 g/dL	6–13 g/L
Urine		
Qualitative	Negative	Negative
Quantitative	50–80 mg/24 h (at rest)	Same
CSF, total	15–50 mg/dL	0.15–0.5 g/dL
Prothrombin time-international normalized ratio	INR: 2.0–3.0	
*Sedimentation rate, erythrocyte		
Westergren		
Male 0–50 y	0–15 mm/h	
Male >50 y	0–20 mm/h	
Female 0–50 y	0–20 mm/h	
Female >50 y	0–30 mm/h	

*Test values depend on laboratory methods.

Test	Conventional Units	SI Units
Sodium		
Serum or plasma (Hep)		
Premature		
Cord	116–140 mEq/L	116–140 mmol/L
48 h	128–148 mEq/L	128–148 mmol/L
Newborn, cord	126–166 mEq/L	126–166 mmol/L
Newborn	133–146 mEq/L	133–146 mmol/L
Infant	139–146 mEq/L	139–146 mmol/L
Child	138–145 mEq/L	138–145 mmol/L
Adult	136–145 mEq/L	136–145 mmol/L
Urine, 24 h	40–220 mEq/d	40–220 mmol/d
	(diet dependent)	(diet dependent)
CSF	138–150 mEq/L	138–150 mmol/L
Specific gravity, urine	1.002–1.030	1.002–1.030
†Testosterone, serum		
Male	300–1200 ng/dL	1.04–41.6 nmol/L
Female	20–80 ng/dL	0.7–2.8 nmol/L
Pregnancy	3–4 × normal	3–4 × normal
Postmenopausal	8–35 ng/dL	0.28–1.22 nmol/L
*Thyroid-stimulating hormone (TSH), serum	0.5–5.0 mcU/mL	0.5–5.0 mU/L
Transferrin, serum		
Newborn	130–275 mg/dL	1.30–2.75 g/L
Adult	200–400 mg/dL	2–4 g/L
>60 yr	190–375 mg/dL	1.9–3.75 g/L
Triglycerides, serum, fasting		
Desirable	<250 mg/dL	<2.83 mmol/L
Borderline high	250–500 mg/dL	2.83–5.67 mmol/L
Hypertriglyceridemia	>500 mg/dL	>5.65 mmol/L
*Triiodothyronine, total (T₃) serum	80–200 ng/mL	1.3–3.8 nmol/L
*Troponin-I, cardiac, serum	<0.4 ng.mL	undetectable
Troponin-T, cardiac, serum	<0.1 ng.mL	undetectable
Urea nitrogen, serum	8–20 mg/dL	2.9–7.1 mmol urea/L
Urea nitrogen:creatinine ratio, serum	12:1 to 20:1	48–80 urea:creatinine mole ratio
*Uric acid		
Serum, enzymatic		
Male	3.5–7.2 mg/dL	208–428 nmol/L
Female	2.6–6.0 mg/dL	155–357 nmol/L
Child	2.0–5.5 mg/dL	0.12–0.32 mmol/L
Urine	250–750 mg/24 h	1.48–4.43 mmol/24 h
	(with normal diet)	(with normal diet)
Urobilinogen, urine	0.1–0.8 Ehrlich unit/2 h	0.1– 3 0.8 Eu/2h
	0.5–4.0 Eu/d	0.5–4.0 Eu/d

*http://www.labcorp.com/datasets/labcorp/html/chapter/mono/he005000.htm;
http://www.utmb.edu/lsg/LabSurvivalGuide/hem/Sedimentation_Rate.htm
†Test values depend on laboratory methods.
ACD, acid-citrate-dextrose; **CHF**, congestive heart failure; **Cit**, citrate; **Cl**, chloride; **CNS**, central nervous system; **CSF**, cerebrospinal fluid; **cyclic AMP**, adenosine 3′, 5′-cyclic phosphate; **EDTA**, ethylenediaminetetraacetic acid; **HDL**, high-density lipoprotein; **Hep**, heparin; **LDL-C**, low-density lipoprotein-cholesterol; **Ox**, oxalate; **RBC**, red blood cell(s); **RIA**, radioimmunoassay; **SD**, standard deviation; **WBC**, white blood cell(s).
Modified from *Stedman's Medical Dictionary for the Health Professions and Nursing, Sixth Edition.* Baltimore: Lippincott Williams & Wilkins, 2008.

Appendix 3

COMMON MEDICAL ABBREVIATIONS

A/C	assist control
ABG	arterial blood gas
ABVD	Adriamycin, bleomycin, vinblastine, and dacarbazine (drug combination)
ACE	angiotensin-converting enzyme
aCL	anticardiolipin
AComA	anterior communicating artery
ACTH	adrenocorticotropic hormone
AD	auris dextra, or right ear
ADH	antidiuretic hormone
ADLs	activities of daily living
ADPKD	autosomal dominant polycystic kidney disease
AFB	acid-fast bacilli
AFP	alpha-fetoprotein
AHDI	Association for Healthcare Documentation Integrity (formerly American Association for Medical Transcription, AAMT)
AHI	apnea-hypopnea index
AHIMA	American Health Information Management Association
AIDS	acquired immunodeficiency syndrome
AK	astigmatic keratotomy
AKA	above-knee amputation
ALL	acute lymphocytic anemia
ALT	alanine aminotransferase
AMD	age-related macular degeneration
AML	acute myelogenous leukemia
ANA	antinuclear antibody
APL	antiphospholipid antibody
APS	antiphospholipid syndrome
ARB	angiotensin II receptor blocker

ARDS	acute respiratory distress syndrome
ARRA	American Recovery and Reinvestment Act of 2009
AS	auris sinistra, or left ear
ASD	atrial septal defect
AST	aspartate aminotransferase
AU	auris utraque, or both ears
AV	arteriovenous
AVN	avascular necrosis
BAER	brainstem auditory evoked response
BAL	bronchoalveolar lavage
BBB	bundle branch block
BG	blood glucose
BiPAP	bi-level positive airway pressure
BI-RADS	Breast Imaging Reporting and Data System
BKA	below-knee amputation
BMD	Becker muscular dystrophy
BMI	body mass index
BMP	basic metabolic panel
BMT	bone marrow transplant
BNP	B-type natriuretic peptide
BPH	benign prostatic hypertrophy
BPPV	benign paroxysmal positional vertigo
BRM	biological response modifier
BSA	body surface area
BSO	bilateral salpingo-oophorectomy
BUN	blood urea nitrogen
BUS	Bartholin, urethra, and Skene (glands)
C&S	culture and sensitivity
C.	*Candida*
CABG	coronary bypass artery graft
CAD	coronary artery disease; computer-aided detection
CBC	complete blood count
CBG	capillary blood glucose
CDIA	Clinical Documentation Industry Association (formerly Medical Transcription Industry Association, MTIA)
CEA	carcinoembryonic antigen
CF	cystic fibrosis
CHF	congestive heart failure
CIN	cervical intraepithelial neoplasia
CK	conductive keratoplasty; creatine kinase
CLL	chronic lymphocytic leukemia
CMG	cystometrogram
CML	chronic myelogenous leukemia
CMP	complete metabolic panel
CMS	Centers for Medicare and Medicaid Services
CMT	Certified Medical Transcriptionist
CMV	cytomegalovirus
CNS	central nervous system
CO2	carbon dioxide
COPD	chronic obstructive pulmonary disease
COPP	cyclophosphamide, Oncovin, prednisone, and procarbazine
COX-2	cyclooxygenase-2 (inhibitors)
CPAP	continuous positive airway pressure
CPK	creatine phosphokinase
CPR	cardiopulmonary resuscitation
CPU	central processing unit
CRP	C-reactive protein, cAMP receptor protein

CRT	cathode-ray tube
CSF	cerebrospinal fluid
CT	computed tomography (scan); calcitonin
CTK	laser thermokeratoplasty
CV	curriculum vitae
CVA	cerebrovascular accident
dB	decibels
DBS	deep brain stimulation
DCIS	ductal carcinoma in situ
DDAVP	desmopressin acetate
DEA	Drug Enforcement Administration
DEXA	dual-energy x-ray absorptiometry
DHHS	Department of Health and Human Services
DHT	dihydroxy testosterone
DJD	degenerative joint disease
DKA	diabetic ketoacidosis
DLCO	diffusing capacity for carbon monoxide
DM	diabetes mellitus
DMARD	disease-modifying antirheumatic drug
DMD	Duchenne muscular dystrophy
DNA	deoxyribonucleic acid
DNR (or DNR/DNI)	do not resuscitate; do not intubate
DOE	dyspnea on exertion
DRE	digital rectal examination
DSL	digital subscriber line
DTRs	deep tendon reflexes
DVT	deep vein (venous) thrombosis
EBL	estimated blood loss
EBV	Epstein-Barr virus
ECC	endocervical curettage
ECOG	Eastern Cooperative Oncology Group
EEG	electroencephalogram; electroencephalography
EG/BUS	external genitalia/Bartholin, urethral, and Skene (glands)
EGD	esophagogastroduodenoscopy
EGFRs	epidermal growth factor receptors
EHR	electronic health record
EKG (also called ECG)	electrocardiogram
ELISA	enzyme-linked immunosorbent assay
EMG	electromyography
EMR	electronic medical record
ENT	ear, nose, and throat
EOMI	extraocular muscles (or movements) intact
ERCP	endoscopic retrograde cholangiopancreatography
ESR	erythrocyte sedimentation rate
ESRD	end-stage renal disease
ESS	endoscopic sinus surgery
ESWL	extracorporeal shock wave lithotripsy
ETOH	alcohol, ethyl alcohol
EUS	endoscopic ultrasound
FAAMT	Fellow of the American Association for Medical Transcription
FDA	Food and Drug Administration
FEF	forced expiratory flow
FEV1	forced expiratory volume measured in one second
FIGO	Federal Internationale de Gynecologie et Obstetrique
FiO2	fraction of inspired oxygen
FNA	fine needle aspiration
FSE	fetal scalp electrode

FSH	follicle-stimulating hormone
FTP	file transfer protocol
FUS	focused ultrasound surgery
FVC	forced vital capacity
GCA	giant cell arteritis
GCS	Glasgow Coma Scale
GERD	gastroesophageal reflux disease
GES	gastric emptying study
GFR	glomerular filtration rate
GH	growth hormone
GHRH	growth hormone-releasing hormone
GI	gastrointestinal
GnRH	gonadotropin releasing hormone
GPA	gravida, para, abortus
GTT	glucose tolerance test
GU	genitourinary
GYN	gynecology
H&P	history and physical
HAART	highly active antiretroviral therapy
HAV	hepatitis A virus
HBOT	hyperbaric oxygen therapy
HBV	hepatitis B virus
hCG	human chorionic gonadotropin
HCO3	abbreviation for bicarbonate ion
Hct	hematocrit
HCV	hepatitis C virus
HDL	high-density lipoprotein, or *good cholesterol*
HEENT	head, eyes, ears, nose, and throat
Hgb	hemoglobin
HIDA	hepatobiliary iminodiacetic acid
HIPAA	Health Insurance Portability and Accountability Act of 1996
HITECH	Health Information Technology for Economic and Clinical Health Act
HIV	human immunodeficiency virus
HLA	human leukocyte antigen
HPI	history of present illness
HPV	human papillomavirus
HSG	hysterosalpingogram
HSV	herpes simplex virus
HSV-1	herpes simplex virus-1
HTN	hypertension
Hx	history
Hz	Hertz
IBD	irritable bowel disease
IBS	irritable bowel syndrome
IC	interstitial cystitis
ICL	implantable Collamer lens
ICSH	interstitial cell-stimulating hormone
ICSI	intracytoplasmic sperm injection
IDC	invasive (infiltrating) ductal carcinoma
IDDM	insulin-dependent diabetes mellitus
IgA	immunoglobulin A
IgD	immunoglobulin D
IgE	immunoglobulin E
IgG	immunoglobulin G
IgM	immunoglobulin M
ILC	invasive (infiltrating) lobular carcinoma
IMV	intermittent mandatory ventilation

INH	isoniazid
INR	international normalized ratio
IOL	intraocular lens
IPAA	ileal pouch anal anastomosis
IR	immediate-release
IRS	Internal Revenue Service
IT	Information Technology
IUPC	intrauterine pregnancy
IUPC	intrauterine pressure catheter
IVF	in vitro fertilization
IVIG	intravenous immunoglobulin
IVP	intravenous pyelogram
JCAHO	The Joint Commission on Accreditation of Healthcare Organizations, now known as The Joint Commission
KOH	chemical abbreviation for potassium hydroxide
KPS	Karnofsky performance status
KS	Kaposi sarcoma
KUB	kidney, ureter, and bladder (x-ray)
LA	lupus anticoagulant
LA	long-acting
LAD	left anterior descending artery
LAN	local area network
LASIK	laser in situ keratomileusis
LAUP	laser-assisted uvulopalatoplasty
LCA	left circumflex artery; left coronary artery
LCD	liquid crystal display
LCIS	lobular carcinoma in situ
LDL	low-density lipoprotein, or *bad cholesterol*
LEEP	loop electrosurgical excision procedure
LFTs	liver function tests
LH	luteinizing hormone
LHRH	leuteinizing hormone releasing hormone
LP	lumbar puncture
LP(a)	lipoprotein (a)
LLQ	left lower quadrant
LRD	laryngopharyngeal reflux disease
LSO	left salpingo-oophorectomy
LUQ	left upper quadrant
MCH	mean corpuscular hemoglobin
MCHC	mean corpuscular hemoglobin concentration
MCV	mean corpuscular volume
MD	muscular dystrophy
MELD	Model for End-Stage Liver Disease
MEN	multiple endocrine neoplasia
METS	metabolic equivalents
MI	myocardial infarction
mmHg	the measurement of blood pressure values
MOPP	mechlorethamine, Oncovin, prednisone, and procarbazine
MRA	magnetic resonance angiography
MRCP	magnetic resonance cholangiopancreatography
MRI	magnetic resonance imaging
MRI/MRA	magnetic resonance imaging/magnetic resonance angiography
MS	multiple sclerosis
MTSO	medical transcription service organization
MUGA	multiple gated acquisition scan
Na	sodium
NAD	no apparent distress

NASH	nonalcoholic steatohepatitis
NCI	National Cancer Institute
NIDDM	non-insulin-dependent diabetes mellitus
NIH	National Institutes of Heath
NPH	intermediate-acting (insulin)
NPO	nothing by mouth
NS	normal saline
NSAID	nonsteroidal antiinflammatory drug
NSVD	normal spontaneous vaginal delivery
O2	oxygen
OAE	otoacoustic emissions
OB	obstetrics
OB/GYN	obstetrics/gynecology
OD	oculus dexter, or right eye
ORIF	open reduction and internal fixation
OS	oculus sinister, or left eye
OSA	obstructive sleep apnea
OT	oxytocin
OTC	over-the-counter
OU	oculus uterque, or both eyes
PA	posteroanterior
PAC	premature atrial contraction
PCN	percutaneous nephrolithotomy
PCO2	partial pressure of carbon dioxide
PComA	posterior communicating artery
PCP	*Pneumocystis carinii* pneumonia
PD	Parkinson disease
PDA	posterior descending artery; patent ductus arteriosus
PDT	photodynamic therapy
PE	pulmonary embolism
PEEP	positive end-expiratory pressure
PEF	peak expiratory flow
PERRLA	pupils equal, round, and reactive to light
PET	positron emission tomography (scan)
PFTs	pulmonary function tests
pH	potential of Hydrogen
PID	pelvic inflammatory disease
PKD	polycystic kidney disease
PLT	platelets
PND	paroxysmal nocturnal dyspnea
PNH	postherpetic neuralgia
PNS	peripheral nervous system
PO2	partial pressure of oxygen
PRK	photorefractive keratectomy
PRL	prolactin
PROM	premature rupture of membranes
PSA	prostate-specific antigen
PTCA	percutaneous transluminal coronary angioplasty
PTH	parathyroid hormone
PUD	peptic ulcer disease
PUVA	psoralen and subsequent exposure to long-wavelength ultraviolet light
PVA	polyvinyl alcohol
PVD	peripheral vascular disease
PVP	photoselective vaporization prostatectomy
RA	rheumatoid arthritis
RAIU	radioactive iodine uptake (test)
RBC	red blood cell; red blood count

RCA	right coronary artery
RDI	respiratory disturbance index
RDW	red (cell) distribution width
REM	rapid eye movement (sleep)
RF	rheumatoid factor
RICE	rest, ice, compression, elevation
RK	radial keratotomy
RLQ	right lower quadrant
RLS	restless leg syndrome
RMT	Registered Medical Transcriptionist
ROM	rupture of membranes
RSO	right salpingo-oophorectomy
RSV	respiratory syncytial virus
RUQ	right upper quadrant
Rx	drug, prescription, therapy
SA	sinoatrial (node)
SAH	subarachnoid hemorrhage
SBA	Small Business Administration
SBE	subacute bacterial endocarditis
SCID	severe combined immunodeficiency disease
SERM	selective estrogen receptor modulator
SG	specific gravity
SHG	sonohysterogram
SIL	squamous intraepithelial lesion
SLE	systemic lupus erythematosus
SLEDAI	SLE disease activity index
SOAP	subjective, objective, assessment, and plan
SPECT	single photon emission computed tomography (scan)
SR	sustained-release
SRT	speech-recognition technology
STD	sexually transmitted disease
T3	triiodothyronine
T4	thyroxine
TAH	total abdominal hysterectomy
TAT	turnaround time
TB	tuberculosis
TCOM	transcutaneous oxygen monitoring
THA	total hip arthroplasty
TIBC	total iron binding capacity
TIMI	thrombolysis in myocardial infarction
TIMs	topical immunomodulators
TIPAL	term infants, premature infants, abortions, living children
TKA	total knee arthroplasty
TLC	total lung capacity
TN	trigeminal neuralgia
TNF	tumor necrosis factor
TNM	tumor, nodes, metastasis
TSH	thyroid-stimulating hormone
TURB	transurethral resection of bladder tumor
TURP	transurethral resection of the prostate
UA	urinalysis
UPPP	uvulopalatopharyngoplasty
USAN	U.S. Adopted Names Council
USB	universal serial bus
UTI	urinary tract infection
UV	ultraviolet
V/Q	ventilation perfusion (scan)

VAC	vacuum-assisted closure
VBAC	vaginal birth after C-section
VBC	visible black character
VCUG	voiding cystourethrogram
VDRL	Venereal Disease Research Laboratory (test)
VPN	virtual private network
VSD	ventricular septal defect
WBC	white blood cell, white blood count
WD	well developed
WHO	World Health Organization
WNL	withing normal limits
WT	work type
WWW	World Wide Web
x	times
YAG	yttrium-alumnium-garnet (laser)

Appendix 4

SUGGESTED WEB SITES

Transcription-Related Sites

Site	Name	Description
http://www.ahdionline.org	Association for Healthcare Documentation Integrity (AHDI)	The organization that sets the standards for education and practice in the field of medical transcription/editing.
http://www.mtjobs.com	MT Jobs	A large source of medical transcription jobs and resumes.
http://www.medicaljobs.com	Medical Jobs	A job board devoted to finding employment in the medical field.
http://mtdaily.com	MT Daily	An Internet MT information and networking community.
http://mtdesk.com	MT Desk	An MT electronic information resource site.

General Medicine-Related Sites

Site	Name	Description
http://www.or-live.com	OR-Live	This site shows videos of actual surgeries, including a demonstration of the equipment used and answers to e-mail questions during the live procedure. The site also contains archives of round table discussions of medical issues and the latest medical news.
http://www.med.umich.edu/ lrc/Hypermuscle/Hyper.html#flex	University of Michigan Health System	*Muscles in Action*. This site uses short videos to demonstrate the muscle actions of the human body.
http://www.sciencedaily.com	Science Daily	The latest medical and research news.
http://www.medscape.com	Medscape	A wealth of medical and drug information, including specialty sites.
http://www.medicalnewstoday.com	Medical News Today	A medical news site from well-regarded sources, updated daily.

Appendix 5

SUGGESTED LIST OF REFERENCES

The Book of Style for Medical Transcription, Third Edition. Modesto, CA: American Association for Medical Transcription, 2008.

Anatomica: The Complete Home Medical Reference. New York: Barnes & Noble Books, 2001.

Bryan, L. *Microsoft Word for Healthcare Documentation, Fourth Edition.* Baltimore: Lippincott Williams & Wilkins, 2011.

Diagnostic Tests Made Incredibly Easy, Second Edition. Springhouse, PA: Springhouse, 2008.

Lilly, LS (Ed.). *Pathophysiology of Heart Disease: A Collaborative Project of Medical Students and Faculty, Fifth Edition.* Baltimore: Lippincott, Williams & Wilkins, 2010.

The Merck Manual of Medical Information: Second Home Edition. New York: Pocket Books, 2003.

Stedman's Medical Abbreviations, Acronyms & Symbols, Fourth Edition. Baltimore, Lippincott Williams & Wilkins, 2008.

Stedman's Medical Dictionary for the Health Professions and Nursing, Sixth Edition. Baltimore: Lippincott Williams & Wilkins, 2007.

Stedman's Word Book Series

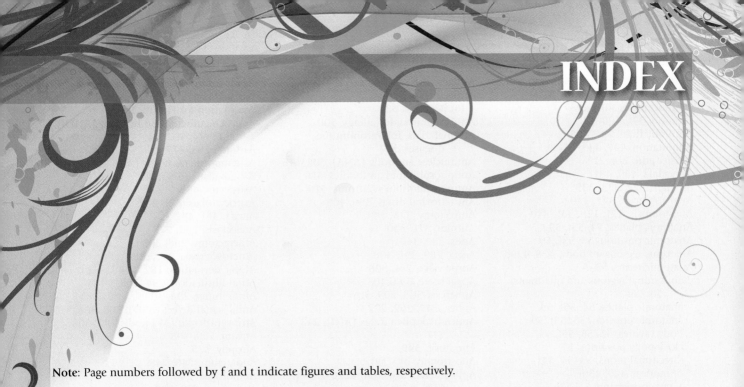

INDEX

Note: Page numbers followed by f and t indicate figures and tables, respectively.

A

A/C mode, 263
Abbreviations
 book of, 31–32
 in cardiology, 307
 in career management, 614
 in dermatology, 194
 in endocrinology, 573
 in gastroenterology, 339
 in imaging, 167
 in immunology, 515
 medical, 51–53
 in neurology, 481
 in obstetrics and gynecology, 407
 in oncology, 548
 in ophthalmology, 219
 in orthopaedics, 444
 in otorhinolaryngology, 247
 in pharmacology, 142
 in pulmonology, 276
 in technology, tools, and techniques, 37–39
 in urology, 374
Abdominal aorta, 354, 375
Abdominal hysterectomy, 398, 408
Abdominal regions and quadrants, 56, 56f
Abdominal ultrasound, 335
Abduct, 234, 247
Ablation, 398, 408
Abortus, 391, 408
Absence seizures, 468, 481
Absorbable sutures, 126, 129
Accelerations (heart rate), 393, 408
Access, 357, 375
Accessory muscles, 262, 277
Accessory organs, 322, 339
Accommodation, 204, 219
Acetabulum, 425, 445
Acetic acid, 408
Acetowhite lesions, 402, 408
Acid-fast bacilli, 267, 277
Acoustic studies, 239–240

Acquired hydrocephalus, 466, 481
Acquired immunodeficiency syndrome (AIDS), 264, 277, 308, 395–396, 501, 516
Acromegaly, 563, 573
Acronyms, 110
 editing and, 106
 physician, 106t
Active immunity, 516
Actual automated speech errors, 30t
Acute hepatitis, 328, 339
Acute lymphocytic leukemia (ALL), 532
Acute myelogenous leukemia (AML), 531, 549
Acute pancreatitis, 328, 339
Acute renal failure, 356–357, 375
Acute respiratory distress syndrome (ARDS), 267–268, 277
Acyclovir (Zovirax), 185–186
Ad-response letter, 598–599
Adaptive immune system, 516
Addison disease, 565, 573
Adduct, 234, 247
Adenocarcinomas, 332, 339, 531, 549
 of prostate, 366
Adenoids, 233, 247, 516
Adenoma, 332, 339
Adhesions, 397, 408
Adjuvant chemotherapy, 269, 277
Adnexa, 390, 408
Adrenal cortex, 561, 573
Adrenal disorders, 564–566
Adrenal glands, 353, 375, 561–562, 574
Adrenocorticotropic hormone (ACTH), 560, 574
Adventitious sounds, 262, 277
Adware, 38
Afferent nerves, 462
Age-related macular degeneration (AMD), 208, 219
Aging eyes. *See* Presbyopia
AHDI. *See* Association for Healthcare Documentation Integrity (AHDI)

AHDI-F. *See* Fellow of the Association for Healthcare Documentation Integrity (AHDI-F)
AHI. *See* Apnea-hypopnea index (AHI)
AHIMA. *See* American Health Information Management Association (AHIMA)
AIDS. *See* Acquired immunodeficiency syndrome (AIDS)
Air and bone conduction tests, 240–241, 247
Air conduction, 247
 in hearing, 234
Ala, nasal, 232, 247
Alanine aminotransferase (ALT), 157, 168
Alcoholic hepatitis, 328, 339
Aldolase, 445
 tests for, 438
Aldosterone, 561, 574
Alimentary canal, 319
Allergen, 500, 516
Allergic salute, 500, 516
Allergic shiner, 500, 516
Allergy, 500–501, 516
 defined, 500
 in medical reports, 69
 medications for, 500–501
 skin test, 510
Allogeneic bone marrow transplant, 508, 516
Allograft, 187, 194
Alpha-fetoprotein (AFP), 537, 549
Alpha-glucosidase inhibitors, 574
 for diabetes, 567
Alveoli, 260, 277
Amblyopia, 206, 219
AMD. *See* Age-related macular degeneration (AMD)
Amenorrhea, 390, 408
American Health Information Management Association (AHIMA), 612

American Recovery and Reinvestment Act of 2009 (ARRA), 10
Amniocentesis, 401, 408
Amnion, 391, 408
Amniotic fluid, 391, 408
Amputation, 437, 445
Amsler grid, 214, 219
Amygdala, 460, 481
Amylase, 322, 333, 339
Anal sphincter, 322, 340
Anastomosis, 121, 129, 331, 340
Anatomic planes, 54, 55f, 59
Anatomic position, 53, 53f, 59
Anatomic regions, of body, 428, 429t
Anatomic terms, 53–57
   abdominal regions and quadrants, 56, 56f
   anatomic planes, 54, 55f, 59
   anatomic position, 53, 53f, 59
   body cavities, 55–56, 55f, 59
   clock body positions, 57
   directional terms, 53–54, 54f
   of motion, 429, 430t
   X-ray positioning, 54–55
Androgen agonists, 375
Androgens, 574
Anemia, 510, 516, 549
Anesthesia, 123, 129
   administration, in surgery, 123, 124t
Anesthesiologist, 123
Aneurysms, 466–467, 481, 505, 516
   intracranial, 467f
   neck, 467
Angina, 296, 308
Angina pectoris, 296
Angiogram, 162, 168
Angiography, 475, 482
Angioplasty, 297, 308, 516
Angiotensin II receptor blockers (ARB), 296–297, 308
Angiotensin-converting enzyme (ACE) inhibitors, 296, 308
Ankle jerk, 474, 482
Antacids, 325
Anterior chamber, of eye, 205, 219
Anterior communicating artery (AComA), 467, 482
Anterior fontanel, 423, 445
Anterior horn, 433, 445
Anterior pituitary gland, 574
Anteroposterior, 53, 55, 161
Anti-double-stranded DNA, 516
Anti-La, 516
Anti-Ro, 516
Anti-Sm, 516
Antiandrogens, 366, 375
Antibiotics, 326, 340
   for pelvic inflammatory disease, 395
   for urinary tract infection, 356
Antibodies, 375, 499, 516
Antibody test, 340
   for hepatitis, 329
Anticardiolipin (aCL), 516
Anticoagulants, 299, 308
   for autoimmune diseases, 507
Antidiuretic hormone (ADH), 356, 375, 560, 574

Antigen, 516
Antigen tests, 340
   for hepatitis, 329
Antihistamines, for allergy, 500
Antimalarials, for autoimmune diseases, 507
Antinuclear antibody (ANA), 502, 516
Antiphospholipid antibodies, 516
Antiphospholipid syndrome, 516
Antiretroviral drugs, 396, 408
Antrectomy, 326, 340
Antrum, 321, 340
Anus, 322, 340
Aorta, 289, 291, 308
Aortic valve, 291, 308
Apgar score, 394, 408
Apheresis, 508–509, 516
Apnea, 247, 262, 277
Apnea-hypopnea index (AHI), 243, 247
Apoptosis, 549
Apostrophe, 100, 110
Appendicular skeleton, 422t, 424–425, 445
Appendix, 516
Applanation tonometry, 215, 220
Application letter, 596–599. *See also* Resumé
   ad-response letter, 598–599
   general distribution letter, 598
   sample, 597f
   tips while sending, 599
Applications
   computer, 20, 24–26, 37
   software, 22, 37
Appositive, 98, 110
Aqueous humor, 205, 220
Arabic numbers, 104, 110
Arachnoid membrane, 461, 482
ARDS. *See* Acute respiratory distress syndrome (ARDS)
Arms, randomized trials, 137, 143
Aromatase inhibitors, 549
ARRA. *See* American Recovery and Reinvestment Act of 2009 (ARRA)
Arrector pili muscles, 179, 194
Arrhythmia, 294, 308
Arterial blood gas test, 271, 277
Arteries, 289, 308
Arterioles, 289, 308
Arteriovenous fistula, 375
Arteriovenous graft, 375
Arthralgia, 516
Arthrocentesis, 445, 512, 517
Arthrodesis, 435, 445
Arthrology, 425, 445
Arthroplasty, 432, 503–504, 517
Arthroscope, 434, 445
Arthroscopy, 445
   for meniscal tears, 433–434
Artificial skin grafts, 187, 194
Arytenoids, 234, 247
Ascending colon, 321, 340
Ascites, 329, 340
Aspartate aminotransferase (AST), 157, 168
Assessment and plan, in medical reports, 70

Assist control mode, 277
Assisted zonal hatching, 393, 408
Association for Healthcare Documentation Integrity (AHDI), 13–14, 16, 614
Asthma, 265, 277
Astigmatic keratotomy (AK), 207, 220
Astigmatism, 206, 220
Astrocytes, 482
Astrocytomas, 471, 482
Ataxia, 461, 482
Atelectasis, 263, 277
Atherectomy, 298, 308
Atherosclerosis, 297, 308
Atopic dermatitis, 182, 194
Atrial fibrillation, 294, 308
Atrial flutter, 294, 308
Atrial septal defect (ASD), 300, 308
Atrioventricular (AV) node, 292, 308
Atrium, 290, 308
Atrophy, 375
Audiogram, 240, 248
Audiologist, 248
Audiology, 229, 248
Audiometer, 240, 248
Audiometry, 240, 248
Auditory system, 230, 248
Aura, 482
Auscultation, 293, 308
Autoantibodies, 502, 517
Autograft, 187, 194
Autoimmune thyroid diseases, 504
Autoimmunity diseases, 502–504, 517
   medications used to treat, 507
   rheumatoid arthritis, 503–504, 503f
   systemic lupus erythematosus, 502–503
   thyroid diseases, 504–505
Autologous blood donation, 121, 129
Autologous bone marrow transplant, 508, 517
Automated perimetry, 214–215
Autonomic nervous system, 463
Autonomic neuropathy, 566, 574
Autosomal dominant polycystic kidney disease (ADPKD), 360, 375
AutoText, 33–34
Avascular, 445
Avascular necrosis (AVN), 432, 445
Axial skeleton, 422–424, 422t, 423f, 445
Azithromycin, for chlamydia, 368
Azotemia, 357

B

B cells, 498, 499, 517
B-type natriuretic peptide (BNP), 308
Babinski test, 474, 482
Back-end SRT, 29, 37
Bacteremia, 482
Bacterial endocarditis, 184, 194, 299, 308
Bacterial infections, 183–184
Bacterial meningitis, 465, 482
Bacterial pneumonia, 263, 277
Bacteruria, 375
BAER. *See* Brainstem auditory evoked response (BAER)

BAL. *See* Bronchoalveolar lavage (BAL)
Band neutrophils, 155, 168
Bandage, 126–127, 129
Barany caloric test, 242, 248
Barium sulfate, 340
Barium swallow, 334
Barrel chest, 267, 277
Barrett esophagus, 324, 340
Bartholin glands, 387, 387f, 388, 408
Basal cell carcinoma, 188, 194
Basal cells, 178, 194
Basal ganglia, 460, 482
Basic metabolic panel (BMP), 155,
    168
Basophils, 155, 168
Becker muscular dystrophy (BMD),
    435
Bell palsy, 470, 482
Benign paroxysmal positional vertigo
    (BPPV), 236, 248
Benign prostatic hyperplasia (BPH), 375
    prostate disorders, 365–366
Benign tumors, 532
Beta hCG, 408t
Beta-blockers, 296, 308
BI-RADS coding system, 403, 403t, 408
Bicarbonate, 271, 277
Biguanides, 574
    for diabetes, 567
Bilateral salpingo-oophorectomies
    (BSO), 398, 408
Bile, 322, 340
Bile salts, 322, 340
Bilevel positive airway pressure (BiPAP)
    machine, 239, 248
Biliary tract, 322, 322f, 340
Bilirubin, 153, 168, 322, 340
Billing, 611–612
Billroth procedure, 326, 340
Biopsy, 149, 168, 517, 549
    in immunology, 511–512
    in neurology, 457–488
    in oncology, 538–539
    in orthopaedics, 438
BiPAP machine. *See* Bilevel positive
    airway pressure (BiPAP) machine
Birth canal, 408
Bisphosphonates, 445
    for osteoporosis, 433
Bladder cancer, 363–364
Bladder disorders, 362–364
    bladder cancer, 363–364
    cystocele, 362–363
    interstitial cystitis, 362
    neurogenic bladder, 363
Bladder distention, 362, 375
Bladder instillation, 362, 375
Bladder neck, 354, 375
Bladder reconstruction, 363, 375
Bleb, 466, 482
Blood, 153
Blood clotting studies, 157–158
Blood culture, 158, 168
Blood glucose (BG), 156, 574
Blood pressure, 295, 308
Blood tests, 333
    in immunology, 510–511
    in oncology, 536

in orthopaedics, 437–438
    in urology, 368
Blood urea nitrogen (BUN), 156, 168,
    368, 375
Blood vessels, 289, 308
Blood-brain barrier, 475, 482
Body cavities, 55–56, 55f, 59
Body directions, 53–54, 54f
Boil, 184, 194
Bone conduction, 248
    in hearing, 234
Bone densitometry, 439, 445
Bone flap, 471, 482
Bone grafting, 445
    in avascular necrosis, 432
Bone health, 157
Bone marrow, 448, 498, 517
Bone marrow aspiration, 438, 445
Bone marrow transplant (BMT), 508,
    517
Bone scan, 439
Bone tumors, 435–437
    benign tumors, 436
    growth of cells in bones causes,
        435
    malignant tumors, 436
    types of, 436
Bones, 445
    of appendicular skeleton, 422t,
        424–425
    of axial skeleton, 422–424, 422t
    defined, 421
    organization and function of, 421
    parts of long, 422f
    remodeling of, 421
    types of, 421–422
Bone marrow, 421
Book of abbreviations, 31–32
Bowman capsule, 353–354, 375
BPPV. *See* Benign paroxysmal positional
    vertigo (BPPV)
Brachytherapy, 269, 277, 366, 375
Bradycardia, 294, 308
Bradykinesia, 468, 482
Brain, 458–461, 482. *See also* Nervous
    system
    brainstem, 461
    cerebellum, 461
    cerebrum, 459–460
    foramen magnum and, 458
    glia in, 459
    limbic system, 460–461
    lobes of, 459f, 460
    meninges and ventricles, 461
    pathways and, 459
    structures of, 459f
Brain tumor, 470–472, 482
    gliomas, 471
    metastatic, 471
    primary, 471, 486
    secondary, 471
    types of, 471
Brain-gut axis, 330, 340
Brainstem, 261, 277, 461, 482
Brainstem auditory evoked response
    (BAER), 241, 248
Brand names, of drugs, 135, 144
BRCA1, 538, 549

BRCA2, 538, 549
Breast cancer, 399, 408
Breech presentation, 394, 408
Bronchi, 259, 277
Bronchial tree, 259–260, 260f
Bronchiectasis, 263, 277
Bronchioles, 259, 277
Bronchiolitis, 263, 277
Bronchitis, 265–266, 277
Bronchoalveolar lavage (BAL), 272,
    277
Bronchodilators, 265, 277
    for allergy, 500
Bronchogenic carcinoma, 268, 277
Bronchopneumonia, 263, 277
Bronchoscope, 272, 277
Bronchoscopy, 272, 277
Bruce protocol, 308
Bruit, 308
Bulb, 179, 194
Bulbourethral glands, 355, 375
Bullae, 184, 194
BUN. *See* Blood urea nitrogen (BUN)
BUN-to-creatinine ratio, 157, 168
Bundle branches, 293, 309
Bundle of His, 293, 309
Burns, 186–187, 194
Bursae, 428, 445
Bursitis, 445
Business associates, 10, 16
Business management, 608–612
    billing in, 611–612
    corporation, 610
    developing client base, 610–611
    entrepreneurship in, 608, 608t
    equipments in, 608–609
    financing in, 609
    insurance in, 609
    partnership, 610
    personality and work preferences in,
        608
    sole proprietorship, 609–610
    taxes in, 610
    type of business, 609–610

C

C corporation, 610, 614
C-reactive protein, 310
C-section. *See* Cesarean section
    (C-section)
CA125, 536–537, 549
CA19-9, 537, 549
CA27.29, 537, 549
CABG. *See* Coronary artery bypass graft
    (CABG)
Cadaver skin, 187
Cadaveric transplant, 358, 375
Calcaneus, 425, 445
Calcitonin (CT), 561, 574
Calcitriol, 353, 376
Calcium channel blockers, 296, 309
Calcium stones, 360
Calyces, 353
Calyx, 376
cAMP receptor protein (CRP), 437,
    445
Canal of Schlemm, 205, 220
Cancellous, 445

Cancer, 549. *See also* Oncology
  as recurrent disease, 534
  defined, 528
  development of, 529-532
  gynecologic, 398-399
  histologic origin of, 531
  invasive, 363
  nanospheres for, 546
  of immune system, 507-510
  ovarian, 398
  pancreatic, 328
  prostate, 366-367
  risk factors, 532-534
  screening tests for, 540-541, 552
  staging by TNM system, 535, 535t
  uterine, 398-399
Cancer classification systems, 534-536
  grade, 534
  performance status, 536
  stage, 534-535
Cancer stage, 534-435, 535t
Candida albicans, 185
Candidiasis, 185, 194
Capillaries, 260, 278, 289, 309
Capitalization, 102-104
Capsules, 138
Carbuncles, 184, 195
Carcinoembryonic antigen (CEA), 537, 549
Carcinogen, 549
Carcinogenesis, 528, 549
Carcinoma in situ, 399, 408
Carcinomas, 531, 549
Cardia, 321, 340
Cardiac arrest, 295, 309
Cardiac catheterization, 309
Cardiac conduction, 292, 309
Cardiac cycle, 292-293, 293f, 309
Cardiac diseases, 295-301. *See also*
    Cardiology
  cardiomyopathy, 298-299
  congenital heart disorders, 300-301
  coronary artery disease, 297-298
  hypertension, 296-297
  pericarditis, 299-300
  valvular heart disease, 299
Cardiac ischemia, 297, 309
Cardiac muscles, 428, 445
Cardiac stress test, 309
Cardiac tamponade, 299, 309
Cardinal numbers, 104, 110
Cardiology, 288-314, 309. *See also*
    Cardiac diseases
  abbreviation in, 307
  blood pressure, 295
  cardiac cycle, 292-293, 293f
  cardiac diseases in, 295-301
  cardiomyopathy, 298-299
  cardiovascular circulation, 291-292
  circulatory system, 289
  combining form in, 306t
  congenital heart disorders, 300-301
  coronary artery disease, 297-298
  defined, 288
  diagnostic studies and procedures in,
    301-304
  heart anatomy, 289-291, 290f
  heart brain in, 304

  heart rate and rhythm, 294-295
  heart sounds, 293-294
  hypertension in, 296-297
  pericarditis, 299-300
  soundalike words in, 305t
  terminology in, 308-314
  valvular heart disease, 299
Cardiomyopathy, 298-299, 309
Cardiopulmonary, 288, 309
Cardiovascular system, 288, 309. *See
    also* Cardiology
  arteries in, 289
  blood vessels in, 289
  circulation in, 291-292
  pathway of blood vessels, 288
Career fairs, 592-593, 614
Career management
  abbreviations in, 614
  application letter in, 596-599
  effective resumés in, 593-596
  entrepreneurship, 608, 608t
  ergonomics benefits in, 613
  industry terminology in, 590-593
  interview success in, 601-603
  job search strategies, 587-590
  medical references in, 606
  medical transcription service
    organization in, 587
  online testing in, 599-601
  owning your own business and,
    608-612
Career management
  personal development in, 603-606
  post-interview thank you note, 603
  professional development in,
    606-607
  terminology in, 614-616
Career profile, 3-17
  electronic medical and health records
    in, 8-9, 8f
  HIPAA in, 9-10
  HITECH Act, 9-10
  Internet in, 606
  knowledge and skills required in,
    4-7, 7t
  medical record keeping in, 7-8, 7f
  medical references in, 606
  medical transcriptionist, 3-4
  overview, 3
  patient confidentiality in, 9-11
  professional affiliation in, 13-14
  terminologies of, 16-17
  work environments and, 11-13
Carina, 259, 278
Carpals, 425, 445
Cartilage, 425, 446
Cartilaginous joints, 425, 446
Casts, 153, 168
Cataract, 208, 220
  visual effect of, 212f
Catecholamines, 561, 574
Catheter, 297, 309
Cathode-ray tube (CRT) monitors,
    21, 37
Cauda equina, 463, 482
Cecum, 321, 340
Cell membrane, 528, 549
Cell saver, 121, 129

Cells, 528-529
  defined, 528
  mitosis, 529
  nucleus, 528-529
  structure, 528-529, 528f
Cellulitis, 184, 195
Central nervous system (CNS),
    458-462, 482
  brain in, 458-461
  spinal cord in, 461-462
Central processing unit (CPU), 21, 37
Centrifuge, 153, 168
Cerebellar function, 473-474
Cerebellum, 461, 482
Cerebral aneurysm, 466, 482
Cerebral angiogram, 475, 482
Cerebral cortex, 459, 482
Cerebrospinal fluid (CSF), 439, 446,
    461, 483
Cerebrovascular disease, 566
Cerebrum, 459-460, 483
Certified Medical Transcriptionist
    (CMT), 13-14, 16, 615
Cerumen, 231, 248
Cervical, 446
Cervical cancer, 399, 399f, 408
Cervical dysplasia, 396-397, 408
Cervical intraepithelial neoplasia (CIN),
    397, 408
Cervical vertebrae, 424
Cervix, 388, 409
Cesarean section (C-section), 394, 409
Chambers, 290-291, 309
Chart note, 72
Chemical name, of drugs, 135, 143
Chemistry panel, 155, 168
Chemoprevention, 549
  in cancer, 538
Chemotherapy, 190, 195, 269, 278, 549
Cheyne-Stokes respirations, 262, 278
Chief complaint, in medical reports, 69
Chlamydia, 368, 376
Chlamydia trachomatis, 368
Cholangiography, 335
Cholangiopancreatography, 335, 340
Cholecystectomy, 120, 129, 327, 340
Cholecystitis, 327, 340
Choledocholithiasis, 327, 340
Cholelithiasis, 326, 340
Cholescintigraphy, 335
Cholesteatoma, 236, 248
Chondrosarcoma, 436, 446
Chordee, 365, 376
Choroid plexus, 461, 483
Chromaffin cells, 565, 574
Chromosomes, 549
Chronic hepatitis, 328, 340
Chronic lymphocytic leukemia (CLL),
    532
Chronic myelogenous leukemia (CML),
    532
Chronic obstructive pulmonary disease
    (COPD), 265-267, 278
  bronchitis, 265-266
Chronic pancreatitis, 328, 341
Chronic renal failure, 357, 376
Chronic sinusitis, 238, 248
Chronological resumé, 593, 615

Chyme, 341
Cigarette smoking
  causes emphysema, 266–267
  causes lung cancer, 269
Cilia, 259, 265, 278
Ciliary body, 204, 220
Cine-esophagram, 334
Circadian rhythm, 560, 574
Circle of Willis, 559, 574
Circulatory system, 288, 289
  defined, 288, 309
Cirrhosis, 329–330, 341
Clark level system, 535, 549
Clavicle, 425, 446
Clean catch, 152, 168, 356, 376
Clear cell carcinoma, 399, 409
Click (heart sound), 294, 309
Click-murmur syndrome, 299
Client base, developing, 610–611
Client/server architecture, 26, 37
Clinic note, 72–73
Clinical radiology, 158
Clinical trials, 549
  of drugs, 136, 143
  phases of, 136–137
  randomized, 137
Clitoris, 387, 387f, 409
Clock body positions, 57
Closed reduction, 431, 446
Clue cells, 409
CMT. See Certified Medical
    Transcriptionist (CMT)
CMV. See Cytomegalovirus (CMV)
Coagulation, 157, 168
Cobblestone, 248
Cobblestoning, 239
Coccyx, 423, 446
Cochlea, 231, 248
Coil embolization, 467, 483
Cold knife cone biopsy, 402–403, 409
Cold spots, 574
Cold sweat, 180, 195
Colectomy, 331, 341
Collagen, 179, 195, 425, 446, 506,
    517
Collateral vessels, 517
Collective nouns, 96, 110
Colon, 99–100, 110, 321
Colonoscope, 335, 341
Colonoscopy, 129, 335, 341
Colorectal cancer, 332, 341
Colostomy, 331, 341
Colostrum, 388, 409
Colposcope, 402, 409
Colposcopy, 403, 409
Combining forms, 44–46, 46t, 59
  in cardiology, 306t
  in dermatology, 193t
  in endocrinology, 572t
  in gastroenterology, 338t
  in imaging, 166t
  in immunology, 514t
  in neurology, 480t
  in obstetrics and gynecology, 406t
  in oncology, 547t
  in ophthalmology, 218t
  in orthopaedics, 443t
  in otorhinolaryngology, 246t

in pulmonology, 275t
in radiologic imaging, 166t
  surgical, 127, 128t
in urology, 373t
Combining vowels, 44–46, 46t, 59
Comma, 98–99, 110
Comma splice, 99, 110
Common bile duct, 322, 341
Communicating hydrocephalus, 466,
    483
Compact bone, 421, 446
  composition of, 422f
Compact disk (CD), 22, 37
Compact Disk-Read Only Memory
    (CD-ROM) drive, 22, 37
Compact Disk-Recordable (CD-R) disk,
    22, 37
Compact Disk-Rewritable (CD-RW)
    disk, 22, 37
Company web sites, 591
Complement, 517
Complete blood count (CBC),
    154–155, 168, 368
  in orthopaedics, 437
Complex partial seizures, 467, 483
Complimentary close, 67–68, 87
Compound adjective, 100, 110
Compound word, 43, 59
Comprehensive metabolic panel
    (CMP), 155–157, 156t, 168, 510
Compression stockings, 270
Computed tomography (CT) scan,
    161–162, 168, 446, 483
  in immunology, 512
  in neurology, 475
  in oncology, 539–540
  in orthopaedics, 439
  of upper abdomen, 161f
Computer applications, 24–26
  medical billing applications, 25–26
  Windows, 24–25
  word-processing applications, 25
Computer processing, 22
Computer programs, 22
Computer skills, 4
Computer systems, 23
Computer-aided detection (CAD), 539,
    549
Concha, 248, 233
Concha bullosa, 233, 248
Conchae, 259, 278
Conduction velocity, 446
  EMG and, 441
Conductive hearing loss, 236, 248
Conductive keratoplasty (CK), 207, 220
Condyloma acuminata, 185, 195
Cone biopsy, 402–403, 409
Cones, 206, 220
Confrontation, 214
Congenital heart disorders, 300–301
Congenital hydrocephalus, 466, 483
Congestion, 297, 309
Congestive heart failure (CHF), 297,
    309
Conjunctiva, 204, 220
Conjunctive adverbs, 96, 110
Conjunctivitis, 204, 220
Connective tissue, 398, 409

Consultation report, 77–79, 87
Continuous positive airway pressure
    (CPAP) machine, 238–239, 248
Contrast material, 161, 168
Controlled substances, 139–141, 143
Convulsive seizure, 483
COPD. See Chronic obstructive
    pulmonary disease (COPD)
Core biopsy, 446, 549
  in oncology, 538
  in orthopaedics, 438
Core decompression, 446
  for avascular necrosis, 432
Cornea, 203–204, 220
Corneal topographer, 215, 220
Corneal topography, 215, 220
Corniculate, 234
Corniculate cartilage, 248
Coronal suture, 446
Coronary angiography, 309
Coronary angioplasty, vascular stent in,
    298f
Coronary arteries, 291, 291f, 309
Coronary artery bypass graft surgery
    (CABG), 298
Coronary artery disease (CAD),
    297–298, 310, 566
Corporate veil, 610, 615
Corporation, 610, 615
Corpus callosotomy, 483
  for seizures, 468
Corpus callosum, 459, 483
Corpus luteum, 389, 409
Correspondence, medical. See Medical
    correspondence
Corticosteroids
  for allergy, 500
  for autoimmune diseases, 507
Corticosterone, 561, 574
Cortisol, 561, 574
Cosmetic surgery, 120
Costal cartilage, 424, 446
Cowper glands, 355, 376
CPAP machine. See Continuous positive
    airway pressure (CPAP) machine
Crackles, 262
Cranial bones, 422, 446
Cranial nerves, 462–463, 483
  assessment of, 473
  functions, and testing modalities of,
    464t–465t
Craniectomy, 483
Craniopharyngiomas, 471, 483
Craniotomy, 467, 471, 483
Creatine kinase (CK), 310
Creatine phosphokinase (CPK) test,
    310, 438, 446
Creatinine, 156, 168, 368, 376
Creatinine clearance, 369, 376
Cricoid, 234, 248
Critical thinking skills, 5
Crohn disease, 330, 341
Crossmatching antigen test, 376
  in kidney transplant, 358–359
CRT monitors. See Cathode-ray tube
    (CRT) monitors
Cryoablation, 366, 376
Cryomyolysis, 409

Cryopreservation, 393, 409
Cryoprobe, 366, 376
Cryosurgery, 189
Cryotherapy, 185, 195, 395, 409
Crystalline lens, 204, 220
Crystals, 153, 168
CT angiogram, 168
CT myelogram, 440, 446
CT-guided biopsy, 539, 549
Culture, 158, 168, 376
    bacteria, 157
    blood, 158
    in orthopaedics, 438
    for STD, 369, 401
    stool, 346
    urine, 158
Culture and sensitivity test, 149, 168
Cuneiform cartilages, 234, 248
Curet, 402, 409
Curettage, 189, 195
Curette, 189
Curriculum vita (CV), 593
Cushing disease, 574
Cushing syndrome, 564–565, 565f, 574
Cutaneous, 177
Cutaneous candidiasis, 185, 195
Cyanosis, 310
Cyclooxygenase-2 (COX-2) inhibitors, 435, 446
Cyclosporine, for autoimmune diseases, 507
Cystic duct, 322, 341
Cystic fibrosis, 267, 278
Cystine, 360, 376
Cystine stones, 360
Cystocele, 362–363, 376
Cystometer, 371, 376
Cystometrogram (CMG), 371, 376
Cystometry, 371, 376
Cystoscope, 363, 376
Cystoscopy, 370, 376
Cytokines, 517
Cytology, 149, 168
Cytomegalovirus (CMV), 278
Cytoplasm, 528, 550

D

Dash, 102, 110
Data, 21, 37
Data storage and transfer, 22–23
Debridement, 121, 129, 187, 195
Debulking, 471, 483
Debulking surgery, 550
Decelerations (heart rate), 393, 409
Decongestants, for allergy, 500
Deep brain stimulation (DBS), 483
    in Parkinson disease, 469
Deep tendon reflexes (DTR), 474, 483
Deep venous thrombosis (DVT), 270, 278, 507, 517
Defecation, 322, 341
Defibrillator, 295
Degenerative joint disease (DJD), 434
Delivery, 394
Demographic information, 70, 87
Demyelination, 469, 483
Deoxyribonucleic acid (DNA), 529, 550
    structure of, 529f

Department of Health and Human Services (DHHS), 10
Dependent clause, 98, 110
Dermatitis, 181–182, 195
Dermatology, 177–198. See also Skin
    abbreviations in, 194
    burns, 186–187
    cellulitis in, 184
    combining forms in, 193t
    dermatitis in, 181–182
    dermis in, 179
    diagnostic studies and procedures in, 190
    diseases and treatment in, 180–190
    epidermis in, 178
    folliculitis in, 184
    frostbite, 187–188
    impetigo in, 184
    integumentary system, anatomy, 177–180
    psoriasis in, 173, 173f
    rosacea in, 182–183
    shingles, 185–186
    skin appearance terminology, 181t
    skin cancer in, 188–190
    skin damage from heat and cold, 186–188
    skin infections in, 183–184
    soundalike words in, 192t
    tinea, 184–185
Dermatomes, 463, 483
Dermatophytes, 184, 195
Dermis, 179, 195
Desaturations, 243, 248
Descending colon, 321, 341
Desiccation, 189, 195
Desktop, 25, 37
Desquamation, 178, 195
Detrusor muscle, 354, 376
Deviated septum, 237–238, 248
DHHS. See Department of Health and Human Services (DHHS)
Diabetes insipidus, 568–569, 574
Diabetes mellitus (DM), 566–568, 574
    chronic complications of, 566–567
    medications for, 567–568
    types of insulin used to control, 567–568
Diabetic ketoacidosis (DKA), 566, 574
Diabetic nephropathy, 566, 574
Diabetic neuropathy, 566, 575
Diabetic retinopathy, 208, 220, 566, 575
Diagonal branches, 291, 310
Dialysis, 376
    during renal failure, 357–358, 357f
Dialysis machine, 357, 376
Diaphoresis, 296, 310
Diaphragm, 56, 59, 260, 278
Diaphysis, 421, 446
Diastole, 292, 310
Diastolic pressure, 295, 310
Dictation, defined, 4, 16
Diet, and risk of cancer, 532
Differential, white blood cell, 155, 168
Diffusing capacity for carbon monoxide (DLCO), 271, 278
Diffusion, 261, 278, 289, 310

Digestion, 323–324, 341
Digestive disorders, 341. See also Gastrointestinal diseases
Digestive process, 323–324
Digestive system, 320, 320f
Digital dictation, 28, 37
    platforms, 28–29, 28f
Digital mammogram, 550
    in oncology, 539
Digital rectal examination (DRE), 365, 376
Digital subscriber line (DSL), 609, 615
Digitalis purpurea, 135
Dihydroxy testosterone (DHT), 366, 376
Dilated cardiomyopathy, 299, 310
Dilated examination, visual, 213
Dilation, 310, 393, 409
Dimethyl sulfoxide (DMSO), 362
Diplopia, 206, 220
Direct laryngoscopy, 242–243, 248
Directory tree, 34, 35f, 37
Discharge summary, 81, 87
Disease-modifying antirheumatic drug (DMARD), 507, 517
Disk, 424, 446
Disk drives, 22, 37
Diskogram, 440
Dislocation, 446
    of joints, 431–432
Distant recurrence, 534, 550
Diuresis, 269, 278
Diuretics, 296, 310
Diverticula, 341
Diverticular disease, 331–332, 341
Diverticulitis, 331, 341
Diverticulosis, 331, 341
Dix-Hallpike maneuver, 242, 248
DLCO. See Diffusing capacity for carbon monoxide (DLCO)
Document management system, 615
Document templates, 32–33
Dopamine, 483
    Parkinson disease and, 468
Doppler ultrasound, 163, 169
    in orthopaedics, 438
Dosage frequency, 139
Double vision. See Diplopia
Dowager hump, 433, 446
Drapes, 120, 129
Dressing changes, 187, 195
Dressings, 121, 126–127, 129, 187, 195
Dressler syndrome, 299, 310
Drug administration, 137–139
    dosage frequency, 139
    drug dosage forms, 138
    drug dosages and frequency, 138–139
    drug forms, 138
Drug book, 31
Drug combinations, for diabetes, 567
Drug dosages, 138–139
    forms, 138
    Latin abbreviations of frequency of, 139t
Drug Enforcement Administration (DEA), 139, 143
Drug forms, 138

Drug regulation and development, 136–137
Drugs, 143. *See also* Pharmacology
defined, 134
dosage frequency, 139
half-life of, 139
knowledge of names of, 135
metric measurement of, 139t
types of, 140t
Drusen, 208, 220
Dry macular degeneration, 208, 220
Dual-energy x-ray absorptiometry (DEXA), 439, 446
Duchenne muscular dystrophy (DMD), 435, 446
Ductal carcinoma in situ (DCIS), 399, 409
Ducts, 179, 195, 409
in breast cancer, 399
Ductus arteriosus, 300, 310
Dukes classification system, 535, 550
Duodenal ulcer, 325, 341
Duodenum, 321, 341
Dura mater, 461, 483
Dutasteride, for prostate disorder, 366
DVT. *See* Deep vein thrombosis (DVT)
Dwarfism, 563, 575
Dysmenorrhea, 390, 409
Dysmetria, 483
Dyspnea, 262, 278, 297, 310
Dystocia, 394, 409
Dystrophin, 435, 446
Dysuria, 376

E

E chart, 213f, 220
E-mail, 26, 37
E-prescriptions, pharmacy automation with, 142
E-Sign Act. *See* Electronic Signatures in Global and National Commerce Act (E-Sign Act)
Ear, 249
anatomy, 230–232, 230f
inner ear, 231–232
middle ear, 231
outer ear, 230–231
disorders, 235–237
cholesteatoma, 236
hearing loss, 236–237
Ménière disease, 236
otitis media, 235
vertigo, 235–236
Eardrum. *See* Tympanic membrane
Earphones, 27–28, 37
EBV. *See* Epstein-Barr virus (EBV)
Ecchymoses, 505, 517
Echocardiogram, 310
Eclampsia, 391, 409
ECOG scale, 550
Ectopic pregnancy, 390, 409
Eczema, 182, 182f, 195
Edema, 181, 195, 296, 310
Editing, 93–111. *See* Proofreading
acronyms in, 106
capitalization in, 102–104
eponyms in, 105–106
grammar review in, 93–96

numbers/numbering systems in, 104–105
overview, 93
proofreading and, 106–109
punctuation marks in, 96–102
symbols in, 105
EEG. *See* Electroencephalography (EEG)
Effacement, 393, 409
Efferent nerves, 462, 483
Effusion, 124, 129
EGFR. *See* Epidermal growth factor receptors (EGFR)
EHR. *See* Electronic health record (EHR)
Elective surgery, 120
Electrocardiogram, 310
Electrocautery, 185, 195, 238, 249, 395, 409
Electroencephalography (EEG), 477f, 483
in neurology, 476–477
video, 476
Electrolytes, 156, 169, 368, 376
Electromyography (EMG), 446
in orthopaedics, 440–441
Electronic charting, 24f
Electronic health record (EHR), 8–9, 16
Electronic medical record (EMR), 8–9, 8f, 16
Electronic signature, 68, 87
Electronic Signatures in Global and National Commerce Act (E-Sign Act), 68, 87
Electronystagmography (ENG), 242, 249
Eligibility criteria, 550
Elixirs, 138, 143
Em dash, 102, 110
Embryo, 391, 410
Embryo transfer, 392–393, 410
Emergency surgery, 120
EMG. *See* Electromyography (EMG)
Emphysema, 266–267, 266f, 278
Employment web site, 591–592, 615
Empyema, 263, 278
EMR. *See* Electronic medical record (EMR)
Encryption, 26, 37
End-stage renal disease (ESRD), 360, 376
Endocardium, 290, 310
Endocervical curettage (ECC), 402, 410
Endocrine gland, 179, 195, 558, 575
Endocrine system, 558–562, 559f. *See also* Endocrinology
adrenal glands, 561–562
anatomy, 558–562
gonads, 562
hypothalamus, 559
pancreas, 562
parathyroid glands, 561
pineal gland, 560
pituitary gland, 559–560
thymus, 561
thyroid gland, 560–561
Endocrinologist, 558, 575
Endocrinology, 558–578, 575. *See also* Endocrinology
abbreviations in, 573

adrenal disorders, 564–566
combining forms in, 572t
defined, 558
diabetes insipidus, 568–569
diabetes mellitus, 566–568
diagnostic studies and procedures in, 569–570
endocrine diseases in, 562–569
endocrine system, anatomy, 558–562
hyperparathyroidism, 564
imaging in, 569–570
laboratory tests in, 569
pituitary disorders, 563–564
soundalike words in, 571t
terminology in, 573–578
Endometrial ablation, 398, 410
Endometrial cancer, 410
Endometriosis, 397–398, 410
Endometritis, 410
Endometrium, 388, 410
Endoscope, 119, 129, 238, 249, 335, 341
Endoscopic retrograde cholangiopancreatography (ERCP), 335, 341
Endoscopic sinus surgery (ESS), 238, 249
Endoscopic ultrasound (EUS), 335, 341
Endoscopy, 119–120, 129, 341, 550
in gastroenterology, 335
in oncology, 538–539
in urology, 370
Endosteum, 422, 446
English language knowledge, MT and, 4
Enteric, 138, 143
Enterovirus, 483
Entrepreneur, 608, 608t, 615
Entrepreneurship, 608, 608t
Environmental exposures, and risk of cancer, 533
Enzymes, 151, 169
Eosinophils, 155, 169
Ependymoma, 471, 484
Epicardium, 290, 310
Epidermal growth factor receptors (EGFR), 269, 278
Epidermis, 178, 195
Epididymis, 355, 376
Epididymitis, 376
Epiglottis, 233, 249, 259, 278, 341
Epilepsy, 468, 483
Epinephrine, 561–562, 575
Epiphysis, 421, 447
Epistaxis, 238, 249
Epithelial carcinomas, 398, 410
Eponyms, 105–106, 110
Epstein-Barr virus (EBV), 278, 517
Equipment, 608–609
Ergonomics, 615
benefits of, 613
Erythema, 181, 195
Erythrocyte count, 154, 169
Erythrocyte sedimentation rate (ESR), 437, 447, 517
Erythrocytes, 531, 550
Erythropoietin, 353, 377
Esophageal sphincter, 321, 323, 341
Esophageal stricture, 341
Esophageal varices, 330, 342

Esophagogastroduodenoscopy (EGD), 335, 342
Esophagoscopy, 342
Esophagram, 334, 342
Esophagus, 321, 342
ESS. *See* Endoscopic sinus surgery (ESS)
Essential hypertension, 297, 310
Estradiol, 575
Estrogen, 388, 410, 562, 575
Ethics, 6, 16
Ethmoid sinuses, 232, 249
Eumelanin, 204, 220
Eustachian tube, 231, 249
Ewing sarcoma, 436, 447
Excise, 189, 195
Excision, 121, 129
Excisional biopsy, 149, 169, 195, 512, 517, 550
    in oncology, 538
Excretory system, 377
Exocrine gland, 179–180, 195
Exocrine pancreas, 328, 342
Exocrine tumor, 328, 342
Exophthalmos, 504, 517
Exploratory surgery, 120
Extensors, 427, 447
External auditory canal, 230, 249
External beam radiation, 189, 195, 269, 278, 550
External fixation, 447
    of fracture, 431
External genital organs, 387, 410
External respiration, 261, 278
External urethral sphincter, 354, 377
Extra-articular, 517
Extracorporeal shock wave lithotripsy (ESWL), 360–362, 377
Extraocular muscles, 204, 204f, 220
Extubation, 121, 129, 263, 278
Eye. *See also* Ophthalmology
    anatomy of, 202–205, 203f
    inner structures, 203–205
    outer structures of, 202–203
    structural diseases of, 208–211
    visual disorders of, 205–208
Eyelashes, 203, 220
Eyelids, 220

F

Falciform ligament, 322, 342
Fallopian tubes, 388, 410
False vocal folds, 234, 249
Famciclovir (Famvir), 186
Family history, in medical reports, 69
Farsightedness, 220. *See* Hyperopia
Fecal fat test, 334, 342
Fecal occult blood test, 334, 342, 537–538
FEF. *See* Forced expiratory flow (FEF)
Fellow of the Association for Healthcare Documentation Integrity (AHDI-F), 14, 16, 614
Female reproductive system, anatomy, 386–390, 387f
    external genital organs, 387
    internal genital organs, 387–388
    mammary glands, 388
    menstrual cycle and, 388–390

Femur, 447
Fern test, 393, 410
Ferritin, 157, 169
Fertility tests, 401
Fertilization, 410
    in humans, 390–392
Fetal heart rate, 393, 410
Fetal scalp electrode (FSE), 393, 410
Fetal well-being, 393
Fetus, 391, 410
FEV1. *See* Forced expiratory volume measured in one second (FEV1)
FEV1-FVC ratio, 271, 278
Fiberoptic laryngoscope, 242, 249
Fibrillation, 294, 310
Fibrillin, 179, 195
Fibroblasts, 187, 195
Fibrosis, 517
Fibrous joints, 425, 447
Fibula, 425, 447
FIGO staging, 535, 550
Figures, 104, 110
File management, 34–35
File server, 23, 37
File Transfer Protocol (FTP), 26, 37
Files, 34, 37
    organizing, 35
Filiform warts, 185, 195
Filtration, 289, 310
Fimbriae, 388, 410
Finasteride, for prostate disorder, 366
Fine needle aspiration (FNA), 149, 169, 517
    in immunology, 511–512
Fine-needle biopsy, 550
    in oncology, 538
Fissures, 260, 278, 331, 342
Fistula, 331, 342, 357, 377
Fixation, 447
    of fracture, 431
Flag, in medical report, 84, 87
Flare, 517
Flaring, 262, 278
Flash drive, 22–23, 23f, 37
Flat bones, 422, 447
Flexible laryngoscopy, 243, 249
Flexors, 427, 447
Flovent, 265
Flow cytometry, 149, 169
Fluids and medications, during surgery, 123–124, 124t
Fluorescein, 215, 220
    angiography, 215, 220
Fluoroscopy, 297, 310, 467, 484
Focal neuropathy, 566, 575
Focal segmental glomerulosclerosis (FSGS), 359, 377
Focused ultrasound surgery (FUS), 398, 410
Folder, 34, 37
    creation, 35
Follicle-stimulating hormone (FSH), 389, 410, 560, 575
Follicles, 179, 195, 388, 410
Follicular aspiration, 392, 410
Folliculitis, 184, 195
Fontanels, 423, 447

Food and Drug Administration (FDA), 135, 143
Foot pedal, 28, 37
Footer, 34, 37
Foramen magnum, 458, 484
Forced expiratory flow (FEF), 271, 278
Forced expiratory volume measured in one second (FEV1), 270, 279
Forced vital capacity (FVC), 270, 279
Forceps, 394, 410
Formalin, 151, 169
Forums, 591, 615
Fourth ventricle, 461, 484
Fovea centralis, 205, 221
Fowler position, during surgery, 123
Fraction of inspired oxygen (FiO$_2$), 263, 279
Fracture, 430–431, 447
    fixation of, 431
    repair, 441
    types of, 431t
Freelancer, 608
Front-end speech recognition, 29, 37
Frontal lobes, 460, 484
Frontal sinuses, 232, 249
Frostbite, 187–188, 195
Frozen embryo transfer, 393
Fulguration, 363, 377
Full-block letter style, 66–67, 67f, 87
Full-thickness burns, 186, 195
Full-thickness skin graft, 187, 196
Function keys, 21, 38
Functional disorder, 330, 342
Functional MRI, 484
Functional resumé, 593, 615
Fundus, 321, 326, 342, 388
Fungal skin infections, 184
Fusion inhibitors, 501, 518
FVC. *See* Forced vital capacity (FVC)

G

Gallbladder, 322, 342
    disease, 326–327
Gallop (heart sound), 294, 310
Gallstones, 326, 342
    in common bile duct, 327
Gamma camera, 311, 575
Gangrene, 184, 196
Gas exchange, 258, 279, 292
Gastric emptying study (GES), 334, 342
Gastric ulcer, 325, 342
Gastric varices, 330, 342
Gastritis, 324, 342
Gastroduodenoscopy, 342
Gastroenterologists, 319, 342
Gastroenterology, 319–346, 342. *See also* Gastrointestinal system
    abbreviations in, 339
    anatomy of gastrointestinal system and, 319–322
    brain-gut axis, 336
    cirrhosis in, 329–330
    colorectal cancer, 332
    combining forms in, 338t
    defined, 319
    diagnostic studies and procedures in, 333–335
    digestive process, 323–324

diverticular disease, 331–332
gallbladder disease in, 326–327
gastrointestinal diseases in, 324–332
hepatitis in, 328–329
inflammatory bowel disease, 330–331
intussusception, 331
irritable bowel syndrome, 330
pancreatic disorders in, 327–328
peptic disorders in, 324–326
soundalike words in, 337t
terminology in, 339–346
Gastroesophageal reflux disease
(GERD), 324, 325f, 342
Gastrointestinal diseases, 324–332
cirrhosis in, 329–330
colorectal cancer, 332
diverticular disease, 331–332
gallbladder disease, 326–327
hepatitis in, 328–329
inflammatory bowel disease, 330–331
intussusception, 331
irritable bowel syndrome, 330
pancreatic disorders, 327–328
peptic disorders, 324–326
Gastrointestinal system, 342. See also
Gastroenterology
accessory organs in, 322
anatomy of, 319–322
esophagus in, 321
large intestine in, 321–322
mouth and throat in, 320–321
small intestine in, 321
stomach in, 321
Gastrojejunostomy, 326
Gastroscopy, 342
Gauze. See Bandage
Gene therapy, in cancer, 538
General anesthesia, 123
General distribution letter, 598
Generalized seizures, 468, 484
Generic name, of drugs, 135, 143
Genes, 529, 550
Genetic factors, and risk of cancer,
532
Genetic testing, in oncology, 538
Genital herpes, 367, 377
Genital tract, 387–388, 410
Genital warts, 195
Genitourinary diseases, 356–368
bladder disorders, 362–364
kidney disorders, 356–362
male genitourinary disorders,
365–368
urinary tract infection, 356
Genitourinary system, 352, 377
anatomy of, 352–355
kidneys, 352–354
male genital organs, 354–355
ureters, 354
urethra, 354
urinary bladder, 354
Genotypes, 329, 342
Germ cell tumors, 398
Gestational diabetes, 392, 410, 567,
575
Giant cell arteritis (GCA), 505, 518
Gigantism, 563, 575
Girdles, 447

Glands, 179–180, 196
Glans penis, 355, 377
Glasgow coma scale (GCS), 473, 484
Glaucoma, 208, 221
Gleason system, 534, 550
Glenoid fossa, 425, 447
Glia, 459, 484
Gliadel, 550
Glioblastoma multiforme, 471, 484
Gliomas, 471, 484, 531, 550
Globus sensation, 324, 342
Glomerular capsule, 353–354, 377
Glomerular filtrate, 355, 377
Glomerular filtration rate (GFR), 368,
377
Glomerulonephritis, 359, 377
Glomerulosclerosis, 359, 377
Glomerulus, 353, 377
Glottis, 234, 249
Glucagon, 562, 575
Glucose, 169, 575
urinary, 153
Glucose tolerance test (GGT), 575
Glycogen, 575
Glycosylated hemoglobin, 575
GnRH agonists. See Gonadotropin
releasing hormone (GnRH)
agonists
Goiter, 518
Gonadotropin releasing hormone
(GnRH) agonists, 397, 410
Gonadotropins, 560, 575
Gonads, 562, 575
Gonio lens, 215, 221
Gonioscopy, 215, 221
Gonorrhea, 368, 377
Gorillapause, 404
Goserelin, 366
GPA system, 391, 410
Grafting, 121, 129
Grafts, 298, 310
Gram stain, 158, 169
Grammar review, 93–96
parts of speech, 94t
sentence fragment, 95
sentence structure, 94–95
subject-verb agreement, 95–96
Graves disease, 504–505, 504f, 518
Gravida, 391, 410
Gray matter, 459, 484
Great longitudinal fissure, 459, 484
Greater saphenous vein, 298, 311
Gross pathology, 149, 169
Growth hormone (GH), 560, 563,
575
Grunting, 263, 279
Gynecologic cancers, 398–399, 411
breast cancer, 399
cervical cancer, 399, 399f
ovarian cancer, 398
uterine cancer, 398–399
Gynecologic disorders, 411
Gynecologic studies, 401–403
colposcopy, 403
cone biopsy, 402–403
laparoscopy, 402
mammography, 403
Gynecologist, 411

Gynecology, 386, 411
Gyri, 459, 484

H

HAART. See Highly active antiretroviral
therapy (HAART)
Haemophilus influenzae, 263, 279
type b, 466
Hair, 179, 196
Half-life of drugs, 139
Hard disk drive, 22, 38
Hard palate, 320, 342
Hardware, 21, 38
Harvesting, of developed eggs, 392
Hashimoto thyroiditis, 505–507, 518
scleroderma, 506–507
Sjögren syndrome, 506
vasculitis, 505–506
Headers, 34, 38
Headings, in medical reports, 68–70
Headsets, 27–28
Health Information Technology for
Economic and Clinical Health
(HITECH) Act, 10–11, 16
Health Insurance Portability and
Accountability Act of 1996
(HIPAA), 9–10, 16, 106
Hearing loss, 236–237, 249
Hearing process, 234–235
air conduction, 234
bone conduction, 235
Heart anatomy, 289–291, 290f
chambers, 290–291
coronary arteries and vessels, 291
layers, 290
valves, 291
Heart attack. See Myocardial infarction
(MI)
Heart block, 295, 311
Heart brain, 304
Heart failure, 297, 311
Heart rate and rhythm, 294–295
Heart sounds, 293–294, 311
lub-dub, 293
murmur, 294
Heart-lung machine, 298, 311
Heartbeat, 292, 311
Helicobacter pylori, 324
Helper T cells, 499, 518
Helping verb, 94, 110
Hematemesis, 325, 343
Hematochezia, 330, 343
Hematocrit, 154–155, 169
Hematologic studies, 153–158, 169
blood clotting studies, 157–158
complete blood count with
differential, 154–155
iron studies, 157
metabolic panel, 155–157
thyroid function tests, 157
Hematology, 153, 169
Hematopoiesis, 421, 447
Hematuria, 152, 169, 377
Hemoccult, 550
Hemochromatosis, 157, 169
Hemodialysis, 357, 377
Hemoglobin, 154, 169
Hemolysis, 411

Hemorrhage, 467, 484
Hemothorax, 263, 279
Hepatic ducts, 322, 343
Hepatic flexure, 321, 343
Hepatic veins, 330, 343
Hepatitis, 328–329, 343
    antigen tests for, 329
Hepatitis A virus, 343
Hepatitis B virus, 329, 343
Hepatitis C virus, 329, 343
Hepatobiliary iminodiacetic acid
        (HIDA) scan, 334–335, 343
Hepatomegaly, 329, 343
HER2/neu, 537, 550
HER2/neu negative, 537, 550
HER2/neu positive, 537, 550
Heredity, 550
Herpes zoster, 185–186, 196
High-density lipoprotein (HDL), 311
High-dose chemotherapy, 550
    with stem cell rescue, 506–507, 518
High-grade astrocytoma, 484
High-grade SIL (HGSIL), 397, 411
Highly active antiretroviral therapy
        (HAART), 501, 518
HIPAA. See Health Insurance Portability
        and Accountability Act of 1996
        (HIPAA)
Hippocampus, 460, 484
Hippocratic oath, 6, 16
Hirsutism, 564, 575
Histamine, 500, 518
Histamine-2 (H2) blockers, 326, 343
Histology, 169
Histopathology, 149, 169
History and physical examination
        (H&P), 74, 75, 87
HITECH Act. See Health Information
        Technology for Economic and
        Clinical Health (HITECH) Act
Hodgkin lymphomas, 508, 518
Homeostasis, 575
    defined, 558
Homocysteine, 311
Homonyms, 48, 49t, 59
Horizontal gaze nystagmus, 204, 221
Hormone therapy, for prostate cancer,
        366
Hormones, 575
Hot spots, 575
Human chorionic gonadotropin (hCG),
        400, 410, 537, 550
Human immunodeficiency virus (HIV),
        264, 279, 395–396, 411, 501, 518
Human leukocyte antigens (HLA), 358,
        377
Human papillomavirus (HPV), 395, 410
Humerus, 425, 447
Hydrocephalus, 466, 484
Hydrothorax, 279
Hyoid, 233, 249
Hyoid bone, 422, 447
Hyperacusis, 470, 484
Hyperbaric therapy, skin wounds, 191
Hypercalcemia, 510, 518, 564, 575
Hyperemesis gravidarum, 392, 410
Hyperglycemia, 562, 575
Hyperkalemia, 357, 377

Hyperopia, 206, 221
Hyperparathyroidism, 561, 564, 576
Hyperplasia, 564, 576
Hypertension, 296–297, 311
Hyperthyroidism, 504, 518
Hypertrophic cardiomyopathy, 299,
        311
Hypertrophy, 299, 311
Hyperventilation, 271, 279
Hyphema, 208, 221
Hyphen, 100–101, 110
Hypochondriac, 56, 59
    regions, 56, 56f
Hypoglycemia, 566, 576
Hypoparathyroidism, 561, 576
Hypopharynx, 233, 249
Hypopituitarism, 564, 576
Hypopnea, 238, 249
Hypospadias, 365, 377
Hypotension, 295, 311
Hypothalamus, 460–461, 484, 559
Hypothyroidism, 505, 518
Hypoventilation, 271, 279
Hysterectomy, 397, 411
Hysterosalpingogram (HSG), 401, 411
Hysteroscopy, 401, 411

I

Ibuprofen, 397
Icons, 25, 38
Icterus, 329, 343
Identical twins, 411
Ileal conduit, 363, 377
Ileal pouch anal anastomosis (IPAA),
        331, 343
Ileostomy, 331, 343
Ileum, 321, 343
Ileus, 343
Ilium, 425, 447
Imaging, 158–159, 169
    abbreviation in, 167
    combining forms, 166t
    in endocrinology, 569–570
    feeling tissue with, 164
    in gastroenterology, 334–335
    in immunology, 512–513
    in neurology, 475–476
    in oncology, 539–541
    in orthopaedics, 438–441
    in otorhinolaryngology, 242
    radiologic, 158–163. See also
        Radiologic imaging
    soundalike words in, 165t
    terminology in, 167–171
Immune response, 518
Immune system, 495, 518. See also
        Immunology
    anatomy of, 497–499
    bone marrow, 498
    cancer of, 507–510
    cells and their products, 498–499
    immunoglobulins role in, 499
    lymphatic vessels and nodes,
        497–498
    lymphoid tissues, 498
    overview of, 496
    spleen, 498
    thymus, 498

Immunodeficiency, 501–502, 518
Immunoelectrophoresis, 518
Immunoglobulins, 499, 518
Immunologic diseases, 500–510
    allergy, 500–501
    autoimmunity diseases, 502–504
    Graves disease, 504–505, 504f
    Hashimoto thyroiditis, 505–507
    immunodeficiency, 501–502
Immunologist, 495, 518
Immunology, 495–521, 518. See also
        Immune system
    abbreviation in, 515
    allergy in, 500–501
    autoimmunity diseases in, 502–504
    combining forms in, 514t
    defined, 495
    diagnostic studies and procedures in,
        510–513
    Graves disease in, 504–505
    Hashimoto thyroiditis in, 505–507
    imaging studies in, 512–513
    immune system in, 496, 497–499
    immunodeficiency in, 501–502
    immunologic diseases, 500–510
    laboratory tests in, 510–512
    self and nonself in, 496–597
    soundalike words in, 514t
    terminology in, 516–521
Immunomodulating drugs, for
        autoimmune diseases, 507
Immunotherapy, 509, 518
    agents, 190, 196
Impetigo, 184, 196
Implantable cardioverter defibrillator
        (ICD), 295, 311
Implantable collamer lens (ICL)
        procedure, 208, 221
Impulses, 458, 484
IMV. See Intermittent mandatory
        ventilation (IMV)
In vitro fertilization (IVF), 392, 411
Incision, 120, 129
Incisional biopsy, 551
    in oncology, 538
Incus, 231, 249
Indefinite pronouns, 96
Independent clause, 94, 110
Indirect laryngoscopy, 249
Ineffective immune response, and risk
        of cancer, 533
Infarction, 518
Inferior vena cava, 270, 279, 292, 311,
        354, 377
Infertility, 392, 411
Infiltration, 123
Inflammatory bowel disease (IBD),
        330–331, 343
Information technology (IT), 24–26
    computer applications in, 24–26
    computer processing in, 22
    computer systems in, 23
    data storage and transfer in, 22–23
    defined, 21, 38
    file management and, 34–35
    hardware and, 21
    Internet and, 26–27
    LAN in, 23

overview, 20–21
software and, 21–22
stand-alone systems in, 23
transcription methods in, 27–29
transcription references and tools in, 30–31
word-processing features in, 32–34
Informed consent, 120, 129
Infundibulum, 388, 411, 559, 576
Infusion, 124, 129
Inhalational dosage, 138
Inhibin, 562, 576
Initialisms, 106, 110
Innate immune system, 496, 518
Inner ear, 231–232, 249
INR. *See* International Normalized Ratio (INR)
Insemination, 392, 411
Insertion, 447
Institute for Safe Medication Practices (ISMP), 53, 59
Instrument tray, 124, 129
Insufflation, 402, 411
Insulin, 562
    resistance, 567, 576
Insurance, 609
Integument, 177, 196
Integumentary system
    anatomy of, 177–180
    defined, 177, 196
Intercostal muscles, 261, 279
Interferon, 329, 343
Interferon alpha, 329, 343
Intermittent mandatory ventilation (IMV), 263, 279
Internal fixation, 447
    of fracture, 431
Internal genital organs, 387–388, 411
Internal radiation therapy, 551
Internal respiration, 261, 279
Internal urethral sphincter, 354, 377
International Normalized Ratio (INR), 169, 334, 343
Internet, 26–27
    in career profile, 606
    for reference, 606
    as transcription tool, 32
Interrupters, 96
Interstitial cell-stimulating hormone (ICSH), 560, 576
Interstitial chemotherapy, 551
Interstitial cystitis (IC), 362, 377
Interstitial nephritis, 359, 377
Intertrigo, 185, 196
Interventricular foramen, 461, 484
Interview success, 601–603
Intracranial aneurysms, 467f
Intracytoplasmic sperm injection (ICSI), 392, 411
Intramuscular dosage, 138, 143
Intraocular lens (IOL), 208, 221
Intrathecal chemotherapy, 551
Intrathecal dosage, 138, 143
Intrauterine pressure catheter (IUPC), 393, 411
Intravenous dosage, 138, 143
Intravenous drugs, to dissolve clot, 270

Intravenous immunoglobulin (IVIG), 507, 518
Intravenous pyelogram (IVP), 369–370, 377
Introductory clause, 98
Introitus, 388, 411
Intubation, 121, 129, 263, 279
Intussusception, 331, 343
Invasion, 551
Invasive cancer, 363, 378
Invasive ductal carcinoma (IDC), 399, 411
Invasive lobular carcinoma (ILC), 399, 411
Invasive procedures, 120
Involuntary muscles, 426, 447
Iris, 204, 221
Iron studies, 157
Irregular bones, 422, 447
Irrigation-aspiration device, 208, 221
Irritable bowel syndrome (IBS), 330, 343
Ischemia, 518
Ischium, 425, 447
Islets of Langerhans, 562, 576
ISMP. *See* Institute for Safe Medication Practices (ISMP)
Isthmus, 560, 576

J

J pouch, 331, 343
Jack-knife prone position, during surgery, 123
Jargon, medical, 51, 52t, 59
Jaundice, 329, 343
Jejunum, 321, 343
Jewett classification, 535, 551
Job search strategies, 587–590
    career fairs, 592–593
    industry terminology in, 590–593
    Internet strategies, 591–592
    network opportunities, 588–590
    newspapers and publications in, 592
    professional associations, 588
    volunteer prospects, 590–591
    word of mouth in, 593
Joint Commission, 53, 59, 615
Joints, 425, 447
    cartilaginous, 425
    dislocation of, 431–432
    fibrous, 425
    synovial, 425
Jump drive, 22

K

Karnofsky performance status (KPS), 536, 551
Kegel exercises, 378
Keratin, 196
Keratinocytes, 178, 196
Ketones, 153, 169
Keyboard, 21, 38
Keyboarding skills, 5
Kidney disorders, 356–362
    kidney failure, 356–359
    kidney stone, 360–362
    nephritis, 359
    polycystic kidney disease, 359–360

Kidney failure. *See* Renal failure
Kidney stone, 360–362, 378
    removal of, 361f
    surgical intervention for, 360–362
    types of, 360
Kidney transplantation, 358–359, 378
    crossmatching antigen test, 358–359
    tissue typing in, 358
Kidney, ureter, and bladder x-ray (KUB), 369
Kidneys, 352–354, 378
Killer T cells, 499, 519
Klebsiella pneumoniae, 263, 279
Knee jerk, 474, 484
Koch pouch, 364, 378
KOH test, 190, 196
Kyphosis, 433, 447

L

Labia, 387, 411
Labia majora, 387, 411
Labia minora, 387, 411
Labor, 393–394, 411
Laboratory data, in medical reports, 70
Laboratory studies, 151–158
    hematologic, 153–158
    laboratory test, 151
    of enzymes, 151
    reference range, 151
    urine tests, 151–153
Laboratory tests, 151, 169
    in endocrinology, 569
    in gastroenterology, 333–334
    in immunology, 510–512
    in neurology, 474
    in obstetrics and gynecology, 400–401
    in oncology, 536–538
    in orthopaedics, 437–438
    in urology, 368–369
Labyrinth, 231, 249
Lacrimal gland, 203, 221
Lactation, 388, 411
LAN. *See* Local area network (LAN)
Landmarks, 236, 249
Laparoscope, 129, 327, 343
Laparoscopic cholecystectomy, 327, 344
Laparoscopy, 120, 129, 397, 402, 412, 551
Laparotomy, 397, 412
    position, during surgery, 123
Large intestine, 321–322, 344
Laryngeal studies, 242–244
    direct laryngoscopy, 242–243
    mirror laryngoscopy, 242
    polysomnography, 243–244
    videostroboscopy, 243
Laryngopharyngeal reflux disease (LRD), 239, 249
Laryngopharynx. *See* Hypopharynx
Laryngoscopy
    direct, 242–243
    flexible, 243
    mirror, 242
    rigid, 243
Laryngospasm, 239, 249
Larynx, 233–234, 234f, 249, 259, 279
Laser in situ keratomileusis (LASIK) surgery, 207, 221

Laser surgery, for vision, 208
Laser therapy, for prostate cancer, 367
Laser thermokeratoplasty (LTK), 207, 221
Laser-assisted uvulopalatoplasty (LAUP), 239, 250
Lateral, 54, 55, 161
Lateral meniscus, 425, 447
Lateral ventricles, 461, 484
LAU. *See* Laser-assisted uvulopalatoplasty (LAU)
Lazarus sign, 463, 484
Lazy eye, 221
LCD monitors. *See* Liquid crystal display (LCD) monitors
Leads, 311
Leaflets, 291, 311
Left anterior descending artery (LAD), 291, 311
Left circumflex artery, 291, 311
Left coronary artery, 291, 311
Left hemisphere, 459, 484
Left internal mammary artery (LIMA), 298, 311
Left lateral decubitus, 161
Left main coronary, 311
Leiomyosarcoma, 398, 412
Lens, 204, 221
Lesion, 531, 551
Leukemia, 531–532, 551
Leukocyte esterase, 153, 169
Leukocytes, 531, 551
Leukopenia, 510, 519
Leukotriene modifiers, for allergy, 500
Leukotriene receptor antagonists, 265, 279
Ligaments, 425, 447
Ligate, 125, 129
Ligation, 121, 129
Light editing, 106, 110
  vs. verbatim transcription, 106–108
Light reflex, 231, 250
Limb salvage surgery, 436, 447
Limbic system, 460–461, 484
Line counts, 590, 615
Lipase, 344
Lipoprotein, 311
Liquid crystal display (LCD) monitors, 21, 38
Listening skills, 5
Lithotripsy, 378
Little dark dots, 109
Liver, 322, 344
Liver enzyme tests, in orthopaedics, 438
Liver function tests (LFT), 157, 169
Living-related transplant (kidney), 358, 378
Lobar pneumonia, 263, 279
Lobectomy, 269, 279
Lobes, 260, 260f, 279, 322, 344, 484, 576
  of brain, 459f, 460
  of pituitary gland, 559
Lobular carcinoma in situ (LCIS), 399, 412
Lobules, 399, 412
Local anesthesia, 123
Local area network (LAN), 23, 38

Local recurrence, 534, 551
Local transanal resection, 332, 344
Localized scleroderma, 506, 519
Long bones, 421, 447
  parts of, 422f
Loop electrosurgical excision procedure (LEEP), 399, 412
Lordotic, 161
Low-density lipoprotein (LDL), 311
Low-grade SIL (LGSIL), 397, 412
Lower gastrointestinal series, 334, 344
Lower respiratory tract, 259–260, 279
LRD. *See* Laryngopharyngeal reflux disease (LRD)
Lub-dub (heart sound), 293, 311
Lumbar, 447
Lumbar diskography, 440
Lumbar puncture (LP), 439, 448, 474–475, 484
Lumbar vertebrae, 424
Lumpectomy, 399, 412
Lung cancer, 268–269, 268f, 279
  smoking causes, 269
  tumor infiltration in, 268f
Lungs, 260, 279
Lunula, 179, 196
Lupus, 502–503
Lupus anticoagulant (LA), 519
Lupus flare, 502, 519
Luteinizing hormone (LH), 389, 412, 560, 576
Luteinizing hormone releasing hormone (LHRH), 366, 378
Lymph, 497, 519
Lymph nodes, 497–498, 519
Lymphadenectomy, 367, 378
Lymphatic system, 497, 497f, 519
Lymphatic vessels, 497, 519
Lymphocytes, 155, 169, 497, 519
Lymphoid organs, 497, 519
Lymphoid tissues, 498
Lymphoma cells, 508, 519
Lymphomas, 519, 531, 551

M

Macrophages, 261, 279, 519
Macros, 33, 38, 615
Macroscopic examination, 152, 170
Macrosomia, 567, 576
Macrovascular disease, 566, 576
Macula, 205, 221
Maculopapular, 181, 196
Magnetic resonance angiography (MRA), 162, 170, 484
  in immunology, 512
  in neurology, 475–476
Magnetic resonance cholangiopancreatography (MRCP), 335, 344
Magnetic resonance elastography (MRE), 164, 170
Magnetic resonance imaging (MRI), 162, 448, 485
  functional, 476
  in immunology, 512
  in neurology, 475–476
  in orthopaedics, 440

Main verb, 95, 110
Malabsorption, 334, 344
Male genital organs, 354–355
Male genitourinary disorders, 365–368
  hypospadias, 365
  prostate disorders, 365–367
  sexually transmitted diseases, 367–368, 380
  testicular torsion, 365
Malignant, 551
Malignant melanoma, 189
Malignant tumors, 532
Malleus, 231, 250
Mammary glands, 180, 196, 388, 412
Mammogram, 403, 412, 539, 551
Mammography, 403
Mandible, 344, 422, 448
Mandibular advance device, 238, 250
Marrow cavity, 421
Mastectomy, 120, 129
Mastication, 323, 344
Mastoid process, 241, 250
Maxilla, 250
Maxillary sinuses, 232, 250
Mean corpuscular hemoglobin (MCH), 155, 170
Mean corpuscular hemoglobin concentration (MCHC), 155, 170
Mean corpuscular volume (MCV), 155, 170
Meatus, 233, 250, 355, 378
Mechanical ventilation, 263, 279
Medial meniscus, 425, 448
Mediastinoscopy, 551
Mediastinum, 260, 279
Medical abbreviations, 51–53
Medical billing applications, 25–26
Medical correspondence, 66–68
Medical dictionary, 30
Medical documentation mistakes, cost of, 36
Medical ethics, 6
Medical history, in medical reports, 69
Medical language, 58
Medical providers, 4, 16
Medical record keeping, 7–8
Medical references, 606
Medical reports, 68–81
  clinic note, 72–73
  consultation report, 77–79
  discharge summary, 81
  formatting guidelines for, 68–71
  history and physical examination, 74, 75
  operative report, 74–77
  progress note, 80
  SOAP note, 73
  time and date stamp, 71
  types of, 71–81
Medical terminology, 42–59
  anatomic terms, 53–57
  defined, 42, 59
  medical abbreviations, 51–53
  slang and medical jargon, 49–50
  word building in, 42–48
  word-confusion problems, 48–49
Medical terminology knowledge, 4–5

Medical transcription service organization (MTSO), 615
Medical transcriptionist (MT)
  defined, 3–4, 16
  knowledge and skills of, 4–7, 7t
  medical record keeping and, 7–8, 7f
  work of, 3–4
Medical word books, 32
Medications, in medical reports, 69
Medicine. *See* Drugs
Medulla, 462f, 561, 576
Medullary cavity, 421, 448
Medulloblastoma, 471, 485
Meibomian glands, 203, 221
Melanin, 178, 196
Melanocytes, 178, 196
Melanomas, 188–190, 196, 531, 551
Melatonin, 560, 576
Melena, 325, 344
Memory stick, 22
Memory T cells, 499, 519
Menarche, 389, 412
Ménière disease, 236, 250
Meninges, 461, 485
Meningiomas, 471, 485
Meningitis, 463–466, 485
  bacterial, 465
  vaccinations for, 466
  viral, 465
Meniscal tears, 433–434
Meniscectomy, 434, 448
Menisci, 425, 448
Menometrorrhagia, 390, 412
Menopause, 389, 412
Menorrhagia, 390, 412
Menses, 389, 412
Menstrual cycle, 388–390, 412
Menstruation, 389, 412
Mental status, 473
Mesothelioma, 269, 280
Mesothelium, 269, 280
Metabolic acidosis, 271, 280
Metabolic alkalosis, 271, 280
Metabolic equivalents (METS), 311
Metabolic panel, 155–157
Metabolism, 519
Metacarpals, 425, 448
Metaphysis, 421, 448
Metaplasia, 324, 344
Metastasis, 485, 551
Metastasize, 196
Metastatic brain tumor, 471, 485
Metatarsals, 425, 448
Microcalcifications, 539, 551
Microkeratome, 207, 221
Microscopic examinations, 152, 170
Microsoft Office, 25
Microsoft Windows, 22, 24
Microsoft Word (MS Word), 25
Microvascular clipping, 467, 485
Microvascular decompression, 470, 485
Midbrain, 462f
Middle ear, 231, 250
Midline, 53, 59
Millimeters of mercury (mmHg), 295, 311
Mirror laryngoscopy, 242, 243f
Misoprostol, 394

Mitosis, 178, 196, 529, 551
Mitral valve, 291, 311
  prolapse, 299, 311
Mixed hearing loss, 237, 250
Model for end-stage liver disease (MELD), 333–334, 344
Modified radical mastectomy, 399, 412
Mohs micrographic surgery, 189, 196
Monitor, 21, 38
Monoclonal antibodies, 190, 196, 509, 519
Monocytes, 155, 170
Monofilament sutures, 126, 130
Mons pubis, 387, 412
Motherboard, 21, 38
Motor examination, 473
Motor nerves, 485
Mouse, 21, 38
Mouth and throat, 320–321, 322
MRA. *See* Magnetic resonance angiography (MRA)
MRE. *See* Magnetic resonance elastography (MRE)
MRI. *See* Magnetic resonance imaging (MRI)
MT. *See* Medical transcriptionist (MT)
Mucus, 233, 250
Multifilament sutures, 130
Multiple endocrine neoplasia (MEN), 565, 576
Multiple gated acquisition scan (MUGA), 311
Multiple myeloma, 436, 448
Multiple sclerosis, 469–470, 485
Murmurs (heart sound), 294, 312
Muscle and flexibility tests, 437, 437t
Muscles, 425–428, 426f, 448. *See also* Musculoskeletal system
  brain controls movement of, 426
  bursae and, 428
  cardiac, 428
  criteria for naming, 427
  involuntary, 426
  organization and function of, 426–427
  skeletal, 427–428
  smooth, 428
  tendons, 428
  types of, 427–428
  voluntary, 426
Muscular dystrophy (MD), 435, 448
Muscularis propria, 354, 378
Musculoskeletal system, 448
  appendicular skeleton in, 424–425, 424t
  axial skeleton, 422–424, 422t
  bones in, 421–425
  bursae in, 428
  cartilage in, 425
  defined, 420
  divisions of skeleton, 422–425
  joints in, 425
  ligaments in, 425
  muscles in, 425–428
  tendons in, 428
Mutation, 530, 551
Mycobacterium, 267
Mycologist, 184, 196

Mycoplasma pneumoniae, 263, 280
Mycoplasmas, 263, 280
Mycosis, 184, 196
Mydriasis, 213, 221
Myelin, 469, 485
Myelogram, 439, 448
Myelography, 439–440
Myelomas, 531, 551
Myocardial band enzymes of creatine phosphokinase, 312
Myocardial infarction (MI), 291, 312
  role hypertension role in, 296
Myocardium, 290, 312
Myoclonic seizures, 468, 485
Myoglobin, 157, 170
Myolysis, 412
Myomectomy, 398, 412
Myometrium, 388, 412
Myopia, 206, 221
Myotonic muscular dystrophy, 435, 448
Myringotomy, 235, 250

N

Nails, 179
Nanospheres, for cancer, 546
Naproxen, 397
Narcotics, 139, 143
Nares, 232, 250
Nasal cavity, 232, 232f, 233
Nasal dorsum, 232, 250
Nasal endoscopy, 242, 250
Nasal mucosa, 233, 250
Nasal polyps, 238, 250
Nasal septum, 232, 250
Nasal sinus, 232, 250
Nasal studies, 242
Nasal turbinate, 233, 248, 259, 278
Nasolacrimal ducts, 203, 221
Nasopharynx, 233, 250
Navigation keys, 21, 38
Nearsightedness, 221. *See* Myopia
Neck, 485
Necrosis, 378
Negative crossmatch, 358, 378
Neisseria gonorrhoeae, 368
Neisseria mengitidis, 320
Neoplasia, 531, 551
Neoplasm, 531, 551
Neoplastic cells, 531, 551
Nephritis, 359, 378
Nephrolithiasis, 360, 378
Nephrology, 352–353, 378
Nephrons, 353, 378
Nephroscope, 362, 378
Nerve conduction studies, 448
Nerve endings, 180
Nerve fiber, 458, 485
Nerve roots, 463, 485
Nerve-conduction studies, 441
Nerves, 458, 485
Nervous system, 485. *See also* Neurology
  anatomy of, 458–463
  central nervous system, 458–462
  defined, 458
  peripheral nervous system, 462–463
Network, 23, 24f
Network contact sheet, 589f
Networking, 615

Neuro-otology, 229, 250
Neurogenic bladder, 363, 378
Neurohormones, 559, 576
Neurologic assessment, 473–474, 485
Neurologic diseases in, 463–472
    aneurysms, 466–467
    Bell palsy, 470
    brain tumor, 470–472
    hydrocephalus, 466
    meningitis, 463–466
    multiple sclerosis, 469–470
    Parkinson disease, 468–469
    seizure disorder/epilepsy, 467–468
    trigeminal neuralgia, 470
Neurologists, 457, 485
Neurology, 457–488, 485
    abbreviations in, 481
    aneurysms in, 466–467
    Bell palsy in, 470
    brain tumor in, 470–472
    combining forms in, 480t
    defined, 457
    diagnostic studies and procedures in,
        472–478
    hydrocephalus in, 466
    laboratory tests in, 474
    meningitis in, 463–466
    multiple sclerosis in, 469–470
    nervous system, anatomy of, 458–463
    neurologic assessment, 473–474
    neurologic diseases in, 463–472
    overview, 457–458
    Parkinson disease in, 468–469
    seizure disorder/epilepsy in, 467–468
    soundalike words in, 479t
    terminology in, 481–488
    trigeminal neuralgia in, 470
Neurons, 458, 485
Neurosonography, 475, 485
Neurosurgery, 457, 485
Neurotransmitters, 486
    epilapsy and, 468
Neutropenia, 510, 519
Neutrophil, 519
Nissen fundoplication, 326, 344
Nitrates, 297, 312
Nitrazine test, 393, 412
Nitrites, 153, 170
Nocturnal, 312
Nodules, 196, 503, 519
Non-Hodgkin lymphoma, 508, 519
Non-small cell lung cancer, 269, 280
Nonabsorbable sutures, 126, 130
Nonalcoholic steatohepatitis (NASH),
    328, 344
Noncommunicating hydrocephalus,
    466, 486
Nonconvulsive seizure, 486
Noninvasive surgery, 120
Nonprescription drugs, 135, 143
Nonsteroidal anti-inflammatory drug
    (NSAID)
    for autoimmune diseases, 507
    for pain, 430
Norepinephrine, 562, 576
Normal, 615
Normal spontaneous vaginal delivery
    (NSVD), 394, 412

Nose, 250
    anatomy of, 232–233
    disorders. See Nose disorders
Nose disorders, 237–238
    chronic sinusitis, 238
    deviated septum, 237–238
    epistaxis, 238
    nasal polyps, 238
Nuclear scan, 312
Nucleoside reverse transcriptase
    inhibitors, 501, 519
Nucleus, 551
Nulligravida, 391, 412
Nullipara, 391, 412
Numbers/numbering systems, 104–105,
    110
Numeric keypad, 21, 38
Nystagmus, 204, 221, 242, 250

O

OAE testing. See Otoacoustic emissions
    (OAE) testing
Oblique, 161
Obstetrician, 386, 412
Obstetrician/gynecologist (OB/GYN),
    386, 412
Obstetrics, 386, 412
Obstetrics and gynecology, 386–415
    cervical dysplasia, 396–397
    combining forms in, 406t
    diagnostic studies and procedures in,
        400–403
    endometriosis, 397–398
    female reproductive system, anatomy,
        386–390, 387f
    gorillapause in, 404
    gynecologic cancers, 398–399
    gynecologic diseases in, 395–399
    human reproduction in, 390–394
    laboratory tests in, 400–401
    menstrual cycle in, 388–390
    sexually transmitted diseases in,
        395–396
    soundalike words in, 405t
    uterine fibroids, 398
Obstetrics studies, 401
Obstipation, 321, 344
Obstructive sleep apnea (OSA),
    238–239, 250
Obtuse marginal branches, 291
Obtuse marginals, 312
Occipital lobes, 460, 486
Occlusion, 519
Occult, 344
Occupational Outlook Handbook, 3
Ocular structural disorders, 209f–211f
Office, Microsoft, 25
Olfactory, 232, 250
Oligodendrocytes, 471, 486
Oligodendrogliomas, 471, 486
Ommaya reservoir, 551
Oncogenes, 530, 551
Oncologist, 527, 551
Oncology, 527–553, 551. See also
    Cancer
    abbreviation in, 548
    biopsy in, 538–539
    cancer classification systems, 534–536

cancer development in, 529–532
cancer risk factors and, 532–534
cancer treatment in, 541–545
cell structure and, 528–529
combining forms in, 547t
defined, 527
diagnostic studies and procedures,
    536–541
imaging in, 539–541
laboratory tests in, 536–538
nanospheres for treating cancer, 546
soundalike words in, 546t
terminology in, 549–553
Online testing, 599–601, 615
Onychomycosis, 179, 196
Oocyte, 413
Oophoritis, 413
Open cholecystectomy, 327, 344
Open reduction, 430, 448
Open reduction and internal fixation
    (ORIF), 431, 448
Operating system, 21–22
Operation, 119, 130
Operative report, 74–77, 87
Ophthalmologist, 202, 221
Ophthalmology, 202–223, 221. See also
    Eye
    abbreviations in, 219
    age-related macular degeneration in,
        208
    amblyopia in, 206
    applanation tonometry in, 215
    astigmatic keratotomy in, 207
    astigmatism, 206
    cataract in, 208
    combining forms in, 218t
    common structural diseases in,
        208–211
    common visual disorders in,
        205–208
    conductive keratoplasty in, 207
    corneal topography, 215
    diabetic retinopathy in, 208
    diagnostic studies and procedures in,
        211
    dilated examination, 213
    diplopia in, 206
    eye anatomy, 202–205
    fluorescein angiography, 215
    glaucoma in, 208
    gonioscopy, 215
    hyperopia in, 206, 207f
    implantable collamer lens procedure
        in, 208
    laser in situ keratomileusis surgery in,
        207
    laser thermokeratoplasty in, 207
    myopia in, 206, 207f
    overview, 202
    photorefractive keratectomy in, 207
    presbyopia in, 206
    radial keratotomy in, 207
    slit lamp examination in, 214
    soundalike words in, 217t
    terminology in, 219–223
    visual acuity assessment in, 211–213
    visual field testing, 214–215
    visual process in, 205

Ophthalmoscope, 213, 221
Opportunistic infections, 264, 280
Optic disc, 205, 221
Optic nerve, 205, 222
Optician, 202, 222
Optometrist, 202, 222
Oral cavity, 320, 344
Orbit, 203, 222
Orchidectomy, 367, 378
Orchiectomy, 378
Orchitis, 378
Ordinal numbers, 104, 110
Organ of Corti, 231, 250
Organelles, 528, 551
Oropharynx, 233, 250, 320, 344
Orotracheal intubation, 121, 130
Orthopaedics, 420–451, 429–437, 448
    abbreviations in, 444
    anatomic regions of body, 428, 429t
    anatomic terms of motion, 429, 430t
    anatomy of musculoskeletal system,
        421–428
    avascular necrosis, 432
    bone tumors, 435–437
    combining forms in, 443t
    diagnostic studies and procedures in,
        437–441
    dislocation, 431–432
    Doppler ultrasound in, 438
    fracture, 430–431
    fracture repair in, 441
    imaging in, 438–441
    laboratory tests in, 437–438
    meniscal tears, 433–434
    muscle and flexibility tests, 437, 437t
    muscular dystrophy, 435
    musculoskeletal diseases, 429–437
    osteoarthritis, 434–435
    osteoporosis, 433
    scoliosis, 432
    soundalike words in, 442t
    sprains, 429–430
    terminologies in, 445–451
Orthopaedist, 420, 448
Orthopnea, 262, 280, 297, 312
Orthostatic hypotension, 295, 312
OSA. See Obstructive sleep apnea
    (OSA)
Oscilloscope, 440, 448
Ossicles, 250
Ossicular chain, 231, 250
Osteoarthritis, 434–435, 434f, 449
Osteoblasts, 421, 449
Osteochondroma, 436, 449
Osteoclasts, 421, 449, 576
Osteocytes, 421, 449
Osteology, 420, 449
Osteonecrosis, 432
Osteophytes, 449
Osteoporosis, 449
Osteosarcoma, 436, 449
Osteotomy, 449
    for avascular necrosis, 432
Ostium, 232, 250
Ostomy bag, 331, 344
Ostomy surgery, 120
Otitis externa, 250
Otitis media, 235, 250

Otoacoustic emissions (OAE) testing,
    241, 250
Otolaryngologists, 229, 251
Otolaryngology, 229, 251
Otologic examination, 240
Otology, 251
Otorhinolaryngology, 229–252, 251
    abbreviations in, 247
    acoustic studies, 239–240
    air and bone conduction tests,
        240–241
    audiometry, 240
    brainstem auditory evoked response
        test in, 241
    cholesteatoma in, 236
    chronic sinusitis in, 238
    combining forms in, 246t
    defined, 229–230
    deviated septum in, 237–238
    diagnostic studies and procedures in,
        239–244
    ear disorders, 235–237
    ear, nose and throat anatomy in,
        230–234
    epistaxis in, 238
    hearing in, 234–235
    hearing loss in, 236–237
    laryngeal studies in, 242–244
    laryngopharyngeal reflux disease in,
        239
    Ménière disease in, 236
    nasal polyps in, 238
    nasal studies in, 242
    nose disorders, 237–238
    obstructive sleep apnea in, 238–239
    otitis externa in, 235
    otitis media in, 235
    otoacoustic emissions testing, 241
    otolaryngologic diseases in, 235–239
    overview, 229
    soundalike words in, 245t
    terminology in, 247–252
    throat disorders, 238–239
    tympanometry, 240
    vertigo in, 235–236
    vestibular studies in, 241–242
    vocal cord paralysis in, 239
Otosclerosis, 251
Otoscope, 251
Otoscopy, 240, 251
Outer ear, 230–231, 251
Outsourcing, 590, 615
Ova and parasites (O&P) test, 334, 344
Oval window, 231, 251
Ovarian cancer, 398, 413
Ovaries, 388, 413, 562, 576
Overflow, 590, 615
Ovulation, 388, 413
Ovulation induction, 392, 413
Ovum, 388, 413
Oxygen saturation, 271, 280
Oxygen use in commercial flight, 273
Oxytocin (OT), 393, 413, 560, 576

P

Pacemaker, 295, 312
Pachydermia, 239, 251
Page numbering, in medical reports, 68

Palate, 320, 344
Palliate, 269, 280
Palliative surgery, 552
Pallor, 296, 312
Palmar erythema, 329, 344
Pancolitis, 330, 344
Pancreas, 322, 344, 562, 577
Pancreatic cancer, 328, 344
Pancreatic disorders, 327–328
Pancreatic duct, 322, 344
Pancreaticoduodenectomy, 328
Pancreatitis, 327–328, 345
Panhypopituitarism, 564, 577
Pap smear, 400, 413
Pap test. See Pap smear
Papilla, 353, 378
Papillary layer, 179, 196
Papillary serous carcinoma, 399, 413
Papilledema, 222
Papillomas, 395, 413
Papillomavirus, 185, 196
Para, 391, 413
Paranasal sinuses, 232, 232f, 251
Parathyroid glands, 561, 577
Parathyroid hormone (PTH), 561, 577
Parathyroidectomy, 564, 577
Parenchyma, 353, 378
Parenteral dosage, 138, 143
Parentheses, 102, 110
Parietal layer, 260, 280
Parietal lobes, 460, 486
Parkinson disease, 468–469, 486
Paronychia, 179, 196
Parotid, 322, 345
Paroxysmal, 312
Paroxysmal atrial tachycardia, 295, 312
Paroxysmal nocturnal dyspnea (PND),
    297, 312
Partial hysterectomy, 398, 413
Partial pressure of carbon dioxide
    (PCO$_2$), 271, 280
Partial pressure of oxygen (PO$_2$), 271,
    280
Partial seizures, 467, 486
Partial thromboplastin time (PTT), 170
Partial-thickness burns, 186, 196
Participants, 136, 143, 552
Partnership, 610, 615
Parts of speech, 94t
Passive immunity, 519
Patella, 425, 449
Patent, 300, 312
    of drugs, 135, 143
Patent ductus arteriosus (PDA), 300,
    312
Pathogen, 519
Pathologist, 170
    defined, 148
    primary work of, 149
    specimen study by, 149
Pathology, 148–151, 170
    defined, 148
    report, 150–151, 170
Pathways, 459, 486
Patient positioning, during surgery,
    122–123, 122f
PCP. See Pneumocystis carinii pneumonia
    (PCP)

Peak expiratory flow (PEF), 272, 280
Peak flow monitoring, 271–272
Peau d'orange, 184, 196
Pectoral girdles, 449
PEF. *See* Peak expiratory flow (PEF)
Pellets/beads, 138
Pelvic girdle, 424, 449
Pelvic inflammatory disease (PID), 395, 413
Penis, 355, 378
Peptic disorders, 324–326, 345
  gastritis, 324
  gastroesophageal reflux disease, 324, 325f
  peptic ulcer disease, 324–326
Peptic ulcer disease (PUD), 324–326, 326f, 345
  surgical procedures for, 327f
Percutaneous nephrolithotomy (PCN), 362, 378
Percutaneous stereotactic rhizotomy, 470, 486
Percutaneous transluminal coronary angioplasty (PTCA), 297, 312
Performance status, 552
  in cancer, 536
Pericardiectomy, 312
Pericardial effusion, 299, 312
Pericardial friction rub, 294
Pericardial window, 300
Pericardiectomy, 300
Pericardiocentesis, 300, 312
Pericarditis, 299–300, 312
Pericardium, 269, 280, 290, 312
Perimetrium, 388, 413
Period, 96–97, 110
Periosteum, 422, 449
Peripheral blood stem cell transplant, 508–509, 519
Peripheral nervous system (PNS), 462–463, 486
  autonomic nervous system, 463
  cranial nerves, 462–463
  spinal nerves, 463
Peripheral neuropathy, 474, 486, 566, 577
Peripheral vascular disease (PVD), 566–567, 577
Peristalsis, 323, 345
Peritoneal dialysis, 357, 358
Peritoneal dialysis peritoneum, 378
Peritoneum, 269, 280, 325, 345, 358
Peritonitis, 325, 345
Pessary, 363, 378
PET scan. *See* Positron emission tomography (PET) scan
Petechiae, 505, 520
Petri dish, 149, 170
Peyer patches, 520
Pfannenstiel incision, 394, 413
Phacoemulsification, 208, 222
Phalanges, 425, 449
Pharmaceutical word book, 31
Pharmacoepidemiology, 135, 143
Pharmacokinetics, 135, 143
Pharmacology, 134–144, 143. *See also* Drugs
  abbreviations in, 142

controlled substances in, 139–141
defined, 134
drug administration in, 137–139
drug regulation and development, 136–137
history of, 135–136
overview, 134–135
terminology in, 143–144
transcribing drug nomenclature and, 141
Pharmacotherapeutics, 135, 143
Pharmacy, 143
  automation, with E-prescriptions, 142
Pharynx, 233, 251, 259, 280, 321, 345
Pheochromocytoma, 565, 577
  chromaffin cells and, 565
  surgical removal of, 566
Pheomelanin, 204, 222
Philadelphia chromosome, 532, 552
Phonemes, 48–49, 51t, 59
Phonosurgery, 239, 251
Phoropter, 213, 222
Photodynamic therapy (PDT), 472, 486
Photoreceptor layer, 205, 222
Photorefractive keratectomy (PRK), 207, 222
Photoselective vaporization prostatectomy (PVP), 367, 379
Photosensitivity, 520
Phototherapy, 182, 196
Physical examination, in medical reports, 69–70
Physical therapy, 449
  in fracture, 431
  in multiple sclerosis, 469
Physician acronyms, 106t
Pia mater, 461, 486
Pineal gland, 560, 577
Pinna, 230–231, 251
Pituitary, 460
Pituitary adenomas, 563, 577
Pituitary disorders, 563–564
Pituitary gland, 486, 559f, 560, 577
Placenta, 390, 413
Placenta abruptio, 391, 413
Placenta previa, 391, 413
Plain film, 159
Plantar warts, 185, 197
Plaques, 183, 197, 297, 312
Plasmapheresis, 469–470, 486
Platelet count (PLT), 155, 170
Platelets, 155, 170, 531, 552
Pleur-evac, 272, 280
Pleura, 260, 280
Pleural effusion, 263, 280
Pleurisy, 262, 280
Plural endings, 46, 47t
PND. *See* Postnasal drip (PND)
Pneumocystis carinii, 265, 280
Pneumocystis carinii pneumonia (PCP), 264–265
Pneumocystis jiroveci, 264
Pneumonectomy, 269, 280
Pneumonia, 263–265, 280
  treatment of, 265
  types of, 264f

viral, 263
walking, 263
Pneumoperitoneum, 402, 413
Pneumothorax, 262, 280
PNH. *See* Postherpetic neuralgia (PNH)
Polyarthritis, 503, 520
Polycystic kidney disease (PKD), 359–360, 379
Polydipsia, 577
Polymer implant wafer, 552
Polyp, 332, 345
Polypectomy, 332, 345
Polyphagia, 577
Polysomnography, 243–244, 251
Polyuria, 379, 577
Polyvinyl alcohol (PVA), 398, 413
Porous bones, 433
Portfolio, 615
Ports, 21, 38
Positional testing, 242
Positive crossmatch, 358, 379
Positive end-expiratory pressure (PEEP), 263, 281
Positron emission tomography (PET) scan, 162, 170, 486
  in immunology, 512–513
  in neurology, 476
  in oncology, 540
Positrons, 162, 170
Posterior chamber, of eye, 205, 222
Posterior communicating artery (PComA), 467, 486
Posterior descending artery (PDA), 291, 312
Posterior fontanel, 423, 449
Posterior horn, 433, 449
Posterior pituitary gland, 577
Posteroanterior, 55, 161
Postherpetic neuralgia (PNH), 186, 197
Postmenopause, 389, 413
Postnasal drip (PND), 238, 251
Postvoid residual, 371, 379
Potential of Hydrogen (pH), 153, 170, 271, 281
Preeclampsia, 391, 413
Prefixes, 43, 44t, 59
  surgical, 127, 128t
Premature atrial contraction, 295, 312
Premature rupture of membranes (PROM), 393, 413
Presbyopia, 206, 222
Prescription drugs, 135, 143
Pressure-equalization tube, 235
Prevnar, 466, 486
Primary brain tumor, 471, 486
Primary cancer, 532, 552
Primary hypertension, 296, 312
Primary tumors, 436, 449
Primigravida, 391, 413
Primitive neuroectodermal tumors (PNET), 471
Privacy rule, HIPAA and, 10, 16
PRK. *See* Photorefractive keratectomy (PRK)
Proctitis, 345
Proctocolectomy, 331, 345
Professional affiliation, 13–14
Professional keyboarding skills, 5

Progesterone, 388, 413, 577
Progress note, 80, 87
Prolactin, 388, 413, 559–560, 577
Pronator muscle, 473, 486
Prone position, 123, 130
Proofreader's marks, 110
Proofreading, 106–109, 110. *See also*
    Editing
    guidelines for, 108–109
    typical items missed in, 108
    verbatim transcription *vs.* light
        editing, 106–108
Prophylactic surgery, in cancer, 538
Prophylaxis, 538, 552
Proprioception, 462, 486
Prostaglandin, 394
Prostate, 355, 379
Prostate cancer, 366–367
Prostate disorders, 365–367
    benign prostatic hyperplasia,
        365–366
    prostate cancer, 366–367
    prostatitis, 365
Prostate-specific antigen (PSA), 379, 552
    in oncology, 536
Prostatitis, 365, 379
Protease inhibitors, 501, 520
Proteins, 153, 552
Proteinuria, 152, 170, 359, 379
Prothrombin time (PT), 170
Protocol, 552
Proton pump inhibitors (PPI), 326, 345
Providers. *See* Medical providers
Proximal neuropathy, 566, 577
Pruritus, 181, 197
Pseudohypertrophy, 435, 449
Psoralen, 182, 197
Psoriasis, 183, 183f, 197
PTT. *See* Partial thromboplastin time
    (PTT)
Pubic symphysis, 387, 413
Pubis, 425, 449
Pulmonary artery, 313
Pulmonary circulation, 292, 312
Pulmonary edema, 269, 281
Pulmonary embolism, 273, 281
Pulmonary function testing (PFT),
    270–271, 281
Pulmonary perfusion, 261, 281
Pulmonary stenosis, 300, 313
Pulmonary valve, 291, 313
Pulmonary veins, 313
Pulmonology, 258–282
    abbreviations in, 276
    acute respiratory distress syndrome,
        267–268
    anatomy of respiratory system,
        259–260
    asthma, 265
    bronchiectasis, 263, 277
    bronchiolitis, 263, 277
    bronchitis, 265–266
    chronic obstructive pulmonary dis-
        ease in, 265–267
    combining forms in, 275t
    cystic fibrosis, 267
    diagnostic studies and procedures,
        270–273

emphysema, 266–267, 266f
lung cancer, 268–269, 268f
mechanical ventilation in, 263
pneumonia, 263–265, 264f
pulmonary edema, 269
pulmonary embolism, 269–270
respiratory disorders in, 263–270
respiratory process in, 260–262
soundalike words in, 274t
terminology in, 277–282
tuberculosis, 267
Pulse oximeter, 271, 281
Pulse oximetry, 271, 281
Punch biopsy, 190, 190f, 197
Punctuation marks, 96–102
    apostrophe, 100
    colon, 99–100
    comma, 98–99
    dash, 102
    hyphen, 100–101
    parentheses, 102
    period, 96–97
    question mark, 97–98
    quotation marks, 102
    semicolon, 99
Pupil, 204, 222
Pure tone audiometry, 240
Purkinje fibers, 293, 313
Purpura, 505, 520
PUVA therapy, 182, 197
Pyelonephritis, 359, 379
Pyloric sphincter, 321, 345
Pylorus, 321, 345
Pyuria, 379

Q

Question marks, 97–98, 110
Quotation marks, 102, 110

R

Radial keratotomy (RK), 207, 222
Radiation oncologist, 552
Radiation therapy, 189, 552
Radical cystectomy, 363, 379
Radical perineal prostatectomy, 367,
    379
Radical prostatectomy, 367, 379
Radical retropubic prostatectomy, 367,
    379
Radioactive iodine uptake (RAIU) test,
    577
Radiograph, 159, 170
Radiography, 552
    in oncology, 539
    in orthopaedics, 439
Radiologic imaging, 158–163
    combining forms in, 166t
    CT scan, 161–162
    MRA, 162
    MRI, 162
    PET scan, 162
    soundalike words, 165t
    ultrasonography, 163, 163f
    in urology, 369–370
    X-ray in, 159–161
Radiologist, 158, 170
Radiology, 158, 170

Radiolucent, 170
Radionuclide scan, 439
Radionuclide thyroid imaging, 577
Radionuclides, 162, 170
Radiopaque, 159, 170
Radius, 449
Rales, 262, 281
Randomized clinical trials, 137, 143,
    552
Rapid ACTH stimulation test, 577
Rash, 180, 197
Raynaud phenomenon, 506, 520
RDI. *See* Respiratory disturbance index
    (RDI)
Receptor, 180, 197, 520
Reconstructive surgery, 552
Rectum, 321–322, 345
Recurrent disease, 534, 552
Red (blood cell) distribution width
    (RDW), 155, 170
Red blood cell indices, 170
Red blood count (RBC), 154, 171
Red marrow, 421, 449
Reduction, 430, 449
Reed-Sternberg cells, 520
Reference range, 151, 171
References and tools, 30–32
    book of abbreviations, 31–32
    Internet resources, 32
    medical dictionary, 30
    medical spell checker software, 30
    medical word books, 32
    pharmaceutical word book, 31
    style book manual, 30
    text-expanding software, 31
Reflex, 474, 487
Reflex testing, 474
Reflux nephropathy, 359, 379
Refraction, 205, 213, 222
Refractive errors, 205, 207f, 222
Regional anesthesia, 123
Registered Medical Transcriptionist
    (RMT), 13, 16
Registered nurse anesthetist, 123, 130
Regurgitation, 299, 313
Rejection, 358, 379
Relapsing-remitting multiple sclerosis,
    469, 487
Remodeling, 449
Renal arteries, 354
Renal artery, 379
Renal calculus, 379
Renal capsule, 353, 379
Renal columns, 353, 379
Renal corpuscle, 379
Renal cortex, 353, 379
Renal failure, 356–359, 379
    acute, 356–357
    chronic, 357
    dialysis in, 357–358
    kidney transplantation in,
        358–359
Renal fascia, 353, 379
Renal hilum, 353, 379
Renal medulla, 353, 379
Renal pelvis, 353, 379
Renal pyramids, 353, 379
Renal sinus, 353, 379

Renal tubule, 354, 379
Renin, 353, 380
Report creation skills, 6
Reports, medical. *See* Medical reports
Reproduction, human, 390–394
  fertility issues in, 392–393
  fertilization, 390–392
  labor and delivery in, 393–394
Resection, 121, 130, 363, 380
Resectoscope, 380
Respiratory acidosis, 271, 281
Respiratory alkalosis, 271, 281
Respiratory disturbance index (RDI),
  244, 251
Respiratory process, 260–263
Respiratory syncytial virus (RSV), 281
Respiratory system, 258, 281
  anatomy of, 259–260
  lower respiratory tract, 259–260
  upper respiratory tract, 259
Restrictive cardiomyopathy, 299, 313
Resumé, 593–596, 616. *See also*
    Application letter
  accomplishments, 596
  chronological, 593, 594f
  education, 596
  functional, 593, 595f
  skills and expertise, 596
  summary/profile, 596
  work experience, 596
Reticulocytes, 155, 171
Retina, 205, 222
Retinal photography. *See* Fluorescein
    angiography
Rh factor incompatibility, 392, 414
Rheumatic fever, 502, 520
Rheumatoid arthritis (RA), 503–504,
  503f, 520
Rheumatoid factor (RF), 510, 520
  in orthopaedics, 438
Rhinoplasty, 130
Rhinoscopy, 242, 251
RhoGAM, 392, 414
Rhonchi, 262, 281
Ribbon, 25
Right coronary artery (RCA), 291, 313
Right hemisphere, 459, 487
Right internal mammary artery (RIMA),
  298, 313
Right lateral decubitus, 161
Right ventricular hypertrophy, 300,
  313
Rigid laryngoscopy, 243, 251
Ringworm, 184–185
Rinne test, 241, 251
Ripening, 393, 414
Risk management, 87
RMT. *See* Registered Medical
    Transcriptionist (RMT)
Robots, in operating theatre, 128
Rods, 206, 222
Roentgenogram, 159
Roman numerals, 104, 110
Romberg test, 487
Root words, 43, 46t, 59
Rosacea, 182–183, 197
Rubor, 180, 197
Rubs, 262, 281, 294, 313

Run-on sentence, 99, 110
Rupture of membranes (ROM), 393,
  414

S

S corporation, 610, 616
Saccule, 232, 251
Sacrum, 449
Salivary glands, 322, 345
Salpingitis, 414
Salpingo-oophorectomy, 398, 414
Salpinx, 388, 414
Saphenous vein graft (SVG), 298, 313
Sarcomas, 531, 552
Scalp, 471
Scapula, 425, 449
Schwannomas, 471, 487
SCL-70, 520
Sclera, 204, 222
Sclerodactyly, 506, 520
Scleroderma, 506–507, 520
Scoliosis, 432, 450
Scotoma, 222
Screening tests, for cancer, 540–541,
  552
Scribes, 7, 16
Scrotum, 380
Sebaceous cyst, 180, 197
Sebaceous glands, 180, 197
Seborrheic dermatitis, 181–182, 197
Sebum, 180, 197
Secondary brain tumor, 471, 487
Secondary cancer, 532, 552
Secondary diabetes, 567, 577
Secondary hypertension, 296, 313
Secondary tumors, 436, 450
Secundigravida, 391, 414
Security rule, HIPAA and, 10, 16
Sedation, 123
Sediments, urine, 153, 171
Segmental cystectomy, 363, 380
Segmented neutrophils, 155, 171
Seizures, 467–468, 487
  classification, 467
  generalized, 468
  status epilepticus, 468
  temporal lobectomy for, 468
Selective estrogen receptor modulators
    (SERM), 450, 552
  in osteoporosis, 433
Self-discipline, in MT, 6
Semicircular canals, 232, 251
Semicolon, 99, 111
Seminal vesicles, 355, 380
Sensorineural hearing loss, 236–237, 251
Sensory examination, 473
Sensory nerves, 463, 487
Sentence fragment, 95, 111
Sentence structure, 94–95
Septoplasty, 237, 251
Serum calcium test, in orthopaedics,
  438
Serum creatinine, 368
Sessile, 436, 450
Severe combined immuno-deficiency
    disease (SCID), 520
Sexually transmitted diseases (STD),
  367–368, 380, 414

AIDS, 395–396
  chlamydia, 368
  genital herpes, 367
  gonorrhea, 368
  human papillomavirus, 395
  in obstetrics and gynecology,
    395–396
  pelvic inflammatory disease, 395
Shave biopsy, 190, 197
Shingles, 185–186, 196
Short bones, 422, 450
Shortcuts, 25, 38
Shoulder girdle, 424, 450
Shunt, 466, 487
Shunt revision, 466, 487
Sigmoid colon, 321, 345
Sigmoidoscopy, 335, 345
Signature, in medical reports, 71
SIL. *See* Squamous intraepithelial lesion
    (SIL)
Silver nitrate, 238, 251
Simple mastectomy, 399, 414
Simple partial seizures, 467, 487
Single photon emission computed
    tomography (SPECT), 487
Singleton, 390, 414
Sinoatrial (SA) node, 292, 313
Sinus, 232, 251, 450
Sinus rhythm, 294, 313
Sjögren syndrome, 506, 520
Skeletal muscles, 427–428, 450
Skene glands, 387, 414
Skin, 177, 197. *See also* Dermatology
  cross-section of, 178f
  dermis, 179
  epidermis, 178
  specialized structures of, 179–180
  subcutaneous layer of, 179
Skin appearance, common terminology
    used in, 181t
Skin biopsy, 190, 197
Skin cancer, 188
Skin graft, 187, 197
Skin infections, 183–184
Skin wounds, hyperbaric therapy, 191
Skull, 422–423, 450
Slang, 49–51, 52t, 59
SLE disease activity index (SLEDAI),
  520
Slit lamp, 214, 222
Small bowel, 321, 345
Small intestine, 321, 345
Small-bowel resection, 331, 345
Small-cell lung cancer, 269, 281
Smear, 400, 414
Smooth muscles, 428, 450
Snellen chart, 212–213, 212f, 222
SOAP note, 73, 87
Social history, in medical reports, 69
Soft palate, 320, 345
Software, 21–22, 38
  applications, 22
  operating system, 21
  systems, 21–22
Sole proprietorship, 609–610, 616
Solution, 138, 143
Somatostatin, 560, 577
Somnoplasty, 239, 251

Sonogram, 163, 171
Sonohysterogram (SHG)
  speculum, 414
  tests, 401
Soundalike words, 48, 50t, 59
  in cardiology, 305t
  in dermatology, 192t
  in endocrinology, 571t
  in gastroenterology, 337t
  in imaging, 165t
  in immunology, 514t
  in neurology, 479t
  in obstetrics and gynecology, 405t
  in oncology, 546t
  in ophthalmology, 217t
  in orthopaedics, 442t
  in otorhinolaryngology, 245t
  in pulmonology, 274t
  in radiologic imaging, 165t
  in urology, 372t
Specific gravity, 153, 171
Speculum, 402
Speech-recognition technology (SRT),
    29–30, 38
Spell-checker software, 30
Spermatic cord, 380
Sphenoid sinuses, 232, 251
Sphygmomanometer, 295, 313
Spider angiomas, 329, 345
Spinal cord, 461–462, 462f, 487
Spinal nerves, 463, 487
Spiral CT scan, 552
Spiral CT scanner, 539
Spirogram, 270, 281
Spirometer, 270, 281
Spirometry, 281. See Pulmonary
    function testing (PFT)
Spleen, 498, 520
Splenic flexure, 321, 345
Split-thickness skin graft, 187, 197
Spongy bone, 421, 450
Sprains, 429–430, 450
Spurs, 434, 450
Spyware, 38
Squamous cell carcinoma, 188, 197,
    363, 380, 399, 414
Squamous intraepithelial lesion (SIL),
    396–397, 414
Squamous skin cells, 178, 197
SRT. See Speech-recognition technology
    (SRT)
Stage, 552
Stand-alone systems, 23, 38
Stapes, 231, 251
Staphylococcus aureus, 184, 263, 281,
    320
Start button, 25, 38
Start menu, 25, 38
Station, 393, 414
Status epilepticus, 468, 487
STD cultures, 369
Steatorrhea, 329, 345
Stem cells, 498, 520
  for restoring eyesight, 216
Stenographer, 7, 17
Stenosis, 297, 313, 487
Stent, 297–298, 298f, 313
Stereotactic biopsy, 540, 552

Stereotactic radiosurgery, 470, 487
Stereotactic surgery, 540, 552
Stereotaxy, 540, 552
Sternum, 260, 281, 298, 313
Stoma, 345
Stomach, 321, 345
Stool, 321, 345
Stool culture, 334, 346
Storage, 22, 38
Stratum corneum, 178, 197
Stratum germinativum, 178, 197
Stratum granulosum, 178, 197
Stratum lucidum, 178, 197
Stratum spinosum, 178, 197
Streptococcus pneumoniae, 263, 281, 320
Striae, 450, 577
Striated muscles, 427, 450
Stricture, 331, 346
Strictureplasty, 331, 346
Stridor, 262, 281
Stroke, 487
Stromal cell tumors, 398, 414
Struvite, 380
Struvite stones, 360
Style book, 30, 38
Subarachnoid hemorrhage (SAH),
    467, 487
Subarachnoid space, 439, 450
Subcutaneous, 179, 197
Subcutaneous dosage, 138, 144
Subcutaneous layer, 179, 197
Subdural space, 461, 487
Subject-verb agreement, 95–96, 111
Sublingual, 322, 346
  dosage, 138, 144
Subluxation, 431–432, 450
Submandibular, 322, 346
Subpial resection, 487
  for seizures, 468
Suffixes, 43–44, 45t, 59
  surgical, 127, 128t
Sulci, 459, 487
Sulfadiazine (Silvadene), 185
Sulfonylureas, 577
  for diabetes, 567
Superficial burn, 186, 197
Superior vena cava, 292, 313
Supine position, 123, 130
Suppositories, 138
Surfactant, 262, 281
Surgeon, 119, 130
Surgery, 119–130, 130
  anesthesia administration in, 123,
    124t
  concept of, 119–120
  defined, 119
  fluids and medications during,
    123–124, 124t
  overview, 119
  patient positioning in, 122–123,
    122f
  procedures, 120
  process, 120–121
  terminology in, 122–127, 129–130
  tools and instruments for, 124–125,
    126t
  wound closures and coverings in,
    125–127

Surgical excision, 189
Surgical history, in medical reports, 69
Surgical procedure, 119
Surgical tools and instruments,
    124–125, 125f
Surgical wound coverings, 127
Suspension, 138, 144
Suspensive hyphen, 101, 111
Sutures, 125–126, 130, 422, 450
  size, 125
  types of, 127t
Suturing, 121, 130
Sweat, 180, 197
Sweat glands, 180, 197
Symbols, 105
Syndrome, 330, 346
Synovectomy, 520
Synovial fluid, 425, 450
Synovial joints, 425, 450
Syrup, 138, 144
System tray, 25, 38
Systemic circulation, 292, 313
Systemic lupus erythematosus (SLE),
    502–503, 520
Systemic scleroderma, 506, 520
Systems software, 21, 38
Systole, 292, 313
Systolic pressure, 295, 313

T

T cells, 498, 520
Tablets, 138, 143
Tachycardia, 294, 313
Takayasu arteritis, 505, 520
Talus, 425, 450
Tarsals, 425, 450
Tarsus, 203, 222
Task bar, 25, 38
Taxes/taxation, 610
Technetium, 313
Technetium-99, 439, 450
Templates, 32–33
  on student CD, 84t
Temporal lobectomy, 487
  for seizures, 468
Temporal lobes, 460, 487
Tendon reconstruction, 504, 521
Tendonitis, 428, 450
Tendons, 428, 450
Tension, in eye, 215, 222
Terminology
  anatomic, 53–57
  in cardiology, 308–314
  in career management, 614–616
  career profile, 16–17
  in correspondence and reports, 87
  in dermatology, 194–198
  of editing, 110–111
  endocrinology, 573–578
  in endocrinology, 573–578
  in gastroenterology, 339–346
  in imaging, 167–171
  in immunology, 516–521
  medical, 42–59
  in neurology, 481–488
  in obstetrics and gynecology,
    408–415
  in oncology, 549–553

Terminology (*Cont.*)
  in ophthalmology, 219–223
  in orthopaedics, 445–451
  in otorhinolaryngology, 247–252
  in pharmacology, 143–144
  in pulmonology, 277–282
  skin appearance, 181t
  in surgery, 122–127, 129–130
  of technology, tools, and techniques, 37–39
  in urology, 375–381
  industrial, 590–593
Terminology, medical. *See* Medical terminology
Test tube baby, 392
Testes, 355, 380, 562, 577
Testicles, 355, 380, 562, 577
Testicular torsion, 365, 380
Testosterone, 562, 577
Tetralogy of Fallot, 300–301, 313
Text, in medical reports, 70–71
Text-expanding software, 31, 605–606
Thalamus, 461, 487
Thallium, 313
The Book of Style for Medical Transcription, 30, 51, 67, 93
Therapeutic surgery, 120
Thiazolidinediones, 577
  for diabetes, 567
Third ventricle, 461
Thoracic, 450
Thoracic cage, 424, 450
Thoracic vertebrae, 424
Thoracoscopy, 552
Thorax, 259, 281
Three-pillow orthopnea, 262, 281
Thrill (heart sound), 294
Throat anatomy, 233–234
  hypopharynx, 233
  larynx, 233–234
  nasopharynx, 233
  oropharynx, 233
Throat disorders, 238–239
  laryngopharyngeal reflux disease, 239
  obstructive sleep apnea, 238–239
  vocal cord paralysis, 239
Thrombocytes, 531
Thrombocytopenia, 510, 521
Thrombolysis in myocardial infarction (TIMI), 313
Thymosin, 561, 578
Thymus, 498, 521, 561, 578
Thyroglobulin, 504, 521
Thyroid, 504, 521
Thyroid cartilage, 233, 251
Thyroid function tests (TFT), 157, 171
Thyroid gland, 560–561, 578
Thyroid hormone, 561, 578
Thyroid-stimulating hormone (TSH), 157, 521, 560, 578
Thyromegaly, 561, 578
Thyroxine (T4), 157, 171, 517, 521, 560, 578
Tibia, 425, 450
Tic douloureux, 470
Tidal volume, 263, 270, 282

TIM. *See* Topical immunomodulators (TIMs)
Tinea, 184–185, 198
Tinea barbae, 185, 198
Tinea capitis, 185, 198
Tinea corporis, 185, 198
Tinea cruris, 185, 198
Tinea pedis, 185, 198
Tinnitus, 232, 251
Tissue chemistry, 149, 171
Tissue typing, 380
  in kidney transplant, 358
Titer, 521
TLC. *See* Total lung capacity (TLC)
TNM system, 552
  for cancer staging, 535, 535t
Tocodynamometer, 393, 414
Tongue, 320, 346
Tongue-retaining device, 239, 252
Tonic-clonic seizures, 468, 487
Tono-Pen, 215
Tonometer, 215, 222
Tonsillectomy, 120, 130
Tonsils, 233, 252, 521
Topical immunomodulators (TIM), 182, 198
Total abdominal hysterectomy (TAH), 398, 414
Total cholesterol test, 333
Total hip arthroplasty (THA), 432
Total hysterectomy, 398, 414
Total iron-binding capacity (TIBC), 157
Total joint replacement, 451
  in avascular necrosis, 432
Total knee arthroplasty (TKA), 432, 451
Total lung capacity (TLC), 271, 282
Tower, 21, 38
TPAL system, 391, 414
Trabeculae, 421, 451
Trabeculectomy, 208, 222
Trabeculoplasty, 208, 223
Trachea, 233, 252, 259, 282
Tracheal bifurcation, 259, 278
Tracheostomy, 120, 130, 259, 282
Traction, 431, 451
Trade name, of drugs, 135, 144
Transcribed, 4, 17
Transcriber, 27, 38
Transcribing drug nomenclature, 141
Transcribing machines, 27–28
Transcription
  risk management, 87
  strategies for success in, 82–84
Transcription instructions, 84–85
Transcription methods, 27–30
  digital dictation in, 28–29, 28f
  earphones, 27–28
  foot pedal, 28
  speech recognition technology in, 29–30
  transcribing machines in, 27–28
Transcription platform, 28, 39
Transcription process, 82
Transcription references and tools, 30–32
  book of abbreviations, 31–32

Internet resources, 32
  medical dictionary, 30
  medical spell checker software, 30
  medical word books, 32
  pharmaceutical word book, 31
  style book manual, 30
  text-expanding software, 31
Transdermal, 138, 144
Transducer, 163, 171
Transfer catheter, 392, 414
Transferrin, 157, 171
Transitional cell carcinoma, 363, 380
Transitional words, 96, 111
Transjugular intrahepatic portosystemic shunt (TIPS), 330, 346
Transplant surgery, 120
Transposition of the great vessels, 300, 313
Transrectal ultrasound, 370, 380
Transsphenoidal, 488
Transsphenoidal adenectomy, 578
  for pituitary disorders, 563–564
Transsphenoidal surgery, for tumor, 471–472
Transurethral resection of bladder (TURB), 363, 380
Transurethral resection of prostate (TURP), 366, 380
Transverse colon, 321, 346
Trendelenburg position, during surgery, 123
Tricuspid valve, 291, 313
Trigeminal neuralgia (TN), 470, 488
Trigone, 354, 380
Triiodothyronine (T3), 157, 171, 521, 560, 578
Troponin, 313
True vocal folds, 234, 252
Tuberculosis, 267, 282
Tubulointerstitial nephritis, 359, 380
Tumor grade, 534
Tumor marker, 536–537, 553
Tumor necrosis factor (TNF) inhibitors
  for autoimmune diseases, 507
Tumor suppressor genes, 530, 553
Tumors, 198, 451, 531
  benign, 532
  malignant, 532
Tuning fork, 240, 252
Tuning fork testing, 240–241, 241f
Tunnels, 26, 39
Turnaround time (TAT), 590, 616
Two-pillow orthopnea, 262, 282
Tympanic membrane, 231, 252
Tympanogram, 240, 252
Tympanometry, 240, 252
Tympanostomy tube, 235, 252
Type 1 diabetes, 567, 578
Type 2 diabetes, 567, 578
Tzanck test, 190, 198

U

Ulcerative colitis, 330, 346
Ulna, 425, 451
Ultrasonography, 163, 163f, 171
Ultrasound studies
  in oncology, 540
  in urology, 370

Ultrasound-guided biopsy, 540, 553
Umbilical cord, 390, 414
Uniform Resource Locator (URL), 26, 39
Universal serial bus (USB), 21, 39
Upper and lower limbs, 424–425
Upper gastrointestinal series, 334, 346
Upper respiratory tract, 259, 282
UPPP. *See* Uvulopalatopharyngoplasty (UPPP)
Urea, 156, 171, 380
Uremia, 357, 380
Ureter, 380
Ureteral orifices, 354, 380
Ureteral sphincter, 354, 380
Ureterolithiasis, 380
Ureteroscope, 370
Ureteroscopy, 370, 380
Ureters, 354
Urethra, 354, 380, 414
Urethritis, 380
Uric acid, 380
    stones, 360
    test, in orthopaedics, 438
Urinalysis, 152, 171, 369
    report, 152t
Urinary bladder, 354, 380
Urinary diversion, 363, 364f, 381
Urinary incontinence, 363, 381
Urinary system, 381
Urinary tract infection (UTI), 356, 381
Urination process, 355–356
Urine, 171, 354, 381
    abnormal components of, 369t
Urine culture, 158, 171, 369
Urine dipstick, 153, 169
Urine test, 368–369
    to diagnose autism, 371
    in immunology, 511
Urobilinogen, 153, 171
Urodynamics, 370–371, 381
Uroflowmetry, 371, 381
Urolithiasis, 360, 381
Urologist, 381
Urology, 352–381
    abbreviations in, 373, 374
    anatomy of genitourinary system, 352–355
    bladder disorders, 362–364
    combining forms in, 373t
    defined, 352, 381
    diagnostic studies and procedures in, 368–371
    endoscopic studies, 370
    genitourinary diseases in, 356–368
    kidney disorders, 356–362. *See also* Kidney disorders
    laboratory tests in, 368–369
    male genitourinary disorders, 365–368
    radiologic studies in, 369–370
    soundalike words in, 372t
    terminology in, 375–381
    ultrasound study in, 370
    urinary tract infection, 356
    urination process in, 355–356

urine test to diagnose autism in, 371
    urodynamic studies, 370–371
Urostomy, 381
Urticaria, 181, 198
Uterine artery embolization, 398, 414
Uterine cancer, 398–399, 414
Uterine fibroids, 398, 414
Uterine sarcoma, 415
Uterus, 388, 415
Utricle, 232, 252
Uvula, 233, 252, 320, 346
Uvulopalatopharyngoplasty (UPPP), 239, 252

V

V/Q ratio, 272, 282
Vacuum extractor, 394, 415
Vagina, 388, 415
Vaginal birth after C-section (VBAC), 394, 415
Vaginal hysterectomy, 398, 415
Vaginal smear, 401
Vaginal wet mount, 401, 415
Vagotomy, 326, 346
Vagus nerve, 326, 346, 488
Valacyclovir (Valtrex), 186
Valsalva maneuver, 231, 240, 252
Valves, 291, 313
Valvular heart disease, 299
Vascular stent, in coronary angioplasty, 298f
Vascular system, structures of, 289f
Vasculitis, 505–506, 521
Vasodilators, 506, 521
Veins, 313
Vena cava filter, 270, 282
Venereal Disease Research Laboratory (VDRL) test, 521
Venereal diseases, 367, 381
Ventilation, 261, 282
Ventilation-perfusion scan (V/Q scan), 272–273, 282
Ventilator, 263, 282
Ventricles, 290, 314, 461, 488
Ventricular fibrillation, 294, 314
Ventricular septal defect (VSD), 300, 314
Ventriculoperitoneal (VP) shunt, 466, 488
Ventriculostomy, 466, 488
Venules, 289
Verbatim transcription, 107, 111
    vs. light editing, 106–108
Veress needle, 402, 415
Vermiform appendix, 321, 346
Verrucae vulgaris, 185, 198
Vertebrae, 423–424, 451
Vertebral column, 423–424, 424f, 451
Vertigo, 235–236, 252
Vesicoureteral reflux, 363, 381
Vesicular, 282
    breath sounds, 262
Vestibular organs, 232, 252
Vestibular studies, 241–242
Vestibular system, 230, 252
Video EEG, 476, 488
Videostroboscopy, 243, 252

Viral hepatitis, 328, 346
Viral load, 396, 415
Viral meningitis, 465, 488
Viral pneumonia, 263
Viral skin infections, 185
Virtual private network (VPN), 26–27, 39
Virus exposure, and risk of cancer, 532–533
Viscera, 488
Visceral layer, 260, 282
Visceral nerves, 463, 488
Visible black character (VBC), 612, 616
Visual acuity, 211, 223
    assessment, 211–213
        refraction, 213
        Snellen chart, 212–213, 212f
Visual effect, of cataracts, 212f
Visual field, 214, 223
    analyzer, 214, 223
    confrontation, 214
    testing, 214, 223
Visual process, 205
Vitrectomy, 208, 223
Vitreous humor, 205, 223
Vocal cords, 234, 252
    paralysis, 239, 252
Voice recognition (VR), 29
Voiding cystourethrogram (VCUG), 370, 381
Voluntary muscles, 426, 451
Vulva, 415

W

Wada test, 477–478
Walking pneumonia, 263, 282
Warts, 185, 198
Waveform, ECG, 314
Weber test, 241, 252
Wedge resection, 269, 282
Wegener granulomatosis, 505, 521
Wet macular degeneration, 208, 223
Wet mount, 401, 415
Wheezes, 262, 282
Whipple procedure, 328, 346
White blood count (WBC), 154, 171
White matter, 460, 488
Widow/orphan control, 33, 39
Windows, 22, 24–25, 39
Womb, 388
Word building, 42–48
    analyzing terms in, 47–48
    combining forms in, 44–46, 46t, 59
    plural endings in, 46, 47t
    prefixes in, 43, 44t
    root word, 43
    suffixes in, 43–44, 45t
Word of mouth, 593
Word-confusion problems, 48–49
    homonyms, 48, 49t, 59
    phonemes, 48–49, 51t
    soundalike words, 48, 50t
    unusual word pronunciations in, 48–49
Word-processing applications, 25, 32–34
    AutoCorrect is feature in, 33
    AutoText feature in, 33–34
    document templates in, 32–33

Word-processing applications (*Cont.*)
    headers and footers in, 34
    macros in, 33
Work environments, 11–13
    at home, 12–13
    in hospitals and clinics, 12
Work type (WT), 590, 616
Workstations, 23
World Wide Web (WWW), 26, 39
Wound closures and coverings,
    125–127, 127t

    dressings and bandages for,
      126–127
    suture for, 125–126, 127t

X

X-ray, 159–161, 171
    in immunology, 512
    in oncology, 539
    of adult human hand, 159f
    positioning, 54–55
Xanthomas, 329, 346

Y

YAG laser, 223
Yellow marrow, 421, 451

Z

Zinger, 602, 616
Zip drives, 22, 39
Zip files, 38
Zoladex, 366
Zona pellucida, 393, 415

CCS1111